Surgery of Spinal Trauma

Surgery of Spinal Trauma

Editors

Jerome M. Cotler, M.D.
Professor and Vice Chairman
Department of Orthopaedic Surgery
Thomas Jefferson University Hospital
Philadelphia, Pennsylvania

J. Michael Simpson, M.D.
Clinical Assistant Professor
Medical College of Virginia
Virginia Commonwealth University
Director of Spine Center
Tuckahoe Orthopaedic Associates
Richmond, Virginia

Howard S. An, M.D.
The Morton International Professor of Orthopaedic Surgery
Rush Medical College
Director of Rush Spine Center and Spine Fellowship Program
Department of Orthopaedic Surgery
Rush-Presbyterian–St. Luke's Medical Center
Chicago, Illinois

Christopher P. Silveri, M.D.
Clinical Assistant Professor
Department of Orthopaedic Surgery
Georgetown University Medical Center
Washington, DC
Clinical Instructor in Orthopaedic Surgery
George Washington University Medical Center
Washington, DC
Spine Surgeon
Fair Oaks Orthopaedics Associates
Fairfax, Virginia

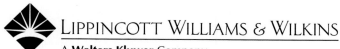

LIPPINCOTT WILLIAMS & WILKINS
A **Wolters Kluwer** Company

Philadelphia • Baltimore • New York • London
Buenos Aires • Hong Kong • Sydney • Tokyo

Acquisitions Editor: Robert Hurley
Developmental Editor: Kristen Kirchner
Production Editor: Kim Yi
Manufacturing Manager: Tim Reynolds
Cover Designer: David Levy
Compositor: Maryland Composition, Inc.
Printer: Maple Press

© 2000 by LIPPINCOTT WILLIAMS & WILKINS
227 East Washington Square
Philadelphia, PA 19106-3780 USA
LWW.com

Printed in the USA

Library of Congress Cataloging-in-Publication Data

Surgery of spinal trauma / edited by Jerome M. Cotler ... [et al.].
    p.   cm.
    Includes bibliographical references and index.
    ISBN 0-683-18108-4
    1. Spine—Wounds and injuries—Treatment.   2. Spine—Surgery.   I. Cotler, Jerome M.
    [DNLM: 1. Spinal Injuries—surgery.   2. Spinal Cord Injuries—surgery. WE 725 S9613 2000]
  RD768.S78 2000
  617.5'6—dc21   99-044551

Care has been taken to confirm the accuracy of the information presented and to describe generally accepted practices. However, the authors, editors, and publisher are not responsible for errors or omissions or for any consequences from application of the information in this book and make no warranty, expressed or implied, with respect to the currency, completeness, or accuracy of the contents of the publication. Application of this information in a particular situation remains the professional responsibility of the practitioner.

The authors, editors, and publisher have exerted every effort to ensure that drug selection and dosage set forth in this text are in accordance with current recommendations and practice at the time of publication. However, in view of ongoing research, changes in government regulations, and the constant flow of information relating to drug therapy and drug reactions, the reader is urged to check the package insert for each drug for any change in indications and dosage and for added warnings and precautions. This is particularly important when the recommended agent is a new or infrequently employed drug.

Some drugs and medical devices presented in this publication have Food and Drug Administration (FDA) clearance for limited use in restricted research settings. It is the responsibility of the health care provider to ascertain the FDA status of each drug or device planned for use in their clinical practice.

10 9 8 7 6 5 4 3 2 1

Contents

Contributing Authors

Howard S. An, M.D.   *The Morton International Professor, Department of Orthopaedic Surgery, Rush University, Rush Medical College, 1725 West Harrison Street, Suite 1063, Chicago, Illinois 60612; and Director of Rush Spine Center and Spine Fellowship Program, Department of Orthopaedic Surgery, Rush-Presbyterian–St. Luke's Medical Center, 1725 West Harrison Street, Chicago, Illinois 60612*

Paul A. Anderson, M.D.   *Clinical Associate Professor, Department of Orthopaedic Surgery, The University of Washington, 1600 East Jefferson Street, #400, Seattle, Washington 98122*

David F. Apple, Jr., M.D.   *Associate Clinical Professor, Department of Orthopaedics, Emory University, 1364 Clifton Road, Atlanta, Georgia 30322; and Medical Director, Shepherd Center, 2020 Peachtree Road, Atlanta, GA 30309*

Wayne B. Bauerle, M.D.   *Strand Orthopaedic Consultants, 849 82nd Parkway, Myrtle Beach, South Carolina 29572*

Johannes Bernbeck, M.D.   *Research Affiliate, Department of Orthopaedics, University of California, Los Angeles, 10833 LeConte Avenue, Room 76-134 CMS, Los Angeles, California 90095-6902; and Staff Physician, Orthopaedics Department, Kaiser Permanente, 1011 Baldwin Park Boulevard, Baldwin Park, California 91706*

Jerome M. Cotler, M.D.   *The Everett J. and Marian Gordon Professor, Department of Orthopaedic Surgery, Jefferson Medical College, Thomas Jefferson University, 130 South 9th Street, Philadelphia, PA 19107; and Orthopaedic Attending, Department of Orthopaedic Surgery, Thomas Jefferson University Hospital, 111 South 11th Street, Philadelphia, Pennsylvania 19107*

Rick B. Delamarter, M.D.   *Associate Clinical Professor, Department of Orthopaedic Surgery, University of California, Los Angeles, 100 UCLA Medical Plaza #755, Los Angeles, California 90077*

Francis Denis, M.D.   *Twin Cities Spine Center, 913 East 26th Street, Suite 600, Minneapolis, Minnesota 55404*

Charles C. Edwards, M.D.   *Division of Orthopaedic Surgery, University of Maryland Hospital, 22 South Greene Street, Baltimore, Maryland 21201*

Steven Falcone, M.D.   *Assistant Professor, Department of Radiology, University of Miami, 1115 NW 14th Street, Miami, Florida 33136; and Assistant Professor, Department of Radiology and Neurological Surgery, Jackson Memorial Hospital, 1611 NW 12th Avenue, Miami, Florida 33136*

Jeffrey S. Fischgrund, M.D.   *Orthopaedic Surgeon, Department of Orthopaedics, William Beaumont Hospital, 3535 West Thirteen Mile Road, Royal Oak, Michigan 48073*

Harry N. Herkowitz, M.D.   *Chairman, Department of Orthopaedic Surgery, William Beaumont Hospital, 3535 West Thirteen Mile Road, Suite 604, Royal Oak, Michigan 48073*

Martin J. Herman, M.D.   *Clinical Instructor, Department of Orthopedic Surgery, UMDNJ-Robert Wood Johnson Medical School, 1 R. Wood Johnson Place—CN19, New Brunswick, New Jersey 08903*

Raymond S. Kirchmier, Jr., M.D.   *Clinical Assistant Professor, Department of Orthopaedic Surgery, Medical College of Virginia, 417 North 11th Street, Richmond, Virginia 23298; and Active Staff, Department of Orthopaedic Surgery, St. Mary's Hospital, 5801 Baremo Road, Richmond, Virginia 23226*

Randall T. Loder, M.D.   *Chief of Staff, Shriners Hospital for Children, Twin Cities, 2025 East River Parkway, Minneapolis, Minnesota 55414*

Paul C. McAfee, M.D.   *Associate Professor of Orthopaedic Surgery, Assistant Professor of Neurosurgery, Johns Hopkins University School of Medicine, 720 Rutland Avenue, Baltimore, Maryland 21205*

Mark C. Nelson, M.D.   *Chief Resident, Department of Orthopaedic Surgery, George Washington University, 2150 Pennsylvania Avenue, NW, Washington, DC 20037*

Stephen J. Pineda, M.D.   *Springfield Clinic, 1025 South 7th Street, Springfield, Illinois 62703*

Peter D. Pizzutillo, M.D.   *Professor, Department of Orthopaedic Surgery, St. Christopher's Hospital for Children, Erie Avenue at Front Street, Philadelphia, Pennsylvania 19134-1095; and Director, Department of Orthopaedic Surgery, MCP/Hahnemann School of Medicine, Broad and Vine Streets, Philadelphia, Pennsylvania 19107*

Armando Ruiz, M.D.   *Assistant Professor, Department of Radiology, University of Miami, 1115 NW 14th Street, Miami, Florida 33136; and Neuroradiologist, Department of Radiology, Jackson Memorial Hospital, 1611 NW 12th Avenue, Miami, Florida 33136*

Christopher P. Silveri, M.D.   *Clinical Assistant Professor, Department of Orthopaedic Surgery, Georgetown University Medical Center; and Spine Surgeon, Fair Oaks Orthopaedic Associates, 3650 Joseph Siewick Drive, Suite 300, Fairfax, Virginia 22033*

J. Michael Simpson, M.D.   *Assistant Clinical Professor, Department of Orthopaedic Surgery, Medical College of Virginia, Virginia Commonwealth University, PO Box 980153, Richmond, Virginia 23298–0153; and Director of Spine Center, Tuckahoe Orthopaedic Associates, PO Box 71690, Richmond, Virginia 23255*

Evelyn M.L. Sklar, M.D.   *Professor of Clinical Radiology and Neurological Surgery, Department of Radiology, University of Miami School of Medicine, 1115 NW 14th Street, Miami, Florida 33136; and Professor of Clinical Radiology and Neurological Surgery, Department of Radiology, Jackson Memorial Hospital, Miami, Florida 33136*

Douglas C. Sutton, M.D.   *486 Golden Gate Drive, Richboro, Pennsylvania 18954*

Allan F. Tencer, Ph.D.   *Professor, Department of Orthopedics, University of Washington, Harborview Medical Center, MS 355798, 325 Ninth Avenue, Seattle, Washington 98104*

Antoine G. Tohmeh, M.D.   *Orthopaedic Surgeon, Department of Surgery, Holy Family Hospital, 5719 North Lidgerwood, Spokane Washington 99207; and Orthopaedic Specialty Clinic, 9631 North Nevada, Spokane Washington 99218*

Alexander R. Vaccaro, M.D.   *Associate Professor, Department of Orthopaedics, Thomas Jefferson University and the Rothman Institute, 925 Chestnut Street, Philadelphia, Pennsylvania 19107; and Co-Director of the Regional Delaware Valley Spinal Cord Injury Center*

Preface

The evaluation and treatment of spinal trauma serves as the cornerstone of knowledge and understanding of all spinal disorders. Appreciation of anatomic integrity, biomechanical stability, utility, and success of nonoperative versus operative intervention, spinal reconstructive techniques and the plethora of instrumentation are essential for the complete spinal surgeon.

In each chapter a thorough review of the subject acts as the platform from which each author delineates finer aspects of diagnostic and therapeutic intervention. While nonoperative and operative options are described for each class of injury, emphasis is placed on technique oriented treatment plans and the nuances of their application. Judicious use of this material will enable the surgeon to formulate a biomechanically sound treatment plan, and provide the most efficient means to obtain successful results. Such a knowledge base will also facilitate the recognition of potential complications and offer mechanisms to avoid these pitfalls.

The sole purpose of this textbook is to provide a definitive resource for the treatment of all categories of spine trauma. The foundation of the book comes from over two decades of enthusiasm, teaching, research, and devoted patient care of our senior editor Dr. Jerome M. Cotler at the Thomas Jefferson University Hospital and Regional Spinal Cord Injury Center of the Delaware Valley. It is, however, punctuated by the expertise of our contributing authors in all fields of spinal disorders.

Jerome M. Cotler
J. Michael Simpson
Howard S. An
Christopher P. Silveri

SURGERY OF SPINAL TRAUMA

Surgery of Spinal Trauma,
edited by J.M. Cotler, J.M. Simpson, H.S. An, and C.P. Silveri.
Lippincott Williams & Wilkins, Philadelphia © 2000.

CHAPTER 1

Anatomy and Surgical Approaches to the Spine

Howard S. An

Prompt diagnosis, proper medical management, and precise surgical techniques comprise the cornerstone of successful surgical procedures in patients with spine trauma. Thorough knowledge of spinal anatomy and related structures is essential in the performance of surgical procedures. The anatomy of the spine, which will include osseous structure and articulations of the cervical, thoracic, and lumbar spine, intervertebral disc and ligaments, muscle and fascia, and neurovascular structures, will be reviewed in this chapter. Review of surgical approaches to both the anterior and posterior aspects of the entire spine will follow.

The human spine is a complex columnar structure that spans from the occiput to the sacrum and protects the spinal cord and nerve roots. The spine provides motions in three dimensions and maintains balance of the head, trunk, and pelvis through the muscles, ligaments, intervertebral disc, and facet joints (Fig. 1). The normal thoracic kyphosis is in the range from 30 to 40 degrees and the normal lumbar lordosis is approximately 55 to 65 degrees. Two thirds of lumbar lordosis is accounted by the angle from L-4 to the sacrum. The magnitude of lumbar lordosis should be about 30 degrees greater than thoracic kyphosis in a given individual. The sacropelvic alignment usually is determined by the sacral inclination angle, which is measured from the vertical axis to the posterior sacral line. The sacral inclination should be about 45 to 50 degrees. A sacrum that is either too verti-

cal or horizontal will affect the sagittal balance of the lumbar spine and the entire trunk. In the stance position, the sagittal vertical axis should fall from the odontoid process through the C7–T1 intervertebral disc and anterior to the thoracic vertebrae. The axis then crosses the spinal column at the T12–L1 intervertebral disc and falls posterior to the lumbar spine. The axis again crosses the spine at the lumbosacral articulation and is located anterior to the second sacral vertebra. This concept of the sagittal vertical axis is important in realignment of sagittal-plane deformities.

NEUROANATOMY

Spinal Cord

From the foramen magnum the spinal cord emerges as a continuation of the medulla oblongata and ends in a cone-shaped structure known as the conus medullaris. The conus medullaris usually is located at the L1–2 intervertebral disc in adults, but may be as high as T-12 or as low as L2–3. In the newborn infant the conus is at the L2–3 region. The cervical cord enlarges maximally at the level of the C-6 vertebra to provide C3–T1 innervation to the upper limbs. The lumbosacral enlargement is present from the T-11 to L-1 vertebral segments, providing L-1 to S-3 cord segments to the lower extremities. It is important to remember the corresponding vertebral segment to the cord segment. For example, the L-1 vertebral segment corresponds to the sacral conus medullaris cord segment as well as the traversing lower lumbar roots.

H.S. An: Department of Orthopaedic Surgery, Rush Medical College, Rush-Presbyterian-St. Luke's Medical Center, Chicago, Illinois 60612.

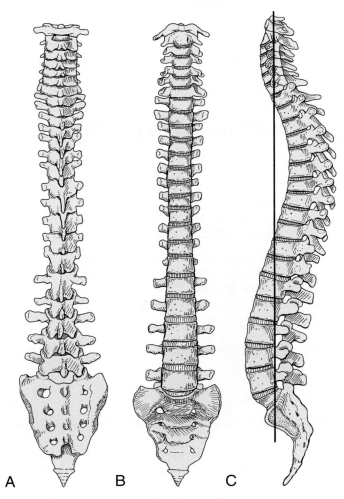

FIG. 1. The human spine. **A:** Posterior view of the entire spine. **B:** Anterior view of the spine. **C:** Lateral view of the spine. The *vertical line* illustrates a plumb line that starts from the odontoid process and crosses the C-7 vertebra and T12–L1 junction and to the posterior aspect of the sacrum. This plumb line is used to assess sagittal imbalance clinically. (Reproduced with permission from An HS: *Principles and Techniques of Spine Surgery*. Baltimore: Williams & Wilkins, 1998.)

Included in the spinal cord is the outer white matter and the inner gray matter (Fig. 2). The white matter of the spinal cord contains nerve fibers and glia divided into three columns: posterior, lateral, and anterior. The posterior column includes the fasciculus cuneatus laterally and fasciculus gracilis medially, mediating proprioceptive, vibratory, and tactile sensations. The lateral column contains the descending motor lateral corticospinal and lateral spinothalamic fasciculi, whereas the anterior funiculus contains the ascending anterior spinothalamic tract and other descending tracts. The lateral spinothalamic tracts cross through the ventral commissure to the contralateral side of the cord, conveying pain and temperature sensations. The anterior spinothalamic tract conveys crude touch sensation.

The gray matter of the spinal cord contains cell bodies of efferent and internuncial neurons. The somatosensory neurons are located in the posterior horn, and the somatomotor neurons are found in the anterior horn of the gray matter. The visceral center of the gray matter is found in the intermediolateral horn. The central ependymal canal is in the center of the spinal cord for the passage of cerebrospinal fluid. The sagittal diameter of the gray matter decreases from C-2 to the upper thoracic levels and remains constant throughout the thoracic levels (1). The sagittal diameter increases again at T-12 and peaks at L-4, gradually diminishing toward the caudad levels. The total cross-sectional area of the spinal cord is greatest at C-6 and decreases markedly to the T2–3 level and remains constant through the thoracic levels. The diameter increases again at L-4 and tapers markedly below S-1. The size of the spinal cord has little or no correlation with age or body habitus.

The pia mater intimately covers the spinal cord and the transparent arachnoid mater that contains the cerebrospinal fluid (Fig. 3). The dura mater is the outermost covering of the spinal cord and is continuous with the inner layer of the cranial dura at the level of the foramen magnum. The spinal cord is anchored to the dura by the dentate ligaments, which project laterally from the lateral side of the cord to the arachnoid and dura at points midway between exiting spinal nerves (Fig. 3). By suspending the spinal cord in the cerebrospinal fluid, the dentate ligaments cushion and protect the cord while minimizing movement of the cord during ranges of motion. The epidural space contains fat, internal vertebral venous plexus, and loose connective tissue. This venous plexus may be involved in spreading infection or neoplasm. The epidural space is about 2 mm at L3–4, 4 mm at L4–5, and 6 mm at L5–S1. Because of this relatively larger epidural space at L5–S1, spinal stenosis is less common at the lumbosacral junction. The plica mediana dorsalis durae matris is a delicate median fold at the lumbosacral epidural region that often blends with the epidural fat. There is a potential space between the dura and arachnoid, and the subarachnoid space is between the arachnoid and pia. The subarachnoid space contains the cerebrospinal fluid, spinal blood vessels, and nerve rootlets from the spinal cord. The dura and arachnoid envelop may terminate between S-1 and S-4 but most commonly at the S-2 region. Distal to the S-2 region, the dura invests the filum terminale and attaches to the coccyx.

The vessels supplying the spinal cord are derived from branches of the vertebral, deep cervical, intercostal, and lumbar arteries and include the anterior spinal artery, lying in the anterior median fissure, and the two posterior spinal arteries, running along the posterolateral sulci (2). These vessels are reinforced by segmental or radicular arteries. The anterior spinal artery in the cervical spine arises from the vertebral artery, which originates from the subclavian arteries. Typically, the vertebral artery enters through the C-6 transverse foramen and courses cephalad within the transverse foramen of each vertebra. It then winds around the lateral mass and

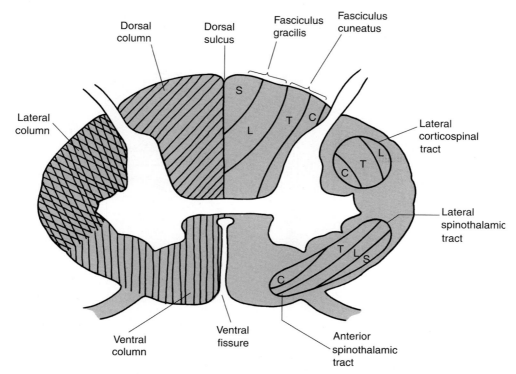

FIG. 2. Cross section of the spinal cord with the outer white matter and the inner gray matter. The white matter of the spinal cord contains nerve fibers and glia and is divided into three columns: posterior, lateral, and anterior. The posterior column includes the fasciculus cuneatus laterally and fasciculus gracilis medially. The lateral column contains the descending motor lateral corticospinal and lateral spinothalamic fasciculi, and the anterior funiculus contains the ascending anterior spinothalamic tract and other descending tracts. The lateral spinothalamic tracts cross through the ventral commissure to the contralateral side of the cord. The gray matter of the spinal cord contains cell bodies of efferent and internuncial neurons. (Reproduced with permission from An HS: *Principles and Techniques of Spine Surgery.* Baltimore: Williams & Wilkins, 1998.)

posterior arch of the atlas and passes through the posterior atlantooccipital membrane into the foramen magnum. The vertebral arteries join together to form the basilar artery beyond the foramen magnum. In the foramen magnum region, the vertebral arteries give branches anteriorly that join together to form the single anterior spinal artery.

The posterior spinal arteries arise either from the inferior cerebellar artery or the vertebral artery. The anterior and posterior spinal arteries are the major blood supply to the spinal cord. The anterior spinal artery supplies the majority of the spinal cord except for the posterior columns. The posterior spinal artery and its branches supply the posterior funiculus, most of the posterior gray columns, and superficial lateral funiculus. The spinal cord also receives blood supplies from radicular arteries and medullary feeders from the vertebral, ascending cervical, posterior intercostal, lumbar, and lateral sacral arteries. These radicular arteries enter the vertebral canal through the intervertebral foramen and divide into anterior and posterior radicular arteries. The anterior radicular arteries supply the anterior spinal artery and the posterior radicular arteries contribute blood to the posterior spinal arteries.

Accompanying the left C-6 spinal nerve root is the most significant radicular artery to the cervical cord, which is an artery originating from the deep cervical artery. Other medullary feeders to the cervical cord are commonly present at C-3 from the left and C-5 and T-1 from the right. There are one or two medullary arteries for the thoracic spinal cord, whereas the radicular artery of Adamkiewicz supplies the lumbosacral spinal cord. This great medullary artery usually accompanies the left ventral root of T9–11, but it may be found anywhere from T-5 to L-5 (2,3). This artery makes a major contribution to the anterior spinal artery and provides the main blood supply to the lower spinal cord. This artery is intradural in its course and crosses over one to three disc spaces before turning to the midline, where it anastomoses with the anterior spinal artery at a mean angle of 20 degrees (3). Venous blood returns from the cord through three veins posteriorly and three veins anteriorly. The venous system within the spinal canal consists of valveless sinuses in the epidural space. The venous plexus is most apparent anteriorly just medial to the pedicles over the midportion of the vertebral bodies. It anastomoses with the veins from the opposite side as well as with the basivertebral sinus, which is located in the space between the posterior longitudinal ligament and the posterior aspect of the vertebral body. The

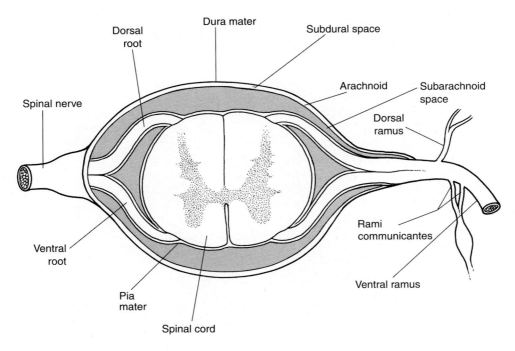

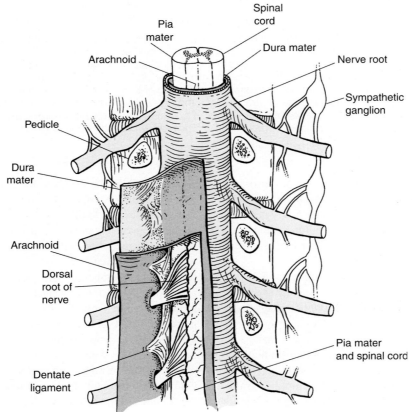

FIG. 3. Cross section of the spinal cord and meninges. The spinal cord is covered by the pia mater, which is the outer lining of the cord, and transparent arachnoid mater that contains the cerebrospinal fluid. The dura mater is the outer covering of the spinal cord. The spinal cord is anchored to the dura by the dentate ligaments that project laterally from the lateral side of the cord to the arachnoid and dura at points midway between exiting spinal nerves. (Reproduced with permission from An HS: *Principles and Techniques of Spine Surgery.* Baltimore: Williams & Wilkins, 1998.)

spinal venous circulation drains primarily into the azygos system and joins directly into the vena cava. Parke et al. (4) and Parke and Watanabe (5) reported on vascularization of the spinal nerve roots and cauda equina. They noted numerous arteriovenous anastomoses throughout the length of the nerve root with many redundant coils along the branches of the radicular arteries. The nerve roots receive their arterial blood supply from anterior and posterior spinal arteries proximally and radicular arteries distally. These vascular cross connections with coiled vessels allow blood flow to be maintained in sections of the root both above and below a point of compression and to resist repeated stretch and relaxation movements of the root.

Spinal Nerves

The spinal nerve roots consist of 8 cervical, 12 thoracic, 5 lumbar, 5 sacral, and 1 coccygeal. The dorsal and ventral roots join to form the spinal nerve. The ventral root and the dorsal root ganglion are within the intervertebral foramen. A pair of spinal nerve roots leaves the dural sac by penetrating the dural sac in an inferolateral direction. This dural sleeve contains the dura mater as well as arachnoid mater and extends as far as the intervertebral foramen, where it becomes the epineurium of the spinal nerve.

The dorsal sensory rootlets in the cervical spine enter the cord through the lateral longitudinal sulcus, and the ventral motor rootlets exit the cord through the ventral lateral sulcus (Fig. 4). There are six or eight rootlets at each level that leave the spinal cord laterally to lie in the lateral subarachnoid space bathed in cerebrospinal fluid. The rootlets join to form the dorsal and ventral roots, which together enter a narrow sleeve of arachnoid and pass through the dura to become a nerve root at each level.

The cervical nerve roots that form from the ventral and dorsal nerve rootlets extend anterolaterally at a 45-degree angle to the coronal plane and inferiorly at about 10 de-grees to the axial plane. The C-5 ventral rootlets are shorter and exit in a more horizontal direction, which may predispose the root to injury during decompressive procedures (6). The cervical nerve roots enter the intervertebral foramina by passing directly laterally from the spinal canal adjacent to the disc and over the top of the corresponding pedicle (Fig. 5A). The anterior root lies anteroinferiorly adjacent to the uncovertebral joint, and the posterior root is close to the superior articular process (Fig. 5B). The cervical nerve root is positioned at the tip of the superior articular process in the medial aspect of the neural foramen. It then courses to a more inferior position over the pedicle in the lateral aspect of the neural foramen. About one third of the foraminal space is occupied by the cervical roots in the normal spine but much more in the degenerative spine. The roots are located in the inferior half of the neural foramen normally, but with the spine fully extended the nerve roots occupy a more cranial part of the foramina and the size of the foramen is decreased. The upper half of the neural foramen contains fat and small veins. The neural foramen is bounded superiorly and inferiorly by pedicles, anteriorly by the uncinate process, the posterolateral aspect of the intervertebral disc, and the inferior portion of the vertebral body above the disc level. The posterior wall of the foramen is formed by the facet joint and superior articular process of the vertebral body below. The dorsal root ganglion in the cervical spine typically is located between the pedicles, but this location may be variable (7). The dorsal root ganglion can be located slightly proximally or distally. The C-7 dorsal root ganglion frequently is located distally. Nerve root injections have been found to be more effective in patients with distally located dorsal root ganglions (7). Degenerative changes of the disc and zygapophyseal joints that bound the intervertebral foramen often compromise the dorsal root ganglion or the spinal nerve.

The thoracic spinal nerves in the thoracic spine are small and occupy about 20% of the intervertebral foramen. Each

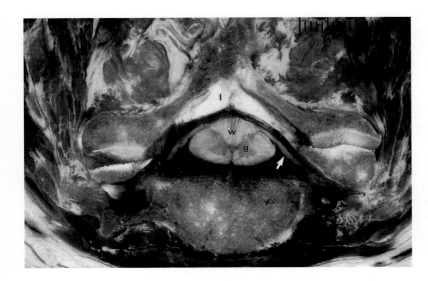

FIG. 4. Cryomicrotome section of the cervical spine showing the dorsal root *(arrow)* and the spinal cord with white matter (w) and gray matter (g) and ligamentum flavum (l). (Reproduced with permission from An HS: *Principles and Techniques of Spine Surgery.* Baltimore: Williams & Wilkins, 1998.)

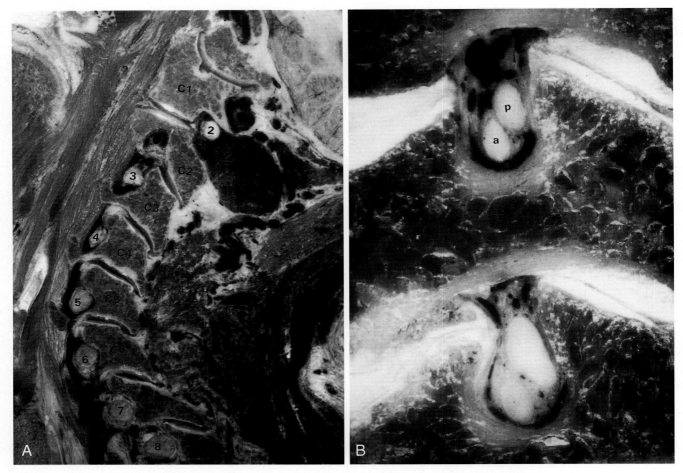

FIG. 5. Cryomicrotome sections of the cervical foramen. **A:** The cervical nerve roots enter the intervertebral foramina by passing directly laterally from the spinal canal adjacent to the corresponding disc and over the top of the corresponding pedicle. **B:** The anterior root lies anteroinferiorly adjacent to the uncovertebral joint, and the posterior root is close to the superior articular process. (Reproduced with permission from An HS: *Principles and Techniques of Spine Surgery.* Baltimore: Williams & Wilkins, 1998.)

thoracic and lumbar spinal nerve exits below the pedicle that bears the same name. The ventral rami of the thoracic nerves do not form plexuses, but each pair runs inferior to the rib as the intercostal nerves. The intercostal nerves give off muscular and cutaneous branches around the back, thorax, and abdomen.

The nerve roots within the lumbar dural sac are arranged loosely with the sacral and coccygeal nerve roots to form the cauda equina (Fig. 6). Each root is covered with its own sleeve of pia mater that is continuous with the pia mater of the spinal cord. The nerve roots within the cauda equina are well organized in a symmetric layering pattern (8). The most posterior nerve elements are the S-5 roots, progressing anteriorly to S-4, S-3, S-2, and S-1 at the L5–S1 level. This arrangement is varied at different levels. For example, at L2–3 level, the L3–S1 roots form an oblique layered pattern with the S2–5 roots occupying the dorsal aspect of the thecal sac. In the lumbar spine, the spinal nerves are larger and occupy about one third of the foramen. The angle formed by each pair of spinal nerve roots and the dural sac gradually be-

comes more acute in the lower lumbar region (7). The angles formed by the L-1 and L-2 roots are about 40 and 32 degrees, respectively, whereas the angle of the L-3 roots is about 30 degrees and those of the L-4 and L-5 roots are 27 degrees (9). The angle for the S-1 root is even more acute at 18 degrees. The length of the nerve roots or the distance from the emerging point of the nerve root from the thecal sac to the dorsal root ganglion increases progressively to a maximum at L-5 and is decreased at S-1. The dorsal root ganglion, which contains the cell bodies of the sensory fibers in the dorsal root, usually lies within the upper, medial part of intervertebral foramen (Fig. 7). The S-1 dorsal root ganglion more frequently is located intraspinally (10). The average dimension of the dorsal root ganglions gradually increases from L-1 to S-1. Using coronal magnetic resonance imaging sections, Hasegawa et al. (11) described the locations of the lumbar dorsal root ganglions in asymptomatic individuals. The nerve root origin was noted to be more cephalad for the caudad nerve roots, particularly S-1.

The lumbar intervertebral foramen is shaped like an in-

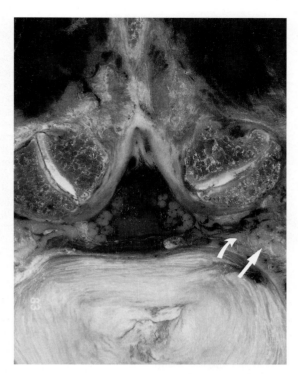

FIG. 6. Cryomicrotome sections of the lumbar spine. Cross section of the lumbar spine at the intervertebral disc level. Nerve roots are arranged in a symmetric pattern. The nerve root in the foramen *(arrow)* is normally surrounded by fat *(curved arrow)*. The facet joints, ligamentum flavum, and epidural fat are well visualized. (Reproduced with permission from An HS: *Principles and Techniques of Spine Surgery.* Baltimore: Williams & Wilkins, 1998.)

verted teardrop and forms a tunnel that connects with the spinal canal. It is bounded superiorly and inferiorly by the pedicle of the adjacent vertebrae. The posterior boundary is formed by the pars interarticularis and ligamentum flavum. The anterior boundary is formed by the posteroinferior margin of the superior vertebral body, the posterior margin of the intervertebral disc, and the posterosuperior margin of the inferior vertebral body. The nerve root normally is surrounded by fat (Fig. 8). In addition, various types of transforaminal ligaments may traverse within the foramen (12).

The spinal nerve divides into dorsal primary rami and ventral primary rami branches. The dorsal primary rami gives medial, lateral, and occasionally intermediate branches to innervate the zygapophyseal joints and the paraspinal musculature (13). The lateral branches of the lumbar dorsal rami innervate the iliocostalis muscle, whereas the intermediate branches supply the longissimus muscle. The medial branches play an important role in the distribution of the zygapophyseal joints. Each medial branch supplies the zygapophyseal joints above and below. For example, the L4–5 zygapophyseal joints are innervated by the L-4 posterior primary rami and the descending branches from the L-3 posterior primary rami. The medial branches of the posterior pri-

mary rami also supply the segmental muscles and interspinous ligaments arising from the spinous process and lamina of the vertebra with the same segmental number as the nerve. For example, the L-2 nerve supplies only those muscles and interspinous ligaments from the L-2 vertebra. The posterior longitudinal ligament and the anterior aspect of the dura are innervated by the sinuvertebral nerve (14,15). This nerve receives contributions from the ventral rami and the gray ramus communicans. The sinuvertebral nerve runs back into the spinal canal through the foramen, running somewhat cranial to the disc. The gray rami from the sympathetic ganglion join the ventral primary rami. The anterior portion of the lumbar intervertebral discs is innervated by sympathetic fibers, whereas the posterior portion of the disc is innervated by the sinuvertebral nerve (16). The sinuvertebral nerves in the lumbar spine are branches of the ventral rami but also receive contributions from the autonomic gray rami. The sinuvertebral nerves innervate the posterior longitudinal ligament, the posterior part of the annulus, and the ventral part of the dura. Peripheral nerve endings consisting of C- and A-delta fibers have been identified in the posterior longitudinal ligament and peripheral layers of the anulus fibrosus (14,15,17). The sinuvertebral nerves typically ascend to innervate the superior disc as well. In other words, the sinuvertebral nerves arising from the L-4 ventral rami innervate the posterolateral part of the L4–5 annulus but also courses

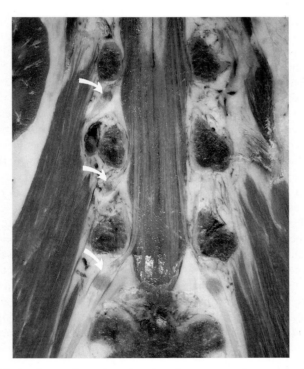

FIG. 7. Coronal section showing the course of nerve roots exiting below the pedicle and joining the dorsal root ganglion *(arrows)* in the intervertebral foramen. (Reproduced with permission from An HS: *Principles and Techniques of Spine Surgery.* Baltimore: Williams & Wilkins, 1998.)

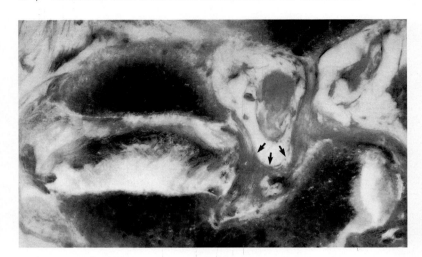

FIG. 8. Sagittal section of the intervertebral foramen with the nerve root surrounded by fat and vascular structures inferiorly. The intervertebral foramen is bounded superiorly and inferiorly by the pedicle of the adjacent vertebrae. The posterior boundary is formed by the pars interarticularis and ligamentum flavum. The anterior boundary is formed by the posteroinferior margin of the superior vertebral body, the posterior margin of the intervertebral disc, and the posterosuperior margin of the inferior vertebral body. Inferiorly, the transforaminal ligament *(arrows)* extend from the posterior margins of the intervertebral disc and superior articular facet. (Reproduced with permission from An HS: *Principles and Techniques of Spine Surgery.* Baltimore: Williams & Wilkins, 1998.)

superiorly to innervate the L3–4 annulus. Sinuvertebral nerves are believed to be derived from the recurrent branch of the spinal nerve and the sympathetic nerve. In animal studies, the posterior portion of the disc and the posterior longitudinal ligament seem to be dually innervated in that both visceral autonomic fibers and somatic nociceptor fibers are present (16,18).

There are interconnections among gray rami, the perivascular plexus around the vertebral artery, and the sympathetic trunk in the cervical spine, all of which contribute to the ventral nerve plexus that innervates the anterior longitudinal ligament, the outer portion of the anulus fibrosis, and the anterior vertebral body (13). The dorsal nerve plexus receives contributions from the sinuvertebral nerves, which originate from the gray rami and perivascular plexus of the vertebral artery in the cervical spine. The first cervical nerve root (suboccipital nerve) exits the vertebral canal above the posterior arch of the atlas and posteromedial to the lateral mass and lies between the vertebral artery and the posterior arch. The posterior primary ramus of the first cervical nerve enters the suboccipital triangle and sends motor fibers to the deep muscles. The anterior primary ramus of the first cervical nerve forms a loop with the second anterior primary ramus and sends fibers to the hypoglossal nerve. The cervical plexus receives fibers from anterior primary rami of C1–4. The cervical plexus is located opposite the C1–3 vertebrae, ventral and lateral to the levator scapulae and middle scalene muscles. The cervical plexus has distributions to the skin and muscles, including the rectus capitis anterior and lateralis, longus capitis and cervicis, levator scapular, and the middle scalene. The cervical plexus also forms loops and branches to supply the sternocleidomastoid and trapezius muscles. The cervical plexus has communications with the hypoglossal nerve from C-1 and C-2 and leaves this trunk as the superior root of the ansa cervicalis, which forms a loop called the ansa cervicalis with the inferior root from C-2 and C-3. The second cervical nerve lies on the lamina of the axis posterior to the lateral mass. The posterior primary ramus (greater occipital nerve) pierces the trapezius about 2 cm below the external occipital protuberance and 2–4 cm from the midline (Fig. 9). Cutaneous branches of the posterior primary rami of C2–5 are consistently present in the skin of the nuchal region. The greater occipital nerve is the largest cutaneous nerve in this region. The lesser occipital nerve is a branch from the anterior cervical plexus and runs upward and lateral to the greater occipital nerve (Fig. 9). The posterior primary ramus of C-3 or third occipital nerve pierces the trapezius more inferiorly about 1 cm medial from the midline (Fig. 9).

The cervical nerve exits over the pedicle that bears the same number, except for the C-8 cervical nerve, which lies between the C-7 and T-1 vertebrae. The posterior primary rami of cervical nerves send motor fibers to the deep muscles and sensory fibers to the skin, but the first cervical nerve has no cutaneous branches. The anterior primary rami of C1–4 form the cervical plexus and those of C5–T1 form the brachial plexus. The lower cervical spinal nerves provide specific dermatomal and motor distributions of the upper extremity, which are essential in the evaluation and treatment of patients with cervical radiculopathy.

The ventral rami of the lumbar spinal nerves in the lumbar region pierce the intertransverse ligament and continue to form the lumbar and lumbosacral plexuses. The L1–4 ventral rami form the lumbar plexus, and the L-4 and L-5 ventral rami join to form the lumbosacral trunk that enters the lumbosacral plexus. The dorsal rami of L-1 or sometimes L-2 and L-3 provide cutaneous branches that cross the posterior iliac crest about 7 to 8 cm from the midline (Fig. 9). These cutaneous branches are the superior cluneal nerves that should be preserved in surgical approaches. Xu et al. (19) reported that the average distances from the posterior superior iliac spine to the superior cluneal nerves, gluteal line, and superior gluteal vessels were 68.8, 26.6, and 62.4 mm, respectively. For posterior iliac crest bone harvesting, the incision should stay within 6.8 cm from the posterior superior iliac spine.

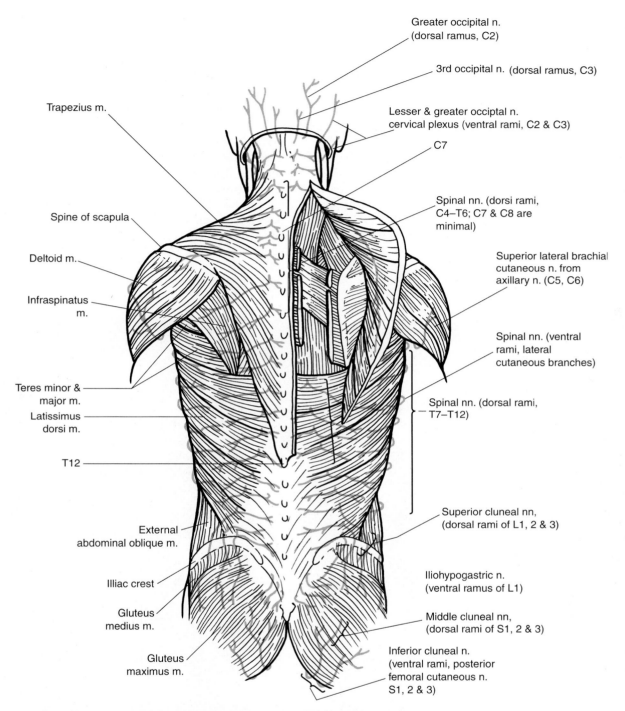

FIG. 9. Cutaneous nerves on the posterior aspect of the neck and back. (Reproduced with permission from An HS: *Principles and Techniques of Spine Surgery.* Baltimore: Williams & Wilkins, 1998.)

The cutaneous branches from both dorsal rami and ventral rami provide sensation in a consistent fashion that is useful clinically. Cutaneous nerves are arranged in a consistent dermatomal pattern. Clinicians should remember when evaluating patients with cervical spine disorders that the C-5 dermatome is present over the deltoid muscle, C-6 dermatome to the thumb, C-7 dermatome to the long finger, and C-8 der-

matome to the small finger. The nipple line corresponds to the T-4 dermatome, and the umbilicus corresponds to the T-8 dermatome. It should be remembered in evaluating the lumbar spine disorders that the L-1 corresponds to the groin, L-2 over the anterior thigh, L-3 over the knee, L-4 over the medial malleolus, L-5 over the great toe, and S-1 over the small toe and bottom of the foot. Sacral dermatomes are located around the perineum, which is important to remember when assessing patients with cauda equina or conus medullaris syndrome as well as when evaluating sacral sparing in incomplete spinal cord syndromes.

Osseous Structures and Articulations

There are osseous structures in the different regions of the vertebral column that have different characteristics aside from the obvious differences in size. The bony anatomy of the atlas and axis in the cervical spine is most unique (Fig. 10). The atlas is a ringlike structure, in which the thick anterior arch blends into the lateral masses. The canal diameters of the atlas were noted to be rather constant at 32 ± 2 mm in the sagittal plane and 29 ± 2 mm in the lateral plane (20). The mean thickness of the anterior ring was 6 ± 1 mm and posteriorly was 8 ± 2 mm. The occipital condyles articulate with the concave superior aspects of the lateral masses as a

cup-shaped joint. The occipital condyles project downward and outward, whereas the superior facet of the atlas faces upward and inward to support the occiput. The atlantooccipital articulation is supported by the anterior and posterior occipital membranes, which are a continuation of anterior longitudinal ligament and ligamentum flavum, respectively (Fig. 10). The atlantooccipital joint mostly allows for flexion, extension, and lateral bending motions. The inferior facets of the atlas are flatter and more circular than the superior facets. They face downward and inward to articulate with the axis (Fig. 10). The atlas has no body, and the anterior tubercle of the anterior arch serves as the attachment site for the longus colli muscle. The posterior tubercle of the atlas serves as the bony attachment site for the rectus minor muscle and suboccipital membrane. The atlas has large transverse processes to which the superior and inferior oblique muscles attach. The transverse foramen is located within the transverse process, through which the vertebral artery passes.

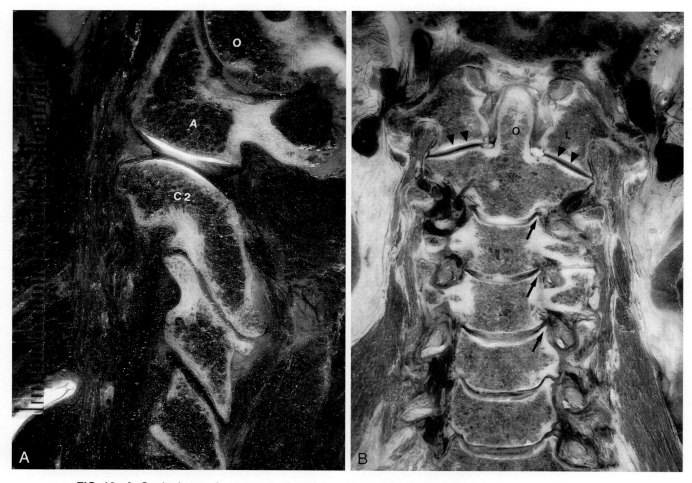

FIG. 10. A: Sagittal cryomicrotome section of the upper cervical spine. The inferior aspect of occiput (o) is convex and articulates with the atlas (A), which is correspondingly concave. The atlas articulates with the axis (C2) below and the joint surface is flat. **B:** Coronal cryomicrotome section of the cervical spine. The atlas articulates with the occipital condyle above and the axis below *(arrowheads)*. The odontoid process (o) projects between the lateral masses (L) of the atlas. The uncovertebral joints are shown with *arrows*. (Reproduced with permission from An HS: *Principles and Techniques of Spine Surgery.* Baltimore: Williams & Wilkins, 1998.)

The axis is unique in its bony anatomy. The odontoid process projects upward, articulating with the posterior aspect of the anterior arch of the atlas as a synovial joint. The projection angle of the odontoid process varies from −2 to 42 degrees, with a mean of 13 degrees (21). The average dens height is about 15 mm (22). The transverse ligament, which spans across the arch of the atlas, holds the odontoid process against the anterior arch of atlas. This transverse ligament is the principal stabilizing structure for atlantoaxial articulation. The transverse ligament has superior and inferior extensions, which form the cruciate ligament of the atlas. Secondary stabilizers of this articulation are the alar ligaments, which arise from the sides of dens to the condyles of the occipital bone and apical ligament (which arise from the apex of the dens to the foramen magnum as a remnant of the notochord). The tectorial membrane is a continuation of the posterior longitudinal ligament. Posteriorly, the axis has the large lamina and bifid spinous process, which serves as the attachment site for the rectus major and inferior oblique muscles. The zone between the lamina and the lateral mass of axis vertebra is indistinct. The pedicles of the axis are large and project medially at 33 degrees and superiorly at 20 degrees (22). The atlantoaxial articulation provides about 50% of the rotatory motion of the cervical spine. The spinal canal at the upper cervical spine is more capacious than the lower cervical spine, with sagittal diameters of 23 mm at C-1 and 20 mm at C-2. When approaching the posterior aspect of the atlas and axis, the surgeon should avoid injuries to the associated neurovascular structures such as the vertebral artery, spinal ganglion of C-2, and spinal cord.

The lower cervical spine bony anatomy from C-3 to C-6 are similar, with slight dimensional increases from C-3 to C-6. C-7 is unique as the transitional vertebra between the cervical and thoracic spine. Posteriorly, spinous processes are bifid from C-3 to C-6 (Fig. 11) and project inferiorly. The C-7 spinous process is quite large and is not bifid. It often is called the vertebra prominens. The lamina blends into the lateral mass, which is the bone between the superior and inferior articular processes. The articular processes oppose each other to form the facet joint. The normal cervical facet joints have articular cartilage and menisci that are surrounded by a capsular ligament and lined by a synovial membrane. Most adult cervical facet joints undergo changes with aging and consist only of a thin layer of cartilage and irregularly thickened subarticular cortical bone. The joint capsules are richly innervated by proprioceptive and pain receptors that may be important in the pathogenesis of neck pain.

The facet joint line is horizontal and slightly circular inferiorly from the posterior aspect. The interfacet distances are relatively constant at different levels, but there are individual variations from 9 to 16 mm, with an average of 13 mm (23). Most posterior lateral mass plate-screw systems are designed to have screw hole distances at 13 mm for this reason. During posterior plate-screw instrumentation, important anatomic considerations include the facet joint lines, lateral mass margins, and joint inclination. There is a definite junction between the lamina and lateral mass, and the lateral edge of the lateral mass forms a ridge down to the transverse process. The facet joint itself is angled about 45 degrees cephalad from the transverse plane (Fig. 11B). The lateral mass of C-7 is more elongated from the superoinferior aspect and thinner than upper levels from the anteroposterior aspect.

A typical cervical vertebra on the anterolateral aspect consists of a body, transverse processes, and pedicles. The body is relatively small and oval in shape, with the mediolateral diameter greater than the anteroposterior diameter (Fig. 11C). From the coronal plane, the superior surface of the vertebral body is concave, and the inferior surface of the body is correspondingly convex. From the sagittal plane, however, the superior surface of the body is slightly convex or straight with the corresponding concave inferior surface of the upper vertebral body.

The anteroinferior edge of the vertebral body is lipped inferiorly. The lateral surfaces of the superior vertebral body project upward, conforming to small grooves in the inferolateral borders of the cephalad vertebra, which forms the uncovertebral joints or joints of Luschka. The vertebral surface average width and depth are 17 and 15 mm, respectively, from C-2 to C-6 and increase to about 20 and 17 mm, respectively, at C-7 (24). Vertebral heights on the posterior wall in the midsagittal plane range from 11 to 13 mm. Projecting laterally from the cephalad aspect of the vertebral body is the anterior tubercle of the transverse process, which joins the posterior tubercle of the transverse process. The anterior tubercle is a costal element, and C-6 anterior tubercle, also known as the carotid tubercle, is prominent as a surgical landmark. Between the posterior tubercle and anterior tubercle is the groove or the costotransverse lamella, which projects inferiorly for the passage of the spinal nerve. The vertebral arterial and venous systems pass through the transverse foramen, which is located medial to the tubercles of the transverse process and lateral to the vertebral body. The transverse processes increase significantly in size at C-6 and C-7. The pedicles project posterolaterally from the vertebral body at a 30- to 45-degree angle and join the lamina to form the vertebral arch. The spinal canal or vertebral foramen is triangular in shape with rounded angles, and the lateral width of the canal is significantly greater than the anteroposterior depth at all levels. Normal sagittal diameters of the cervical spine are 17 to 18 mm at C3–6, and 15 mm at C-7 (24). The cross-sectional area of the spinal canal is largest at C-2 and smallest at C-7. The height of the pedicle is about 7 mm, and the width is about 5 to 6 mm, with a slight increase from C-3 to C-7 (24). As mentioned before, the C-2 pedicle is larger, with a height of 10 mm and width of 8 mm. From C-3 to C-7, the angulation of the pedicles varies from 8 degrees below to 11 degrees above the transverse plane. The pedicle angle in the sagittal plane decreases from about 45 to 30 degrees from C-3 to C-7. Despite some successful clinical reports, transpedicular screw placement in the cervical spine should be regarded as difficult and perhaps dangerous due to the small size of the pedicle from C3–6 (25–27).

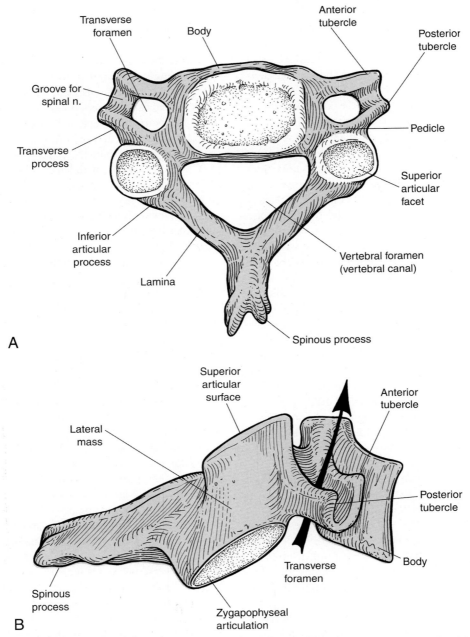

FIG. 11. Bony anatomy of the lower cervical spine. **A:** View from the top shows the vertebral foramen, superior articular facet, transverse process, transverse foramen, and the body. **B:** Side view shows the spinous process, superior and inferior articular surfaces, tubercles of the transverse process, and the body.

The cervical nerve roots emerge from the vertebral canal via the intervertebral foramen, which is bordered by the uncinate process anteriorly, the superior facet posteriorly, and the adjacent pedicles superiorly and inferiorly (9). The intervertebral foramen was measured by Ebraheim et al. (28) to be an average of 7.5 to 8.5 mm in height and 4.5 to 7 mm in width. The foraminal height and width gradually increase from C-3 to C-7. Ebraheim et al. (28) studied the cervical nerve root groove that extends about 1.5 to 2 cm from the medial aspect of the pedicle to the lateral end of the trans-

verse process and associated costal process, where it is bounded by the anterior and posterior tubercles. The nerve root groove was divided into three zones, and the medial zone or the intervertebral foramen is important in the etiology of cervical radiculopathy.

There is a transition region at the cervicothoracic junction, with C-7 having similar anatomic characteristics at T-1 and T-2. The dimensions of the vertebral body transverse and spinous processes are larger at C-6 and C-7 as well. In addition, dimensions of the spinal canal decrease at C-6 and C-7,

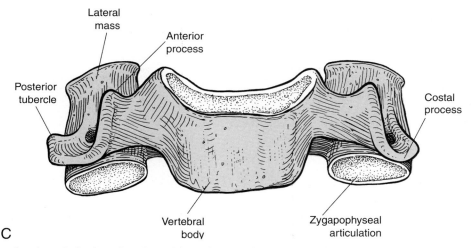

Lateral mass
Anterior process
Posterior tubercle
Costal process
Vertebral body
Zygapophyseal articulation

C

FIG. 11. *Continued.* **C:** Anterior view shows the vertebral body, transverse processes, lateral mass, and articular processes. (Reproduced with permission from An HS: *Principles and Techniques of Spine Surgery.* Baltimore: Williams & Wilkins, 1998.)

representing a distinct transition to the thoracic region. The articulating facet joint between C-7 and T-1 resembles a thoracic facet joint, and the lateral mass of C-7 is thinner than that of upper levels. Inner diameters of the pedicles at C-7, T-1, and T-2 from medial to lateral plane average 5.2, 6.3, and 5.5 mm, respectively. Medial angulations of the pedicle are 34, 30, and 26 degrees at C-7, T-1, and T-2, respectively (23). The diameter of the pedicle is relatively large at the C7–T1 region as compared to the cervical and upper thoracic regions (29). The morphologic characteristics should be remembered when performing transpedicular procedures in the cervicothoracic region.

The thoracic vertebrae are unique in their articulation with the ribs. They have heart-shaped bodies and a circular spinal canal (Fig. 12). This round spinal canal has less free space for the spinal cord than the cervical and lumbar regions. The articular facets for the ribs are located in the body and transverse process. The radiate and costovertebral ligaments are between the body and rib, whereas the costotransverse and intertransverse ligaments are between the transverse process and rib. The spinous processes are long and slender and overlap to the lower vertebral arches. The thoracic column is mechanically stiffer and less mobile because of the rib attachment. The upper and middle thoracic vertebrae have inherent stability against anteroposterior translation, whereas the lower thoracic vertebrae have greater stability against rotation due to the orientation of the facet joint. T-1 is atypical in that it has a long horizontal transverse process. The size of the transverse processes gradually decreases from T-1 to T-10. T-9 to T-12 vertebrae have tubercles similar to those of the lumbar vertebrae. The pedicle of the thoracic vertebrae measures in height about 10 mm at T-4 and 14 mm at T-12 and in width about 4.5 mm at T-4 and 7.8 mm at T-12 (30). The pedicles incline anteromedially ranging from 0.3 degrees at T-12 to 13.9 degrees at T-4. The pedicle wall is thicker medially than laterally (31).

In the lumbar spine the vertebral body is largest at L-5, which transmits the body weight to the base of the sacrum (Fig. 13). The pedicles connect between the body and the posterior elements. The transverse pedicle width averages 18 mm at L-5 and becomes smaller in the upper lumbar spine, with an average of 9 mm at L-1. The medial angulation or transverse pedicle angle is about 30 degrees at L-5 and only 12 degrees at L-1 (32). From the posterior aspect, the pedicle is located about 1 mm inferior to the tip of the inferior articular process or in the middle of the transverse processes horizontally and the most posterior prominence of the superior articular process vertically. Near the transverse process and pedicle attachment, the accessory process is present as an irregular bony prominence. In the lumbar spine the facet joints are more sagittally oriented to resist axial rotation. The lumbosacral facet is oriented more coronally to resist anteroposterior translation. Mamillary processes are prominences on the posterior edge of the superior articular processes. The lumbar spinal canal is oval in the upper lumbar region and becomes triangular in the lower lumbar region.

The nerve root takes off from the thecal sac, courses under the lateral recess, and travels through the intervertebral foramen (33,34). Lee et al. (35) subdivided the lateral lumbar spinal canal into three anatomic zones: entrance zone, mid zone, and exit zone. The entrance zone is the subarticular area just medial to the pedicle and is synonymous with the lateral recess area. The mid zone is located under the pars interarticularis and the pedicle, and the exit zone is synonymous with the intervertebral foramen. The entrance zone is located underneath the superior articular process of the facet joint medial to the pedicle. The entrance zone is the cephalad aspect of the more commonly known lateral recess, which begins at the lateral aspect of the thecal sac and runs obliquely downward and laterally toward the intervertebral foramen. Anatomically, the lateral recess is bordered laterally by the pedicle, posteriorly by the superior articular facet, and anteriorly by the postero-

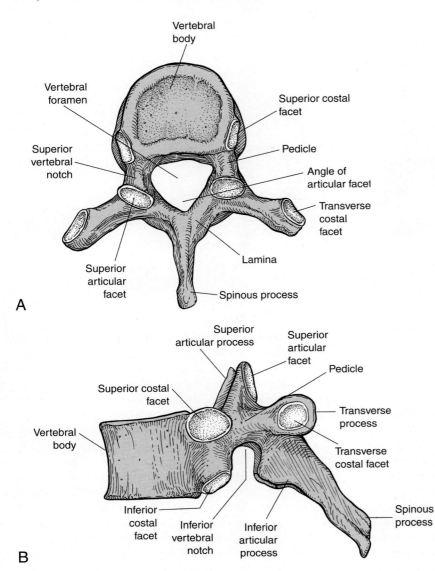

Vertebral
body

Vertebral
foramen

Superior costal
facet

Superior
vertebral
notch

Pedicle

Angle of
articular facet

Transverse
costal
facet

Superior
articular
facet

Lamina

Spinous process

A

Superior
articular process

Superior
articular
facet

Pedicle

Superior costal
facet

Transverse
process

Vertebral
body

Transverse
costal facet

Inferior
costal
facet

Inferior
vertebral
notch

Inferior
articular
process

Spinous
process

B

FIG. 12. The thoracic vertebra. **A:** Top view shows articulation with the rib. The vertebra has a heart-shaped body and circular vertebral canal. **B:** Side view shows the vertebral body, facets for the rib, pedicle, and inferiorly projecting spinous process. (Reproduced with permission from An HS: *Principles and Techniques of Spine Surgery*. Baltimore: Williams & Wilkins, 1998.)

lateral surface of the vertebral body and adjacent intervertebral disc. The medial border of the lateral recess is formed by the thecal sac. The narrowest portion of the lateral recess is between the superior border of the pedicle and the broad portion of the superior articular facet. The nerve root in this region is covered by the root sleeve and surrounded by cerebrospinal fluid. The lateral margin of the nerve root sleeve contacts the medial cortical bone of the pedicle, and the medial margin of the nerve root is surrounded by epidural fatty tissue. The normal lateral recess measurements have been well delineated by computed tomography (36). A lateral recess height of 5 mm or more is normal, a height of 2 mm or less is pathologic, and a height of 3 to 4 mm is suggestive of lateral recess stenosis. The mid zone is located under the pars interarticularis just below the pedicle. It is bounded anteriorly by the posterior aspect of the vertebral body and posteriorly by the pars interarticularis. The medial boundary is open to the central spinal canal. The nerve roots normally run obliquely downward through the lateral recess into the intervertebral foramen. The nerve root

travels around the subpedicular notch and contacts posteriorly with the ventral wall of the pars interarticularis, where the ligamentum flavum is attached. The exit zone is formed by the intervertebral foramen. The lumbar intervertebral foramen is shaped like an inverted teardrop and forms a tunnel that connects with the spinal canal. It is bounded superiorly and inferiorly by the pedicles of the adjacent vertebrae. The posterior boundary is formed by the pars interarticularis and the ligamentum flavum. The anterior boundary is formed by the posteroinferior margin of the superior vertebral body, the posterior margin of the intervertebral disc, and the posterosuperior margin of the inferior vertebral body. The normal foraminal height varies from 20 to 23 mm and the width at the upper foraminal area varies from 8 to 10 mm (11). The ventral and dorsal nerve roots occupy 23% to 30% of the area of the foramen and lie anterior to the dorsal root ganglion. The dorsal root ganglion normally lies within the superior lateral portion of the lumbar intervertebral foramen and directly below the pedicle in 90% of lumbar levels. Foraminal height less than 15

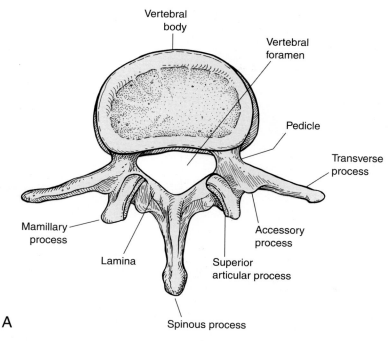

Vertebral body

Vertebral foramen

Pedicle

Transverse process

Mamillary process

Lamina

Accessory process

Superior articular process

Spinous process

A

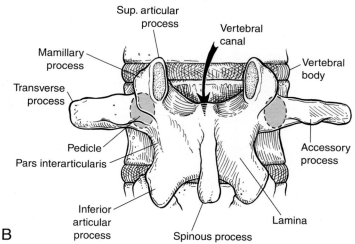

Sup. articular process

Vertebral canal

Mamillary process

Vertebral body

Transverse process

Pedicle

Pars interarticularis

Accessory process

Inferior articular process

Lamina

Spinous process

B

FIG. 13. The lumbar vertebra. **A:** Top views show the larger vertebral body, pedicles that connect between the body, and posterior elements. The vertebral foramen is more triangular in shape. **B:** Posterior view shows the lamina, pars interarticularis, transverse process, and articular processes. The pedicle region is outlined by the *oval*. (Reproduced with permission from An HS: *Principles and Techniques of Spine Surgery.* Baltimore: Williams & Wilkins, 1998.)

mm and posterior disc height less than 4 mm is associated with nerve root compression 80% of the time (37).

Included in the bony structures of the sacrum are the ala, promontory, sacral crests, sacral foramina, and articular surfaces (Fig. 14). The sacrum is composed of five fused sacral vertebrae that provide strength and stability to the pelvis while transmitting the body weight to the pelvis. The four pairs of sacral foramina contain ventral and dorsal divisions of the sacral nerves. The anterior sacral foramina are larger than the dorsal sacral foramina. The median sacral crest represents fused spinous processes, and S-5 has no spinous process. The intermediate sacral crests represent the fused articular processes, and the lateral sacral crests are the tips of the transverse processes of the sacral vertebrae. The sacral hiatus leads to the sacral canal, which contains fatty connective tissue, the filum terminale, S-5 nerve, and coccygeal nerve. The sacral cornu is the inferior articular process of the S-5 vertebra and projects

laterally. The coccyx consists of four rudimentary vertebrae. The coccygeal cornu articulates with the sacral cornua. The coccyx provides attachments for parts of the gluteus maximus and coccygeus muscles, and anococcygeal ligament.

The sacroiliac joint consists of the sacral articular process with hyaline cartilage and the iliac surface with fibrocartilage. The sacroiliac joint is stabilized by interosseous sacroiliac, posterior sacroiliac, and anterior sacroiliac ligaments (Fig. 14). Connecting ligaments in the lumbosacral junction and the pelvis include the sacrotuberous ligament from the sacrum to the ischial tuberosity, the sacrospinous ligament that divides the pelvis into greater and lesser sciatic notches, and the iliolumbar ligaments that connect the L-5 transverse processes to the ala of sacrum. The iliolumbar ligaments connect the transverse process of the fifth lumbar vertebra to the ilium. The iliolumbar ligament can be divided into different parts based on anatomic location, such as ante-

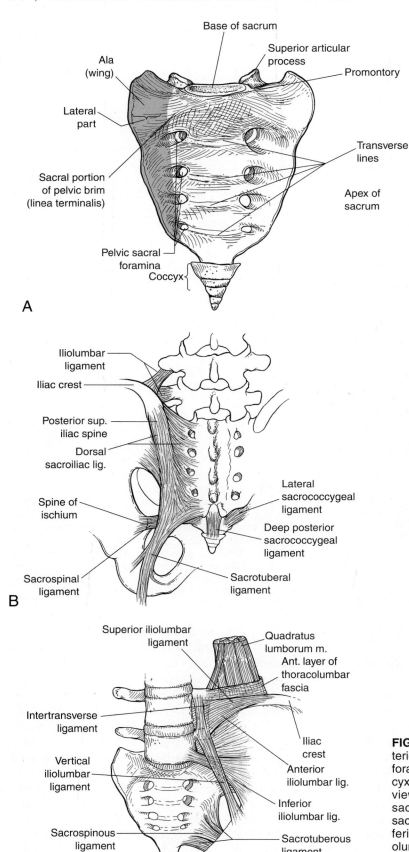

FIG. 14. The sacrum and sacroiliac articulation. **A:** Anterior view of the sacrum. The ala, promontory, sacral foramina, and articular surfaces are shown. The coccyx consists of four rudimentary vertebrae. **B:** Posterior view shows the iliolumbar, posterior sacroiliac, and sacrotuberous ligaments. **C:** Anterior view of the sacroiliac articulation shows the anterior iliolumbar, inferior iliolumbar, vertical iliolumbar, and superior iliolumbar ligaments. (Reproduced with permission from An HS: *Principles and Techniques of Spine Surgery*. Baltimore: Williams & Wilkins, 1998.)

rior, superior, posterior, inferior, and vertical. The iliolumbar ligament is important in resisting forward translation of the L-5 vertebra on the sacrum.

Intervertebral Disc and Ligaments

The intervertebral disc is an avascular structure that includes the nucleus pulposus at the interior of the disc, the outer anulus fibrosus, and the cartilaginous endplates adjacent to the vertebral surfaces. The nucleus pulposus is derived from the primitive notochord and functions as a shock absorber. The anulus fibrosus maintains the stability of the motion segment along with ligaments and articulations. The nucleus pulposus is bordered clearly by the anulus fibrosus in infancy, but in the adult the margin between the nucleus pulposus and anulus fibrosus becomes less distinct (Fig. 15). After 50 years of age, the nucleus pulposus becomes more difficult to distinguish from the anulus fibrosus, and the nucleus pulposus becomes a fibrocartilaginous mass similar to the inner zone of the anulus fibrosus (Fig. 15). The anulus fibrosus has an outer collagenous layer in which the fibers are arranged in oblique layers of lamellae. The fibers of lamella run perpendicular to the fibers of the adjacent lamella. This oblique arrangement can offer resistance to motion in all directions. The collagen fibers in the posterior portion of the disc run more vertical than oblique, which may account for the rela-

tive frequency of annular tears seen clinically. The anulus fibrosus is firmly attached to the adjacent vertebral endplates. The cartilaginous endplate is a layer of hyaline cartilage that rests on the subchondral bone and serves as a barrier between the pressure of the nucleus pulposus and the adjacent vertebral bodies. This cartilage is a growth plate and is responsible for endochondral ossification during growth. The cartilaginous endplates also serve as the insertion site for the inner fibers of the anulus fibrosus and the diffusion of nutrients from the subchondral bone to the disc.

Some translatory movement in the sagittal plane is allowed by the cervical intervertebral disc, but lateral movement is resisted by the uncinate process, which is located at the posterolateral aspect of the disc and may help prevent disc herniation in this area. Degeneration of the anulus fibrosus in the cervical region is similar to that of the lumbar spine in that concentric, transverse, and radial tears of the anulus fibrosus can occur. Radial tears in the anulus fibrosus portion of the disc may be clinically significant (Fig. 15). The discs are thinnest in the thoracic region and thickest in the lumbar region, where they constitute one third of its length. The discs are thicker anteriorly in the lumbar spine because of lordotic curvature, and the vertebral endplates of L-3 are parallel and horizontal (Fig. 15). Normally the lumbar discs are concave or straight posteriorly, but the L5–S1 disc normally is slightly convex.

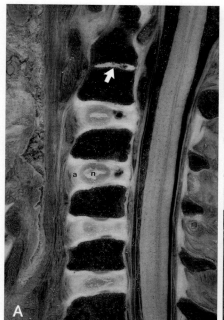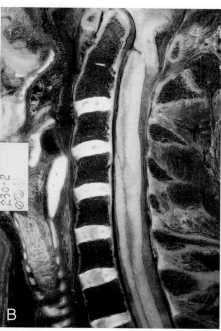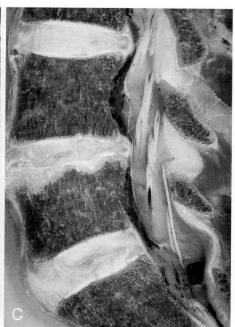

FIG. 15. Sagittal cryomicrotome sections of the spine. **A:** Sagittal cryomicrotome of a skeletally immature cervical spine showing the intervertebral disc with clear margin between the nucleus pulposus and anulus fibrosus. The *arrow* indicates the synchondrosis between the odontoid process and the body. **B:** Sagittal cryomicrotome section in an adult showing indistinct margin between the nucleus pulposus and the anulus fibrosus as the nucleus pulposus becomes a fibrocartilaginous mass similar to the inner zone of the anulus fibrosus. **C:** Sagittal cryomicrotome section of the lower lumbar spine showing the degenerative disc with bulging anulus fibrosus and loss of height at L4–5. (Reproduced with permission from An HS: *Principles and Techniques of Spine Surgery.* Baltimore: Williams & Wilkins, 1998.)

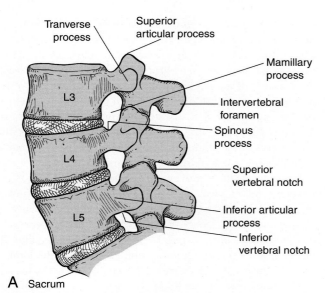

Tranverse process

Superior articular process

Mamillary process

Intervertebral foramen

Spinous process

Superior vertebral notch

Inferior articular process

Inferior vertebral notch

L3

L4

L5

A Sacrum

FIG. 16. Sagittal cryomicrotome of the lumbar spine. The anterior and posterior longitudinal ligaments are shown *(arrows)*. The ligamentum flavum *(curved arrow)* is located just above the epidural fat. (Reproduced with permission from An HS: *Principles and Techniques of Spine Surgery.* Baltimore: Williams & Wilkins, 1998.)

The outermost fibers of the anulus fibrosus are contiguous with the anterior and posterior longitudinal ligaments (Fig. 16). The anterior longitudinal ligament is a strong band that attaches from the skull as the anterior atlantooccipital membrane and continues caudally over the entire length of the spine down to the sacrum. The anterior longitudinal ligament is thinner and more closely attached at the intervertebral disc margins than at the concave anterior vertebral surfaces. In the upper cervical spine the posterior longitudinal ligament is wider than the lower cervical spine and wider over the intervertebral disc than over the vertebral bodies. The posterior longitudinal ligament in the cervical spine is double layered. The deep layer sends fibers to the anulus fibrosus and continues laterally to the region of the intervertebral foramina (38). The anterior longitudinal ligament also sweeps around and envelops the lateral aspects of the vertebral bodies under the longus colli muscle with the lateral extension continuous with the deep layer of the posterior longitudinal ligament in the region of the intervertebral foramina (38). The superficial or more dorsal layer of the posterior longitudinal ligament is adjacent to the dura mater and continues as a connective tissue membrane that envelops the dura mater, nerve roots, and vertebral artery, suggesting that this membrane may serve as a protective barrier.

The transverse process in the thoracic spine and the body have articulations with the rib and connecting costotransverse ligaments and radiate ligament. The thoracic spine is inherently more stable than the cervical or lumbar spine due to the attachment of the ribs. The posterior longitudinal ligament is broad in the thoracic and lumbar regions, where it is attached to the intervertebral discs and helps to prevent hy-

perflexion of the vertebral column and resist posterior protrusion of the intervertebral disc. Dural ligaments have been reported in the lumbar spine, namely, Spencer's ligament that courses from the dural tube to the posterior longitudinal ligament and Hoffmann's ligament that courses from the nerve root sheath to the inferior aspect of the pedicle with the neural canal (39,40). Wiltse et al. (41) also described a peridural membrane that lies anterior to the posterior longitudinal ligament at the level of the vertebral body. Yaszemski and White (42) described the discectomy membrane that is between the posterior longitudinal ligament and the nerve root at the level of the disc. It is important to recognize these membranes, particularly during surgical approaches.

The ligamentum flavum is a short ligament that joins the laminae of adjacent vertebrae, attaching to the anterior surface of the lamina above to the superior margin of the lamina below, extending laterally to the articular processes, and contributing to the boundary of the intervertebral foramen (Fig. 16). The ligamentum flavum consists primarily of elastic fibers, but the elasticity lessens with aging. Anterior buckling or hypertrophy may contribute to spinal stenosis. There is a gap in the midline of the ligamentum flavum for the exit of veins.

The ligaments between the vertebral arches include the interspinous ligament that connects adjacent spinal processes and the supraspinous ligament that stretches across the tips of the spinous process (Fig. 16). In the cervical spine the interspinous ligament is thin and less well developed than in the lumbar region. The interspinous ligaments attach in an oblique orientation from the posterior superior aspect to the anterior inferior aspect of the spinous process. The supraspinous ligament extends in the cervical region as the ligamentum nuchae, which spans from the external occipital protuberance to the seventh cervical vertebrae. The ligamentum nuchae is a fibroelastic septum for the attachment of adjacent muscles. The supraspinous ligament consists largely of tendinous fibers derived from the back muscles. It is better developed in the upper lumbar region and often absent in the lower lumbar region.

Muscles

The three groups of muscles in the back can be divided into superficial, intermediate, and deep intrinsic groups (Fig. 17). The superficial group consists of the trapezius and latissimus dorsi muscles (Fig. 17A). The trapezius originates from the external occipital protuberance and the medial nuchal line of C-7 to T-12 spinous processes and inserts on the spine of the scapula, acromion, and lateral aspect of the clavicle. The trapezius is innervated by the eleventh cranial nerve and functions to extend the head. The latissimus dorsi arises from the lumbar aponeurosis and the posterior iliac crest and lower four ribs and inserts on the bottom of the intertubercular groove of the humerus to extend, adduct, and rotate the arm medially. Its innervation is the thoracodorsal nerve.

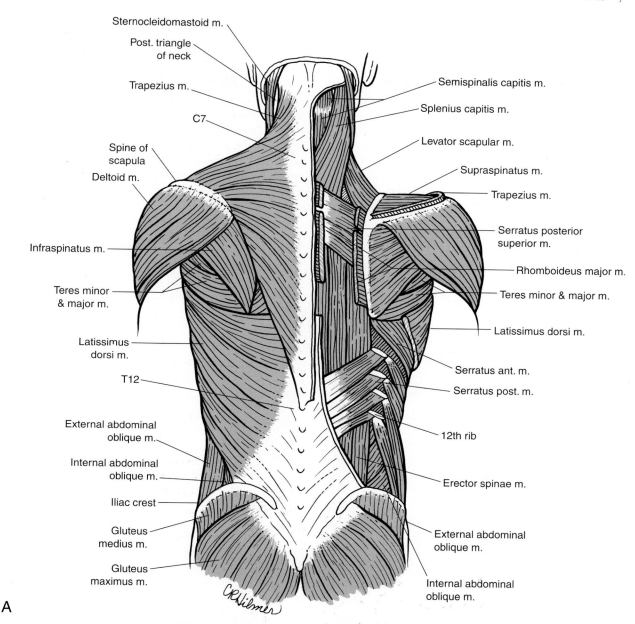

FIG. 17. Muscles of the back. **A:** Superficial layer.

The serratus posterior superior forms the intermediate layer, arises from the lower part of the ligamentum nuchae and the spinous processes of the seventh and upper thoracic vertebrae, and inserts on the upper second to fifth ribs. The serratus posterior inferior arises from the lower thoracic and upper two lumbar spinous processes and inserts on the lower four ribs. The serratus posterior muscles are innervated by the ventral rami of spinal nerves or intercostal nerves. Their function is to enlarge the thorax during respiration.

The intrinsic muscles are involved with movements of the vertebral column. The intrinsic muscles of the back are subdivided into superficial, intermediate, and deep layers. The posterior muscles of the back are innervated by the dorsal rami of the spinal nerves. The superficial muscles are longer and span many vertebrae, whereas the deepest muscles span only one vertebral segment. In the cervical spine, deep to the trapezius and the rhomboids, unlike the muscles in the thoracic and lumbar regions, the splenius capitis and splenius cervicis muscles arise medially and pass laterally as they are traced upward. These muscles comprise the superficial group of the intrinsic back muscles. They originate from the spinous processes of the lower cervical and upper thoracic spines, insert on the transverse processes of the upper cervical spine and the mastoid process, and aid in lateral bending and extension of the head and cervical vertebral column.

In the intermediate layer of intrinsic deep muscles, the erector spinal muscles lie within a fascial compartment between the posterior and middle layers of the thoracolumbar fascia (Fig. 17B). The erector spinae is arranged in three vertical columns: iliocostalis laterally, longissimus intermediately, and spinalis medially. The erector spinae arises from the posterior part of the iliac crest, the posterior aspect of the sacrum, the sacroiliac ligaments, and the sacral and inferior lumbar spinous processes. The iliocostalis muscle is subdivided into lumbar, thoracic, and cervical portions. The intermediate longissimus arises from the transverse processes of the thoracic and cervical vertebrae and the mastoid process of the skull. The longissimus muscle is subdivided into longissimus thoracic, cervicis, and capitis. The spinalis muscle is narrow and insignificant. It extends from the spinous processes of the superior thoracic region. The erector spinae muscle is the primary extensor of the vertebral column.

Several short muscles are found in the deepest layer of the intrinsic back muscles between the transverse and spinous processes, namely, semispinalis, multifidus, and rotatores (Fig. 17C). This deep group of muscles is collectively known as the transversospinalis muscle. The semispinalis muscle is divided into thoracis, cervicis, and capitis according to the insertion of the muscle bundles. Deep to the semispinalis are the multifidus muscles that span from one to three vertebral segments. The muscle bundles run upward and medially from the transverse processes to spinal processes, covering laminae of

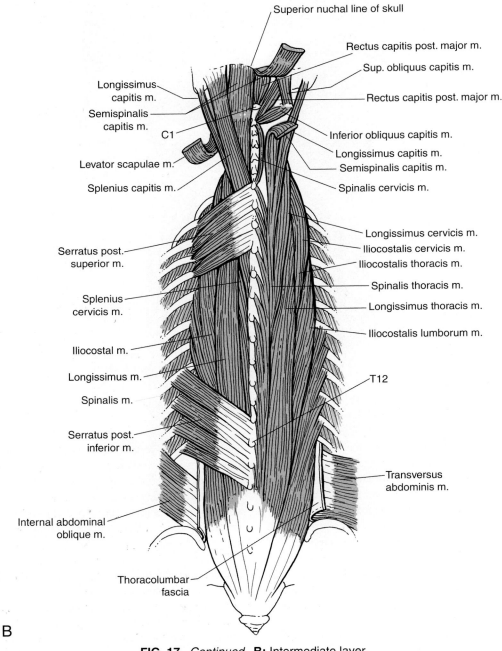

FIG. 17. *Continued.* **B:** Intermediate layer.

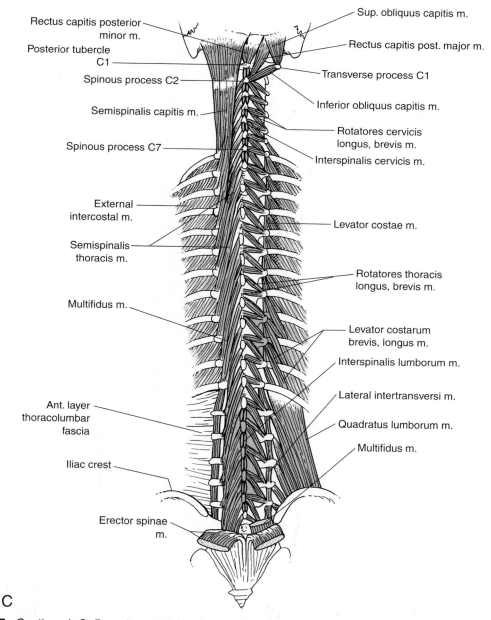

Rectus capitis posterior minor m.
Posterior tubercle C1
Spinous process C2
Semispinalis capitis m.
Spinous process C7
External intercostal m.
Semispinalis thoracis m.
Multifidus m.
Ant. layer thoracolumbar fascia
Iliac crest
Erector spinae m.

Sup. obliquus capitis m.
Rectus capitis post. major m.
Transverse process C1
Inferior obliquus capitis m.
Rotatores cervicis longus, brevis m.
Interspinalis cervicis m.
Levator costae m.
Rotatores thoracis longus, brevis m.
Levator costarum brevis, longus m.
Interspinalis lumborum m.
Lateral intertransversi m.
Quadratus lumborum m.
Multifidus m.

C

FIG. 17. *Continued.* **C:** Deep layer. (Reproduced with permission from An HS: *Principles and Techniques of Spine Surgery.* Baltimore: Williams & Wilkins, 1998.)

S-4 to C-2 vertebrae. The rotatores muscles arise from the transverse process of one vertebra and insert into the base of the spinous process of the second vertebra above. The interspinales and intertransversalis muscles, also known as short rotators, pass from one vertebra to the next vertebra above.

The suboccipital muscles in the upper cervical spine attach from the occiput to the second vertebra. Rectus capitis posterior major originates from the C-2 spinous process and inserts on the inferior nuchal line of the occiput. Rectus capitis posterior minor originates from the posterior tubercle of the atlas and inserts on the occiput. Obliquus capitis inferior originates from the C-2 spinous process and inserts on the

transverse process of atlas. Obliquus capitis superior originates from the transverse process of the atlas and inserts on the occiput between the superior and inferior nuchal lines.

SURGICAL APPROACHES

Posterior Exposure of the Upper Cervical Spine

The upper cervical spine can be surgically approached anteriorly or posteriorly. Several posterior occipitocervical fusion techniques have been described in the literature (43–47). Posterior atlantoaxial stabilization and fusion also can be accomplished with wires and iliac bone graft in the majority of cases (48,49). Newer techniques utilize screw fixation between the lateral mass of C-1 and C-2 (45,50). Complications associated with posterior occipitocervical or atlantoaxial fusion may be devastating. Extreme care is required during passage of the wires to prevent injuries to the brainstem or spinal cord. The vertebral artery must be protected during exposure and instrumentation. The use of somatosensory evoked potential monitoring is routine in myelopathic cases. Postoperative external support with a halo vest is recommended in the majority of wiring cases.

Generally, a halo vest is applied preoperatively. Anesthesia and intubation must be done cautiously; awake intubation using fiberoptic light is recommended in all unstable cases to minimize neck manipulation. If traction is not required and preoperative alignment is acceptable, surgery can be performed in the halo vest on the routine operating table. If traction or spinal realignment is necessary during the procedure, the halo ring should be attached to a traction device on the Stryker table. To facilitate exposure of the occiput and upper cervical spine, a halo ring with a posterior opening is recommended.

A reverse Trendelenburg position allows for venous drainage and less bleeding during the procedure (Fig. 18). A midline incision is made from the external occipital protuberance to the spinous process of C-2. Surgical dissection on the occiput and the ring of the atlas must be completed in a gentle manner, as excess pressure may result in a fracture of the atlas or slippage of the instrument. The ring of the atlas should not be dissected more than 1.5 cm laterally because the vertebral artery is at risk beyond this margin. Dissection of the foramen magnum from the inferior edge of the foramen should be avoided to prevent uncontrollable venous bleeding. Wiring and other methods for stabilization of the upper cervical spine are well described elsewhere in the book.

Posterior Exposure of the Lower Cervical Spine and Fusion

Exposing the posterior elements of the lower cervical spine is simple. Either Mayfield tongs or Gardner-Wells tongs are used for positioning. Venous drainage is allowed with reverse Trendelenburg positioning. A midline incision is followed by subperiosteal dissection, exposing the spinous processes, lamina, and facet joints. Only the levels to be fused should be exposed, as creeping fusion extension is common. In performing a cervical laminectomy, the junction between the lamina and facet is thinned with a power burr, and a small curette or thin Kerrison rongeur is used to finish the cut. Meticulous hemostasis is mandatory to prevent hematoma formation. Posterior fusion and stabilization of the cervical spine is a well-established procedure. The standard triple wiring and fusion with bone graft is performed in the majority of cases. If laminectomy has been performed, facet wiring, Luque rodding, or lateral mass plating can be performed (23,51–54).

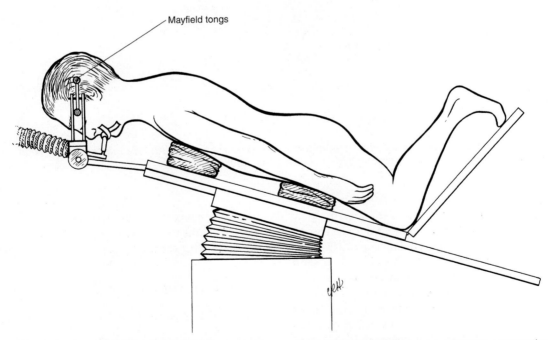

FIG. 18. Operating position for posterior cervical procedures. The Mayfield tongs and frame secure the head in position and the reverse Trendelenburg position allows venous drainage and less bleeding during the procedure. (Reproduced with permission from An HS: *Principles and Techniques of Spine Surgery.* Baltimore: Williams & Wilkins, 1998.)

Anterior Exposure of the Upper Cervical Spine

Anterior approaches to the upper part of the cervical spine include dislocation of the temporomandibular joint (55), osteotomy of the mandible (56), transoral approach (57–59), and anterior retropharyngeal approaches (60–63). There are advantages and disadvantages to each procedure, and the surgeon should be thoroughly familiar with the anatomy and potential complications associated with the particular procedure before undertaking this formidable task.

The transoral approach allows exposure of the midline between the arch of the atlas and C-2 (57,58). The exposure may be extended cephalad by dividing the soft and hard palate to allow access to the foramen magnum and lower half of the clivus. The transoral procedure is a technically demanding operation with limited surgical indications. Any oropharyngeal or dental infections must be treated prior to elective transoral surgery. Somatosensory evoked potential monitoring, fiberoptic nasotracheal intubation, and nasogastric tube are used. The patient is placed in the supine position with the head held in slight extension using the Mayfield frame. The oral cavity is cleansed with chlorhexidine, and perioperative antibiotics including an intravenous cephalosporin and metronidazole are given for 72 hours as prophylaxis against wound infection. The key surgical landmark is the anterior tubercle on the atlas to which the anterior longitudinal ligament and longus colli muscles are attached. The vertebral artery is a minimum of 2 cm from this point in the midline. The transoral retractors then are inserted, exposing the posterior oropharynx. The area of the incision is infiltrated with 1:200,000 epinephrine. A midline 3-cm vertical incision centered on the anterior tubercle is made through the pharyngeal mucosa and muscle. The mucosa and muscle are closed later in separate layers. The tubercle of the atlas and anterior longitudinal ligament are exposed superiosteally, and the longus colli muscles are mobilized laterally. A high-speed burr may be used to remove the anterior arch of the atlas to expose the odontoid process.

An anteromedial retropharyngeal approach to the upper cervical spine, which is an extension of Smith-Robinson approach to the lower cervical spine, has been described by DeAndrade and Macnab (60). The neck is hyperextended and the chin turned to the opposite side. The degree of neck hyperextension should be assessed preoperatively, as too much hyperextension may produce cord compression and neurologic injury. A skin incision is made along the anterior aspect of the sternocleidomastoid muscle and curved toward the mastoid process. The platysma and the superficial layer of the deep cervical fascia are divided in the line of the incision to expose the anterior border of the sternocleidomastoid. The sternocleidomastoid muscle is retracted anteriorly and the carotid artery laterally. The superior thyroid artery and lingual vessels are ligated. The facial artery is identified at the upper portion of the incision, which helps to locate the hypoglossal nerve adjacent to the digastric muscle. The superior laryngeal nerve is in close proximity to the superior thyroid artery. Excessive retraction of this nerve may cause hoarseness or inability to sing high notes. Stripping of the longus colli muscle exposes the anterior aspect of the upper cervical spine and basiocciput.

McAfee et al. (62) described another technique of retropharyngeal anterior exposure of the upper cervical spine. A right-sided submandibular transverse incision and division of the platysma leads to the sternocleidomastoid muscle and its deep cervical fascia. With the aid of a nerve stimulator, the mandibular branch of the facial nerve should be identified and the retromandibular vein ligated during the initial stage of dissection. The anterior border of the sternocleidomastoid muscle is mobilized. The submandibular salivary gland and the jugular digastric lymph nodes are resected. To prevent a salivary fistula, care should be taken to suture the duct in the salivary gland. The digastric tendon is divided and tagged for later repair. The hypoglossal nerve is identified and mobilized. To mobilize the carotid contents laterally, the carotid sheath is opened and arterial and venous branches ligated. These include the superior thyroid artery and vein, lingual artery and vein, ascending pharyngeal artery and vein, and facial artery and vein, beginning inferiorly and progressing superiorly. The superior laryngeal nerve also is identified with the aid of a nerve stimulator and mobilized. The prevertebral fasciae are transected longitudinally to expose and dissect the longus colli muscles.

Whitesides and Kelley (63) described the anterolateral retropharyngeal approach, which also provides exposure of the upper cervical spine but not of the basiocciput. This approach involves dissection anterior to the sternocleidomastoid but posterior to the carotid sheath. The skin incision is made from the mastoid along the anterior aspect of the sternocleidomastoid. The external jugular vein is ligated, and the greater auricular nerve is spared if possible. The sternocleidomastoid and splenius capitus muscles are detached from the mastoid, leaving a fascial edge for later repair. The spinal accessory nerve should be identified and protected. The carotid contents along with the hypoglossal nerve anteriorly are retracted, while retracting the sternocleidomastoid posteriorly. Blunt dissection leads to the transverse processes and anterior aspect of C-1 to C-3. Potential complications of this approach include injuries to the spinal accessory nerve, sympathetic ganglion, and vertebral artery.

Anterior Exposure of the Lower Cervical Spine

The anterior approach to the lower cervical spine has been well described in the literature (55,64,65). The patient is placed in a supine and slight reverse Trendelenburg position to minimize venous pooling in the surgical area (Fig. 19). Traction is applied to the head by using Gardner-Wells tongs or a halter device. Caudally directed countertraction is applied to the shoulders using adhesive tape. The right-handed surgeon prefers the right-sided approach, but to minimize injury to the recurrent laryngeal nerve, the cervical spine often is approached from the left, particularly for the C6–T1 re-

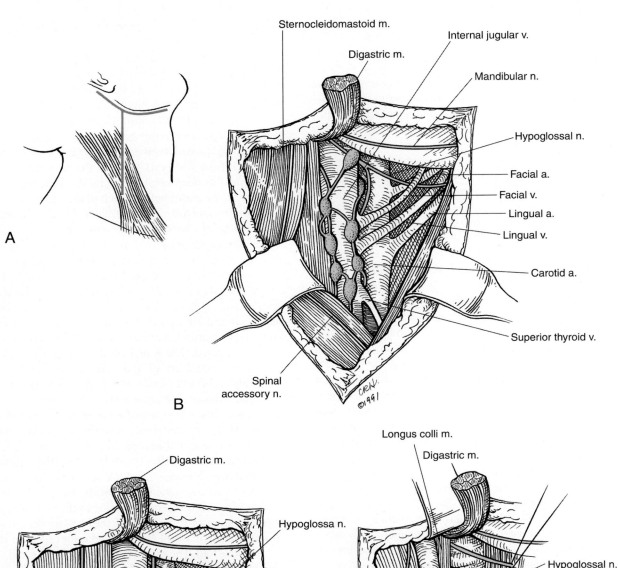

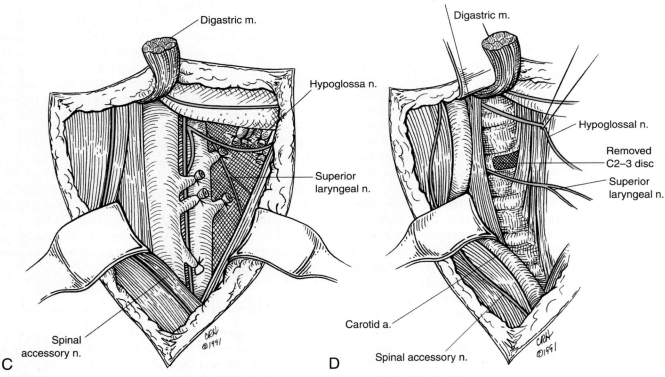

FIG. 19. McAfee's retroperitoneal approach to the upper cervical spine. **A:** Right-sided submandibular T-shaped incision is made. **B:** Division of the platysma leads to the sternocleidomastoid muscle and its deep cervical fascia. The mandibular branch of the facial nerve should be preserved. The digastric tendon is divided and tagged for later repair. The hypoglossal nerve is next identified and mobilized. **C:** The carotid contents are mobilized laterally by ligating arterial and venous branches. These include the superior thyroid artery and vein, lingual artery and vein, ascending pharyngeal artery and vein, and facial artery and vein, beginning inferiorly and progressing superiorly. The superior laryngeal nerve is identified and mobilized. **D:** The prevertebral fasciae are transected longitudinally to expose and dissect the longus colli muscles. (Reproduced with permission from An HS: *Principles and Techniques of Spine Surgery.* Baltimore: Williams & Wilkins, 1998.)

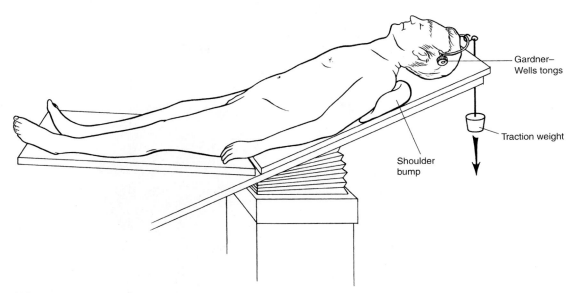

Gardner–Wells tongs

Traction weight

Shoulder bump

FIG. 20. Supine position for the anterior cervical procedures. The patient is placed in a supine and slight reverse Trendelenburg position to minimize venous pooling in the surgical area. Traction is applied to the head using Gardner-Wells tongs or halter device, and a bump in the upper thoracic area is placed to extend the cervical spine. (Reproduced with permission from An HS: *Principles and Techniques of Spine Surgery.* Baltimore: Williams & Wilkins, 1998.)

gion. On the right side, the recurrent laryngeal nerve may leave the carotid sheath at a higher level, and the surgeon must take caution during dissection, especially below C-6. A horizontal incision is used depending on the level. The hyoid bone overlies the third vertebra, the thyroid cartilage over the C4–5 intervertebral disc space, and the cricoid ring is located at the C-6 vertebra (Fig. 20). Placement of a needle on the skin coupled with intraoperative radiographs or fluoroscopy may guide the skin incision. A vertical incision anterior to the sternocleidomastoid may be necessary in cases where multiple levels must be exposed. The transverse incision is used most commonly and usually made in line with the skin crease from the midline to the middle of the sternocleidomastoid muscle. The skin and subcutaneous tissue are undermined, followed by division of the platysma muscle. The sternocleidomastoid muscle is retracted laterally and strap muscles medially. The deep cervical fascia is divided between the sternocleidomastoid muscle and strap muscles, and blunt finger dissection is performed through the pretracheal fascia along the medial border of the carotid sheath (Fig. 21). A self-retaining retractor is positioned to expose the prevertebral fascia and longus colli muscles (Fig. 21).

Care must be taken not to enter the carotid sheath laterally to avoid injury to the carotid artery, internal jugular vein, or vagus nerve. Extreme caution should be taken medially, as the strap muscles surround the thyroid gland, trachea, and esophagus. The surgical dissection should not enter the plane between the trachea and esophagus because the recurrent laryngeal nerve is at risk. A sharp self-retaining retractor should be avoided to prevent perforation of the esophagus

medially. It is important to check for the temporal arterial pulse once the retractor is spread. Prolonged occlusion of the carotid artery may cause brain ischemia and stroke. The superior thyroid artery is encountered above C-4 and the inferior thyroid artery is seen below C-6. These vessels should be identified and ligated as necessary. During the left-sided approach, one should be aware of the thoracic duct below C-7. Further dissection is performed by palpating the prominent disc margins ("hills") and concave anterior vertebral bodies ("valleys"). A bent 18-gauge needle is placed in the disc space, and a lateral radiograph taken to confirm the correct level. Inadvertent penetration to the spinal cord is prevented by this bent needle. To minimize bleeding and prevent injury to the sympathetic chain, the prevertebral fascia and the anterior longitudinal ligament must be divided in the midline and subperiosteal mobilization of the longus colli muscles completed.

In the majority of cases, this anteromedial approach to the cervical spine is utilized. However, in special circumstances, lateral approaches described by Hodgson (66) and Verbiest (67) may be used. Hodgson (66) first described an approach to the lower cervical spine, dissecting posterior to the carotid sheath exposing the anterior and lateral aspect of the cervical spine. This approach avoids the thyroid vessel, vagus nerve, and superior laryngeal nerve. Verbiest (67) modified the approach for exposure of the vertebral artery. His modification involves dissecting anteriorly to the carotid sheath and exposing the vertebral artery and nerve roots posterior to the transverse processes. These lateral approaches may be better in cases where the lesion is localized laterally or if the vertebral artery must be exposed (Fig. 22).

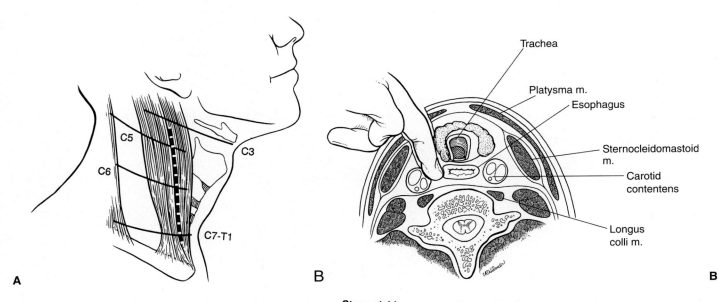

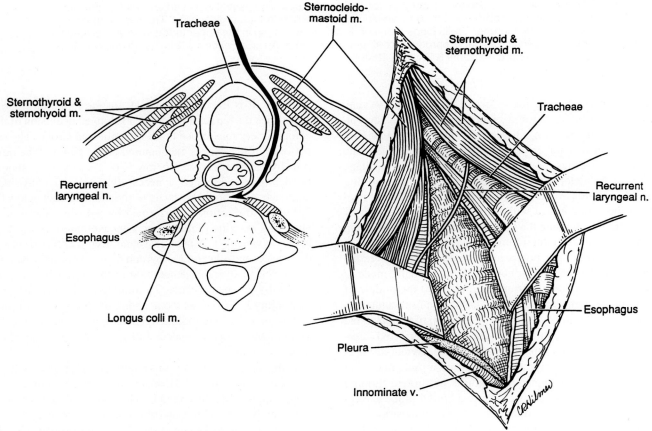

FIG. 21. Smith-Robinson anteromedial approach to the lower cervical spine. **A:** Skin incisions used for anterior cervical approaches. A horizontal incision is used at the level of the hyoid bone for C3–4, the thyroid cartilage for C4–5, and the cricoid ring for C-6. **B:** Division of the platysma muscle is followed by lateral retraction of the sternocleidomastoid muscle. The deep cervical fascia is divided between the sternocleidomastoid muscle and strap muscles, and blunt finger dissection is performed through the pre-tracheal fascia along the medial border of the carotid sheath. **C:** A self-retaining retractor is positioned to expose the prevertebral fascia and longus colli muscles. (Reproduced with permission from An HS: *Principles and Techniques of Spine Surgery.* Baltimore: Williams & Wilkins, 1998.)

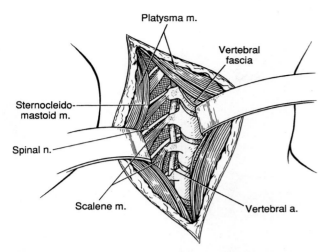

FIG. 22. Lateral approach used by Verbiest. This approach exposed the transverse processes and the vertebral artery. The dissection is done anterior to the carotid sheath, exposing the vertebral artery and nerve roots posterior to the transverse processes. (Reproduced with permission from An HS, Cotler JM: *Spinal Instrumentation.* Baltimore: Williams & Wilkins, 1992.)

CERVICOTHORACIC JUNCTION

Surgical approaches to the upper thoracic vertebrae present a challenge to the spinal surgeon. Anterior exposure of the upper thoracic vertebrae may be accomplished through the low cervical, supraclavicular, sternum-splitting, or transthoracic approach (68). The low cervical approach is simply an extension of the anteromedial approach to the lower cervical spine (69). Starting 4 cm below the mastoid process, an oblique cervical incision is made extending to the sternoclavicular joint. Alternatively, a horizontal incision can be made at the base of the neck. After division of the platysma muscle, the dissection is completed between the sternocleidomastoid muscle laterally and the esophagus and trachea medially to reach the spine. The inferior thyroid artery and vein are ligated. The recurrent laryngeal nerve must be identified from the right-sided approach, whereas the thoracic duct must be spared from the left-sided approach.

The supraclavicular approach utilizes a transverse incision above the clavicle with deep dissection kept posterior to the carotid sheath. After incision of the platysma muscles, division of the clavicular head of the sternocleidomastoid is completed. The internal jugular vein, subclavian veins, and carotid artery must be protected from injury during division of the sternocleidomastoid muscle. After division of the sternocleidomastoid muscle, the fascia beneath is divided to release the omohyoid from its pulley. The subclavian artery and its branches, which include the thyrocervical trunk, suprascapular artery, and transcervical artery, must be identified. Ligation of the suprascapular and transcervical arteries may be necessary. The dome of the lung and the phrenic nerve are in close proximity to the scalenus anterior muscle. The phrenic nerve should be identified and

retracted before division of the scalenus anterior muscle. The brachial plexus and supraclavicular nerves are more superficial at the lateral border of the scalenus anterior muscle. Division of the scalenus anterior muscle exposes Sibson's fascia in the floor of the wound, which covers the dome of the lung. Sibson's fascia is divided transversely using scissors, and the visceral pleura and lung are retracted inferiorly. The trachea, esophagus, and recurrent laryngeal nerve must be protected during medial retraction. The posterior thorax, stellate ganglion, and upper thoracic vertebral bodies are now visible looking from downward through the thoracic inlet. The inferior thyroid artery and vertebral artery should be identified. If approach is made from the left, the thoracic duct should be identified. If damaged, the thoracic duct should be doubly ligated both proximally and distally to prevent chylothorax.

The low cervical and supraclavicular approaches usually allow for exposure of the lower cervical spine and the first and second thoracic vertebrae. However, the distal extent of the exposure may be limited by the size and position of the anterior thorax. Additionally, obese or muscular patients with short necks would be poor candidates for these approaches due to limited visibility at the distal extent of the exposure. Generally, low cervical or supraclavicular approaches do not provide extensile exposure of the upper thoracic spine. All complications discussed in association with the anteromedial approach to the low cervical spine apply to these two approaches, particularly injury to the recurrent laryngeal nerve, thoracic duct, lung, or great vessels.

The upper thoracic vertebrae also may be approached through a standard thoracotomy entering the chest through the bed of the third rib. However, access to the low cervical region is restricted by the scapular and remaining ribs. Turner and Webb (70) described a more extensile surgical approach to the upper thoracic spine from T-1 to T-3. The right-sided approach is preferred to avoid the left subclavian artery, which is more curved than the right brachiocephalic artery. The incision is made medial and inferior to the scapula. The scapula is retracted laterally by dividing the trapezius, latissimus dorsi, rhomboids, and levator scapulae muscles. The posterior 7 to 10 cm of each of the second, third, fourth, and fifth ribs are removed. If T-1 is involved, 2 to 3 cm of the first rib also also are excised. Exposure of the vertebrae is made with an L-shaped incision in the pleura and intercostal muscles. Potential complications of this approach include potential restriction of scapular movement and paralysis of the intercostal muscles due to the muscle-splitting aspects of this dissection.

The best access to the cervicothoracic junction from C-4 to T-4, particularly in the obese patient, is provided by the sternal-splitting approach (Fig. 23) (71–73). The skin incision is made anterior to the left sternocleidomastoid muscle and extends along the midsternal area down to the xiphoid process. Following division of the platysma muscle and superficial cervical fascia, blunt dissection is completed between the laterally situated neurovascular bundle and medial

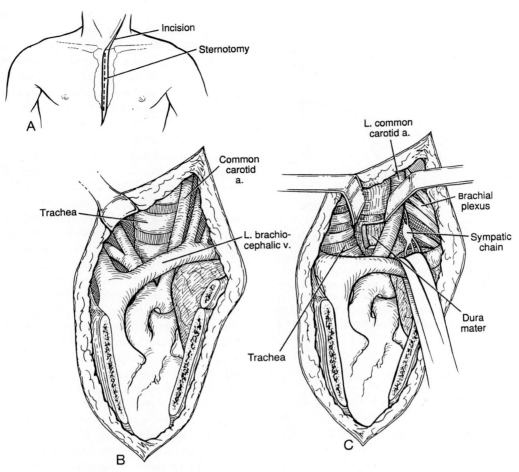

FIG. 23. Sternum-splitting approach. **A:** Skin incision is made anterior to the left sternoclei-domastoid muscle and extends along the midsternal area down to the xiphoid process. **B:** Neck dissection is the same for the Smith-Robinson approach. Retrosternal adipose and thymus tissues are retracted from the manubrium. Median sternotomy exposes the left brachiocephalic vein and the common carotid artery. **C:** Retraction of the left brachiocephalic vein and common carotid exposes from C-4 to T-4. (Reproduced with permission from An HS, Cotler JM: *Spinal Instrumentation.* Baltimore: Williams & Wilkins, 1992.)

visceral structures. The retrosternal adipose and thymus tissues are retracted from the manubrium. Medial sternotomy should be performed carefully to prevent injury to the pleura. Sternohyoid, sternothyroid, and omohyoid muscles are identified and transected as necessary. The inferior thyroid artery is ligated and transected. Blunt dissection is completed in a cranial to caudal direction until the left brachiocephalic vein is exposed. The brachiocephalic vein may be ligated and transected if necessary, but postoperative edema of the left upper extremity may be a problem.

Great caution should be taken to avoid injuries to the sympathetic nerves, cupula of the pleura, great vessels, and thoracic duct, which passes into the left venous angle between the subclavian artery, and common carotid artery. Because there is significant perioperative mortality associated with this approach, modified approaches to the cervicothoracic junction have been reported (74–76). A less aggressive T-shaped incision on the anterior chest wall was reported by

Sundaresan et al. (76) (Fig. 24). Dissection is taken down to the level of the body manubrium and clavicle with ligation of the anterior jugular venous arch and medial supraclavicular nerves. The left-sided approach is preferred because the recurrent laryngeal nerve is less variable on the left and farther from the midline than the right. At the level of the manubrium and clavicle, the sternal and clavicular heads of the sternocleidomastoid muscle are detached and retracted. The strap muscles are similarly detached and retracted. After clearing the fatty and areolar tissues in the suprasternal space, the sternal origin of the pectoralis major is stripped laterally. The medial half of the clavicle then is stripped subperiosteally with removal of the medial third of the clavicle with a Gigli's wire saw. A rectangular piece of the manubrium is removed along with its posterior periosteum. At this point, the exposed inferior thyroid vein and the innominate vein (if necessary) may be ligated. Dissection is continued between the left carotid artery on the left and the

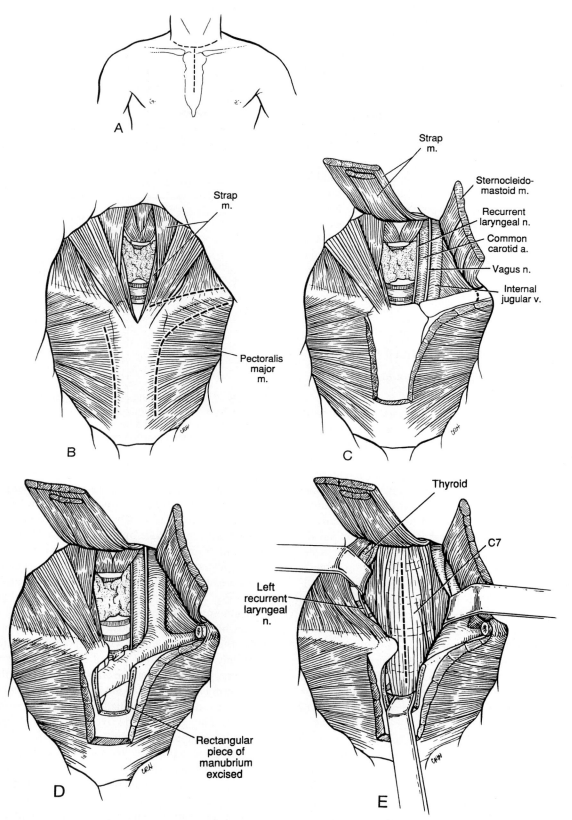

FIG. 24. Modified approach to the anterior cervicothoracic junction used by Sundaresan et al. **A:** T-shaped incision on the anterior chest wall. **B:** Dissection is taken down to the level of the body manubrium and clavicle. **C:** The sternal and clavicular heads of the sternocleidomastoid muscle are detached and retracted. The strap muscles on the ipsilateral side of approach are similarly detached and retracted. **D:** The sternal origin of the pectoralis major is stripped laterally, and the medial third of the clavicle and a rectangular piece of the manubrium are removed. **E:** Dissection is continued between the left carotid artery on the left and the innominate artery, trachea, and esophagus on the right. (Reproduced with permission from An HS, Cotler JM: *Spinal Instrumentation.* Baltimore: Williams & Wilkins, 1992.)

29

innominate artery, trachea, and esophagus on the right. Special attention must be given to protection of the thoracic duct and left recurrent laryngeal nerve.

Kurz et al. (75) reported a modified anterior approach to the cervicothoracic junction by removing the medial one third of the clavicle. They reported no complications in four patients with tumors, but one patient had recurrence of tumor.

Darling et al. (74) reported on four patients who underwent a modified anterior approach to the cervicothoracic spine involving a transverse osteotomy between the body of the sternum and the manubrium. Using this technique, excellent exposure of the cervicothoracic junction from C-3 to T-4 is possible without the need to resect the clavicle or the manubrium. A combined low cervical and transthoracic approach also has been described to gain greater access to the cervicothoracic junction in patients with severe kyphoscoliosis (77).

THORACIC AND THORACOLUMBAR SPINE

Posterior Approaches to the Thoracic and Thoracolumbar Spine

It is relatively simple to expose the posterior of the thoracic and thoracolumbar spine, but meticulous techniques are required to avoid pseudarthrosis. The patient usually is positioned on the four-poster or Relton-Hall frame. By adjusting all posters with regard to the patient's width and height, pressure points are distributed evenly on the chest and proximal thighs, while obtaining some reduction of the deformity. Pressure on the brachial plexus and ulnar nerves must be avoided for obvious reasons. It is important to keep the abdomen free of pressure to allow for venous drainage of the lower extremities and to decrease blood loss during surgery. Initial subperiosteal dissection is completed with a Cobb elevator, exposing the spinous processes, lamina, facets, and tips of the transverse processes. Facet excision is completed with instruments such as an osteotome, rongeur, or power burr. Decortication should be completed meticulously using gouges, rongeur, or power burr. Power instruments should be held in both hands, resting both wrists or forearms on the patient to provide proprioceptive feedback to the surgeon and to minimize risk of unexpected wayward deviation of the instrument.

Laminectomy may be indicated occasionally for epidural lesions or intradural tumors. Thoracic laminectomy should be completed by thinning the lateral margins of the lamina using a power burr and finishing the cut using a curet or Kerrison rongeur. The transpedicular approach is useful for biopsy or decompression in the thoracic and thoracolumbar spine. Transpedicular biopsy or decompression requires a thorough knowledge of thoracic pedicle anatomy. The thoracic pedicle is located by crossing a horizontal line at the midportion of the transverse process and a vertical line at the junction between the lamina and transverse process (Fig. 25). A power burr is used to remove the outer cortex. A pin

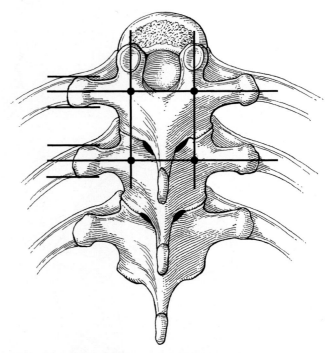

FIG. 25. Thoracic pedicle entry point. The thoracic pedicle is located by crossing a horizontal line at the midportion of the transverse process and a vertical line at the junction between the lamina and transverse process.

is placed to confirm the location of the pedicle with a roentgenogram. An angle-tipped curette can be used to remove tissue from the vertebral body. Decompression of the spinal cord can be done by excising the pedicle and removing tissue from a posterolateral direction (78).

The posterolateral costotransversectomy technique allows exposure of the anterior and lateral aspect of the thoracic vertebra (Fig. 26). This approach is less extensive than a formal thoracotomy and may be preferred for lesions in the lateral aspect of the vertebral body, lesions that do not require a long strut graft, or patients who cannot tolerate a formal thoracotomy. The patient is placed halfway between a lateral decubitus and prone position with a pad in the axilla, and the upper arm is slightly extended and securely supported. A C-shaped curved incision is made along the paraspinous muscles, spanning about four to five ribs. The middle portion of the incision should be about 2.5 inches from the midline at the paraspinal depression. By undermining the skin and subcutaneous tissue, exposure of the paraspinous muscles and posterior elements of the spine is completed. The trapezius and latissimus dorsi muscles are divided either longitudinally or transversely. The rib and transverse process are resected at one to four levels, depending on the extent of the lesion. The rib is exposed subperiosteally and excised approximately 3.5 inches lateral to the vertebra and disarticulated at the costovertebral junction. Careful retraction of the pleura will lead to the vertebrae. The pedicles, neural foramina, and spinal nerves should be identified. For neural de-

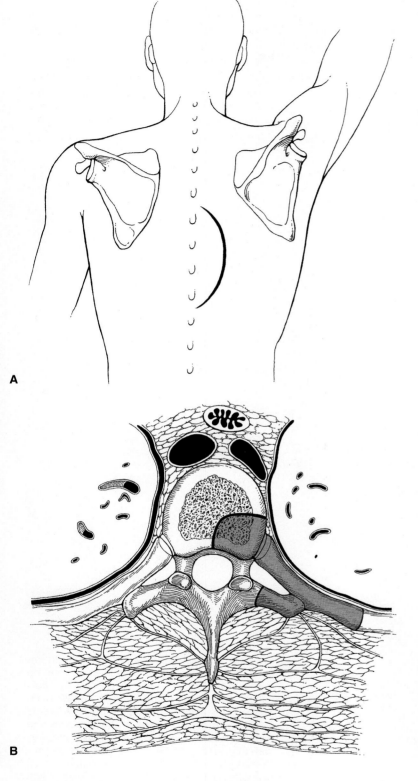

A

B

FIG. 26. Posterolateral costotransversectomy technique. **A:** C-shaped curved skin incision is made along the paraspinous muscles, spanning about four to five ribs. **B:** The rib and transverse process are resected at one to four levels, depending on the extent of the lesion. The rib is excised approximately 3.5 inches lateral to the vertebra and disarticulated at the costovertebral junction. Careful retraction of the pleura expose the vertebral bodies, pedicles, neural foramina, and spinal nerves.

compression, the pedicles may be widened or excised to expose the dura. A strut bone graft may be inserted if necessary.

In similar fashion, a posterolateral approach can be used to expose the anterolateral aspect of the vertebral body in the thoracolumbar region (Fig. 27) (79,80). The patient is placed prone or in the lateral decubitus and rolled slightly toward the anterior side. A left-sided or right-sided approach can be done, depending on the pathologic anatomy of the lesion. The skin incision may be in a C or J shape to expose the dorsolumbar fascia and latissimus dorsi fasciae. These fasciae are incised, and the erector spinae muscle group is retracted medially from the surface of the eleventh and twelfth ribs. These ribs are isolated subperiosteally and resected. The transverse processes of L-1 and L-2 may be resected to gain exposure. The T-12 or L-1 nerve is identified and traced back to its foramen. The pedicle of the appropriate vertebra is resected using a Kerrison punch and the dura is exposed laterally. Discectomy or vertebrectomy and fusion then can be performed.

Total spondylectomy through the posterolateral approach has been described for lesions that require *en bloc* excision (40,81,82). This is a formidable procedure and should be performed only by those with prior experience.

The kneeling position is preferred for posterior exposure of the lumbar spine to lessen blood loss by reducing intraabdominal venous pressure. For lumbar fusion cases, a midline incision is made and subperiosteal dissection of the paraspinous muscles is completed, exposing the spinous process, lamina, facet joint capsules, pars interarticularis, and

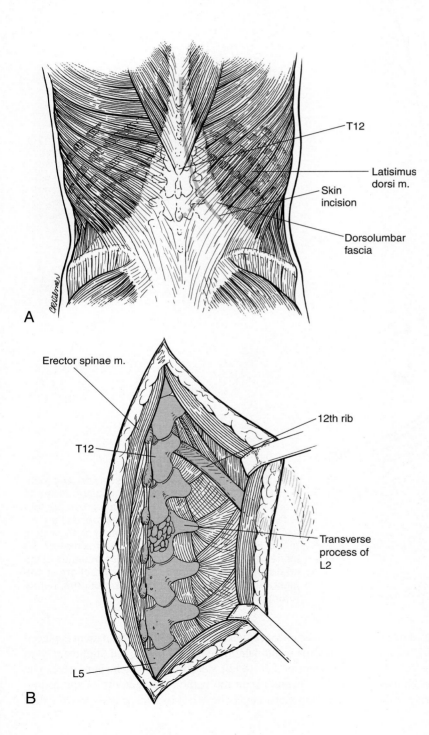

A

T12

Latisimus dorsi m.

Skin incision

Dorsolumbar fascia

Erector spinae m.

T12

12th rib

Transverse process of L2

L5

B

FIG. 27. Posterolateral approach to the thoracolumbar spine. **A:** The skin incision may be made in a C or J shape to expose the dorsolumbar fascia and latissimus dorsi fascia. **B:** The erector spinae muscle group is retracted medially from the surface of the eleventh and twelfth ribs. These ribs are isolated subperiosteally and resected. The transverse processes of L-1 and L-2 may be resected to gain exposure. The twelfth or L-1 nerve is identified and traced back to its foramen. The pedicle of the appropriate vertebra is resected for exposure of the dura laterally. (Reproduced with permission from An HS: *Principles and Techniques of Spine Surgery.* Baltimore: Williams & Wilkins, 1998.)

transverse processes. Care should be taken to avoid destroying the facet capsule above the planned fusion site. The facet joints to be fused should be prepared meticulously by excising the cartilage from the joints and removing the cortical bone from the lateral portion of the superior articular process. Decortication of the transverse process, lateral gutter, and sacral ala is performed carefully, using a power burr. Morselized bone from the iliac crest is placed in the prepared gutter. Posterior lumbar interbody fusion is a technique that involves insertion of the bone grafts into the disc space after carefully retraction of the nerve roots. Great care must be taken to avoid damage to the nerve roots.

The paraspinal muscle-splitting approach described by Wiltse (83) is useful for patients who require exposure of the transverse processes and the intervertebral foramen without the need for central laminectomy. A far lateral herniated disc or foraminal herniated disc is a typical case for utilizing this approach. The patient is placed in the kneeling position. For bilateral exposures, either two paraspinal incisions or a longer midline incision can be made. The author prefers the paraspinal incision for unilateral exposure and the midline incision for bilateral exposure. The lateral incision is made approximately two finger breaths or 1.75 inches from the midline. This incision should be made at the junction between the multifidus and longissimus muscles. These muscles are well identified on computed tomographic or magnetic resonance imaging axial views, and the exact distance from the midline may be calculated preoperatively. Following mobilization of the skin and subcutaneous tissue, a fascial incision is made over the junction between the multifidus and longissimus muscles. The index finger is used to dissect between the longissimus and multifidus muscles toward the edge of the facet capsule and transverse processes. A periosteal Cobb elevator is used to expose the transverse processes or the ala of the sacrum. Two Gelpi retractors or other self-retaining retractors are placed. Procedures such as foraminotomy, discectomy, partial pedicle resection, or intertransverse fusion can be performed through this approach.

The transpedicular approach is useful for biopsy, decompression, or screw insertion (84–86). Knowledge of the pedicle anatomy in relation to neural structures is crucial. The entry point to the pedicle from the posterior approach is located at the crossing of two lines (Fig. 28). The vertical line is represented as an extension of the facet joint in line with the bony crest coming from the superior articular facet. The horizontal line passes through the midportion of the transverse process at its base or 1 mm below the joint line. The sacral entrance point is at the lower point of the L5–S1 articulation. The nerve root is situated just medial and inferior to the pedicle as it exits the canal into the intervertebral foramen. Therefore, one must avoid the area medial and inferior to the pedicle to prevent damage of the nerve root. A small rongeur or burr is used to decorticate the pedicle entrance. A Steinmann pin with roentgenographic imaging can be used to confirm the location of the pedicle. A blunt instrument is advanced carefully through the pedicle into the vertebral body.

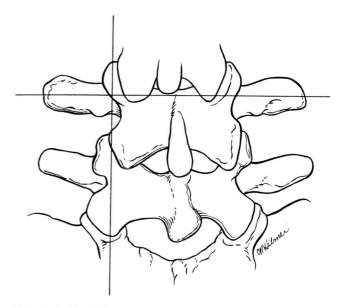

FIG. 28. The pedicle entrance point of the lumbar spine is located at the crossing of two lines. The *vertical line* is the extension of the facet joint in line with the bony crest coming from the inferior articular facet. The *horizontal line* passes through the middle of the insertion of the transverse process, or 1 mm below the joint line. The sacral entrance point is at the lower point of the L5–S1 articulation. (Reproduced with permission from An HS, Cotler JM: *Spinal Instrumentation.* Baltimore: Williams & Wilkins, 1992.)

The amount of medial angulation varies, depending on the level and entry point. Preoperative imaging studies should be used to determine exact angulations, depth, and size of the pedicle.

Posterior exposure of the sacrum and coccyx is done through a vertical midline incision. One must be careful to avoid a dural tear in the midline, particularly in patients with an occult spinal bifida. The posterior sacral foramina are richly surrounded by venous structures and can be sources of significant bleeding. Subperiosteal dissection around the coccyx should be done carefully to avoid injury to the rectum anteriorly. Posterior laminectomy of the sacrum for exposures of the nerve roots along with anterior exposure of the sacrum may be necessary for resection of certain sacral tumors.

Anterior Approaches to the Thoracic and Thoracolumbar Spine

Anterior Exposure of the Thoracic Spine

The anterior transthoracic approach is best to obtain wide exposure of the thoracic vertebral bodies (Fig. 29) (87). A right-sided thoracotomy is preferred for exposure of the upper thoracic spine to avoid the subclavian and carotid arteries in the left superior mediastinum. In the lower thoracic spine, a left-sided thoracotomy is preferred to avoid the liver. Because dissection is easier from above downward, the rib at

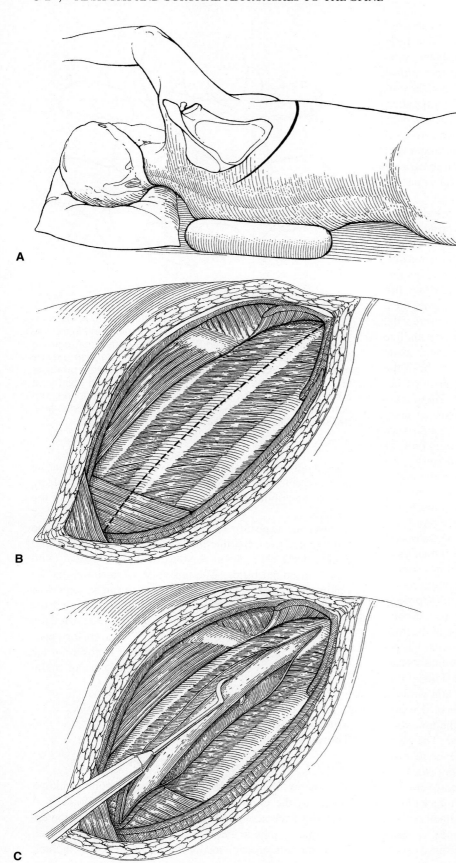

FIG. 29. Anterior exposure of the thoracic spine. **A:** The patient is in the lateral decubitus position with a roll under the axilla. The skin incision is made along the rib intended for removal from the anterior margin of the latissimus muscle anteriorly to the costochondral junction. **B:** The anterior aspect of the latissimus muscle can be undermined or minimally incised, and the posterior border of the serratus anterior muscle is mobilized or transected. **C:** Rib resection is performed by incising the overlying periosteum and using a rib stripper to dissect off the intercostal musculature. Care is taken not to damage the neurovascular bundle that travels along the inferior margin of the rib.

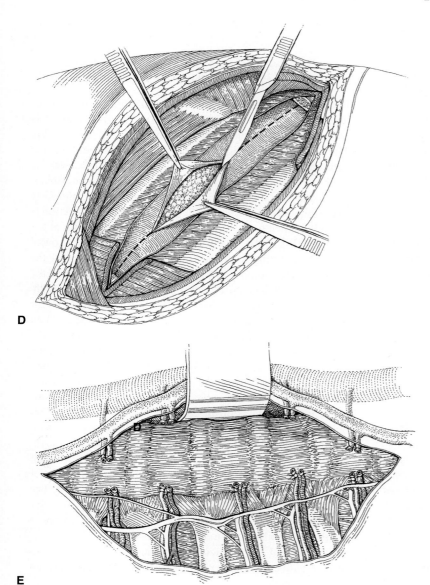

D

E

FIG. 29. *Continued.* **D:** Rib resection is followed by division of the pleura in the thoracic cavity. **E:** Segmental vessels are ligated as needed in the middle of the vertebral bodies. (**E:** Reproduced with permission from An HS, Cotler JM: *Spinal Instrumentation.* Baltimore: Williams & Wilkins, 1992.)

one or two levels above the lesion should be removed, particularly if multiple levels are involved. For the thoracotomy approach, place the patient in the lateral decubitus position, moving the arm forward (Fig. 29A). Insertion of a double-branched endotracheal tube into the right and left main stem bronchi is helpful to allow selective collapse of the lung. An axillary roll under the down arm is important to prevent compression of axillary neurovascular structures. The skin incision is made along the rib intended for removal from the anterior margin of the latissimus muscle anteriorly to the costochondral junction. The anterior aspect of the latissimus muscle can be undermined or minimally incised, and the posterior border of the serratus anterior muscle is mobilized or transected (Fig. 29B). The lateral margin of the trapezius muscle is mobilized and transected if necessary (Fig. 29C).

Palpation of the ribs is done between the rib cage and serratus anterior muscle to verify the correct rib level. Rib resection is performed by first incising the overlying periosteum in the midportion of the rib using electrocautery (Fig. 29C). A rib stripper is used to dissect off the intercostal musculature, and care is taken to prevent damage to the neurovascular bundle that travels along the inferior margin of the rib (Fig. 29D). Once the rib has been exposed, it is divided at the costochondral junction anteriorly, elevated, and resected as far posteriorly as the exposure will allow. This rib can be saved for bone grafting. The chest is sharply entered in the center of the rib bed, and the lung is retracted anteriorly and inferiorly. The pleura overlying the vertebral bodies is incised, and the segmental vessels are ligated as needed in the middle of the vertebral bodies (Fig. 29E). Blunt dissection is performed beginning over the disc spaces in a plane that is developed and includes the ligated segmental vessels and carried to the opposite pedicle. A moist lap and malleable retractor are placed on the opposite side of the vertebral body to retract and protect the great vessels and esophagus (Fig. 29E).

Recently, thoracoscopic techniques instead of formal thoracotomy procedures have been used in some patients (88). Thoracoscopic procedures can reduce postoperative pain, minimize respiratory difficulties, shorten hospital stays, and improve shoulder girdle function easily compared to formal thoracotomy procedures. These video thoracoscopic surgery techniques have been applied to treat multiple diseases of the thoracic spine, such as disc herniation, vertebral abscess, tumor, fractures, and spinal deformities. General anesthesia with double-lumen intubation is recommended. The patient is placed in a lateral position, and the ipsilateral lung is collapsed. The table is flexed to widen the intercostal spaces. The entire chest should be prepped to allow conversion to an open thoracotomy should the need arise during the procedure. The surgeon and the assistant should view separate monitors. Typically a 1-cm incision is made in the midaxillary line over the sixth intercostal space. The skin and the intercostal muscles are spread using a hemostat. Blunt dissection with a finger creates an opening into the pleural space. Any pleural adhesions should be released prior to insertion of the trocar. A 1-cm trocar is placed through the intercostal opening for insertion of the thoracoscope into the chest cavity. Placement of the initial trocar is variable depending on the level of the thoracic spine to be accessed. A 1-cm, rigid, 30-degree angled scope is placed, and exploratory thoracoscopy is performed. In those patients in whom complete resorptive atelectasis and lung collapse does not occur, temporary CO_2 insufflation can expedite and enhance collapse for better visualization. Use of gravity by Trendelenburg or reverse Trendelenburg positioning or tilting the table forward can enhance retraction of the lung. Working ports are placed in the posterior axillary line and higher in the anterior axillary line. A fan retractor may be placed through a separate portal to retract the lung. The upper and lower thoracic regions can be approached thoracoscopically by placing the portals at appropriate levels. Once the thoracic spine is visualized through the parietal pleura and the correct level is ascertained by counting the ribs and verified with a radiograph after placing a laparoscopic needle into the disc space, the pleura is divided over the portion of the spine to be exposed. Thoracoscopic electrocautery is used to divide the pleura. The segmental vessels are mobilized, clipped, and ligated. For spinal cord decompression in thoracic herniated disc cases, a rib osteotomy is first performed. A 3-cm piece of the rib is removed by dividing the costovertebral and costotransverse ligaments and cutting the rib. The superior portion of the pedicle is removed to expose the lateral aspect of the thecal sac. Discectomy is completed by removing the herniated disc away from the thecal sac. In addition to discectomy, other procedures such as corpectomy, fusion, and even instru-

mentation may be performed through this thoracoscopic approach.

Anterior Exposure of the Thoracolumbar Junction

For exposure of the thoracolumbar junction, a thoracoabdominal approach is used (Fig. 30) (87). The patient is placed in a lateral decubitus position with the left side up. The left-sided approach is preferred to avoid the liver and vena cava on the right side. A skin incision is made over the tenth rib from the lateral border of the paraspinous musculature to the costal cartilage. The incision is curved anteriorly to the edge of the rectus sheath (Fig. 30A). The dissection is extended down to the muscle layers to the periosteum of the tenth rib (Fig. 30B). The key is to access the retroperitoneal space by splitting the costal cartilage after removal of the tenth rib. After removing the rib, the pleura is incised and the lung retracted. The costal cartilage is split along its length. Under the retracted split tips of costal cartilage, the retroperitoneal space is identified by the light areolar tissue. Blunt dissection is performed to mobilize the peritoneum from the undersurface of the diaphragm and abdominal wall. After the peritoneum is retracted, the external oblique, internal oblique, and the transverse abdominis muscles of the abdomen are divided one layer at a time. The next step entails circumferential incision in the muscular portion of the diaphragm adjacent to the costal margin. The diaphragm is incised circumferentially 1 inch from the peripheral attachment to the chest wall. Marker stitches or clips are placed for resuturing the diaphragm later. For exposure of the T12–L1 region, the crus of the diaphragm is cut and mobilized. The segmental vessels are tied and ligated as necessary to mobilize the aorta. Malleable retractors are positioned to expose the thoracolumbar junction.

Exposure of the thoracolumbar junction may be accomplished with either an eleventh or twelfth rib approach while remaining in the extrapleural and retroperitoneal spaces (50). These exposures entail splitting the tip of the costal cartilage and mobilizing the parietal pleura from the undersurface of the rib bed. The peritoneum is mobilized anteriorly, and the retroperitoneal space is bluntly dissected toward the spine. These approaches give less extensile exposure of the thoracolumbar junction as compared with the thoracoabdominal approach.

Anterior Exposure of the Lumbar Spine

There are several techniques for anterior exposure of the lumbar spine (Fig. 31).

A standard retroperitoneal flank approach is used in the lower lumbar region (Fig. 32A) (87). The patient is placed in the right lateral decubitus position, exposing the left flank. This retroperitoneal exposure utilizes division of the abdominal muscles and blunt dissection through the retroperitoneal space toward the psoas muscle and the spine (Fig. 32B). The

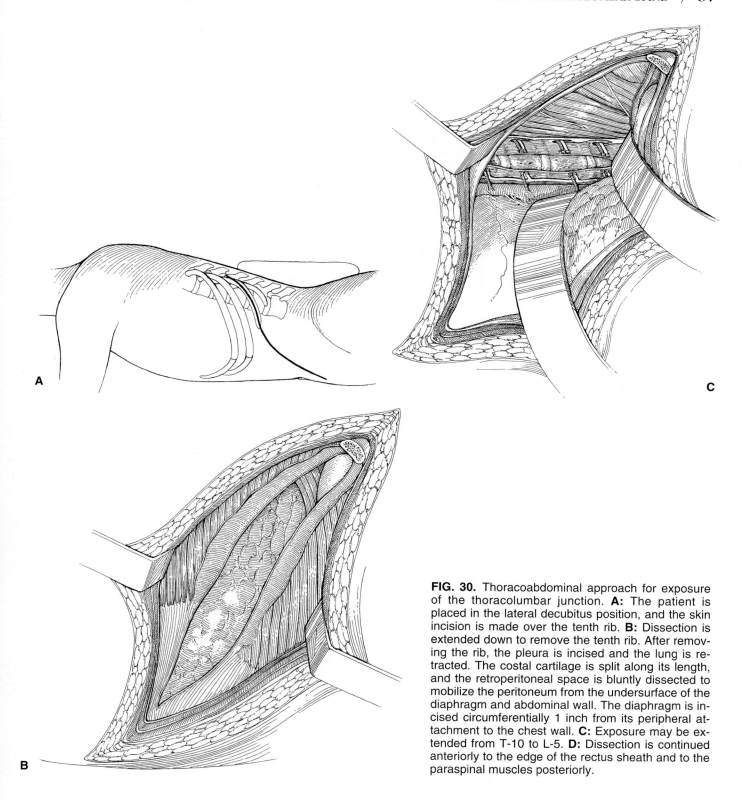

FIG. 30. Thoracoabdominal approach for exposure of the thoracolumbar junction. **A:** The patient is placed in the lateral decubitus position, and the skin incision is made over the tenth rib. **B:** Dissection is extended down to remove the tenth rib. After removing the rib, the pleura is incised and the lung is retracted. The costal cartilage is split along its length, and the retroperitoneal space is bluntly dissected to mobilize the peritoneum from the undersurface of the diaphragm and abdominal wall. The diaphragm is incised circumferentially 1 inch from its peripheral attachment to the chest wall. **C:** Exposure may be extended from T-10 to L-5. **D:** Dissection is continued anteriorly to the edge of the rectus sheath and to the paraspinal muscles posteriorly.

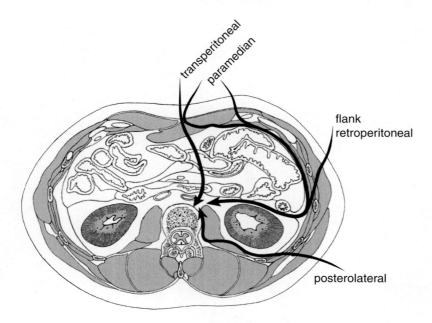

FIG. 31. Different approaches to the lumbar spine. The transperitoneal approach is used to expose the anterior aspect of the lower lumbar spine. The paramedian approach also exposes the anterior aspect of the lower spine, but it utilized a retroperitoneal dissection. Flank retroperitoneal approaches expose the anterolateral aspect of the lumbar spine. The posterolateral approach is limited to the posterolateral aspect of the spine.

incision extends from the midaxillary line to the edge of the rectus sheath. The level of the incision varies according to the level of the spine approached. Dissection is through the external oblique, internal oblique, and transversus abdominis muscles (Fig. 32B). The retroperitoneal space is entered laterally by identifying the retroperitoneal fat, taking care to avoid penetration of the peritoneum just lateral to the rectus sheath. Blunt finger dissection anterior to the psoas muscle will lead to the spine. The genitofemoral nerve on the ante-

rior surface of the psoas muscle and the sympathetic chains medial to the muscle should be identified (Fig. 32C). Extreme caution should be taken to avoid injury to the ureter, which can be identified medially along the undersurface of the peritoneum, and the pulsating aorta, which is easily palpated. The aorta is mobilized and a retractor positioned around the vertebral body (Fig. 32D). The segmental vessels are ligated to expose the valleys of the vertebral bodies. At the L4–5 region, the iliolumbar vein should be identified and

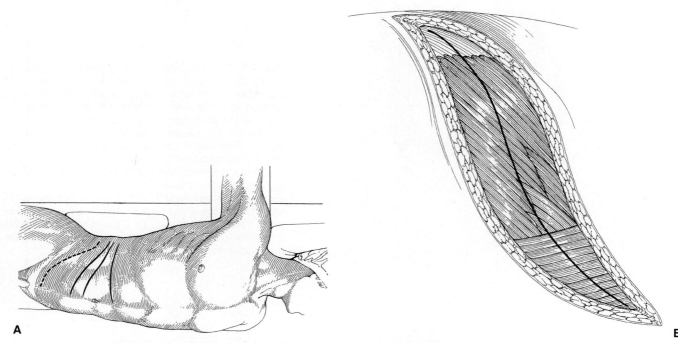

A   B

FIG. 32. Retroperitoneal flank approach to the lumbar spine. **A:** The patient is placed in the right lateral decubitus position, and the incision depends on the level of exposure required. **B:** Retroperitoneal exposure utilizes division of the abdominal muscles and blunt dissection through the retroperitoneal space.

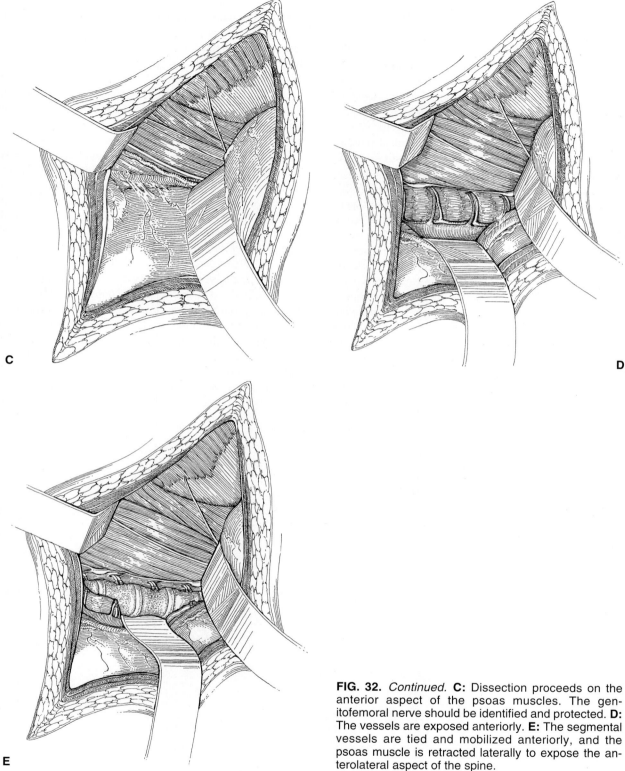

C

D

E

FIG. 32. *Continued.* **C:** Dissection proceeds on the anterior aspect of the psoas muscles. The genitofemoral nerve should be identified and protected. **D:** The vessels are exposed anteriorly. **E:** The segmental vessels are tied and mobilized anteriorly, and the psoas muscle is retracted laterally to expose the anterolateral aspect of the spine.

ligated to mobilize the great vessels. For exposure of L5–S1, the midline within the vascular bifurcation should be palpated by passing the finger over the left common iliac artery. The left common iliac vein is retracted to the left and cephalad, while the middle sacral vein and the superior hypogastric plexus are retracted to the right bluntly.

For exposure of the anterior aspect of the L3–S1 vertebrae, the paramedian retroperitoneal approach may be used. For this approach, the patient is placed in the supine position. The anterior exposure of the lower lumbar vertebrae and the sacrum is better with this technique then the lateral approach. The lateral edge of the rectus abdominal muscle is palpated, and a vertical incision is made. The length of the incision depends on the number of vertebrae to be exposed. The dissection is made to the level of abdominal fascia. The lateral border of the rectus abdominal muscle is palpated, and an incision is made in the anterior rectus sheath along the lateral edge of the muscle. The fibers of the rectus muscle are retracted medially to expose the posterior rectus sheath and the arcuate line. The inferior aspect of exposure should not go beyond the level of inferior epigastric vessels. Great caution is taken to preserve these vessels and to preserve innervation to the rectus abdominal muscle. The linea arcuata divides the posterior rectus fascia proximally and the transversalis fascia distally.

The preperitoneal space can be entered and blunt dissection leads to the retroperitoneal space and the anterior aspect of the spine. The peritoneum is mobilized medially while the dissection is carried down to the iliac vessels. The psoas muscle, aorta, iliac artery and vein, genitofemoral nerve, ureter, sympathetic chain, and superior hypogastric plexus are identified. For exposure of L3–5, the psoas muscle is mobilized laterally off the vertebral bodies, the left segmental vessels are identified and ligated, and the aorta and iliac vessels are mobilized medially. The iliolumbar vein should be ligated for exposure of L4–5. For exposure of L5–S1 disc, the aortic bifurcation at L4–5 is dissected further and the vessels retracted laterally to enter the disc. Alternatively, a smaller midline incision can be made, followed by division of the linea alba (89). The left rectus abdominis

muscle is retracted laterally to divide the posterior rectus sheath from the linea arcuata at the lateral edge of the muscle. Blunt dissection is completed to mobilize the peritoneum and maintain the extraperitoneal approach to the lumbosacral junction. With special retractors or video assistance, the anterior approach to the lower lumbar region can be performed with minimally invasive techniques without the need to use CO_2 insufflation (63). The transperitoneal approach also provides excellent exposure to the lumbosacral junction using a vertical or transverse incision in the lower abdomen (Fig. 33A). This approach also may be accomplished with a mini incision technique (90). The patient is placed in the supine position with the lumbosacral spine hyperextended. The transverse incision requires transection of the rectus abdominis muscle while the vertical incision splits the rectus abdominis muscles in the midline linea alba. Following division of the anterior rectus sheath, the conjoined fascia of the posterior rectus sheath and abdominal fascia is opened to the peritoneum. The peritoneum is carefully divided, and the bowel contents mobilized away from the aorta and iliac vessels. The aortic bifurcation is palpated at the L4–5 region (Fig. 33B). Saline infiltration of the tissue over the anterior surface of the sacral promontory may be done to elevate the posterior peritoneum off the vascular structures. The posterior peritoneum is opened and the L5–S1 disc identified (Fig. 33C). The sacral artery runs down along the anterior aspect of the sacrum and may be

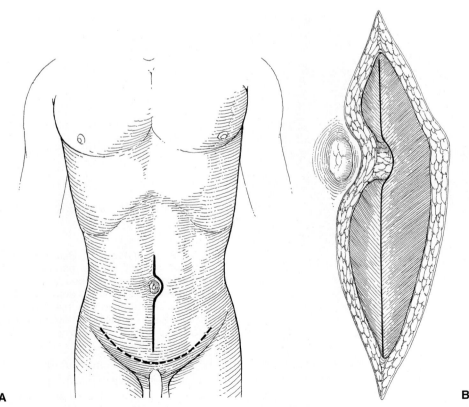

FIG. 33. Transperitoneal approach to the lower lumbar spine and the sacrum. **A:** Skin incision is through a vertical or transverse incision made in the lower abdomen. **B:** The rectus sheaths are divided in the middle line or the linea alba.

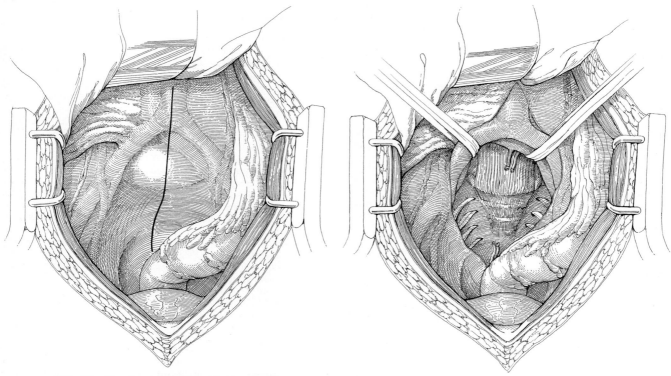

FIG. 33. *Continued.* **C:** The peritoneum is divided carefully, and the bowel contents are mobilized away from the aorta and iliac vessels. The posterior peritoneum is carefully separated and divided. **D:** The aortic bifurcation is palpated and mobilized for exposure of the L5–S1 intervertebral disc.

ligated for distal exposure purposes (Fig. 33D). Extreme caution should be taken to protect the left iliac vein in the aortic bifurcation and to preserve the superior hypogastric plexus, which is important for sexual function. Electrocautery must be avoided to prevent damage to the hypogastric plexus. The left common iliac artery and left common iliac vein are retracted to the left, while the hypogastric plexus and right iliac vessels are retracted to the right. Retractors or Steinmann pins can be used to expose the L5–S1 region. Exposure can be extended to the L4–5 region by mobilizing the great vessels to the right after ligating the L4–5 segmental vessels and the iliolumbar vein. Care must be taken not to injure the left ureter, which crosses the left common iliac vessels over the sacroiliac joint.

In summary, this chapter outlined the anatomy of bone and joints, intervertebral disc, ligaments, muscles, and related structures of the spine. This chapter also has reviewed the basic surgical approaches to the spine, with reference to more detailed information available in the literature. Knowledge of the anatomy is the first step toward better understanding of pathology of the spine, imaging studies, and surgical approaches.

REFERENCES

1. Kameyama T, Hashizume Y, Sobue G. Morphologic features of the normal human cadaveric spinal cord. *Spine* 1996;21:1285–1290.
2. Dommisse GF. The blood supply of the spinal cord. *J Bone Joint Surg* 1974;56B:225.
3. Lu J, Ebraheim NA, Biyani A, Brown JA, Yeasting RA. Vulnerability of great medullary artery. *Spine* 1996;21:1852–1855.
4. Parke WW, Gammell K, Rothman RH. Arterial vascularization of the cauda equina. *J Bone Joint Surg* 1981;63A:53–62.
5. Parke WW, Watanabe R. The intrinsic vasculature of the lumbosacral spinal nerve roots. *Spine* 1985;10:508–515.
6. Shinomiya K, Okawa A, Nakao K, et al. Morphology of C5 ventral nerve rootlets as part of dissociated motor loss of deltoid muscle. *Spine* 1994;19:2501–2504.
7. Yabuki S, Kikuchi S. Positions of dorsal root ganglia in the cervical spine. An anatomic and clinical study. *Spine* 1996;21:1513–1511.
8. Cohen MS, Wall EJ, Brown RA, Massie JB, Rydevik B, Garfin SR. Cauda equina anatomy I: intrathecal nerve root organization. *Spine* 1990;15:1244–1251.
9. An HS. Anatomy of the cervical spine. In: An HS, Simpson JM (eds). *Surgery of the Cervical Spine*. London: Martin-Dunitz, 1994:1–40.
10. Kikuchi S, Sato K, Konno S, Hasue M. Anatomic and radiographic study of dorsal root ganglia. *Spine* 1994;19:6–11.
11. Hasegawa T, Mikawa Y, Watanabe R, An HS. Morphometric analysis of the lumbosacral nerve roots and dorsal root ganglia by magnetic resonance imaging. *Spine* 1996;21:1005–1009.
12. Nowicki BH, Haughton VM. Ligaments of the lumbar neural foramina. *Clin Anat* 1992;5:126–135.
13. Gerbrand JG, Baljet B, Drukker J. Nerves and nerve plexuses of the human vertebral column. *Am J Anat* 1990;188:282–296.
14. Bogduk N. The innervation of the lumbar spine. *Spine* 1983;8:286–293.
15. Bogduk N, Tynan W, Wilson A. The nerve supply to the human intervertebral discs. *J Anat* 1981;132:39–56.
16. Nakamura S, Takahashi K, Takahashi Y, Morinaga T, Shimada Y, Moriya H. Origin of nerves supplying the posterior portion of lumbar intervertebral discs. *Spine* 1996;21:917–924.
17. Cavanaugh JM, Kallakuri S, Ozaktay C. Innervation of the rabbit lumbar intervertebral disc and posterior longitudinal ligament. *Spine* 1995;20:2080–2085.
18. Imai S, Hukuda S, Maeda T. Dually innervating nociceptive networks in the rat lumbar posterior longitudinal ligament. *Spine* 1995;20:2086–2092.

19. Xu R, Ebraheim NA, Yeasting RA, Jackson WT. Anatomic consideration for posterior iliac bone harvesting. *Spine* 1996;21:1017–1020.
20. Doherty B, Heggeness MH. The quantitative anatomy of the atlas. *Spine* 1994;19:2497–2500.
21. Doherty B, Heggeness MH. Quantitative anatomy of the second cervical vertebra. *Spine* 1995;20:513–517.
22. Xu R, Naudaud MC, Ebraheim NA, Yeasting RA. Morphology of the second cervical vertebra and the posterior projection of the C2 pedicle axis. *Spine* 1995;20:259–263.
23. An HS, Gordin R, Renner K. Anatomic considerations for plate-screw fixation of the cervical spine. *Spine* 1991;16:S548–S551.
24. Panjabi MM, Duranceau J, Goel V, Oxland T, Takata K. Cervical human vertebrae. Quantitative three-dimensional anatomy of the middle and lower regions. *Spine* 1993;16:861–874.
25. Abumi K, Itoh H, Taneichi H, Kaneda K. Transpedicular screw fixation for traumatic lesions of the middle and lower cervical spine: description of the techniques and preliminary report. *J Spinal Disord* 1994;7:19–28.
26. Jeanneret B, Gebhard JS, Magerl F. Transpedicular screw fixation of articular mass fracture-separation: results of an anatomic study and operative technique. *J Spinal Disord* 1994;7:222–229.
27. Miller RM, Ebraheim NA, Xu R, Yeasting RA. Anatomic consideration of transpedicular screw placement in the cervical spine. 1996;21:2317–2322.
28. Ebraheim NA, An HS, Xu R, Ahmad M, Yeasting RA. The quantitative anatomy of the cervical nerve root groove and the intervertebral foramen. *Spine* 1996;21:1619–1623.
29. Bailey AS, Stanescu S, Yeasting RA, Ebraheim NA, Jackson WT. Anatomic relationship of the cervicothoracic junction. *Spine* 1995;13:1431–1439.
30. Vaccaro AR, Rizzolo SJ, Allardyce TJ, et al. Placement of pedicle screws in the thoracic spine. *J Bone Joint Surg* 1995;77A:1193–1199.
31. Kothe R, O'Holleran JD, Liu W, Panjabi MM. Internal architecture of the thoracic pedicle. *Spine* 1996;21:264–270.
32. Zindrick M, Wiltse LL, Doornik A. Analysis of the morphometric characteristics of the thoracic and lumbar pedicles. *Spine* 1987;12:160–166.
33. An HS, Glover JM. Lumbar spinal stenosis: historical perspectives, classification, and pathoanatomy. *Semin Spine Surg* 1994;6:69–77.
34. Bose K, Balasubramaniam P. Nerve root canals of the lumbar spine. *Spine* 1984;9:16–18.
35. Lee CK, Rauschning W, Glenn W. Lateral lumbar spinal canal stenosis: classification, pathologic anatomy and surgical decompression. *Spine* 1980;13:313–320.
36. Rauschning W. Normal and pathologic anatomy of the lumbar root canals. *Spine* 1987;12:1008–1019.
37. Hasegawa T, An HS, Haughton VM, Nowicki B. Lumbar foraminal stenosis: critical heights of the intervertebral discs and foramina. *J Bone Joint Surg* 1995;77A:32–38.
38. Hayashi K, Yabuki T, Kurokawa T, Seki H, Hogaki M, Minoura S. The anterior and the posterior longitudinal ligaments of the lower cervical spine. *J Anat* 1977;124:633–636.
39. Hoffmann M. Die befestigung der dura mater im wirbelcanal. *Arch Anat Physiol (Anat Ab)* 1898: 403.
40. Spencer DL, Irwin GS, Miller JAA. Anatomy and significance of the lumbosacral nerve roots in sciatica. *Spine* 1983;8:672.
41. Wiltse LL, Fonseca AS, Amster J, Dimartino P, Ravessoud FA. Relationship of the dura, Hoffmann's ligaments, Batson's plexus, and a fibrovascular membrane lying on the posterior surface of the vertebral bodies and attaching to the deep layer of the posterior longitudinal ligament: an anatomical, radiologic, and clinical study. *Spine* 1993;18: 1030.
42. Yaszemski M, White AA. The discectomy membrane (nerve root fibrovascular membrane): its anatomic description and its surgical importance. *J Spinal Disord* 1994;7:230–235.
43. Grantham SA, Dick HM, Thompson KC, Stinchfield FE. Occipitocervical arthrodesis. *Clin Orthop* 1969;65:118.
44. Grob D, Dvorak J, Panjabi M, Froehlich M, Hayek J. Posterior occipitocervical fusion. A preliminary report of a new technique. *Spine* 1991;16S:S17–S24.
45. Grob D, Jeanneret B, Aebi M, Markwalder TM. Atlantoaxial fusion with transarticular screw fixation. *J Bone Joint Surg* 1991;73B:972–976.
46. Smith MD, Anderson P, Grady S. Occipitocervical arthrodesis using contoured plate fixation. *Spine* 1993;18:1984–1990.
47. Wertheim SB, Bohlman HH. Occipitocervical fusion. *J Bone Joint Surg* 1987;69A:833–836.
48. Brooks AL, Jenkins EB. Atlanto-axial arthrodesis by the wedge compression method. *J Bone Joint Surg* 1978;60A:279–284.
49. Griswold DM, Albright JA, Schiffman E, et al. Atlanto-axial fusion for instability. *J Bone Joint Surg* 1978;60A:285–292.
50. Magerl F, Seeman PS. Stable posterior fusion of the atlas and axis by transarticular screw fixation. In: Kehr P, Weidner A (eds). *Cervical Spine.* Wien: Springer-Verlag, 1987:322–327.
51. Anderson PA, Henley MB, Grady MS, Montesano PX, Winn HR. Posterior cervical arthrodesis with AO reconstruction plates and bone graft. *Spine* 1991;16S:S72–S79.
52. Callahan RA, Johnson KM, Margolis RN, et al. Cervical facet fusion for control of instability following laminectomy. *J Bone Joint Surg* 1977;59A:991–1002.
53. Ebraheim NA, An HS, Jackson WT, et al. Internal fixation of the unstable cervical spine using posterior Roy-Camille plates: preliminary report. *J Orthop Trauma* 1989;3:23–28.
54. Roy-Camille R, Saillant G, Mazel C. Internal fixation of the unstable cervical spine by a posterior osteosynthesis with plates and screws. In: Sherk HH (ed). *The Cervical Spine.* Philadelphia: JB Lippincott, 1989:390–421.
55. Riley LH Jr. Surgical approaches to the anterior structures of the cervical spine. *Clin Orthop* 1973;91:16–20.
56. Hall JE, Denis F, Murray J. Exposure of the upper cervical spine for spinal decompression. *J Bone Joint Surg* 1977;59A:121–123.
57. Crockard HA. Anterior approaches to lesions of the upper cervical spine. *Clin Neurosurg* 1988;34:389–416.
58. Crockard HA, Calder I, Ransford AO. One stage transoral decompression and posterior fixation in rheumatoid atlanto-axial subluxation. *J Bone Joint Surg* 1990;72B:682–685.
59. Fang HSY, Ong GB. Direct anterior approach to the upper cervical spine. *J Bone Joint Surg* 1962;44:158.
60. DeAndrade JR, Macnab I. Anterior occipitocervical fusion using an extra-pharyngeal exposure. *J Bone Joint Surg* 1969;51A:1621–1626.
61. Laus M, Pignatti G, Malaguti MC, Alfonso C, Zappoli FA, Giunti A. Anterior extroral surgery to the upper cervical spine. *Spine* 1996;21:1687–1693.
62. McAfee PC, Bohlman HH, Riley LH, et al. The anterior retropharyngeal approach to the upper pan of the cervical spine. *J Bone Joint Surg* 1987;69A:1371–1383.
63. Whitesides TE Jr, Kelley RP. Lateral approach to the upper cervical spine for anterior fusion. *South Med J* 1966;59:879–883.
64. Robinson RA, Walker E, Ferlic DC, Wiecking DK. The results of anterior interbody fusion of the cervical spine. *J Bone Joint Surg* 1962;44A:1569–1578.
65. Smith GW, Robinson RA. The treatment of certain cervical spine disorders by anterior removal of the intervertebral disc and interbody fusion. *J Bone Joint Surg* 1958;40A:607.
66. Hodgson AR. An approach to the cervical spine (C3–7). *Clin Orthop* 1965;39:129.
67. Verbiest H. Anterolateral operations for fractures and dislocations in the middle and lower parts of the cervical spine. *J Bone Joint Surg* 1969;51A:1489–1530.
68. Charles R. Anterior approach to the upper thoracic vertebrae. *J Bone Joint Surg* 1989;71B:81–84.
69. Fielding JW, Stillwell WT. Anterior cervical approach to the upper thoracic spine. A case report. *Spine* 1976;1:158–161.
70. Turner PL, Webb JK. A surgical approach to the upper thoracic spine. *J Bone Joint Surg* 1987;69B:542–544.
71. An HS, Vaccaro A, Cotler JM. Spinal disorders at the cervico-thoracic junction. *Spine* 1994;15:2557–2564.
72. Hodgson AK, Stock FE, Fang HSY, et al. Anterior spinal fusion: the operative approach and pathologic findings in 412 patients with Pott's disease of the spine. *Br J Surg* 1960;48:172–178.
73. Lehman RM, Grunwerg B, Hall T. Anterior approach to the cervicothoracic junction: an anatomic dissection. *J Spinal Disord* 1997;10:33–39.
74. Darling GE, McBroom R, Perrin R. Modified anterior approach to the cervicothoracic junction. *Spine* 1995;13:1519–1521.
75. Kurz LT, Pursel SE, Herkowitz HN. Modified anterior approach to the cervicothoracic junction. *Spine* 1991;16:542–547.
76. Sundaresan N, Shah I, Foley KM, et al. An anterior surgical approach to the upper thoracic vertebrae. *J Neurosurg* 1984;61:686–690.

77. Micheli JJ, Hood RW. Anterior exposure of the cervicothoracic spine using a combined cervical and thoracic approach. *J Bone Joint Surg* 1983;65A:992–997.

78. Ahlgren BD, Herkowitz HN. A modified posterolateral approach to the thoracic spine. *J Spinal Disord* 1995;8:69–75.

79. Larson SJ, Hoist RA, Hemmy DC, et al. Lateral extracavity, approach to traumatic lesions of the thoracic and lumbar spine. *J Neurosurg* 1976;4S:628–637.

80. Lesoin F, Rousseaux M, Lozes G, et al. Posterolateral approach to tumours of the dorsolumbar spine. *Acta Neurochir (Wien)* 1986;81:40–44.

81. Roy-Camille R, Mazel C, Saillant G, et al. Treatment of malignant tumors of the spine with posterior instrumentation. In: Sudaresan N, Schmidek HH, Schiller AL, et al. (eds). *Tumors of the Spine.* Philadelphia: WB Saunders, 1990:473–487.

82. Stener B. Total spondylectomy in chondrosarcoma arising from the seventh thoracic vertebra. *J Bone Joint Surg* 1971;53AB:288–295.

83. Wiltse LL. The paraspinal sacrospinalis-splitting approach to the lumbar spine. *Clin Orthop* 1973;91:48–57.

84. Fidler MW, Niers BBAM. Open transpedicular biopsy of the vertebral body. *J Bone Joint Surg* 1990;72B:884–885.

85. Jelinek JS, Kransdorf MJ, Gray R, Aboulafia AJ, Malawer MM. Percutaneous transpedicular biopsy of vertebral lesions. *Spine* 1996;21:2035–2040.

86. Roy-Camille R, Saillant G, Mazel C. Internal fixation of the lumbar spine with pedicle screw plating. *Clin Orthop* 1986;203:7–17.

87. An HS, Riley LH III. *An Atlas of Surgery of the Spine.* London: Martin Dunitz, 1998.

88. Regan JJ, Mack MJ, Picetti GD. A technical report on video-assisted thoracoscopy in thoracic spinal surgery. *Spine* 1995;20:831–837.

89. Onimus M, Papin P, Gangloff S. Extraperitoneal approach to the lumbar spine with video assistance. *Spine* 1996;21:2491–2494.

90. Mayer HM. A new microsurgical technique for minimally invasive anterior lumbar interbody fusion. *Spine* 1997;22:691–700.

Surgery of Spinal Trauma,
edited by J.M. Cotler, J.M. Simpson, H.S. An, and C.P. Silveri.
Lippincott Williams & Wilkins, Philadelphia © 2000.

CHAPTER 2

Pathophysiology and Initial Treatment of Acute Spinal Cord Injuries

Johannes Bernbeck and Rick B. Delamarter

In the United States, 7,600 to 10,000 people sustain and survive spinal cord injury (SCI) each year. The incidence of traumatic SCI is declining due to preventive measures, including the development of safer automobiles with better restraint systems, higher occupational safety standards, regulation of sports (e.g., no spear tackling in football), as well as improvements in the emergency medical systems and acute trauma care. These advances have led to a declining incidence of SCI, but the proportion of SCI due to domestic violence is on the rise. A greater number of patients are surviving their acute trauma. The proportion of patients with incomplete paraplegia is increasing, while the proportion of patients with complete tetraplegia is decreasing (1).

Several trends in the subacute period are emerging. Improvements in SCI rehabilitation are leading to shorter hospitalization. From 1974 to 1994, the average initial hospital stay (acute and rehab combined) for paraplegics decreased from 122 to 53 days, and for tetraplegics it has been halved from 150 to 75 days. The life expectancy for SCI patients is still below the average population, but it is improving. Ninety-two percent of SCI patients are discharged to independent or residential living with assistance (1).

Despite this progress, the impact of SCI on the patient, the patient's family, and society is staggering. There are 183,000 to 203,000 people with SCI living in the United States today. Lifetime costs for health care and living expenses vary depending on severity of injury and age. A 25-year-old high

J. Bernbeck and R.B. Delamarter: Department of Orthopaedic Surgery, UCLA University Spine Associates, Los Angeles, California 90024.

tetraplegic is estimated to incur lifetime costs of $1.35 million, whereas in the 50-year-old paraplegic this figure is closer to $326,000 (1).

Patients with SCI undergo dramatic quality-of-life changes that sometimes are devastating. These areas of change encompass independence, lifestyle, body image, personal goals, career goals, economic security, and interpersonal relationships. At postinjury year 8, only 36.2% of paraplegics and 27.4% of tetraplegics are employed (1). Marriage is much less likely to succeed in the face of SCI.

Most of the recent medical progress in SCI has been in injury prevention and rehabilitation, leading to a lower incidence of SCI and higher function for individuals affected by SCI. The emphasis of this chapter is on the pathophysiologic processes in early SCI and the acute management of the SCI patient to diminish the potential for subsequent mechanical or ischemic insult to the injured spinal cord.

PATHOPHYSIOLOGIC MECHANISMS OF TRAUMATIC NEUROLOGIC INJURY

Spinal Cord

The initial spinal cord trauma may involve compression, contusion, laceration, blast injury, and ischemic injury to the spinal cord components. These components include the axons, cell bodies, myelin, and blood vessels. The spinal cord usually is injured by a primary mechanical insult that triggers hemorrhage, edema, and ischemia. This injury usually occurs when the skeletal structures fail to dissipate the energy of trauma and this energy then is imparted directly on the cord.

The injury may occur directly by flexion, extension, axial loading, or rotation forces, or it may occur indirectly by displaced disc or bone fragments. The most common cause of SCI is cervical fracture-dislocation (2), but SCI may occur without radiographic evidence of injury. These secondary effects lead to expansion of the zone of injury in the spinal cord and further neurologic loss (Fig. 1). When the primary injury is cord compression from bone, ligaments, hematoma, intervertebral disc, or a foreign body, the neural injury is a function of both the time and degree of compression. Prolonged compression can cause further neurologic loss.

The cascade of complex biochemical events leading to secondary injury is only partially understood. Following the initial injury, there is hemorrhage and inflammation in the central gray matter of the cord. Autonomic dysfunction, hypotension, and bradycardia further jeopardize spinal cord perfusion and compound the ischemic insult. Studies on animal SCI models have shown an increase in tissue sodium, lactate, and water content along with decreased extracellular calcium, tissue oxygenation, pyruvate, and adenosine triphosphate. This is consistent with a scenario of ischemia and hypoxia with an uncoupling of oxidative phosphorylation and aerobic glycolysis (3).

Histologic, electron microscopic, and electrophysiologic findings in spinal cord compression have been defined in a dog model (4). These changes in the spinal cord, dorsal root ganglia, and cauda equina adjacent to the injury progress in direct proportion to the duration of compression. Delamarter et al. (4) compressed the lower spinal cord at the L-4 level in 30 beagle dogs. All dogs were paraplegic initially. Decompression immediately or after 1 hour of compression led to recovery of ambulation (Tarlov 4 and 5) as well as bowel and bladder control. These groups also recovered 85% to 72% of their baseline somatosensory evoked potential amplitude (Fig. 2). Histologically, discrete areas of Wallerian degeneration and demyelination could be seen in the immediate and 1-hour decompression groups. No central cord necrosis was seen in these animals. The animals in which the spinal cord

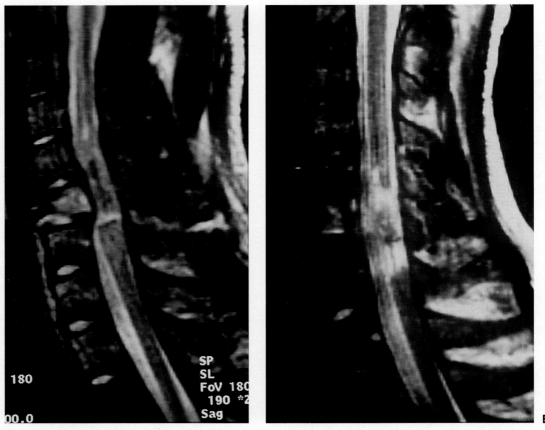

FIG. 1. A 17-year-old surfer suffered a severe C6–7 fracture-dislocation with complete quadriplegia. **A:** Lateral magnetic resonance imaging (MRI) scan taken approximately 90 minutes after injury. Note the damaged spinal cord with hemorrhage and edema as well as transection of the spinal cord at the level of the C6–7 disc space. The patient was taken to the operating room and had urgent spinal cord decompression with vertebrectomy and fusion, approximately 2.5 hours after the initial injury. **B:** Lateral MRI taken 3 days after decompressive surgery. Note the spinal canal is completely decompressed. There is severe spinal cord damage with increased signal over the entire vertebral bodies of C6–7, with a clear expansion of the zone of injury in the spinal cord. This patient recovered some C6 nerve root function postoperatively, but there was no further neurologic improvement.

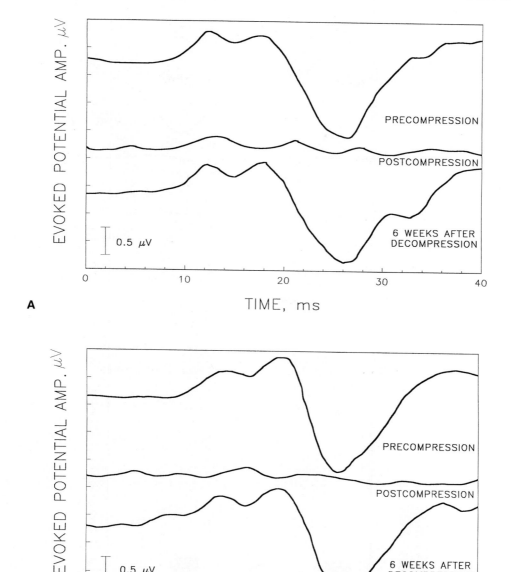

FIG. 2. Delamarter et al. compressed the lower spinal cord at the L-4 level in 30 beagle dogs. All dogs were paraplegic initially, and decompression was done immediately, at 1 hour, 6 hours, 24 hours, and 1 week. Decompression immediately or after 1 hour led to recovery of ambulation as well as bowel and bladder control and substantial somatosensory evoked potential improvement. The animals in which the spinal cord was decompressed after 6 or more hours had no neurologic recovery, and their evoked potential amplitudes recovered only 10% to 29%. **A:** Somatosensory evoked potential of a dog with initial paraplegia and immediate decompression of the spinal cord. Note the normal precompression evoked potential waveform, the essentially flat-lined postcompression waveform, and the near-normal waveform 6 weeks after decompression. **B:** Somatosensory evoked potential with initial complete paraplegia and decompression 1 hour following injury. Note the flat-line postcompression evoked potential waveform and the near-normal waveform 6 weeks after decompression.

(continued)

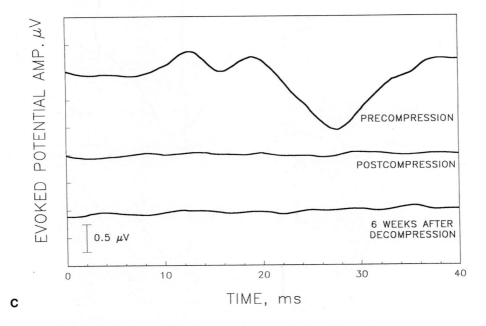

C

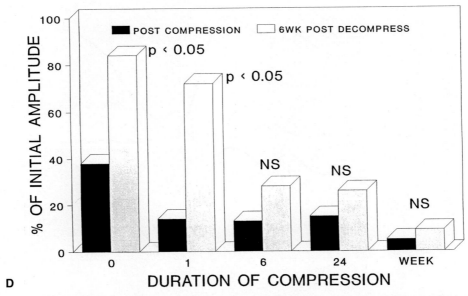

D

FIG. 2. *Continued.* **C:** Somatosensory evoked potentials in a dog with initial paraplegia and decompression 6 hours following injury. Note the flat-line postcompression waveform and the flat-line waveform 6 weeks after decompression. **D:** Bar graph showing somatosensory evoked potential recovery following decompression at the various time intervals. Note the substantial improvement in evoked potentials with dogs decompressed immediately or at 1 hour (statistically significant). The animals decompressed at 6 hours or later had no significant improvement in their evoked potentials or neurologic recovery. These results indicate a brief window of opportunity for decompression of an injured spinal cord.

was decompressed after 6 or more hours had no neurologic recovery. They remained paraplegic and incontinent, and their evoked potential amplitudes recovered only 10% to 29%. The histology on these animals showed central necrosis, loss of axonal architecture, and fibrosis (Fig. 3). These results indicate a brief "window of opportunity" for reduction and decompression of the spinal cord; as secondary injury takes place, there is less potential for recovery.

Four theories have been advanced to address the mechanism of secondary injury. Each theory explains some facets of the complex process, and there is evidence of close synergism between the mechanisms of secondary injury.

The free radical theory suggests that oxygen free radicals accumulate in the injured central nervous system tissues due to rapid depletion of antioxidants. The free radicals attack membrane lipids, proteins, and nucleic acids, producing lipid peroxides that cause cell membrane failure.

The calcium influx theory cites the intracellular flow of calcium ions into neurons as the propagator of secondary injury. Calcium ions activate phospholipases, proteases, and phosphatases, which results in disruption of mitochondrial activity and cell membrane dysfunction.

The opiate receptor theory is based on evidence that endorphins may be involved in promoting secondary SCI. Some experimental SCI models have indicated that naloxone may enhance neurologic recovery, but other studies are in conflict with these results. The therapeutic effect of opioid antagonists may be dose dependent.

The inflammatory theory proposes that inflammatory mediators are released in the acutely traumatized spinal cord, thus causing further tissue damage and neurologic loss. These mediators include prostaglandins, leukotrienes, platelet-activating factor, and serotonin (5).

The acute histologic findings in SCI are central cord gray matter necrosis in the first few hours after injury, followed by cystic degeneration and eventually scar tissue along the axonal long tracts. This scarring takes place over the ensuing weeks in areas where axonal integrity has been interrupted.

Cauda Equina

The cauda equina is more resilient to mechanical insult than the spinal cord. This appears to be partially attributable to the anatomy of the cauda equina and partially due to the difference in the neural tissue involved. The neural tissue in the spinal cord consists mostly of cell bodies and presynaptic neural structures, whereas the cauda equina is composed of postsynaptic myelinated axons.

Pedowitz et al. (6) and Olmarker et al. (7) showed that there is a relationship between the way compression is applied to the cauda equina of pigs and degree of neural injury. Less than 50 mm Hg of pressure does not appear to cause neural injury regardless of how long this pressure is applied to the cauda equina. Four hours of compression at 100 mm Hg results in a marked decrease in both afferent and efferent conduction, with partial recovery after 1.5 hours. Compression at 200 mm Hg causes a complete afferent conduction block after 2 hours and a near-complete efferent conduction block after 3 hours. After this injury at 200 mm Hg, there is no afferent recovery and only partial efferent recovery 1.5 hours after the compression is released (7). Delamarter et al. (8) demonstrated in an animal model of cauda equina compression that decompression allows significant improvement in neurologic function with no significant difference in the evoked potentials, clinical examination, or histology whether the cauda equina has been compressed momentarily, for 1 hour, 6 hours, 24 hours, or 1 week.

The space available for the cauda equina and conus medullaris in lumbar spine trauma can be described by several measurements. The midsagittal diameter (MSD) describes the anteroposterior diameter in the midline at a given level. It is a one-dimensional measurement and does not correlate with neurologic injury. The transverse spinal area (TSA) is measured on a computed tomographic (CT) scan with the aid of a computer-aided design program. It is a two-dimensional measurement that is technically involved and correlates with neurologic injury. The percentage patency is the TSA at the injury level divided by the average TSA of a normal area. This measurement has no units and is based on two-dimensional measurement. It does not correlate well with neurologic injury. A calculated TSA can easily be derived from a CT scan without the aid of a computer. It approximates the true TSA and correlates well with neurologic injury (9).

The calculated TSA is derived as follows:

$$TSA = 0.8[\pi(\tfrac{1}{2}MSD \times \tfrac{1}{2}transverse\ diameter)] + 0.1.$$

Rasmussen et al. (9) found that a TSA at L-1 of 1.25 cm^2 or greater will not result in conus medullaris or cauda equina injury. A TSA between 1.25 and 1.0 cm^2 results in some patients becoming paraplegic. A TSA below 1.0 cm^2 results in paraplegia in all patients. Each more caudal level tolerates progressively greater canal compromise without neurologic injury. Theoretically, each level tolerates 0.06 cm^2 more compression than the level above it, but this has not been shown with statistically significant subject numbers (9).

Cauda equina syndrome is characterized by bowel and bladder dysfunction, perineal anesthesia, and variable sensory and motor loss in the lower limbs. In a model measuring bladder function by cystometrograms and lower limb function with cortical evoked potentials, lower limb function has been shown to be more labile than bladder function when the cauda equina is compressed 50%. At 75% compression, bladder detrusor function is consistently and profoundly impaired (10).

In penetrating injury to the cauda equina due to gunshot wounds and stab wounds, surgical intervention has not been shown to be of benefit (11). In a retrospective study, 29 patients with penetrating injuries to the cauda equina had incomplete injuries. Fifteen patients were treated surgically (laminectomy, debridement, and dural exploration). Of these, 7 improved, 7 remained unchanged, and 1 deteriorated

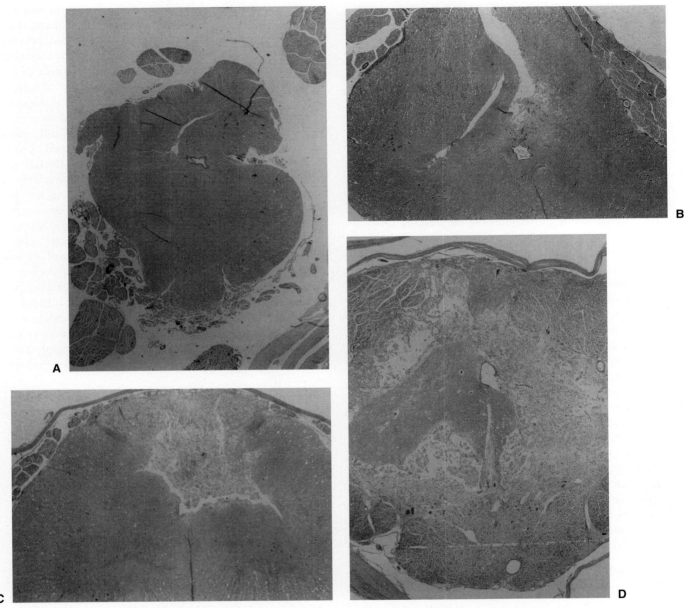

FIG. 3. A: Dog that had 1 hour of compression. The section at the level of the spinal cord injury shows distortion of the spinal cord with some damage to both the central and lateral structures, but maintenance of considerable neural tissue [hematoxylin and eosin (H&E) stain, original magnification × 4]. **B:** Dog with 6 hours of spinal compression. The section shows further residual distortion, central necrosis, and demyelination with some cystic changes and wallerian degeneration (H&E stain, original magnfication × 6). **C:** Dog that had 6 hours of compression with neurologic recovery, following decompression. The section, approximately 1 cm above the spinal cord injury, shows cystic degeneration in the central and posterior columns. The longer the spinal cord compression was maintained, the higher up the spinal cord degenerative changes occurred (H&E stain, original magnification × 6). **D:** Dog that had 24 hours of spinal cord compression. No neurologic recovery followed decompression. This section, approximately 5 mm above the injury site, shows severe destructive changes in both the anterior and posterior columns, significant Wallerian degeneration, and cystic changes (H&E stain, original magnification × 6).

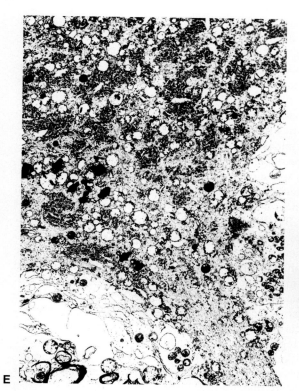

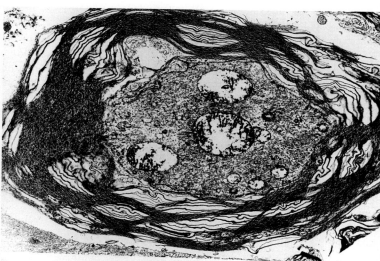

E

F

FIG. 3. *Continued.* **E:** After 6 hours of compression. This section of neural fragment with exiting dendrite was taken from 5 mm below the level of spinal cord injury. Note significant degenerative changes in the mitochondria and disorganization of the neuropil on both sides of the exiting dendrite (original magnification × 6,000). **F:** Section from a dog with 24 hours of compression. This nerve fiber section was taken 5 mm above the level of spinal cord injury from the anterior cord. Note the unraveling and loosening of myelin laminae, with significant distortion of the myelin and moderate degeneration of the mitochondrial contents (original magnification × ~14,000).

neurologically. Fourteen patients were treated nonoperatively. Of these, 10 improved and 4 remained neurologically unchanged. Of the ten patients in the study who had bowel or bladder dysfunction, none improved (regardless of treatment). Twenty-eight percent of surgical patients had major complications (cerebrospinal fluid leak, pseudomeningocoele, or wound infection), whereas none of the nonoperatively managed patients had these complications (11).

PRINCIPLES OF ACUTE SPINAL CORD INJURY CARE

Initial Management

The primary goals in the initial management of SCI is prevention of secondary injury, clinical assessment, and radiographic evaluation of the spine. Today, most SCI patients are transported from the field to the trauma center by emergency medical service personnel who are trained to immobilize any polytraumatized patient in a rigid collar on a backboard. A backboard aids greatly in transferring the patient, but the patient should be moved to a padded but firm surface on arrival to the hospital. Prolonged immobilization on a backboard decreases forced vital capacity by 20% and can cause decu-

bitus ulcers, especially in the face of sensory loss (12–14). Spinal precautions should be observed until instability can be ruled out or until the spine is definitively stabilized. Spinal immobilization should not interfere with life-saving measures, and American Trauma Life Support guidelines should be followed (15). The evaluation of life-threatening injuries must not be delayed to "clear the spine."

If SCI is suspected and the patient is seen within 3 hours of injury, the current standard practice [National Acute Spinal Cord Injury Study (NASCIS) III] is to administer methylprednisolone (MPS) 30 mg/kg as a loading dose, followed by a 23-hour infusion at a rate of 5.4 mg/kg/h (16). If the patient is seen within 3 to 8 hours, the infusion continues for 48 hours. Supplemental oxygen should be administered to all acute SCI patients to maintain O_2 saturation at 100%. Patients with high cervical injuries may require intubation to maintain ventilation.

Spinal cord injury is accompanied by disruption of sympathetic outflow. The unopposed vagal tone causes vasodilatation and bradycardia. These ultimately may lead to hypotension and neurogenic shock. Patients with neurogenic shock generally have a heart rate of 50 to 70. This must be differentiated from hypovolemic shock, which is the most common cause of circulatory system failure in trauma patients. Hypovolemic shock presents with hypotension and tachycardia. Neurogenic shock is managed with an initial fluid challenge, Trendelenburg positioning, vasopressors (e.g., dopamine and phenylephrine), atropine (to treat bradyarrhythmias), inotropic agents, and placement of a Swan-Ganz catheter for hemodynamic monitoring.

Appropriate management of SCI and prevention of secondary injury and further neurologic loss can have a major impact on decreasing the morbidity of SCI and improving patient outcomes. One regional SCI system reports that in 1972 the incidence of SCI in patients with structural spine injuries was 81%. By 1992 this figure dropped to 57% (17). Another study showed a decrease in complete SCI from 64% to 46% of all SCI (18).

Spinal cord injury frequently is accompanied by significant associated injuries. Spinal cord injury due to motor vehicle accidents is accompanied by extremity fractures in 40%, loss of consciousness in 42.5%, and pneumothorax/hemothorax in 16.6% of cases (19). The evaluation and treatment of life-threatening injuries sometimes compromises acute SCI evaluation and treatment. In this early period the spine should be stabilized and protected from further injury. Radiographic and neurologic assessment of SCI is part of the secondary trauma survey. The assessment and therapeutic interventions for SCI may not interfere with life-saving measures. It should, nevertheless, be remembered that when the patient survives the acute trauma, SCI is the most enduring determinant of future quality of life. Early intervention and prevention of further SCI can have a favorable effect on this outcome.

Patients presenting with a neurologic deficit and evidence of cervical spine injury generally should be placed in cervical traction. The exceptions to this are atlantooccipital distraction injuries and type IIA hangman's fractures, in which case cervical traction is contraindicated. When traction is indicated, it is applied either with tongs or a halo ring. Each of these devices has advantages. Tongs (e.g., Gardner-Wells tongs) are placed 1 cm above the ear and manually tightened. They are easily applied by one person, without wrenches. Halo application is somewhat more involved. requiring tools, four pins, and proper alignment in three planes. The halo gives three-dimensional control, which can aid greatly in the reduction of facet dislocations. After cervical alignment is achieved, the halo can be incorporated into a halo vest. Ideally, the traction device should be compatible with magnetic resonance imaging (MRI). The most important factor in the selection of traction device often is availability. Expeditious reduction can significantly improve a patient's neurologic outcome. In general, traction should not wait until after a CT myelogram or MRI has been completed. A lateral C-spine x-ray film is obtained prior to applying traction and repeated after each incremental increase in traction. Intravenous midazolam (Versed; 1 to 4 mg) is used for sedation and cervical muscle relaxation. Initial traction may start with 10 lb of weight and increased in 5-lb increments. This process is interrupted in the event of neurologic deterioration or disc distraction of more than 1 cm. Up to 140 lb of traction has been reported (20). The objectives are early stabilization, decompression, and realignment of the spinal canal.

A detailed standardized initial neurologic examination, as well as follow-up examinations, should be obtained. These examinations are helpful in planning interventions and in monitoring recovery.

The initial neurologic examination determines the level and type of neurologic injury as well as any pattern of neurologic sparing distally. The examination is repeated at regular intervals and additionally after patient transfer, traction adjustment, intubation, surgery. or other interventions that could affect the spinal cord. Marshall et al. (21) prospectively evaluated 283 patients admitted to five trauma centers. Fourteen patients deteriorated neurologically during acute hospitalization. In 12 patients the event could be associated with a management intervention, e.g., traction, halo vest application, surgery, or Stryker frame/rotabed rotation. These findings emphasize the importance of a detailed standardized neurologic examination of the SCI patient on admission and at regular intervals thereafter.

The American Spinal Injury Association (ASIA) has developed a form for the standardized documentation of motor and sensory findings in SCI. The sensory function is graded as follows: 0 = insensate, 1 = impaired sensation, 2 = normal sensation, NT = not testable. The motor function is graded on a seven-point scale: 0 = total paralysis, 1 = palpable or visible contraction, 2 = active movement with full range of motion (ROM) but not against gravity, 3 = active movement (full ROM) against gravity, 4 = active movement (full ROM) against moderate resistance, 5 = active movement (full ROM) against full resistance, NT = not testable.

To ensure accurate, complete, and reproducible documentation, we use the ASIA scoring form for SCI at our institution (Fig. 4). Initial and subsequent examinations are documented on these forms with date, time, and examiner. Any subtle neurologic change is clearly and reliably documented by this method.

There are anecdotal reports of patients presenting acutely with complete neurologic deficits who recovered significant function when the injury was reduced rapidly, thus restoring canal alignment. In one of the earliest reviews of SCI outcomes, Frankel and colleagues (22) reported retrospectively on 682 patients who had postural reduction at the National Spinal Injuries Centre in Stoke Mandeville Hospital, England, between 1951 and 1968. These patients had fractures and fracture dislocations in all regions of the spine.

"Throughout the tables a small number of initially complete neurological lesions become incomplete and a larger number of incomplete lesions improve."

No correlation was established between the timing of reduction, the severity of the initial neurologic lesion, the amount of reduction, and neurologic recovery.

In their series of 68 patients with cervical facet fracture-dislocations, Hadley et al. (23) presented two patients with

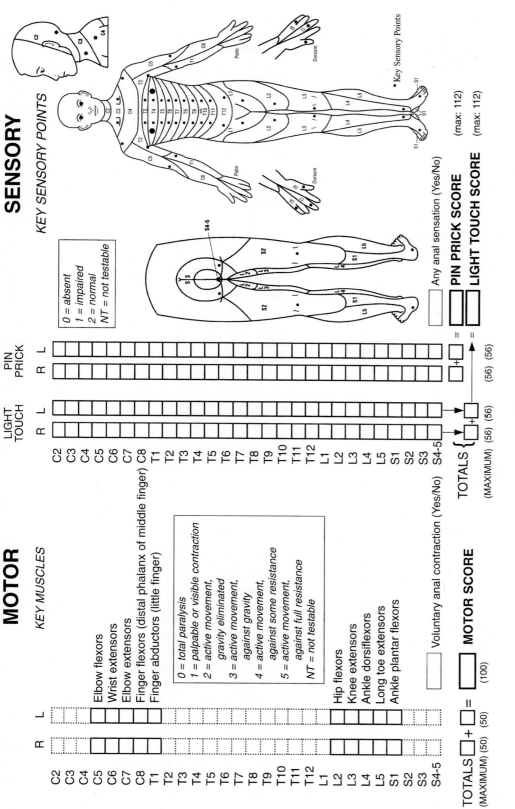

FIG. 4. Neurologic classification of spinal cord injury.

complete injuries who recovered significant function. One patient presented with a unilateral dislocation and a complete neurologic deficit. The dislocation was reduced, and at 94 months the patient had some residual deficits but was ambulatory with arm braces. The other patient presented with complete neurologic loss due to bilateral facet dislocation. The spine was reduced within 4 hours of injury, and the patient regained normal neurologic function.

The results of timely reduction in patients with incomplete neurologic injury are more promising. Aebi et al. (24) reported neurologic improvement in 31% of patients with incomplete quadriplegia due to cervical trauma when this was reduced (surgically or nonsurgically) within 6 hours of injury.

These clinical observations are corroborated by the experimental conclusions established by Delamarter et al. (4) in their canine spinal cord compression model. In this model, neurologic recovery was enhanced by early decompression. Anderson and Bohlman (25) reviewed 58 patients with incomplete SCI secondary to fractures or dislocations of the cervical spine. In this retrospective study, they found some improvement in neurologic function even if operative decompression was carried out more than 1 year after the injury. Other authors have shown that the energy imparted to the spinal cord and the timing of decompression influence the prognosis for recovery (26).

Pharmacologic Therapy

Based on an understanding of the biochemical events in SCI, pharmacologic regimens have been developed to halt the progression of neurologic damage after the primary injury. Numerous ongoing efforts in the laboratory and in clinical studies are aimed at optimizing neurologic outcome through pharmacologic intervention. Research is centered on corticosteroids, 21-aminosteroids, free radical scavengers, opiate antagonists, calcium channel blockers, and neurotrophic factors. Some of these agents are classified in Table 1.

The most promising agents currently are MPS, tirilazad, and GM_1 ganglioside. They are all being evaluated in an ongoing clinical trial.

The efficacy of glucocorticoids in the treatment of cerebral edema due to closed head injury and brain tumors led to the investigation of these agents in the treatment of SCI. It was thought that if these agents were effective in treating

cerebral swelling, they may be beneficial by decreasing spinal cord swelling. Subsequently, MPS has been shown to reduce excitatory amino acid neurotoxicity, inhibit lipid peroxidation, increase spinal tissue blood perfusion, and inhibit traumatic ion shifts (27).

In 1990, Bracken et al. (16) reported on the results of NASCIS II, a multicenter, prospective, randomized, placebo-controlled, double-blinded clinical trial. They showed that high-dose intravenous MPS improved clinical outcome. This is the only study to date that has suggested neurologic injury reversal by pharmacologic means.

NASCIS II studied acute SCI patients for the efficacy and safety of MPS and naloxone with placebo controls. Ninety-five percent of these patients were treated within 14 hours of injury. Methylprednisolone was given intravenously as an initial bolus dose of 30 mg/kg followed by an infusion of 5.4 mg/kg/h for 23 hours. Naloxone was given intravenously as a 5.4 mg/kg bolus followed by 4.0 mg/kg/h for 23 hours. There were 487 patients enrolled in the study: 162 patients received MPS, 154 patients received naloxone, and 171 patients received placebo. The results showed that MPS given within 8 hours of SCI increased the neurologic recovery seen at 6 weeks, 6 months, and 1 year after injury. Both incomplete and complete SCIs improved more with the administration of MPS. The amount of recovery also correlated to the severity of the initial injury. There was no significant difference in the mortality of the MPS group compared with the other groups. Patients treated with MPS later than 8 hours after injury had less neurologic recovery than placebo or naloxone-treated patients (i.e., MPS may actually be detrimental if given more than 8 hours after SCI). Naloxone did not significantly improve neurologic recovery compared to placebo (16).

NASCIS II has been criticized for errors in experimental design and incomplete data. Descriptions of the radiographic findings as well as the details of medical and surgical protocols were not reported. The initial neurologic injuries within each group were not described. The neurologic grading did not include functional outcomes, so there was no clinically useful measure of recovery (28,29).

NASCIS III was similar in its design to its predecessor. The three groups in NASCIS III were as follows: (i) MPS bolus 30 mg/kg followed by MPS 5.4 mg/kg/h for 23 hours; (ii) MPS bolus 30 mg/kg followed by MPS 5.4 mg/kg/h for 47 hours; and (iii) MPS bolus 30 mg/kg followed by tirilazad every 6 hours for 48 hours. NASCIS III concluded and recommends MPS 30 mg/kg followed by 5.4 mg/kg/h for 23 hours if started within 3 hours of injury and continuing for 48 hours if started 3 to 8 hours after injury.

Tirilazad is a synthetic 21-aminosteroid (lazeroid). The 21-aminosteroids are potent antioxidants that exhibit neuroprotective effects by a variety of means. They improve spinal cord blood flow and membrane stabilization. Lazeroids also have fewer side effects than MPS. NASCIS II suggested no increased complications from MPS, but NASCIS I demonstrated that a 10-day glucocorticoid treatment was associated

TABLE 1. *Classification of pharmacologic agents used in spinal cord injury therapy*

Agent	Class
Naloxone	Mu-opioid receptor antagonist
Methylprednisolone	Corticosteroid
Nimodipine	Calcium channel blocker
4-Aminopyridine	Potassium channel blocker
GM_1 ganglioside	Glycolipid (neurotrophic factor)
Tirilazad (lazeroid)	Lipid peroxidase inhibitor
Vitamin E	Free radical scavenger

with an increase risk of complications (29). Other studies have reported an increased risk of pneumonia, wound infection, and prolonged hospital stay in patients treated with glucocorticoids for acute SCI (30).

Gangliosides are a major component of cell membranes in central nervous system tissue. They have been shown to stimulate neuronal regeneration in injured tissue (31). Their mechanism of action is thought to be the enhanced survival of residual axonal tracts that pass through the site of injury, thereby facilitating the recovery of useful motor function distally. They also inhibit amino acid-induced neurotoxicity.

Geisler et al. (32) demonstrated statistically significant neurologic improvement in SCI patients given systemic GM_1 ganglioside sodium salt (Sygen). At 1 year after injury, a significant enhancement of neurologic recovery was demonstrated using both the ASIA and Frankel grading systems (32). The improvement in functional outcome occurred in initially paralyzed rather than in weak (paretic) muscles (32). A large multicenter study is in progress to validate these preliminary findings and to establish the safety and efficacy of two different dosing regimens (33).

4-Aminopyridine is a fast potassium channel blocker that prolongs the duration of action potentials, thereby enhancing nerve conduction.

4-Aminopyridine has been given to a small cohort of patients with incomplete SCI. These patients demonstrated temporary neurologic improvements lasting several days after administration of this agent (34). Further studies are in progress.

Surgical Therapy

Early decompression and stabilization of patients with incomplete SCI has been shown to be beneficial in numerous studies (35–38). Nonoperative treatment of incomplete SCI due to thoracic fractures has repeatedly been shown to give inferior results. Frankel et al. (22) reported 17 patients with thoracic fractures and Frankel B or C neurologic findings. All patients were treated nonsurgically. Eight improved to grade D or better. The average improvement was 1.1 Frankel grade (22). Burke and Murray (37) nonoperatively treated 16 Frankel B patients; 13 improved to grade D or better. Their overall results show an average improvement of 1.3 Frankel grades per patient.

Bradford et al. (36) treated 13 Frankel B or C patients with posterior stabilization; 11 of them had decompressions acutely. The stabilization procedure was done at an average of 4 months after injury. All improved at least one Frankel grade and 11 improved to Frankel grade D for an average improvement of 1.5 Frankel grades per patient. Bohlman et al. (35) reported on eight Frankel B and C patients treated with late anterior decompression and fusion. All improved to at least Frankel D for an average improvement of 2.0 Frankel grades. Krengel et al. (38) studied 14 patients with thoracic incomplete SCI. They found that this group comprised 1.2% of all spinal injuries. All were treated by operative reduction, stabilization, or decompression. Twelve had surgery within 24 hours. Average neurologic improvement was 2.2 Frankel grades per patient.

The surgical treatment of SCI varies with the type of neurologic and skeletal injury, the acuity of the injury, and the severity of associated injuries. Surgical priorities are realignment, decompression, and stabilization. If there is adequate space for the cord after realignment, then decompression often is unnecessary and only stabilization and fusion may be needed. The majority of SCI patients with instability probably are best treated with surgical stabilization. The choice of instrumentation is based on the status of the posterior elements, the presence or absence of anterior column support, and the vertebral levels affected. Cervical facet dislocations generally can be reduced and stabilized with simple wiring or lateral mass plates (Fig. 5). In facet fracture-dislocations, greater rotational stability may be achieved by the addition of lateral mass plates. When anterior cervical decompression is indicated, a bone strut alone often fails to provide adequate stability, and anterior cervical plating or posterior instrumentation may be necessary to achieve stability (Fig. 6).

The choice of cervical orthotics includes halo vest, cervical thoracic orthosis, rigid cervical orthosis, or soft collar. The soft collar is an ineffective means of immobilization, whereas the rigid cervical orthosis and cervical thoracic orthosis are progressively more effective in limiting flexion and extension. The halo vest is the only cervical orthosis that provides significant rotational stabilization. For the thoracolumbar spine, a thoracolumbosacral orthosis effectively immobilizes the spine.

Acutely, spinal cord compression in thoracolumbar burst fractures may be treated by posterior instrumentation and indirect reduction through ligamentotaxis. This is most effectively done within the first 2 to 3 days after injury. A posterior approach is indicated in the patient with a lumbar burst fracture with a lamina fracture. Cammisa et al. reported a 37% incidence of dural tears with lamina fractures. In patients with a burst fracture, a lamina fracture, and neurologic injury, the incidence of dural laceration is 69%; 25% of these patients have nerve roots entrapped in the lamina fracture. An anterior approach does not allow reduction of these roots or repair of the posterior dural laceration (39). A posterior approach usually is indicated in patients who are neurologically intact with thoracolumbar fracture and significant segmental deformity. The most straightforward means of correcting this deformity and maintaining correction is with posterior instrumentation (40), unless there is severe crushing of the vertebral body, which may require a vertebrectomy and anterior fusion.

Relative indications for posterior reduction and stabilization include neurologically intact patients with unstable fractures. Generally, this should be carried out within 1 to 2 weeks of injury. A posterior approach can be used within 48 hours of a burst fracture with neurologic deficit to achieve an indirect reduction of the fracture fragments and decompres-

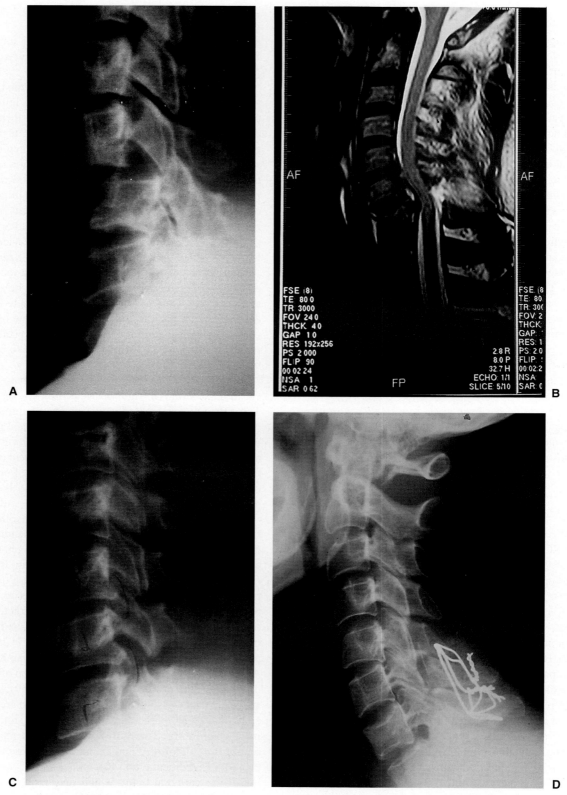

FIG. 5. A 28-year-old woman was involved in a head-on motor vehicle accident. She was brought into the emergency room unable to move her arms or legs. **A:** Lateral cervical spine x-ray film shows a bilateral facet dislocation at C6–7. **B:** Immediate magnetic resonance image reveals C6–7 subluxation. Note distortion and compression of the spinal cord at the dislocated level. **C:** Gardner-Wells tong traction was immediately applied. With 75 pounds of traction, reduction of the facet dislocation was easily accomplished. The patient noticed almost immediate improvement in her neurologic examination. She was taken to surgery for cervical stabilization. **D:** Postoperative lateral x-ray film shows Bohlman triple wire fusion of the reduced facet dislocation. Over a 3-month time period the patient had complete neurologic recovery.

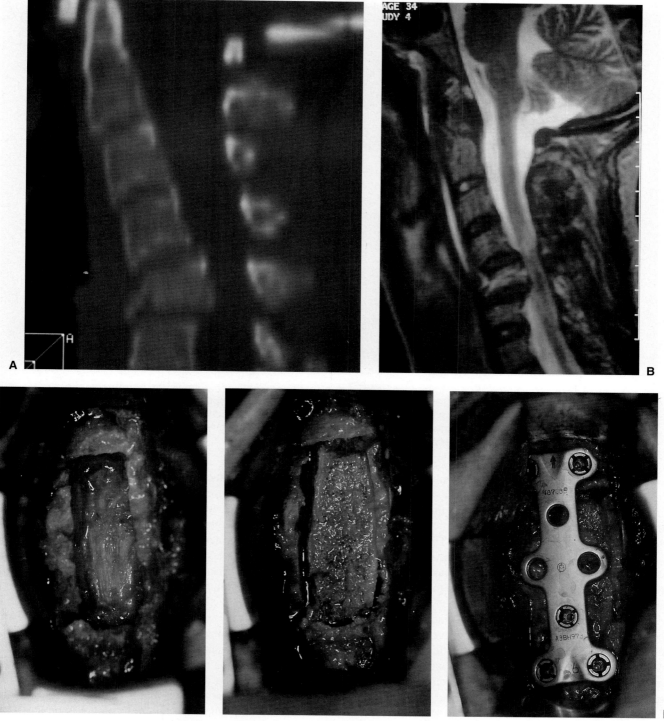

FIG. 6. A 24-year-old woman was brought into the emergency room following a rollerblading accident. Immediate neurologic evaluation revealed a complete C5 quadriplegia. **A:** Lateral x-ray film reveals flexion compression injury with retropulsion of the C5 vertebral body and kyphotic angulation. **B:** Emergent magnetic resonance imaging with the patient in halo traction reveals significant fracture of the C5 vertebral body. Note severe compression of the spinal cord with edema and hemorrhage of the neural tissue. The patient was taken for immediate surgical decompression and underwent a C5 vertebrectomy. **C:** Intraoperative photograph taken after the C5 vertebrectomy and exposure of the decompressed dural sac. **D:** Intraoperative photograph shows the iliac crest strut graft in place at C4–6. **E:** Interoperative photograph shows the anterior cervical plate fixation and stabilization.

(continued)

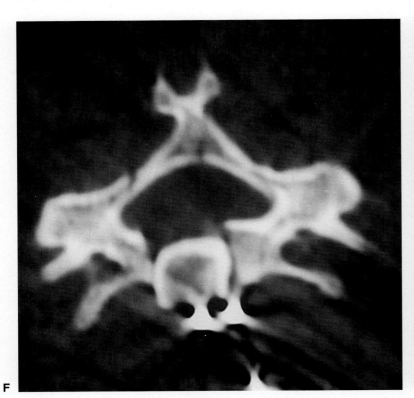
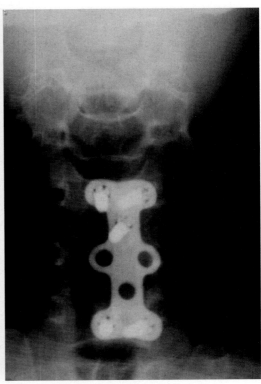

F

G

FIG. 6. *Continued.* **F:** Postoperative computed axial tomographic scan shows the vertebrectomy and strut graft fusion of the C5 vertebral body. Note complete decompression of the spinal canal. **G:** Anteroposterior x-ray film shows the anterior plate fusion. This patient recovered the C5 and C6 nerve roots, but she remained quadriplegic from the C7 level. Recovery from complete quadriplegia is rare, although root recovery, following surgical decompression, is observed frequently.

sion of the neural elements. In 85% of patients with this injury, this approach gives adequate decompression (40,41).

Posterior indirect reduction and instrumentation is contraindicated in patients with incomplete neurologic deficits who are more than 10 days after injury. This approach also is contraindicated where CT shows minimal vertebral body compression with significant retropulsion, or where the retropulsed fragment is flipped around so that the cancellous surface faces posteriorly (40).

Anterior decompression and fusion is indicated in a number of SCIs. It is seldom indicated in upper cervical injuries due to the space available for the cord in this region. If, after realignment of the lower cervical spine, anterior cord compression is still present, then anterior decompression is indicated. Anderson and Bohlman (42) noted improvement in 63% of patients with complete neurologic deficits after cervical fracture if they had anterior decompression and arthrodesis. Fourteen percent of these patients recovered two new functional motor root levels and 35% recovered one level. Neurologic improvement was seen even if this surgery was performed after 18 months (42). In patients with cervical fractures and incomplete neurologic deficits, 53% became functional ambulators after anterior decompression and arthrodesis (25). Improvement was diminished if operative intervention was delayed for more than 1 year after injury.

If, after a thoracolumbar posterior indirect reduction, significant anterior compression remains, then anterior decompression is indicated. If it is noted that a retropulsed fragment is rotated 180 degrees or is detached, then anterior decompression is indicated. Based on the aforementioned studies, neurologic recovery is optimized if decompression is carried out promptly. Also, in the presence of cord compression, thoracolumbar injuries that are more than 1.5 weeks old are treated most effectively by anterior decompression due to immobility of the fracture fragments. The goal with anterior surgery is to achieve an open reduction of the spinal canal under direct visualization. This is done through a retroperitoneal approach, a transthoracic approach, or a standard anterior cervical approach, depending on the level of the injury (40). The first priority is spinal cord decompression. After this is accomplished, the anterior column is reconstituted with strut graft as needed and instrumentation is performed when there is residual instability.

Low lumbar fractures (L3–5) account for less than 4% of all spine fractures. The cauda equina, which occupies the spinal canal in this region, is more resistant to injury than the spinal cord, which ends in the conus medullaris at L-1. Nonetheless, when there is a fracture in this region with neurologic compromise, expeditious decompression of the cauda equina frequently is indicated (43).

RECOVERY OF FUNCTION

The prognosis for recovery depends on the type of neurologic injury. Sometimes, the terms used to describe these injuries vary from the standardized terminology, and this can lead to confusion.

The American Spinal Injury Association has established terminology and definitions for the description of SCI. Tetraplegia (preferred to "quadriplegia") describes cervical cord injury affecting arms, trunk, pelvic organs, and legs. Paraplegia describes injury to thoracic, lumbar, and sacral cord injuries as well as cauda equina injuries. Paraplegia spares arm function but can affect the trunk, pelvic organs, and lower extremities, depending on the level of injury. Quadriparesis and paraparesis are no longer used. Neurologic level (sensory and motor level) refers to the most caudal segment of the spinal cord with useful sensory and motor function on both sides of the body. Skeletal level describes the level that is radiographically found to have the greatest vertebral damage. When there is partial sensory or motor preservation below the neurologic level and sacral segments are preserved, the injury is described as incomplete. The absence of motor and sensory function in the lowest sacral segment defines a complete neurologic injury by the ASIA standards. The zone of partial preservation describes the dermatomes caudal to the neurologic level that are partially innervated.

Incomplete injuries often present as characteristic clinical syndromes (i.e., anterior cord syndrome, posterior cord syndrome, central cord syndrome, Brown-Séquard syndrome, conus medullaris syndrome). Anterior cord syndrome presents with a loss of motor function, sharp/dull sensation, light touch sensation, and temperature sensation below the level of injury. Deep pressure sensation and proprioception are preserved below the level of injury. The anterior horn cells and anterolateral long tracts are damaged at the level of injury. The posterior gray matter horns and posterior columns are spared by this injury. This injury is seen most commonly in the cervical region; the mechanism typically is compression or flexion. The prognosis for anterior cord syndrome is worst of all the incomplete syndromes, with rare return of any muscle function.

Posterior cord syndrome is rare. It involves the posterior columns and causes sensory loss below the level of injury.

Central cord syndrome occurs almost exclusively in the cervical spine. It occurs in patients with underlying stenosis or often in older patients with more rigid spines. It is characterized by injury to the central gray matter of the cord, which contains the motor horn cells for the upper extremities. Central cord syndrome presents clinically as upper extremity weakness that is greater than the lower extremity weakness. The sacral sensory levels are spared from injury. Bowel, bladder, and lower extremity function usually return significantly, whereas upper extremity function improves only modestly.

Conus medullaris injury typically is associated with a skeletal injury level at the thoracolumbar junction. It gener-

ally presents with a loss of perirectal sensation, poor rectal tone, and a loss of bowel and bladder control. The prognosis for improvement of these symptoms is poor.

A number of studies are in progress to examine the regeneration of axonal tracts following traumatic SCI. Swiss researchers transected the thoracic spinal cord of young adult rats. This was followed by administration of antibodies (inhibitory neurite factor −1, IN-1) to neutralize myelin-associated neurite growth inhibitory factor (44). This treatment resulted in growth of corticospinal axons into spinal cord levels caudal to the injury site.

Cheng et al. (45) reported a rat model in which they transected the spinal cord at T-8. They then used peripheral nerve grafts to bridge individual axonal tracts. Acidic fibroblast growth factor was mixed with fibrin glue and used to stabilize the anastomoses. Over the next 6 months, hind limb function in these rats improved compared to controls. This study is far removed from the treatment of human SCI, but it does show that regeneration is possible in a completely transected adult animal spinal cord. This type of research may eventually discover protocols that have similar effects in the human spinal cord.

Even with all of the surgical and pharmacologic sophistication available, the most positive impact on SCI can be effected with preventive measures to decrease the incidence of these devastating injuries. Surgical decompression can improve the neurologic outcome of patients with incomplete injuries. Surgical stabilization of unstable spine injuries may prevent neurologic deterioration and aids in rehabilitation of these patients. The role of pharmacologic therapy has not been rigorously defined. A wide variety of agents show promise in preventing neurologic deterioration and regaining function. This is an area of intense research and shows great promise for the future.

REFERENCES

1. UAB National Spinal Cord Injury Statistical Center. *Spinal Cord Injury Facts and Figures at a Glance.* Birmingham: University of Alabama, Birmingham, 1996.
2. Riggins R, Kraus J. The risk of neurologic damage with fractures of the vertebrae. *J Trauma* 1977;17:126–133.
3. Jannsen L, Hansebout R. Pathogenesis of spinal cord injury and newer treatments: a review. *Spine* 1989;14:23–32.
4. Delamarter RB, Sherman J, Carr J. Pathophysiology of spinal cord injury. *Bone Joint Surg Am* 1995;77A:1042–1049.
5. Young W, Huang P, Kume-Kick J. Cellular ionic and biomolecular mechanisms of the injury process. In: Benzel E, Tator C, eds: *Contemporary Management of Spinal Cord Injury.* AANS, 1995:28–31.
6. Pedowitz R, Garfin S, Massie J, et al. Effects of magnitude and duration of compression on spinal nerve root conduction. *Spine* 1992;17;194–199.
7. Olmarker K, Rydevik B. Holm S. Edema formation in spinal nerve roots induced by experimental graded compression: an experimental study on the pig cauda equina with special reference to differences in effects between rapid and slow onset of compression. *Spine* 1989;14:569–573.
8. Delamarter R, Sherman J, Carr J. 1991 Volvo award in experimental studies: cauda equina syndrome: neurologic recovery following immediate, early, or late decompression. *Spine* 1991;16:1022–1029.
9. Rasmussen P, Rabin M, Mann D, Perl J, Lorenz M, Vrbos L. Reduced transverse spinal area secondary to burst fractures: is there a relationship to neurologic injury. *J Neurotrauma* 1994;11:711–720.

10. Delamarter R, Bohlman H, Bodner D, Biro C. Urologic function after experimental cauda equina compression, cystometrograms versus cortical evoked potentials. *Spine* 1990;15:864–870.

11. Robertson D, Simpson R. Penetrating injuries restricted to the cauda equina: a retrospective review. *Neurosurgery* 1992;31:265–270.

12. Chan D, Goldberg R, Tascone A, Harmon S, Chan L. The effects of spinal immobilization on healthy volunteers. *Ann Emerg Med* 1994;23:48–51.

13. Linares H, Mawson A, Suarez E, et al. Association between pressure sores and immobilization in the immediate post-injury period. *Orthopedics* 1987;10:571–573.

14. Schafermeyer R, Ribbeck B, Gaskins J, et al. Respiratory effects of spinal immobilization in children. *Ann Emerg Med* 1991;20:1017–1019.

15. American College of Surgeons Committee on Trauma. *Advanced Trauma Life Support Manual,* 5th edition. Chicago: American College of Surgeons, 1993.

16. Bracken M, Shepard MJ, Collins, W, et al. A randomized, controlled trial of methylprednisolone or naloxone in the treatment of acute spinal cord injury. *N Engl J Med* 1990;322(20):1405–1411.

17. Waters RL, Apple DF, Meyer PR, Cotler JM, Adkins RH. Emergency and acute management of spine trauma. In: Stover SL, DeLisa JA, Whiteneck GG (eds). *Spinal Cord Injury: Clinical Outcomes from the Model Systems.* Maryland: Aspen Publication, 1995:56–57.

18. Slucky AV, Eismont FJ. Treatment of acute injury of the cervical spine. *J Bone Joint Surg Am* 1994;76A:1882–1896.

19. Go BK, DeVivo MJ, Richards JS. The epidemiology of spinal cord injury. In: Stover SL, DeLisa JA, Whiteneck GG (eds). *Spinal Cord Injury: Clinical Outcomes from the Model Systems.* Maryland: Aspen Publishers, 1995:21–51.

20. Cotler JM, Herbison GJ, Nasuti JF, Ditunno JF, An H, Wolff BE. Closed reduction of traumatic cervical spine dislocation using traction weights up to 140 pounds. *Spine* 1993;18:386–390.

21. Marshall L, Knowlton S, Garfin SR, Klauber MR, Eisenberg HM, Kopaniky D, et al. Deterioration following spinal cord injury: a multicenter study. *J Neurosurg* 1987;66:400–404.

22. Frankel HL, Hancock DO, Hyslop G, et al. The value of postural reduction in the initial management of closed injuries of the spine with paraplegia and tetraplegia. *Paraplegia* 1969;7:179–192.

23. Hadley MN, Fitzpatrick BC, Sonntag VK, Browner CM. Facet fracture-dislocation injuries of the cervical spine. *Neurosurgery* 1992;30:661–666.

24. Aebi M, Mohler J, Zach GA, Morscher E. Indication, surgical technique, and results of 100 surgically-treated fractures and fracture-dislocations of the cervical spine. *Clin Orthop* 1986;203:244–257.

25. Anderson P, Bohlman H. Anterior decompression and arthrodesis of the cervical spine: long-term motor improvement (part 1). *J Bone Joint Surg* 1992;74A:671–682.

26. Guha A, Tator CH, Endrenyi L, Piper I. Decompression of the spinal cord improves recovery after acute experimental spinal cord compression injury. *Paraplegia* 1987;25:324–339.

27. Greene K, Marciano, F, Sonntag V. Pharmacological management of spinal cord injury: current status of drugs designed to augment functional recovery of the injured human spinal cord. *J Spinal Dis* 1996;9:355–366.

28. Geisler F. Prevention of spinal cord injury. In: Benzel E, Tator C (eds). *Contemporary Management of Spinal Cord Injury.* AANS, 1995:255–260.

29. Zeidman SM, Ling GS-F, Ducker TB, Ellenbogen RG. Clinical applications of pharmacologic therapies. *J Spinal Dis* 1996;9(5):367–380.

30. Galandiuk S, Rague G, Appel S, Polk HC. The two-edged sword of large dose steroids for spinal cord trauma. *Ann Surg* 1993; 218:419–425, 425–427 (disc).

31. Rengachary S, Alton S. Resuscitation and early medical management of the spinal cord injury patient. In: Benzel E, Tator C (eds). *Contemporary Management of Spinal Cord Injury.* AANS, 1995:60–61.

32. Geisler FH, Dorsey FC, Coleman WP. Recovery of motor function after spinal cord injury—a randomized, placebo-controlled trial with GM-1 ganglioside. *N Engl J Med* 1991;324:1829–1838, 1991; 325:1659–1660.

33. Geisler FH, Dorsey FC, Coleman WP. Past and current clinical studies with GM-1 ganglioside in acute spinal cord injury. *Ann Emerg Med* 1993;22:1041–1047.

34. Hansebout RR, Blight AR, Fawcett S, Reddy K. 4-Aminopyridine in chronic spinal cord injury: a controlled, double blind, crossover study in eight patients. *J Neurotrauma* 1993;10:1–18.

35. Bohlman H, Freehafer A, Dejak J. The results of treatment of acute injuries of the upper thoracic spine with paralysis. *J Bone Joint Surg* 1985;67A:360–369.

36. Bradford D, Akbarnia B, Winter R, et al. Surgical stabilization of fracture and fracture-dislocations of the thoracic spine. *Spine* 1977; 2:185–196.

37. Burke D, Murray D. The management of thoracic and thoraco-lumbar injuries of the spine with neurologic involvement. *J Bone Joint Surg* 1976;58B:72–78.

38. Krengel W, Anderson P, Henley B. Early stabilization and decompression for incomplete paraplegia due to a thoracic-level spinal cord injury. *Spine* 1993;18:2080–2087.

39. Cammisa F, Eismont F, Green B. Dural laceration occurring with burst fractures and associated laminar fractures. *J Bone Joint Surg* 1989;71A:1044–1052.

40. McAfee P, Levine A, Anderson P. Surgical management of thoracolumbar fractures. *Instrum Course Lectures* 1995;44:47–55.

41. Dickson F, Harrington P, Erwin W. Results of reduction and stabilization of the severely fractured thoracic and lumbar spine. *J Bone Joint Surg* 1978;60A:799–805.

42. Anderson P, Bohlman H. Anterior decompression and arthrodesis of the cervical spine: long-term motor improvement (part 2). *J Bone Joint Surg* 1992;74A:683–692.

43. Delamarter R, Wang J. Surgical and non-surgical management of fractures of the lumbar spine. In: Capen D (ed). *Comprehensive Management of Spine Trauma.* Missouri: Mosby, 1998:214–234.

44. Bregman B, Kunkel-Bogden E, Schnell L, Dai HN, Gao D, Schwab ME. Recovery from spinal cord injury mediated by antibodies to neurite growth inhibitors. *Nature* 1995;378:498–501.

45. Cheng H, Cao Y, Olson L. Spinal cord repair in adult paraplegic rats: partial restoration of hind limb function. *Science* 1996; 273: 510–513.

Surgery of Spinal Trauma,
edited by J.M. Cotler, J.M. Simpson, H.S. An, and C.P. Silveri.
Lippincott Williams & Wilkins, Philadelphia © 2000.

CHAPTER 3

Biomechanics of Spinal Trauma

Mechanisms, Tissue Tolerance, and Implant Performance

Allan F. Tencer

Understanding the biomechanics of spinal trauma provides several important practical benefits. Knowledge of the response and tolerance of the spine to loads in different directions allows the design of effective equipment that can reduce the potential for injury. Appreciation of the remaining stability and load carrying capacity of the injured spine yields insight into methods of stabilization that allow healing without further injury. Comparisons of different implant systems permits selection of the appropriate device for the clinical problem being addressed. This chapter first introduces some basic concepts of biomechanics that are necessary for understanding the mechanical response of the spine. Then mechanisms, tolerance levels, and resulting injuries, as well as the mechanical performance of various fixation techniques, are presented for four major regions of the spine: the axial-atlanto-occipital region, the cervical spine and cervicothoracic junction, the thoracic and lumbar spine, and the lumbosacral junction. The focus of this chapter will be on clinically relevant information derived from

biomechanical testing that can be applied to the treatment of these injuries.

BIOMECHANICS OF INDIVIDUAL COMPONENTS OF THE SPINE

Basic Definitions

Force has direction and magnitude. The action of a force is to change the direction of motion of a body and its velocity (either increasing or decreasing it). Multiple forces acting on an object can be replaced by their sum, a single force or *resultant* having a *line of action* or specific direction in which it acts (Fig. 1). A *moment* results from a force acting at a distance from a fulcrum or *center of rotation*. The result is bending or rotation of the body about the center. A common example is the effect of body weight on the spine (Fig. 2), which both compresses the spine and creates forward flexion. Although many forces and moments in different directions act on the spine, they can be resolved into the basic loads (Fig. 3). These are *compressive and tensile forces* acting along the axis of the spine, anteroposterior and mediolateral *shearing forces* that directly displace the vertebrae in these directions, *sagittal plane bending* causing flexion or

A.F. Tencer: Harborview Biomechanics Laboratory, Department of Orthopaedics, Harborview Medical Center, Seattle, Washington 98104.

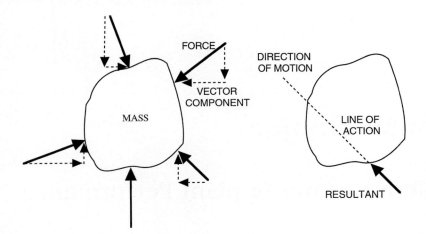

FIG. 1. Left: Multiple forces can act on a body. These forces can be resolved into components (in this case, vertically and horizontally) and added together. **Right:** The sum of these multiple forces is a single resultant force acting in a defined direction, the line of action.

extension, *lateral bending*, and *torsion* or rotation about the longitudinal axis of the spine.

Under load, a spinal motion segment (two vertebrae and their interconnecting soft tissues) displaces in a characteristic way. As shown in Fig. 4, the motion segment has a *neutral zone* or region where it can be displaced with little force. Beyond the neutral zone, as the tensions in the tissues increase, it enters an *elastic zone* where increasing force is required to produce greater displacement in any direction. Finally, the *zone of failure* is reached, where tissue tearing and/or bony fracture result. The neutral zone has been shown to be the most sensitive parameter in defining a spinal injury (1). Release of the applied load, after loading into the dam-

age region, results in the motion segment remaining in some deformed position, because of tissue damage. However, total stability may not be lost because some remaining tissues are available to carry load. Examples of characteristic fracture patterns having *residual stability* will be provided in the section discussing lumbar spine injuries.

The spine exhibits *viscoelastic behavior*. This means that it has an *elastic* or displacement-related response and a *viscous* or time-related response to applied force. An example of the elastic response is a spring under compressive load deforming in direct proportion to the force applied, regardless of how fast the load is applied. Pushing liquid out of a syringe demonstrates the viscous response. For fluid to be pushed out faster requires considerably higher force than when the fluid is allowed to exit slowly. The viscosity or re-

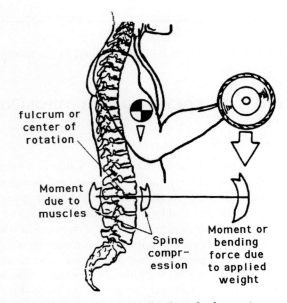

FIG. 2. A moment, due to application of a force at some distance from a fulcrum, causes both compression and bending. In this example, the fulcrum is within the disc, and both body weight and the weight being held cause forward bending that is counteracted by the erector spinae muscles, resulting in significant compression of the spine. (Adapted from Smith TJ, Fernie GR. Functional biomechanics of the spine. *Spine* 1991;16:1197–1203.)

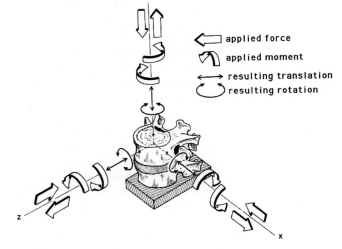

FIG. 3. Basic loads acting on the spine (forces and moments) and the resulting motions of the vertebrae (translations and rotations), forces; tension-compression, anteroposterior, or transverse shearing causing subluxation of the vertebra, moments; flexion/extension, lateral bending, and axial torsion. (Adapted with permission White AA III, Panjabi MM. *Clinical Biomechanics of the Spine*, 2nd edition. Philadelphia: JB Lippincott, 1990.)

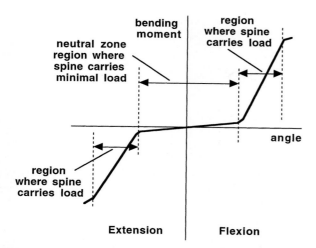

FIG. 4. Typical load-displacement (applied bending moment in flexion or extension and resulting angulation) behavior of a spinal motion segment (two vertebrae and interconnected soft tissues) showing neutral zone region (angular motion under minimal load) and elastic region with increasing resistance to motion under load.

sistance to flow of the fluid governs the response. These concepts have direct practical significance. At higher rates of force application in compression, vertebrae are stronger because of the *hydraulic stiffening* effect of the fat and marrow in trabecular bone. This will be discussed in detail in the section on burst fractures of the lumbar spine. Another example of the effect of viscosity is the *creep* response of the spine to load. Creep occurs when a motion segment is under a constant load and continues to deform progressively, although at a slower and slower rate (Fig. 5). This behavior explains why we become shorter in stature throughout the day. Conversely, if the motion segment is loaded to some deformation and then held in constant position, the internal stresses in the tissues will decrease, resulting in stress relaxation. This can be felt in the tissues during stretching before exercise, when holding some fixed position for a period of time. A practical application concerns the use of distraction instrumentation, for example, in scoliosis correction. The force of distraction drops rapidly at first, then more slowly in patients over time (Fig. 6).

Kinematics defines the motion response of the spine to load. Although the actual response is complex, including motions in directions other than that in which the load is applied (*coupled motions*), reasonable estimates of the response of the spine and the tissues that would be involved in resisting the applied load can be determined from estimation of *the center and axis of rotation* of the motion segment (Fig. 7). The center of rotation is a fixed point that may translate with the complete motion segment, but does not move relative to the motion segment. In other words, this is the fixed point around which the vertebra rotates in response to the applied load. The center of rotation concept applies to planar or two-dimensional motions. For three-dimensional motions, an axis of rotation must be defined. This axis may not be per-

pendicular to the plane of motion. An example of this is the asymmetric effect on motion of the fracture of one facet. Appreciating the location of the center of rotation is particularly important when considering where to place spinal instrumentation, as will be discussed later. In general, the farther the implant is from the center of rotation, the less load it experiences or the greater stiffness it produces.

Vertebra

The basic biomechanical properties of the major individual elements, that is. the vertebral body, the disc, the major ligaments, and the facets are first presented. The vertebral body dimensions at various levels are shown in Fig. 8, as this may be of assistance in sizing implants for stabilization (2,3). The vertebral body is principally formed of trabecular bone with a thin cortex and superior and inferior endplates (Fig. 9). The vertical columns of trabecular bone are the principal load-bearing structures, transferring load from the annulus and endplate above to that below (4). The cross ties (horizontal trabeculae) assist in load bearing by preventing the vertical columns from buckling. Buckling of a long slender column is a common mechanism of failure under compressive loading, and loss of cross tie support is more critical than loss of area of the trabecular column. This is because the load causing buckling failure decreases as column cross-sectional area decreases but as the square of the length of the column increases (5). Practically speaking, it has been well demonstrated that a direct relationship exists between quantitative computerized tomography and vertebral bone strength (Fig. 10) (6,7). Quantitative computerized tomography provides a measure of the mean density of the vertebra; however, the density of the vertebra is not uniform throughout. Samples from different regions of the same vertebral body show that the greatest trabecular bone strength occurs in the center, followed by the middle posterior region (Fig. 11) (8). This information has important implications for the attachment of implants, because the pullout strength of screws is directly related to the density of the material (actually its shear strength) into which they are placed (9). Loading rate also affects the strength of vertebral motion segments, changing both the strength and the mode of failure under compressive loading (10).

Disc-Nucleus-Endplate

One can think of the disc as a structure consisting of three major components: the annulus, which resists tensile (hoop) stresses along with bulk compression of its material; the nucleus, which converts some of the compressive force to internal pressure that creates disc bulging and hoop or expansion (tensile) stresses; and the endplates, which form a flexible seal on the vertebral body and prevent extrusion of the nucleus (Fig. 12). Classic studies by Nachemson (11) demonstrated *in vivo* that pressure in the nucleus is 1.3 to 1.6 times the vertical load per unit area applied to the vertebra,

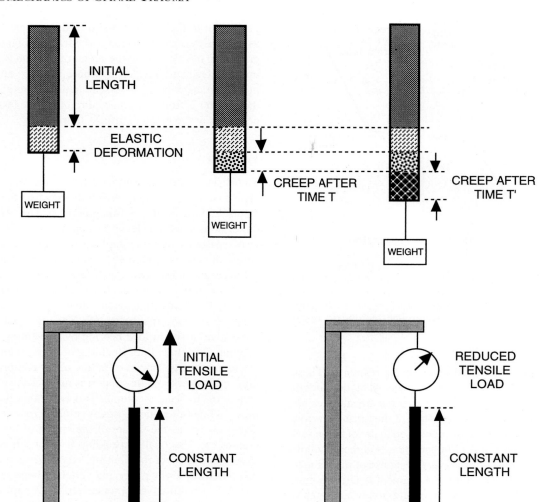

FIG. 5. Basic concepts of tissue creep and stress relaxation. **Top:** In creep, a weight hung from a biologic tissue first will drop due to the elastic stretching of the tissue, then continue to descend because of the creep or viscous response. **Bottom:** If a tissue is stretched and then held in position, the force within the tissue will decrease over time, resulting in stress relaxation.

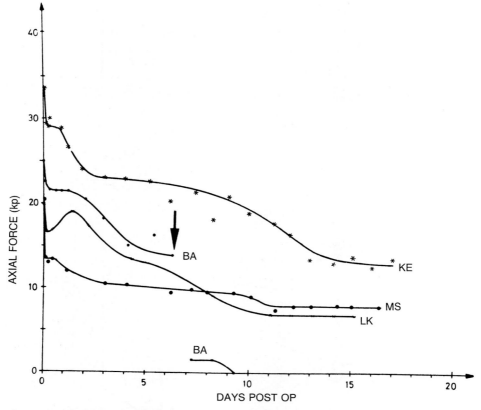

FIG. 6. An example of the time-related creep behavior of the spine. Instrumented distraction rods were applied to several patients undergoing scoliotic correction, and the distractive force was monitored over time showing significant decreases from the initial force values. (Reproduced with permission from Nachemsen A, Elfstrom G. Intravital wireless telemetry of axial forces in Harrington distraction rods in patients with idiopathic scoliosis. *J Bone Joint Surg* 1971;53A:445–465.)

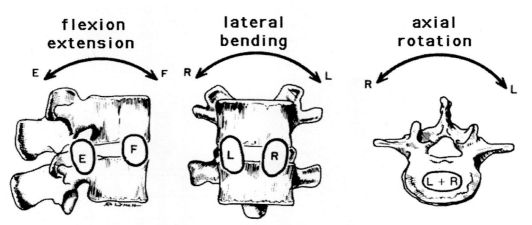

FIG. 7. The approximate centers of rotation of the lumbar spine in flexion/extension, lateral bending, and axial rotation. (Reproduced with permission from White AA III, Panjabi MM. *Clinical Biomechanics of the Spine,* 2nd edition. Philadelphia: JB Lippincott, 1990.)

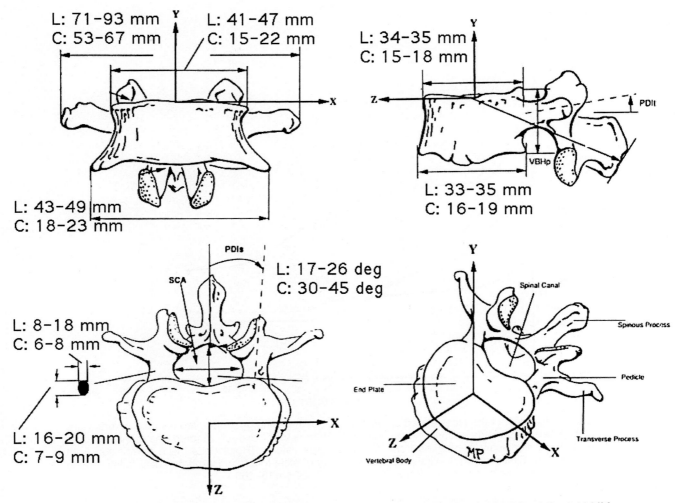

FIG. 8. Some basic dimensions of lumbar (L) and cervical vertebrae (C). (Adapted from Panjabi MM, Duranceau J, Goel V, Oxland T, Takata K. Cervical human vertebrae. Quantitative three dimensional anatomy of the middle and lower regions. *Spine* 1991;16:861–869; and Panjabi MM, Goel V, Oxland T, Takata K, et al. Quantitative three dimensional anatomy. *Spine* 1992;17:299–306.)

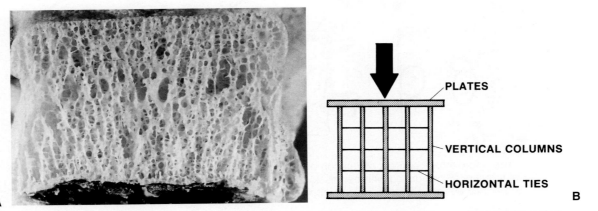

FIG. 9. Architecture of the vertebral body showing the trabecular bone (**A**) as vertical load-bearing columns with horizontal ties to prevent buckling (**B**). (Reproduced with permission from White AA III, Panjabi MM. *Clinical Biomechanics of the Spine,* 2nd edition. Philadelphia: JB Lippincott, 1990.)

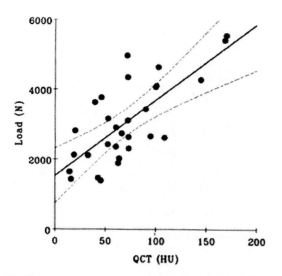

FIG. 10. Quantitative computerized tomography (QCT) measurements in Haunsfield units (HU) versus whole lumbar vertebral strength in compression. (Reproduced with permission from Mow VC, Hayes WC. *Basic Orthopedic Biomechanics.* New York: Raven Press, 1991.)

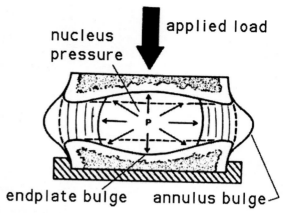

FIG. 12. Structure and conceptual function of the disc-nucleus-endplate unit under load. Compressive load is converted into a hydrostatic pressure in the nucleus pulposus, which in turn gives rise to bulging of the disc annulus and endplate. The annulus bulge causes the fibers of the annulus to experience tensile stress. (Reproduced with permission from Mow VC, Hayes WC. *Basic Orthopedic Biomechanics.* New York: Raven Press, 1991.)

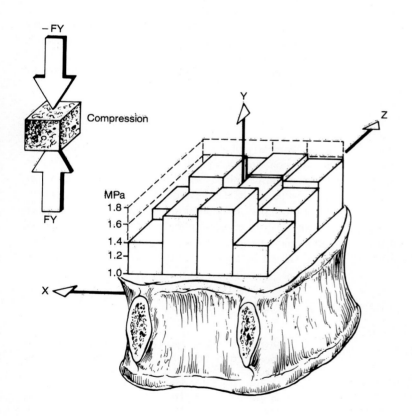

FIG. 11. Relative strengths of trabecular material in compression from various parts of the vertebral body. (Reproduced with permission from Mow VC, Hayes WC. *Basic Orthopedic Biomechanics.* New York: Raven Press, 1991.)

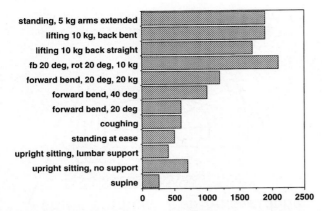

FIG. 13. Measured pressure in the nucleus pulposus *in vivo* and resulting compressive load on the L-3 lumbar disc due to various body positions and activities for a person weighing 70 kg. (Adapted from Nachemson AL. Disc pressure measurements. *Spine* 1981;6:93–97.)

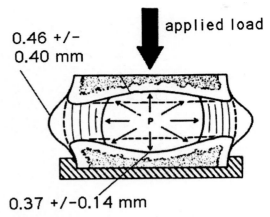

FIG. 14. Bulging of the disc and endplates in response to a compressive load applied to the vertebral body. (Data adapted from Doherty BJ, Heggeness MH. Vertebral body endplates deform under physiological axial loading. Transactions of the 39th Annual Meeting of the Orthopedic Research Society, 1993:88.)

and it is significantly affected by the vertical compressive load applied, which is determined by body position and activity (Fig. 13).

The pressure generated in the nucleus acts to bulge the endplates upward and the disc outward (Fig. 14) (12–14). Knowledge of the tensile properties of the annulus are important, because the disc tends to fail in tension, either by stretching of fibers as the vertebra angulates and/or by tensile stresses caused by bulging (Fig. 15). The fiber failure tensile stress is greatest in the outer anterior ring of the annulus, and, significantly, the posterior annulus fibers are only about 50% as strong (15). This is important because the posterior annulus is also thinner than the anterior annulus, therefore predisposing the posterior region to fail at considerably lower load than the anterior region. It is interesting to note that there is considerable load sharing among the posterior part of the disc, the posterior longitudinal ligament (PLL), and the posterior elements in flexion and that the disc itself can withstand less than half of the flexion failure load

of the intact vertebral motion segment (Fig. 16) (16). In addition to the tensile stresses caused by separation of the vertebral bodies at the posterior border of the disc, considerable nucleus pressure is generated, which adds to the tensile stresses experienced by the posterior disc tissue in flexion due to disc bulging. Typical disc failures due to flexion are shown in Fig. 17.

Facet Joints

The facets clearly play a role in limiting motion in various planes by bony interaction, and these motions vary in different regions of the spine. From Fig. 18, directions of motion limited by the facets can be deduced, being anterior translation (of the superior vertebra) and compression in the cervical spine, anterior translation in the thoracic spine, and axial rotation and anterior translation in the lumbar spine. However, it should be appreciated that the facets also are sur-

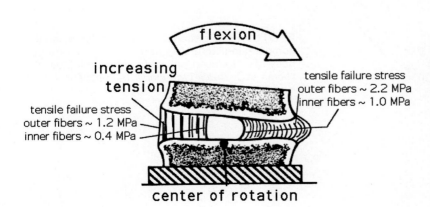

FIG. 15. Flexion generates tensile stresses in the posterior fibers of the disc annulus, with the greatest stress at the outermost fibers that are furthest from the center of rotation. Note the difference in tensile strength between anterior and posterior disc fibers. (Adapted from White AA III, Panjabi MM. *Clinical Biomechanics of the Spine,* 2nd edition. Philadelphia: JB Lippincott, 1990; and Acaroglu ER, Iatridis JC, Setton LA, Foster RJ, Mow VC, Weidenbaum M. Degeneration and aging affect the tensile behavior of human lumbar anulus fibrosus. *Spine* 1995;20: 2690–2701.)

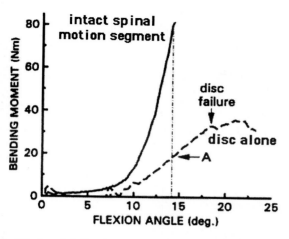

FIG. 16. Load-deflection plot (vertebral flexion moment vs. flexion angle) of an intact motion segment and of an isolated disc. (Reproduced with permission from Adams MA, Green TP, Dolan P. The strength in anterior bending of lumbar intervertebral discs. *Spine* 1994;19:2197–2203.)

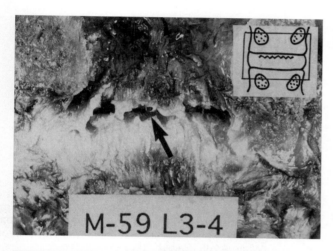

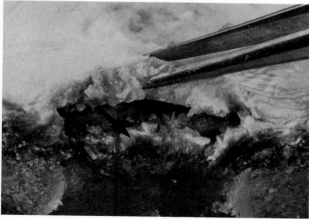

FIG. 17. Typical appearance of disc tissue after flexion failure demonstrating tensile tearing of the posterior disc tissue. (Reproduced with permission from Adams MA, Green TP, Dolan P. The strength in anterior bending of lumbar intervertebral discs. *Spine* 1994;19:2197–2203.)

rounded by a very tight fibrous capsule; therefore, loads that tend to separate the facet surfaces also contribute to loading the facets and limiting spinal motion (Fig. 19). The resulting contributions of the facets to load sharing have been investigated in a number of studies (17–23). In the lumbar motion segments, loss of facets had the greatest effect on motion in posterior shear (posterior translation of the inferior vertebra relative to the superior one), flexion, extension, lateral bending, and axial torsion loading.

Spinal Ligaments

The spinal ligaments have well-defined structural functions. These functions can be deduced by considering the known paths of motion of two adjacent vertebrae of a spinal motion segment, the locations of attachment of the ligaments, their orientations, their states of prestress, and their elastic stiffness properties. The response of any ligament under tension shows three particular features (Fig. 20), a toe region where relatively large deformations occur under low loads, an elastic region, and a failure region that defines the range of maximum load capacity. Figure 21 demonstrates, based on elongation, how different ligaments contribute to resisting spinal motion. Note that this does not take into account the elastic stiffness of the ligaments, which must be known to determine the actual loads they support. Many posterior ligaments, based on elongation, contribute to resisting flexion, especially the supraspinous, interspinous, and facet capsules. Similarly, the anterior longitudinal and capsular ligaments resist extension, and the intertransverse ligaments and facet capsules resist lateral bending. The major strain during torsion occurs in the capsule of the facet whose faces are separating (24,25). The ligamentum flavum appears to have lower strain, but again the stiffness of the ligament must be defined to yield information about the actual contributions of the soft tissue elements.

Some stiffness properties of individual ligaments have been tested and are shown in Table 1 (26–31). It is clear that ligament properties are governed by a number of variables (Fig. 22, namely, bone mineral content of the vertebra, rate of loading (28), and age of the specimen (27). By considering the stiffness data presented in Table 1, it becomes clear that even though the posterior ligaments closer to the center of rotation of the motion segment, such as the ligamentum flavum, exhibit less strain, they have considerably greater stiffness. Therefore, the posterior elements appear to resist loads, at least in flexion, fairly uniformly.

Neurologic Tissues

Although the neurologic tissue (nerve root sleeves and dura) are not structural in terms of carrying significant loads dur-

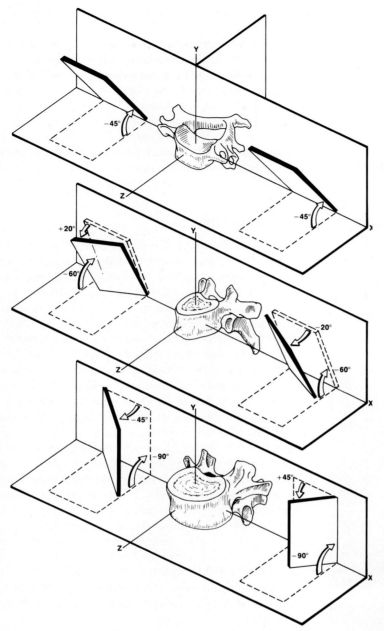

FIG. 18. Schematic diagram of the orientation of the facet joints of different regions of the spine. **Top:** Cervical spine. **Middle:** Thoracic spine. **Bottom:** Lumbar spine. (Reproduced with permission from White AA III, Panjabi MM. *Clinical Biomechanics of the Spine,* 2nd edition. Philadelphia: JB Lippincott, 1990.)

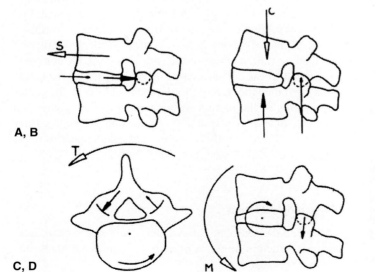

FIG. 19. Loading directions that create loads in the facets include those that bring the surfaces together causing impingement and those that separate them causing stretching of the fibrous capsules. **A:** Anterior shear of the superior vertebra. **B:** Compression. **C:** Axial torsion. **D:** Flexion or extension. (Reproduced with permission from Adams MA, Hutton WC. The mechanical function of the lumbar apophyseal joints. *Spine* 1983;8:327–330.)

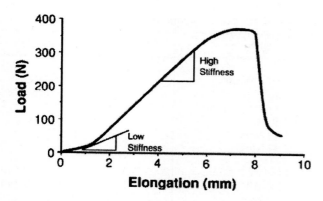

FIG. 20. Characteristic load-elongation properties of a typical ligament under tensile loading, low stiffness or toe region, high stiffness or elastic region, and failure region. (Reproduced with permission from Woo SL-Y, An K-N, Arnoczky SP, Wayne JS, Fithian DC, Myers BS. Anatomy, biology and biomechanics of tendon, ligament, and meniscus. In: Simon SR (ed). *Orthopedic Basic Science.* Chicago: American Academy of Orthopedic Surgeons, 1994:45–87.)

ing a traumatic event, it is important to appreciate the elasticity of these tissues in determining how much stability must be restored to the injured spine to prevent further injury. The elongation of the nerve trunk at its elastic limit is about 20%, with elongation at failure, about 30% (32). The dura is tethered within the spinal canal by thin anterior ligaments and by the nerve roots themselves. Head and neck flexion create strain in this structure. The strain on the posterior surface of the dura varies with spinal level, increasing caudally. The strain in the dural tissue between C-2 and C-5 can reach 15% by flexion of the spine within its normal range of motion with the posterior elements removed (Fig. 23). The mean tensile strain to failure of the dura ranges from 30% to 40% (33). This implies that doubling the flexion angular range, especially in the cervical region, due to for example instability, may produce significant damage to the dura.

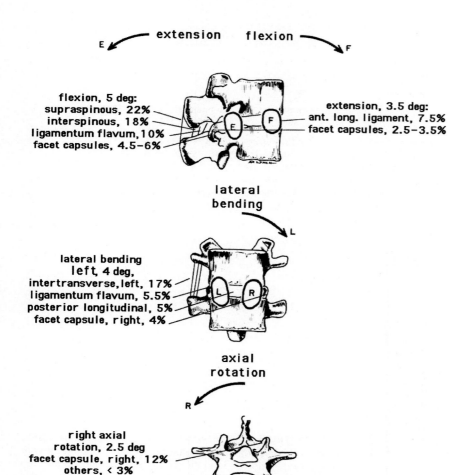

FIG. 21. Estimated centers of rotation of spinal motion segments and resulting strains (change in length/ligament resting length) in the principal ligamentous tissues for the lumbar spine. (Adapted from Tencer AF, Mayer TG. Soft tissue strain and facet face interaction in the lumbar intervertebral joint: part II. Calculated results and comparison with experimental data. *J Biomech Eng* 1983;105:210–215; Panjabi MM, Goel VK, Takata K. Physiological strains in the lumbar spinal ligaments. *Spine* 1982;7:192–203; and White AA III, Panjabi MM. *Clinical Biomechanics of the Spine,* 2nd edition. Philadelphia: JB Lippincott, 1990.)

TABLE 1. *Stiffness, strength, and elongation of various isolated tissues of the vertebral motion segment*

Source	Ligament	Stiffness	Strength	Elongation
Lumbar				
Waters and Morris (26)	Interspinous	113 N/mm^2		25%
Nachemson and Evans (27)	Ligamentum flavum	49.4 N/mm^2	440 kg/cm^2	46%
Neumann et al. (28)	Anterior longitudinal	74–214 N/mm	599–1572 N	
Dumas et al. (29)	Ligamentum flavum	350 N/mm		
	Facet capsules	259 N/mm		
	Interspinous	94 N/mm		
Cervical				
Yoganandan et al. (30)	Anterior longitudinal	14.9–82.7 N/mm	120.5–349.5 N	7.5–6.3 mm
	Ligamentum flavum	21.9–92.9 N/mm	130.6–335 N	7.6–7.9 mm
Fielding et al. (31)	Transverse ligament C1–2		72–111 Kp	

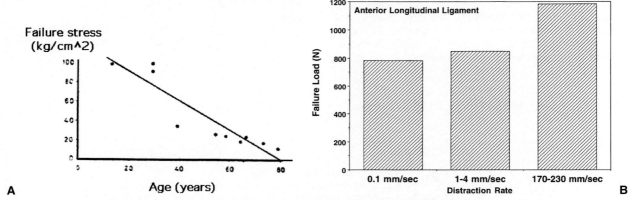

FIG. 22. Effect of some variables on tensile properties of individual spinal ligaments. **A**: Effect of specimen age. (Reproduced with permission from Nachemson AL, Evans JH. Some mechanical properties of the third human lumbar interlaminar ligament (ligamentum flavum). *J Biomech* 1968;1:211–220.) **B**: Effect of rate of loading. (Data adapted from Neumann P, Keller TS, Ekstrom L, Hansson T. Effect of strain rate and bone mineral content on the structural properties of the human anterior longitudinal ligament. *Spine* 1994;19:205–211.)

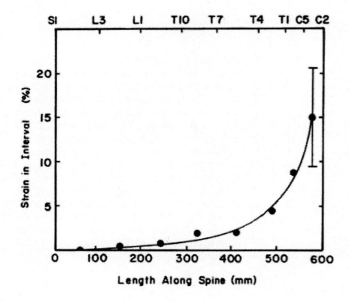

FIG. 23. Distribution of strain in the posterior dura due to head and neck flexion as measured in the midpoints of various intervals along the spine. (Reproduced with permission from Tencer AF, Ferguson RL, Allen BL Jr. A biomechanical study of thoracolumbar spine fractures with bone in the canal: part III. Mechanical properties of the dura and its tethering ligaments. *Spine* 1985;10:741–747.)

OCCIPITO-ATLANTO-AXIAL JOINTS

Normal Motion and Function of Components

The function of the C0-C1-C2 joint complex can be appreciated by observing the arrangement of its bony surfaces (Fig. 24). The articulation of the skull with the first cervical vertebra (C0–1) allows about 13 degrees of flexion/extension and 8 degrees of lateral bending. In contrast, C1–2, because of the orientation of the odontoid process, permits a significant amount of axial rotation (47 degrees) and some lateral bend-ing (10 degrees), but negligible flexion and extension (34). The center of axial rotation is aligned with the longitudinal axis of the odontoid. The odontoid functions not only as a guiding axis for head rotation, but resists shearing (horizontal transverse forces) and bending of the head in the posterior and lateral directions, and, indirectly through the transverse ligament, in flexion.

Ligaments function to limit motion as their internal tension increases; therefore, if the center of rotation of the joint and the orientation and attachment sites of the liga-

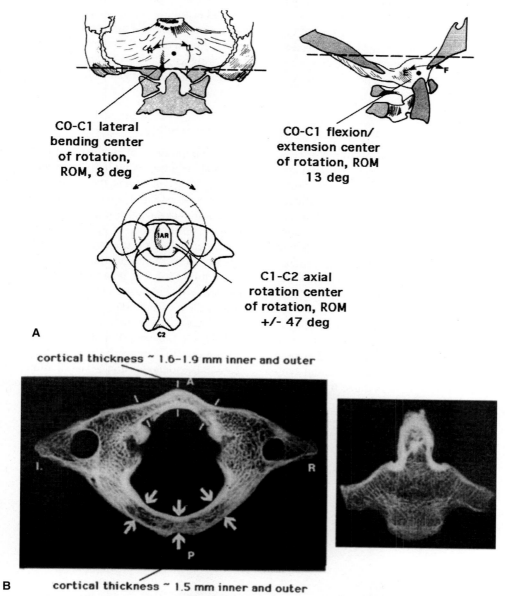

CO-C1 lateral bending center of rotation, ROM, 8 deg

CO-C1 flexion/ extension center of rotation, ROM 13 deg

C1-C2 axial rotation center of rotation, ROM +/- 47 deg

A

cortical thickness ~ 1.6-1.9 mm inner and outer

B cortical thickness ~ 1.5 mm inner and outer

FIG. 24. A: Geometry of the atlanto-occipital and atlanto-axial joints of the upper end of the cervical spine, showing major bony structures, mean ranges of motion, and approximate centers of rotation. (Reproduced with permission from Doherty BJ, Heggeness MH, Esses SI. A biomechanical study of odontoid fractures and fracture fixation. *Spine* 1993;18:178–184; and Heggeness MH, Doherty BJ. The trabecular anatomy of the axis. *Spine* 1993;18:1945–1949.) **B:** Cortical thicknesses of the ring of C-1 and the odontoid process of C-2 indicating regions of higher and lower stresses. (Adapted from White AA III, Panjabi MM. *Clinical Biomechanics of the Spine,* 2nd edition. Philadelphia: JB Lippincott, 1990.)

ment are known, its approximate motion-limiting functions can be deduced. Experimental studies have been helpful in quantifying these observations, especially when multiple ligaments have similar functions. The transverse ligament restrains flexion and anterior motion of the head, as shown by Fielding et al. (35), since this ligament was always torn with the C0-C1-C2 complex loaded to failure in these directions, Figure 25. Crisco, et al (36) showed that the capsular ligaments of C1–2 act as backups to the alar and transverse ligaments, especially in axial rotation. Injury to one or both capsular ligaments in isolation does not increase joint motion in any direction. However, injury to an alar ligament first increases the rotational angle at failure by about 10%, followed by a similar increase with loss of the second alar ligament. Once these ligaments have been sectioned, the capsules play the significant role in resisting rotation, with progressive increases in motion as they are sectioned.

Mechanism of Injury and Load Tolerance

The loads applied to the C0-C1-C2 joints are complex, typically resulting from a blow to the head or by differential motion between the head and the torso. Nonetheless, certain structures typically are injured due to loading in specific directions. For example, as shown in Fig. 26, flexion of the occiput, without compression, produces mainly type III odontoid fractures [inferior to the base of the odontoid, including bone of C-2 (37)] at a mean load of 2,033 lb, lateral bending results in type II fractures (at the base of the odontoid), and extension creates mainly type II fractures at similar loads (38,39).

That the odontoid acts as a cantilever, resisting bending by the head, necessitates its particular cortical and trabecular anatomy (40). The odontoid has very thick cortical bone at its base (Fig. 24), which explains its considerable and symmetric strength in different loading directions. It should be appreciated that although the strength characteristics of the odontoid are similar in these different directions of loading, the mechanism of load transfer is not the same. Extension of the occiput loads the surface of C-1 against the odontoid, whereas flexion loads the transverse ligament, which, because of its band arrangement, transfers load to the odontoid. The consequence of this is certain failure of the transverse ligament in flexion-type injuries (35). As discussed earlier, loss of the transverse and alar ligaments significantly increases the axial rotational instability of the joint.

The application of compression may result in fracture of the posterior or anterior arch of the atlas (Fig. 26) (41), along with other injuries such as separation of the lateral masses and ligament failure. Cadaveric specimens demonstrated anterior or posterior arch failure under axial loading resulting from weights of 3 to 6 kg dropped from a height of 1 m. These resulted in a mean failure load of 3,050 N, with the specimen in neutral position (42).

Residual Stability

Of great importance clinically is an understanding of the mechanical stability remaining after injury. Mechanically, the stability of a joint (that is, the displacement of the bony components) can be expressed in several forms. As shown in Fig. 4, the joint has a neutral zone or range of motion that occurs with very little load. In addition, there may be an elastic zone, depending on the structures that have been injured. The sum of these motions defines the overall range of motion of the joint (36). The neutral zone has been found to be the more sensitive indicator of the effect of injury. Again, this is simply the measured range of motion of the joint in a particular direction under minimal load.

Jefferson fractures (fractures of the ring of the atlas) have been shown to increase the neutral zone motion by a mean of 27% in flexion/extension. Axial rotation and lateral bending were minimally affected. The effect of odontoid fracture has

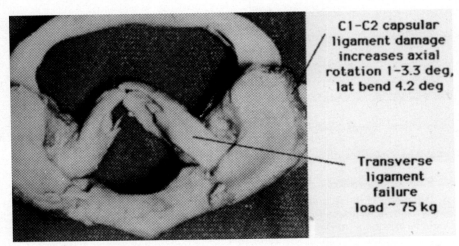

FIG. 25. Structural function of the major ligaments of the C0-C1-C2 complex. (Adapted from Fielding JW, Cochran GVB, Lawsing JF III, Hohl M. Tears of the transverse ligament of the atlas. *J Bone Joint Surg* 1974;56A:1683–1691.)

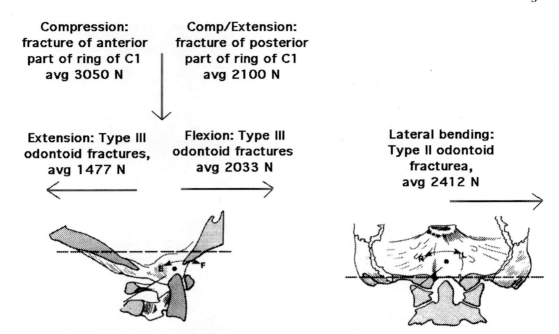

Compression:
fracture of anterior
part of ring of C1
avg 3050 N

Comp/Extension:
fracture of posterior
part of ring of C1
avg 2100 N

Extension: Type III
odontoid fractures,
avg 1477 N

Flexion: Type III
odontoid fractures
avg 2033 N

Lateral bending:
Type II odontoid
fracturea,
avg 2412 N

FIG. 26. Directions of loading and some typical resulting injuries, along with mean loads required to produce these injuries in the C0-C1-C2 joints. (Adapted from White AA III, Panjabi MM. *Clinical Biomechanics of the Spine,* 2nd edition. Philadelphia: JB Lippincott, 1990.)

not been specifically measured. However, if the alar or transverse ligaments are damaged, there will clearly be significant increases in rotational instability as well as translation, which could cause cord occlusion.

Fixation Biomechanics

Doherty et al. (39) and Sasso et al. (43) showed that the strength of fixation of type II fractures of the odontoid using 3.5-mm diameter cortical screws and loaded either in extension or obliquely, ranged from 512 to 1,157 N (mean 687 N) compared to a force range of 979 to 2,225 N (mean 1,510 N), which was required in the same direction to create the fracture in those specimens. Therefore, the strength of odontoid screw fixation is about 45% that of the intact odontoid. A second screw of the same diameter did not increase fixation strength.

The atlanto-axial joint of C1–2 provides a unique problem in spinal fixation because of the lack of a vertebral body at C-1. Stability at this level is provided by ligamentous connections and interaction of the ring of C-1 on the odontoid as described earlier. Four methods have been commonly used for posterior fixation of fractures in this region (Fig. 27). The Gallie type fixation (44) uses a single posterior bone graft between the arch of the atlas and the spinous process of C-2, which is wired in place. The Brooks fixation (45) uses double wires placed anterior to the arch of C-1 and the lamina of C-2, which capture double bone grafts fit between the arch and the lamina, as well as providing compression across the injury. In the Magerl transarticular screw technique (46,47) the screws are placed from the junction of the lamina and articu-

lar mass of C-2 into the mass of C-1. Additionally, small grafts are placed posteriorly between the arch and lamina of C1–2 and are wired in place. The Halifax method (48) uses clamps placed between the arch of C-1 and the lamina of C-2. In a study by Grob et al. (49), these four methods were compared biomechanically in terms of their ability to limit angulation (the mean of flexion, extension, lateral bending, and axial rotation motions) as well as anteroposterior translation at C1–2. The relative motions allowed between C-1 and C-2 with fixation are shown in Fig. 27. These observations were confirmed by Hajek et al. (50), who found mean flexion stiffnesses of 3.1, 2.3, and 0.8 Nm/deg for the Halifax, Brooks, and Gallie constructs. To put these stiffness values in perspective, consider that when the head is not controlled by muscle forces, its dead weight produces a bending moment (rotational force) around the occiput of about 2.7 Nm.

CERVICAL SPINE

Normal Motion and Function of Components

The estimated flexion and extension centers of rotation (51), as well as normal cervical ranges of motion (52), are shown in Fig. 28. It can be appreciated that the centers of rotation lie close to the facet articulations (51), demonstrating the motion-limiting role of the facets (because the center of rotation by definition is the point on the object where no rotation occurs). The measured flexion/extension, lateral bending, and rotational motions in the normal spine demonstrate fairly uniform ranges of about 10 degrees from C2–3 to C7–T1, in each direction for each level (Fig. 28).

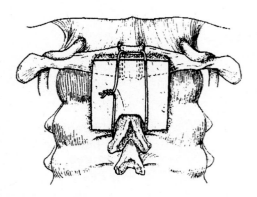

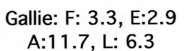

Gallie: F: 3.3, E:2.9
A:11.7, L: 6.3

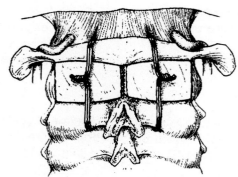

Brooks: F: 1.0, E:0.7
A:3.3, L: 0.7

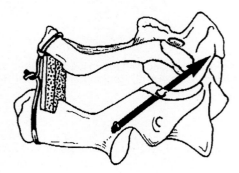

Magerl: F: 1.1, E:1.1
A:0.7, L: 0.7

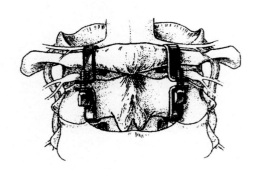

Halifax: F: 0.6, E:0.6
A:5.3, L: 0.8

FIG. 27. Four common methods of fixation of the atlanto-axial (C1–2) articulation. Gallie (44) posterior bone graft notched to fit the spinous process of C-2 and wired in place. Brooks technique (45) has bone graft placed between the posterior arches of C-1 and C-2 with double wires compressing the graft. Magerl (46,47) transarticular screws between C-2 and C-1 with posterior bone grafts secured by wire loops. Halifax clamps (48) around the posterior arches of C-1 and C-2. A, axial rotation; E, extension; F, flexion; L, lateral bending. Numerical values indicate average motions (in degrees) between fixed vertebrae under loads in the specific directions. (Reproduced with permission from Grob D, Crisco JJ III, Panjabi MM, Wang P, Dvorak J. Biomechanical evaluation of four different posterior atlantoaxial fixation techniques. *Spine* 1992;17:480–490.)

The major stabilizers of the spine are the surrounding muscles. Magnetic resonance imaging has the advantage of noninvasive quantification of *in vivo* muscle activity. It has been used to identify the active cross sections of cervical spine muscles during flexion and extension (Fig. 29). Flexion results mainly from the actions of the splenius capitus, semispinalis capitus. semispinalis cervicis and multifidus, and lateral bending from the sternocleidomastoid longus capitis and colli (53).

The vertebra is the main structure supporting compression of the spine. However, compressive load has been shown to be distributed approximately two thirds on the vertebral body itself and one third through the lateral masses (54). Further, the uncinate processes serve mainly to limit axial rota-

tion (removal increased rotation by 25%) and lateral bending (14%) (55). Isolated facet capsule sectioning showed that these structures contribute about 25% of resistance in axial rotation and 30% in flexion/extension (Fig. 30) (56). Progressive transection of ligamentous components and the disc followed by mechanical loading has shown how the applied load is shared between them. Only small increases in flexion angle occur in specimens loaded in flexion as the structures are progressively sectioned from a posterior to an anterior direction, until only the disc and anterior longitudinal ligament remain intact. Similarly, loading in flexion and cutting structures from anterior demonstrates stability until the facets are removed, leaving only the ligamentum flavum and posterior ligaments. In extension, loss of the anterior longitudinal lig-

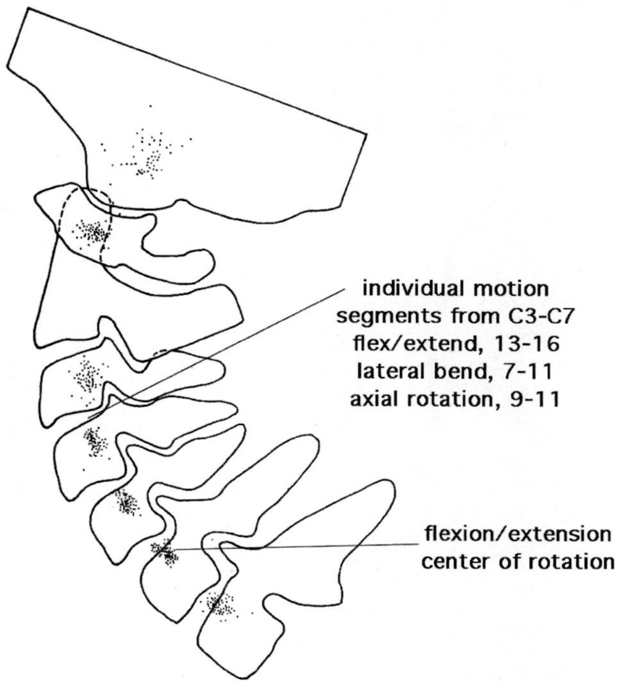
individual motion
segments from C3-C7
flex/extend, 13-16
lateral bend, 7-11
axial rotation, 9-11
flexion/extension
center of rotation

FIG. 28. Measured flexion/extension center of rotation and range of motion of individual segments of the cervical spine (in degrees) (C3–7). (Adapted from van Mameren H, Sanches H, Beursgens J, Drukker J. Cervical spine motion in the sagittal plane: II. Position of segmental averaged instantaneous centers of rotation, a cineradiographic study. *Spine* 1992;17:467–474.)

ament and the anterior half of the disc was sufficient to increase extension angle beyond the normal, whereas sectioning of the posterior half of the disc after cutting all posterior ligaments resulted in increased motion (57). This demonstrates the important role of the disc in flexion/extension stability, followed by the facet joints.

Mechanism of Injury and Load Tolerance

Cervical spine injuries occur typically during certain athletic activities, such as diving into shallow water (58), and in motor vehicle accidents. In vehicle accidents, the primary spinal levels injured are C-5 and C-6, and the most prevalent type of injury is combined compression and flexion, followed by facet dislocation. Cervical spinal injuries accounted for 44% of all spinal injuries with cord involvement and comprised 14% of the total number of spinal injuries in records of the National Accident Sampling System. In contrast, thoracolumbar injuries accounted for 31%, and only 1% were thoracolumbar cord injuries. The primary mechanism, as will be discussed in detail later, was frontal impact for serious injuries (abbreviated injury score, AIS, >3), and all directions of impact (frontal, rear, side) for less serious injuries (AIS = 1) (59).

The mechanics of injury to the cervical spine are complex, because the cervical spine is essentially an unstable column with a large weight (the head) on its upper end. Without the action of the muscles to stabilize it, it tends to collapse into extension, unless the head is bent forward, locking the spine

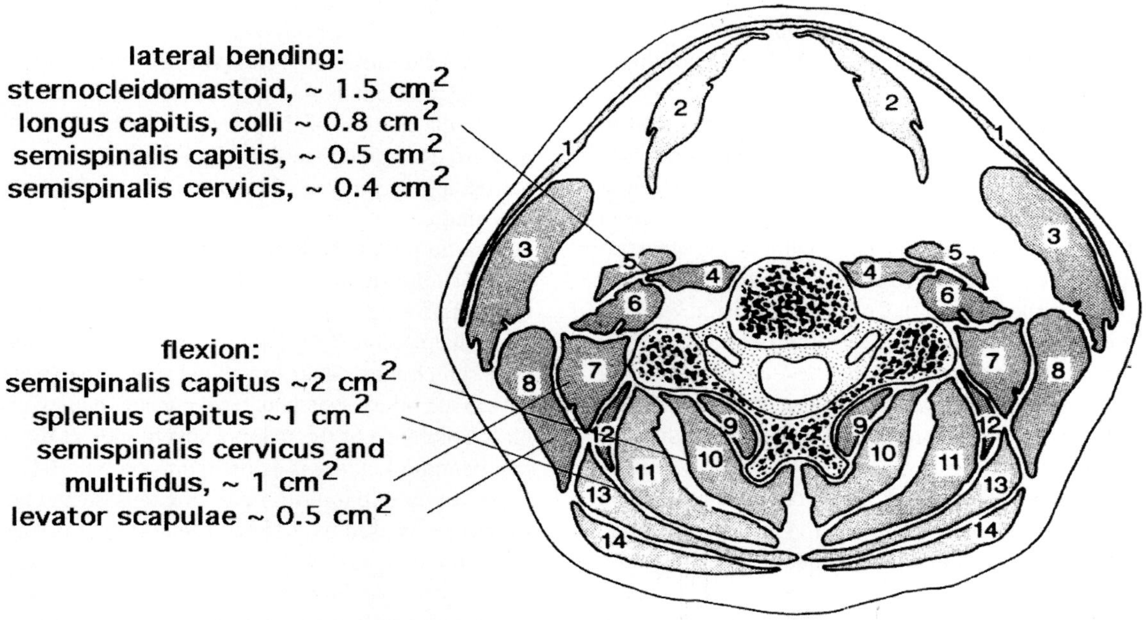
lateral bending:
sternocleidomastoid, ~ 1.5 cm2
longus capitis, colli ~ 0.8 cm2
semispinalis capitis, ~ 0.5 cm2
semispinalis cervicis, ~ 0.4 cm2
flexion:
semispinalis capitus ~2 cm2
splenius capitus ~1 cm2
semispinalis cervicus and
multifidus, ~ 1 cm2
levator scapulae ~ 0.5 cm2
1
2
3
4
5
6
7
8
9
10
11
12
13
14

FIG. 29. Cross section of the cervical spine and skull indicating major muscle groups and resulting activity of each based on active cross-sectional area as measured from magnetic resonance imaging. Groups of muscles with the greatest active cross-sectional area (in cm^2) are shown for flexion and lateral bending. (Adapted from Conley MS, Meyer RA, Bloomberg JJ, Feeback DL, Dudley GA. Noninvasive analysis of human neck muscle function. *Spine* 1995;20:2506–2512.)

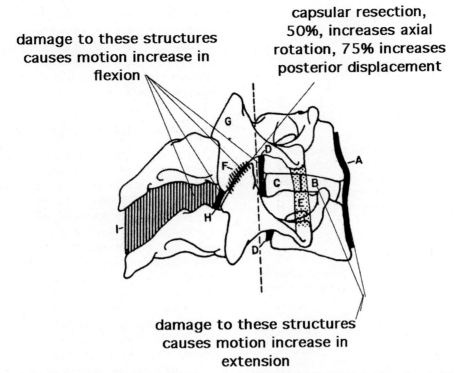

damage to these structures
cause motion increase in
flexion

capsular resection,
50%, increases axial
rotation, 75% increases
posterior displacement

damage to these structures
causes motion increase in
extension

FIG. 30. Contributions of various passive tissue components of the cervical spine to loading in different directions. (Adapted from Zdeblick TA, Abitbol JJ, Kunz DN, McCabe RP, Garfin S. Cervical stability after sequential capsule resection. *Spine* 1993;18:2005–2008; and Panjabi MM, White AA III, Johnson RM. Cervical spine mechanics as a function of transection of components. *J Biomech* 1975;8:327–336.)

in flexion (60). Injuries to the cervical spine may be grossly grouped as tension or compression based, in both cases coupled with bending. Direct tension, such as occurs in judicial hanging, creates cervical dislocation, typically at C2–3, with an approximate energy of 132 Nm required to create injury (61).

Differential motions between the head and torso tend to create significant neck tensile forces combined with bending, even without direct impact. This may occur in automobile crashes, for example, where the torso is restrained from moving by the seat and shoulder belts while high accelerations are applied to the head, causing combined bending and tension injuries to the neck (62). Combining tension with extension typically results in a combination of posterior element fracture, along with anterior disc and anterior longitudinal ligament damage. A common mechanism of tension/extension injury occurs during rear-end collisions in vehicles without head rests, where the torso motion is stopped by the seat back while the head continues to extend posteriorly over the top of the seat (Fig. 31) (63). This may even occur in vehicles with head rests due to a combination of a flexible seat that bends backward allowing the occupant to slide up the seat back during impact, a tall occupant, and/or a poorly adjusted (too low) or collapsing head rest. Kornhauser (64) estimated the approximate tolerance of the neck to extension as about 57 Nm in bending around the occipital condyles. Tension combined with flexion can result

again from rear-end impacts. It is accentuated by complex interactions among the torso, seat back, head, and head rest. For example, a flexible seat with a head rest controls the primary motion of the body, that is, backward into the seat during rear-end impact, but it returns the energy to the head and torso as it rebounds forward off the seat. If the shoulder belt arrests the motion of the torso, the head is still free to flex forward and rotate, resulting in a flexion moment applied to the occipital condyles. Estimated thresholds for flexion injury that cause pain are in the range of 61 Nm (for fiftieth percentile males) and that result in tissue injury, about 120 Nm (64). Injuries can include soft tissue damage, typically to the posterior ligaments combined with, at higher load levels, facet dislocation (65). Lateral bending combined with tension, which may occur in vehicle side impacts, can result in soft tissue injuries such as facet capsule damage and disc injury. Tolerance of the passive soft tissues of the neck to lateral bending loading is estimated as 54 Nm (64).

As opposed to injuries involving tension and bending, that is, injuries caused by differential motion of the head relative to the torso, a second type of injury occurs by direct impact to the head. A small difference in location of the impact load vector can result in significantly different injuries to the cervical spine (Fig. 31). When the head is flexed forward so that the cervical spine is not in its normal lordotic posture, the cervical spine tends to lock and not allow further flexion. Compression applied in this case likely will result in a burst

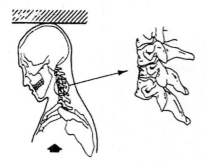

**compression-flexion
wedge fracture,
~ 7000 N**

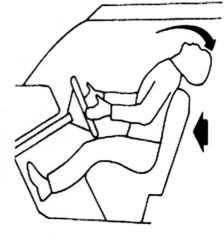

**hyperextension, 57 N-m
hyperflexion, 120 N-m
lateral flexion, 54 N-m**

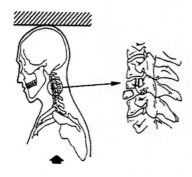

**compression
burst fracture,
~ 4800-6800 N**

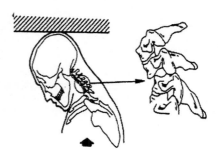

**compression flexion
anterior dislocation**

FIG. 31. Some common mechanisms of cervical spine injury with approximate tolerance levels. **Upper left:** Anterior wedge fracture due to blow on the vertex of the head just anterior to the anterior surface of the cervical spine. **Lower left:** Burst fracture due to impact on the vertex of the head with the load vector aligned with the cervical vertebral bodies. **Upper right:** Inertial injuries, due to difference in velocity and position between the head and torso, such as hyperextension of neck in a rear-end impact without a headrest, (hyperflexion and lateral flexion injury mechanisms not shown). **Lower right:** Anterior dislocation due to flexion combined with compression. (Reproduced with permission from States J. Soft tissue injuries of the neck. Transactions of the Society of Automotive Engineers, Paper 790135, 1979; and McElhaney JH, Myers BS. Biomechanical aspects of cervical trauma. In: Nahum AM, Melvin JW (eds). *Accidental Injury.* New York: Springer Verlag, 1993.)

injury, with vertical fracture lines in the vertebra and the possible retropulsion of bone into the canal (Fig. 32) (60). When the impact is located progressively more anteriorly, the resulting injury changes first to a wedge compression fracture, then to facet dislocation (66). Although these observations generally are true, the complexity of the spine makes the specific responses to load more difficult to predict. For example, Fig. 33 demonstrates the resultant motions of the spine under

axial loading, even when the motions of both ends of the cervical spine, that is, the skull and the cervicothoracic junction, are controlled. Extension, flexion, and buckling are all evident under compressive loading (67).

Although the experiment just discussed placed constraints to motion at the ends of the cervical spine, an excellent study by Nightingale et al. (68) recently showed how padding, designed to reduce trauma to the head in a fall, can affect cer-

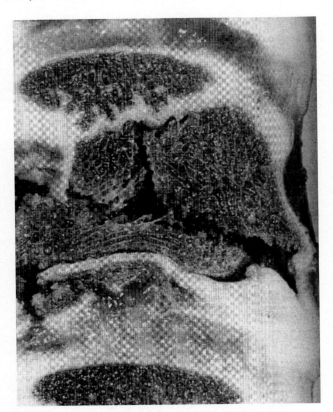

FIG. 32. Example of a cervical spine burst injury due to compression in a calf spine model. (Reproduced with permission from Shono Y, McAfee PC, Cunningham BW. The pathomechanics of compression injuries in the cervical spine. *Spine* 1993;18:2009–2019.)

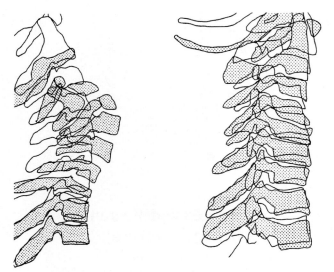

FIG. 33. Initial *(outline)* and final *(shaded)* position of the cervical spine to axial compressive impact loading. **Left:** This spine shows buckling into extension along with compression. **Right:** A second spine shows failure mainly in compression. (Reproduced with permission from Pintar FA, Yoganandan N, Sances A Jr, Reinart J, Harris G, Larson SJ. Kinematic and anatomical analysis of the human cervical spinal column under axial loading. Transactions of the Society of Automotive Engineers, Paper 892436, 1989.)

vical spine response to impact. In the case of direct impact to the head, for example, during a fall on the head, padding acts to pocket the head, resisting its ability to move out of the path of the descending torso. The result is that the descending torso loads the cervical spine. They showed, particularly for posterior impacts, that a significantly greater number of cervical spinal injuries resulted when head motion was restrained by padding. Whereas it is clear that padding reduces the magnitude of impact load on the head, additional consideration will have to be given to its role in cervical spine injuries.

An important aspect to cervical spinal injury is the effect of fracture on the spinal cord during and after impact, because injury to the cord clearly increases the severity of the injury. Recent studies using cervical spines containing a transducer placed into the spinal canal to measure cross-sectional dimension and height changes during the impact event showed that maximum transient canal occlusion in clinical burst fractures averaged 70.5% occlusion of the midsagittal diameter of the canal, whereas after injury the mean canal occlusion was only 9.4% (60). This observa-

tion, that the occlusion of the cord is on average 7.5 times greater during impact than that observed after injury may help explain why cord injury symptoms, observed in victims of neck injury, may not correspond to the observed postinjury canal intrusion. It was interesting to note that of a mean of 13.1-mm height loss of the cervical spine with impact, only about 5% was recovered after impact. This implies that canal occlusion must occur by other mechanisms in addition to vertebral bone retropulsion. A second mechanism of canal occlusion is shown in Fig. 34. Extension of the spine, along with height loss, causes anterior bulging of the ligamentum flavum. After burst fracture injury, flexion of the spine tends to decrease canal occlusion, whereas extension accentuates it considerably (69). This may have important implications for postinjury transport of patients with neck injuries. They usually are immobilized in an upward gaze position (Fig. 35), which tends to extend the cervical spine.

Residual Stability

"Clinical instability has been defined as the loss of the ability of the spine under physiologic loads to maintain its patterns of displacement so there is no initial or additional neurologic deficit, no major deformity, and no incapacitating pain" (70). Determination of the stability offered by remaining intact structures can offer insight into biomechanically effective

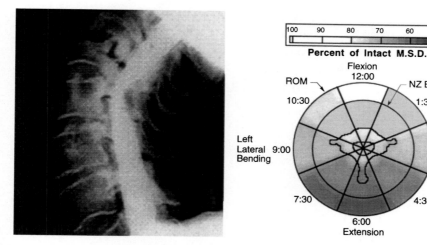

FIG. 34. Effect of extension on canal occlusion after cervical burst fracture. **Left:** Radiograph demonstrating occlusion of the canal in a burst fracture cervical spine having height loss, with extension due to ligamentum flavum bulge. **Right:** Effect of variation of cervical spine position on measured spinal canal occlusion. ROM = range of motion; MSD = midsagittal diameter. (Reproduced with permission from Ching RA, Watson NA, Carter JW, Tencer AF. The effect of post injury spinal position on canal occlusion in a cervical spine burst fracture model. *Spine* 1997;22:1710–1715.

methods of cervical spine fixation. For example, in the case of ligamentous injuries, Panjabi et al. (57) showed that loss of posterior ligaments does not significantly affect flexion or extension if the disc remains intact. However, loss of the anterior half of the disc, although not affecting flexion, does significantly increase extension motion compared to the intact spine under the same load. In injuries caused by combined compression and flexion loading, axial rotation, flexion, and extension were all affected (Fig. 36). Injuries involving compression and extension show the greatest effect on axial rotation, whereas pure compression had little effect on motion in any direction (71). It should be appreciated that any injury that involves vertebral fracture results obviously in less ability of the vertebra to carry load, but that a second effect is reduction in the tensions of the surrounding ligaments, even if they are not damaged, creating increased laxity of the motion segment.

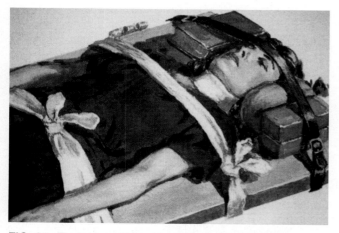

FIG. 35. Typical position of transport of the spinal injury patient, which places the spine in extension.

Fixation Biomechanics

External Orthoses

During transport of a cervical spine fracture patient to the hospital, protection against spinal cord injury is accomplished by immobilization of the cervical spine. Comparison of various methods for immobilization demonstrates that supporting the cervical spine with sandbags and taping significantly reduces motion and is by far superior to the use of any type of cervical orthosis (Figs. 35 and 37) (72). In addition, the motion-restricting abilities of six commonly used othoses for the management of cervical spine instability have been compared by Wolf and Johnson (73). In comparison to the normal cervical spine, the soft collar permitted all flexion and rotation, the halo allowed very little, and other external devices permitted between 13% and 66% of normal cervical spine motion (Fig. 38).

Halo Orthosis

Controversy exists over the ability of the halo apparatus to stabilize the cervical spine. Cervical spine motion with the halo in place has been reported to be as low as 1% to 4% of normal (73); however, other laboratory studies (74) and clinical observations (75,76) describe significant displacements occurring in the cervical spine stabilized with this device. This discrepancy may be explained by consideration of the factors affecting halo stability and by the specific movements of patients studied. The restriction of motion by the halo apparatus has been found to be least in the lower cervical spine and greatest in the upper cervical spine (74). Because the halo device is not rigidly attached to the thorax, and the thorax can change shape depending on activity, both the restriction of cervical motion and the distraction force

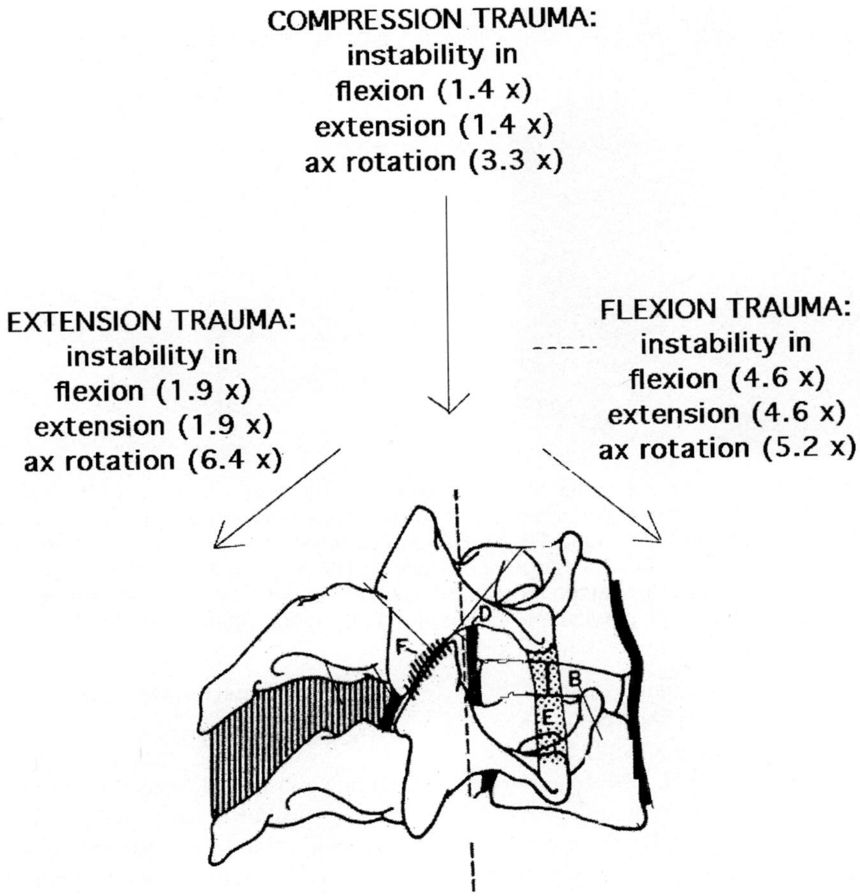

COMPRESSION TRAUMA:
instability in
flexion (1.4 x)
extension (1.4 x)
ax rotation (3.3 x)

EXTENSION TRAUMA:
instability in
flexion (1.9 x)
extension (1.9 x)
ax rotation (6.4 x)

FLEXION TRAUMA:
instability in
flexion (4.6 x)
extension (4.6 x)
ax rotation (5.2 x)

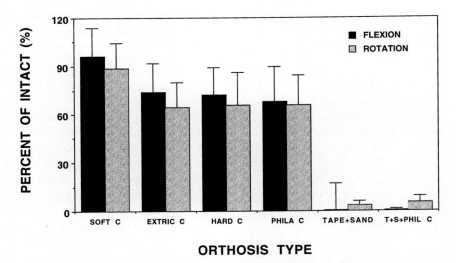

FIG. 36. Effects of injury on cervical spine stability demonstrating the effects of flexion, extension, and compression trauma in terms of increase in the neutral zone range of motion (neutral zone is the range where little force is required to cause movement). (Adapted from Panjabi MM, Duranceau JS, Oxland TR, Bowen CE. Multidirectional instabilities of traumatic cervical spine injuries in a porcine model. *Spine* 1989;14:1111–1115.)

FIG. 37. Comparison of the total cervical motion compared with the intact spine (100% = normal motion) without immobilization, and with various methods of restricting motion in four directions of motion. SOFT C, soft collar; EXTRIC C, extrication collar; HARD C, hard collar; PHILA C, Philadelphia collar; TAPE+SAND, tape and sandbags; T+S+PHIL C, tape and sandbags and Philadelphia collar. (Data adapted from Podolsky S, Baraff LJ, Simon RR, Hoffman JR, Larmon B, Ablon W. Efficacy of cervical spine immobilization methods. *J Trauma* 1983;23:461–464.)

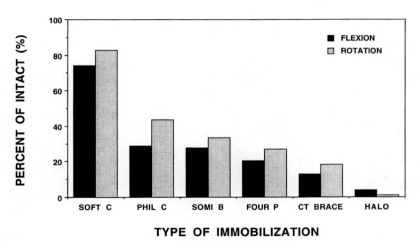

FIG. 38. Cervical spine motions in flexion and axial rotation allowed with any of six external cervical orthoses in comparison to normal spine motion: Soft collar (SC) of stockinette filled with foam; Philadelphia collar (PC) of Plastizote reinforced with anterior and posterior plastic struts; four-poster brace (FB) with mandibular and occipital supports connected to anterior and posterior thoracic plates; Guilford brace (GB) with mandibular and occipital supports rigidly connected to each other and to thoracic plates that are themselves connected; SOMI orthosis (SO) consists of a rigid anterior thoracic plate supported from the shoulders and connected by straps. This device has both mandibular and occipital supports and an optional headpiece; molded cervicothoracic orthosis (MO) with long anterior and posterior thoracic plates, and halo orthosis (HO) has a ring fastened to the skull by percutaneous pins. (Data adapted from Wolf JW Jr, Johnson RM. Cervical orthoses. In: *The Cervical Spine. The Cervical Spine Research Society.* Philadelphia: JB Lippincott, 1990:33–103.)

applied on the neck to help maintain axial alignment of the spine can change with different activities of the patient (74). Distraction forces on the spine due to the halo were noted to be greatest when the patients studied were supine and least when sitting, which was partly attributed to the weight of the head counteracting the distractive force along the spine when the patient was seated upright (77).

Several factors related to the halo and its interface with the thorax affect the stability that it contributes to the cervical spine. One is the vest–thorax interface, with spinal motion governed by (i) vest–thorax fit, (ii) vest–thorax interface friction, (iii) tightness of the vest straps, and (iv) changes in shape of the thorax (Fig. 39). Krag and Benynon (78) demonstrated the validity of increasing vest–thorax contact area in relatively rigid areas of the thorax such as the sternum anteriorly, the lateral aspects of the trunk, and the interscapular region posteriorly, while decreasing contact in mobile areas, such as the upper aspect of the shoulder girdle, the pectoralis major muscles, the upper part of the abdomen, and the posterior aspects of the scapula. Further, permitting adjustability of the trunk contact pads and maintaining rigid connections between them enhances fit and decreases vest flexibility, thereby reducing vest–trunk motion. Lengthening the vest has been demonstrated not to be effective in reducing cervical motion because extending it over the flexible abdomen does not provide increased contact surface (79).

Even with an effective vest–thorax interface, cervical spinal motion can occur due other factors related to the vest–thorax interface. Strap tightness, vest–thorax friction, and vest deformability all significantly affect cervical spinal stability (Fig. 40). Probably the most effective way to increase the stabilizing properties of the halo is selection of a stiffer vest. The halo superstructure is sufficiently stiff in most vests such that increasing its rigidity by tightening couplings beyond recommended settings or adding additional bars has no effect (80). With respect to the pin connection to

the skull, applying the same torque to the pin when passed through halo rings of different materials does not result in the same axial load being applied to the skull, because of distortion of the threads within the ring. Tightening the locking nut can further decrease the pin/skull axial force by up to 71% (Fig. 41) (81,82). Considering all the described variables, there are no consistent differences in the stabilizing abilities of commercially available vests, although, in specific directions, some vests allow significantly greater motion of the injured spine than do others (Fig. 42) (80).

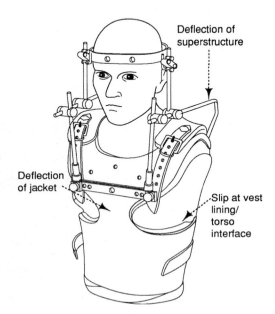

FIG. 39. Potential sources of motion in the halo apparatus that can cause cervical spine motion. (Adapted from Mirza S, Anderson PAA, Tencer AF. Biomechanical factors controlling intervertebral motion in cervical spine injuries fixed with a halo vest. *Spine* 1997.)

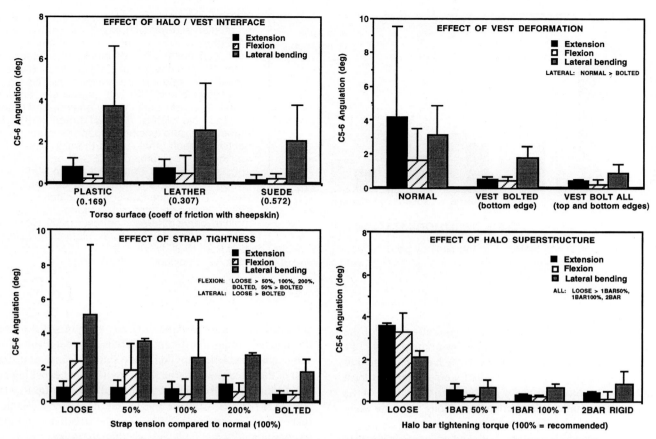

FIG. 40. Relative motion at the C3–4 level with complete transection, except for the anterior longitudinal ligament, after stabilization with the halo apparatus due to various effects. **Upper left:** Effects of different frictional interfaces between the vest and halo. SHP/plastic, sheepskin-plastic is less than the skin frictional coefficient; SHP/leather, sheepskin-leather equals the skin frictional coefficient; SHP/suede, sheepskin-suede is greater than the skin frictional coefficient. **Upper right:** Contribution of vest deformation. **Lower left:** Effect of vest side strap tightness with a sheepskin- leather interface. 100% = normal orthotist application tightness. **Lower right:** Effect of changing halo bar nut torque. (Reproduced with permission from Mirza S, Moquin RR, Anderson PA, Tencer AF, Steinmann J, Oamau D. Stabilizing properties of the halo apparatus. *Spine* 1997;22:727–733.

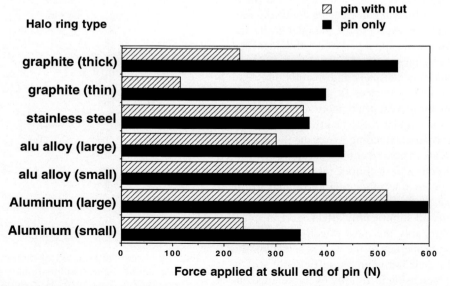

FIG. 41. Effect of halo ring type and the locking nut on the force transferred to the skull by the pin. (Adapted from Kerwin GA, Chou KL, White DB, Shen KL, Salciccioli GG, Yang KH. Investigation of how different halo influence pin forces. *Spine* 1994;19:1078–1081.)

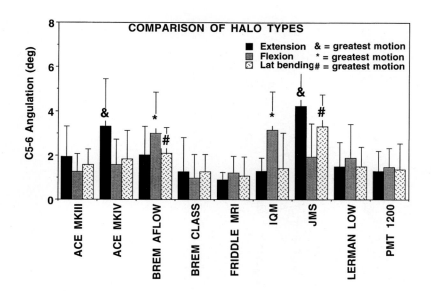

FIG. 42. Mean rank of eight halo vest designs in terms of vest–thorax motions for loads applied to the vest and the vest–halo ring structure in various directions. Depuy (Warsaw IN); JMS (Mt. Laural, NJ); Pope (Greenwood, SC); PMT (Minneapolis, MN); Ace (Jacksonville, FL); Camp (Jackson, MI); Bremer (Jacksonville, FL). (Reproduced with permission from Mirza S et al. Stabilizing properties of the halo apparatus. *Spine* 1997;22:84.)

Internal Fixation

As discussed in the section on residual stability, an appreciation of the loads that the injured motion segment can support can be useful in determining the type of fixation that can be used. For example, injury to the posterior elements without disc and facet damage may not, from a biomechanical viewpoint, require internal stabilization. Vertebral damage results in loss of stability in all load directions except for lateral bending. Appreciating the location of the center of rotation is important for improving the stability in fixation (Fig. 43) (83). The further from the center of rotation the fixator is located, the lower the forces on the implant and at the implant–bone interface and the greater the moments (bending loads) it will be capable of resisting.

A number of techniques have been used for fixation of cervical spine fractures and have been compared biomechanically for resistance to motion under load. When comparing test results it is important to note both the direction of loading and the type of injury being simulated. Pelker et

al. (84) compared the stabilizing potential of some common techniques including spinous process wiring (85), laminectomy with facet fusion (86), H grafting (87), H grafting with facetectomy (88), anterior plating (89), and posterior plating (90). Of the methods tested, they found that the most effective was an H graft wired to the vertebrae, with polymethyl methacrylate placed over the wires, graft, and spinous processes. In a more recent comparison using a model of single- or two-level, posterior column or three column injuries, Kotani et al. (91) concluded that anterior plating provided less stability than posterior constructs, and that posterior constructs could not provide torsional stability in multiple column injuries (Fig. 44). Overall, the most effective constructs were combined anterior and posterior fixations or transpedicular screws. With cervical corpectomy and placement of an anterior methacrylate graft, Richman et al. (92) similarly found that posterior lateral mass plating was significantly more stable than anterior plate fixation.

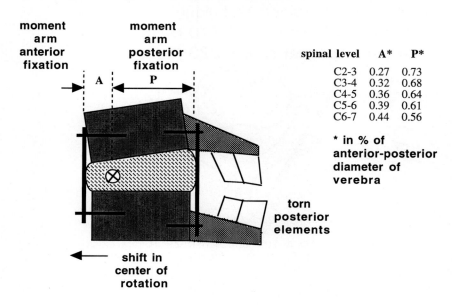

spinal level	A*	P*
C2-3	0.27	0.73
C3-4	0.32	0.68
C4-5	0.36	0.64
C5-6	0.39	0.61
C6-7	0.44	0.56

* in % of anterior-posterior diameter of verebra

FIG. 43. Lateral view of a cervical motion segment with flexion/extension center of rotation location. (Adapted from Amevo B, Aprill C, Bogduk N. Abnormal instantaneous axes of rotation in patients with neck pain. *Spine* 1992;17:748–756.) In this example, a posterior fixation device would be more effective in limiting flexion/extension motions than one placed anteriorly, because of its longer moment arm (distance of the points of fixation of the implant to the spine center of rotation).

Posterior wiring:
compression: 110% of intact
torsion: 120% of intact
flexion: 130% of intact
extension: 130% of intact

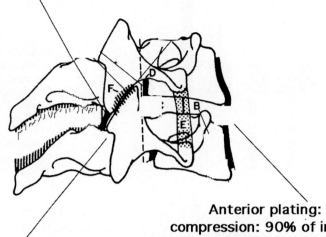

Anterior plating:
compression: 90% of intact
torsion: 82% of intact
flexion: 80% of intact
extension: 120% of intact

Posterior plating:
compression: 118% of intact
torsion: 112% of intact
flexion: 90% of intact
extension: 145% of intact

FIG. 44. Comparison of representative fixation techniques in stabilizing three column cervical spinal injuries compared to intact stiffness, expressed as a percentage of intact motion. (Adapted from Kotani Y, Cunningham BW, Abumi K, McAfee PC. Biomechanical analysis of cervical stabilization systems. An assessment of transpedicular screw fixation in the cervical spine. Spine 1994;19:2529–2539.)

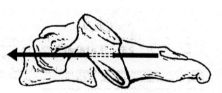

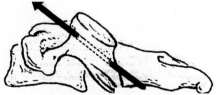

Roy-Camille technique
inferior screw, 382 N-cm
superior screw, 184 N-cm

Magerl technique
inferior screw, 310 N-cm
superior screw, 223 N-cm

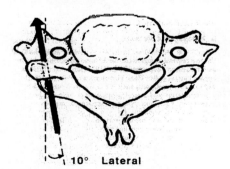

10° Lateral

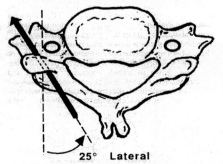

25° Lateral

FIG. 45. Comparison of flexion bending moments supported by two different techniques of lateral mass screw fixation. (Adapted from Choueka J, Spivak JM, Kummer FJ, Steger T. Flexion failure of posterior cervical lateral mass screws. *Spine* 1996; 21:462–468.)

TABLE 2. *Reported ranges in observed motion (in degrees) of individual lumbar segments*

Direction	L1–2	L2–3	L3–4	L4–5	L5–S1
Flexion extension	5.6–13.0	7.6–15.8	8.6–15.9	12.2–19.0	8.2–18.7
Lateral bending	4.9–10.0	7.0–12.4	5.7–12.4	5.7–9.5	2.3–5.5
Axial rotation	0.6–4.5	1.2–4.6	0.9–4.0	0.8–4.7	0.6–2.1

Reproduced with permission from Dvorak J, Panjabi MM, Novotny JE, Chang DG, Grob D. Clinical validation of functional flexion-extension roentgenograms of the lumbar spine. *Spine* 1991; 16:943–950; and White AA III, Panjabi MM. *Clinical Biomechanics of the Spine*, 2nd edition. Philadelphia: JB Lippincott, 1990.

With regard to individual fixation methods, for example, anterior plating in simulated cervical spine flexion compression injuries, the Synthes CSLP plate produced higher flexion and torsional stiffnesses than the Caspar plate with unicortical fixation and the same plate with bicortical fixation (93). A comparison of lateral mass screw fixation showed that the Magerl technique of screw placement provides greater strength in flexion loading as well as not violating unfused facet joints inferiorly (Fig. 45) (94). Considering the use of threaded cylinders placed into the disc space to promote fusion, Brantley et al. (95) found that, in cervical fusion, single and double cylinders were similar in their ability to reduce motion segment range of motion to a tricortical bone graft, and that the overall decrease in motion was about 50% that of the intact spinal segment. It should be emphasized that this construct can replace the tricortical bone graft but is not effective alone in stabilizing severely injured motion segments because it gains purchase mainly through tensioning of the soft tissues of the spine.

LUMBAR AND LUMBOSACRAL SPINE

Normal Motion and Function of Components

Lumbar spine flexion/extension range of motion *in vivo* averages about 11.9 degrees at L1–2, increasing to 17 degrees at L5–S1 (Table 2), and in lateral bending, ranges from 7.9 degrees at T12–L1 to 12.4 degrees at L3–4, and decreases again to 5.1 degrees at L5–S1 (96). At least 55% of a sample population may have at least one hypomobile motion segment, with only 9% having a hypermobile segment in flexion/extension (97). In addition, men as a group have a somewhat greater flexion/extension range in the lumbar spine compared to women (58.4 degrees vs. 53.4 degrees) and range of motion decreases with age (98). Intersegmental lumbar axial rotation is quite small, averaging only about 2 degrees per motion segment (99).

Muscles are the primary stabilizers of the lumbar spine. The major muscles demonstrate patterns of co-contraction, for example, between the erector spinae and latissimus dorsi in flexion, and the right and left external obliques along with the right and left latissimus dorsi in lateral bending (100). The net result of muscles with short moment arms (101) (distance of muscle line of action to the center of rotation of the spine) is a high compressive force acting on the spine

(Fig. 46), reaching nearly 2,500 N (about 3.5 times body weight) when holding a weight with outstretched arms (102). In addition, it should be appreciated that this compressive force can result in high shear forces, especially in the lower lumbar motion segments that are oriented at an oblique angle to the line of action of the compressive force (Fig. 47) (103).

Progressive transection of spinal soft tissues in cadaveric motion segments provides insights into their functions. With flexion, each posterior structure contributes a small amount to resisting the applied load, but once only the posterior lon-

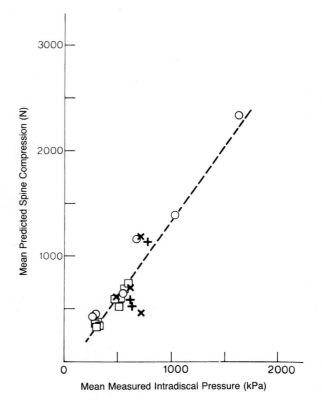

FIG. 46. Predicted compressive force on the third lumbar vertebra for different tasks and its relation to measured intradiscal pressure. (Reproduced with permission from Schultz A, Andersson G, Ortengren R, Haderspeck K, Nachemson A. Loads on the lumbar spine. Validation of a biomechanical analysis by measurements of intradiscal pressures and myoelectric signals. *J Bone Joint Surg* 1982; 64A:713–720.)

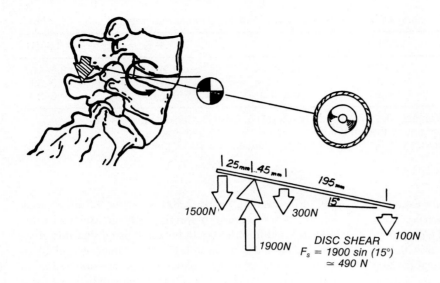

FIG. 47. In the case where a body weight of 300 N acts 45 mm from the fulcrum (center of flexion/extension of the vertebra) and an external weight of 100 N acts 240 mm anteriorly, the erector spinae muscles must generate a counteracting force of 1,500 N to balance the flexion moment produced by the anterior loads. The 1,900-N load acting on the vertebral body, inclined at 15 degrees, results in a 490-N shear force (Fs) at the disc. (Reproduced with permission from Smith TJ, Fernie GR. Functional biomechanics of the spine. *Spine* 1991;16:1197–1203.)

gitudinal, the disc, and the anterior longitudinal remain, angulation increases significantly. In extension, loss of the anterior longitudinal and the anterior part of the disc is sufficient to significantly increase extension (104). This demonstrates the roles of various lumbar spinal structures (Fig. 48).

Mechanism of Injury

In contrast to the cervical spine, the lumbar spine is a stable column; therefore, its motions under load and the resulting injuries are more predictable. As shown by Holdsworth (105) (Fig. 49) and defined by Ferguson and Allen (106), combinations of forces cause typical injuries, such as compression and flexion loading causing anterior wedge fractures, and torsion resulting in disc and facet damage. A classic mechanism of lumbar injury occurs with occupants of vehicles in frontal collisions wearing seat belts without shoulder restraints. This restrains the lower part of the body

while allowing the upper part to pivot forward, resulting in a Chance fracture (all three columns fail in tension with hyperflexion) or a flexion distraction injury (posterior elements fail in tension while anterior and middle elements fail in compression) (Fig. 50) (107).

Another common injury is the burst fracture of the spine. Roaf (108) postulated that bursting may be the result of the fluid component in the vertebra, which is composed of fat and marrow (109). Kazarian and Graves (110) demonstrated that the fluid component (fat and marrow) caused stiffening of vertebrae subjected to rapid compressive loading as opposed to slow loading. This mechanism was well demonstrated by Tran et al. (10), who subjected spinal specimens to the same energy of fracture (same average force and vertebral height loss) but at distinctly different rates of loading. The rapidly loaded specimens had a mean canal occlusion of about 48% compared with the slowly loaded specimens at 7%. The proposed mechanism of the burst fracture is shown in Fig. 51. During loading, the nucleus is pressurized, acting

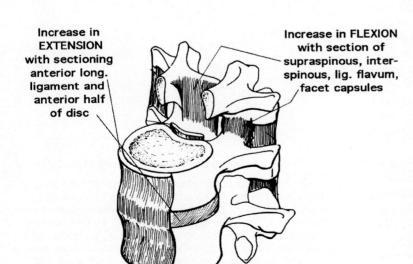

FIG. 48. Schematic diagram showing the functions of various structures of the lumbar spine in resisting flexion and extension. (Adapted from White AA III, Panjabi MM. *Clinical Biomechanics of the Spine,* 2nd edition. Philadelphia: JB Lippincott, 1990; and Posner I, White AA III, Edwards WT, Hayes WC. A biomechanical analysis of the clinical stability of the lumbar and lumbosacral spine. *Spine* 1982;7:374–388.)

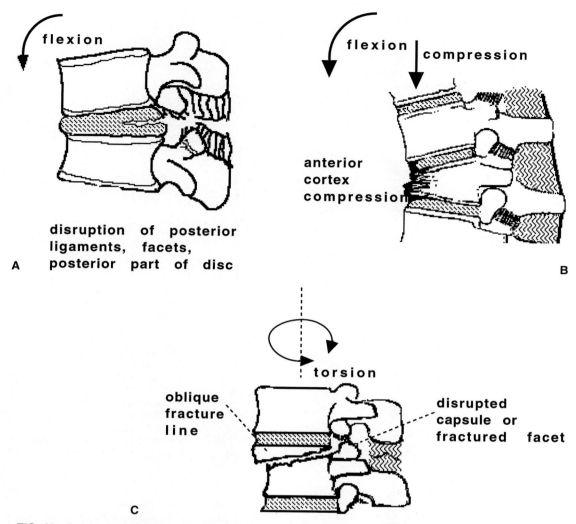

FIG. 49. A: Injury caused by a flexion moment results in progressive tearing of posterior ligaments, possible fracture of the pedicle or lamina or tearing of the facet capsules, and damage to the posterior part of the disc. **B:** Failure of the spine due to the application of a compressive load in the anterior part of the vertebra causes crushing of the anterior cortex, as well as a flexion moment that can disrupt the posterior elements. **C:** Failure of the vertebral column due to a torsional load, with characteristic fracture of a facet, and a spiral to oblique fracture line in the vertebra due to tensile failure as would occur in a long bone. (Adapted from Holdsworth F. Fractures, dislocations, and fracture-dislocations of the spine. *J Bone Joint Surg* 1970;52A:1534–1551.)

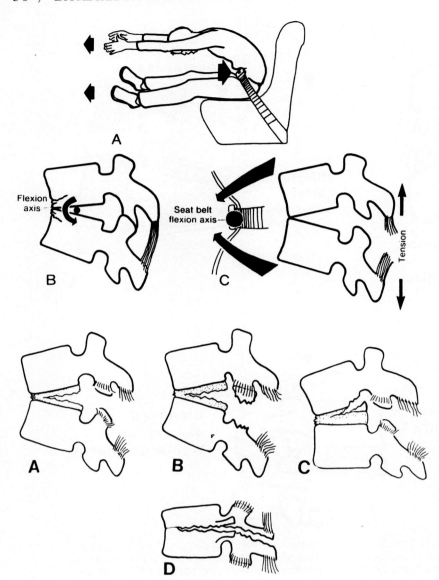

FIG. 50. Top, A–C: Mechanism for the creation of a flexion-distraction injury to the lumbar spine due to the restraining effect of a seat belt without shoulder belt. **Bottom:** Various types of injuries resulting from flexion-distraction, including tearing of posterior elements, facet capsules, and the disc **(A)**, tearing of posterior ligaments and disc and fracture of the facets **(B)**, disruption of posterior elements and fracture of the posterior wall of the vertebra **(C)**, and Chance fracture through the spinous process and vertebral body **(D)**. (Reproduced with permission from Evans DC. Biomechanics of spinal injury. In: Gonza ER, Harrington IJ (eds). *Biomechanics of Musculoskeletal Injury.* Baltimore: Williams & Wilkins, 1982:31–86.)

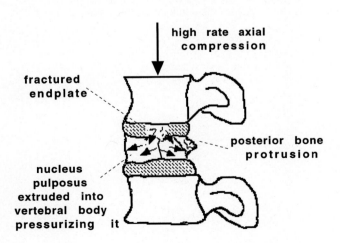

FIG. 51. Schematic diagram of the characteristics of the compressive burst fracture of the lumbar spine, characterized by vertical cracking of the vertebra and retropulsion of bone into the spinal canal. A possible mechanism is displacement of the nucleus pulposus through the fractured endplate into the vertebral bone, which along with deformation of the vertebra, pressurizes the fat and marrow contents. This internal pressurization may result in explosion of the vertebra and posterior retropulsion of bone into the spinal canal.

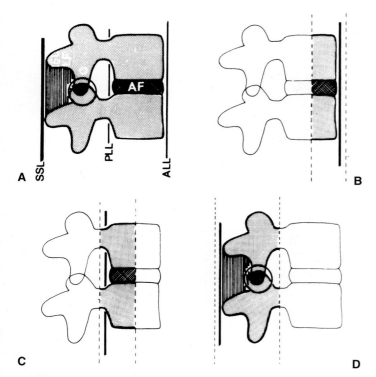

FIG. 52. Concept of the three columns of the spine. **A:** Intact spine motion segment. **B:** Anterior column consists of the anterior half of the disc and the anterior longitudinal ligament (ALL). **C:** Middle column consists of the posterior half of the disc and the posterior longitudinal ligament (PLL). **D:** Posterior column consists of the facet joints and the posterior ligaments (SSL). (Reproduced with permission from Denis F. The three column spine and its significance in the classification of acute thoracolumbar injuries. *Spine* 1983;8:817–831.)

on the endplates, which are known to bulge. This inward bulging followed by penetration of the nucleus through the endplate causes the fat and marrow within the vertebra to displace. At a slow crush rate, the trapped marrow can exit the vertebral body. At a high rate, the fluid cannot escape rapidly enough through pores or fissures (109), the pressure within the vertebra increases, and the body explodes. This mechanism explains the vertical fracture lines seen in the vertebra compared with the crushed appearance one might expect due to direct compressive failure.

Residual Stability

Denis (111) introduced the concept of the three "columns" of the spine to assist in visualizing the mechanical effects of injury. As shown in Fig. 52, the anterior column consists of the anterior part of the disc and anterior longitudinal ligament, the middle column is comprised of the posterior part of the disc and the PLL, and the posterior column, the facets and posterior ligaments. Although the original theory was based on clinical observations, Panjabi et al. (112) demonstrated

that the theory is biomechanically valid and that the middle column is the primary determinant of mechanical stability of the lumbar motion segment.

Haher et al. (113) demonstrated how injury to the different columns affects the center of rotation of the injured spine in flexion/extension. As with the cervical spine, appreciation of the location of the center of rotation for various motions can help in selection of the location of the fixation which is likely to produce the greatest stability or alternatively, the lowest forces in the implant, particularly at the bone/implant interface. As shown in Figure 53, in the intact spine, the instant center of rotation in flexion is located in the anterior part of the disc, and posterior muscle forces balance the weight of the trunk which acts through its center of gravity, located anterior to the spine. With loss of the anterior column (anterior longitudinal ligament and anterior half of the disc), the center of rotation moves posteriorly, to the region of the facets, increasing the moment arm of the trunk weight and decreasing that of the posterior muscles. This implies that the compressive force on the spine will increase in this situation. When both anterior and middle columns are compromised, the center of rotation moves posterior to the spinal musculature, and there is no effective way for muscle forces to counteract the trunk moment. Destruction of the posterior column, with the anterior and middle columns intact, shifts the center of flexion/extension to the anterior border of the vertebra, Figure 53.

Haher, et al. (114) also demonstrated the effect of injury on the location of the axis of axial rotation of the lumbar motion segment, due to torsional loading. Both the facet joints and the disc affect the position of the axis of axial rotation, Figure 54. Loss of the facets moves the axis to the midpart of the disc. Conversely, injury to the disc and facets shifts the axis posterior to the facets, to a point which is approximately at the location of the intersection of the perpendiculars from the surfaces of the facet joints. If the axis of rotation changes, the effective moment arms of muscles, soft tissue stabilizers, and any applied instrumentation are altered as well. Of most importance is maximizing the moment arms of the forces applied by spinal instrumentation in order to lower the forces they must exert to maintain stability of the injured spine. Lower force in the instrumentation results in lower stresses on implant components and at the bone-implant interface.

Since the spine is subjected to loads in three dimensions, it is imperative to define the three dimensional instability of the spine. Ching, et al. (115) liken the mechanical stability of the spine conceptually to a ball in a flat bottom dish. As shown in Figure 55, the ball may move freely within a neutral equilibrium zone, which is equivalent to the normal mobility of the spinal intervertebral joint. If displaced excessively in any direction, the ball rises up the side of the dish, and when the load is released, returns to the neutral zone. This simulates the restraining effects of the disc and ligaments at the ends of the range of motion. If an injury occurs, a part of the dish is broken, increasing the range of the neutral zone. Although the spine may still be able to support external load, its range of mobility is abnormally large, result-

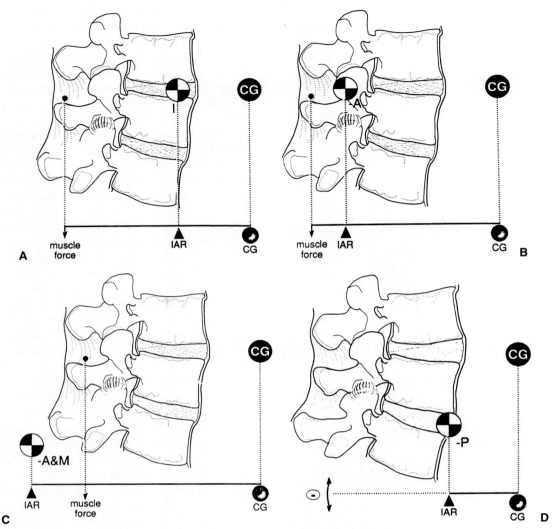

FIG. 53. Sagittal plane view of a lumbar motion segment showing the location of the flexion/extension axis of rotation (IAR) in various conditions. **A:** Intact (I) spine and the balance between muscle forces and body weight acting through the center of gravity (CG) of the upper body. **B:** After loss of the anterior column (−A). **C:** After loss of the anterior and middle columns (−A&M). The center of rotation is shifted posterior to the line of action of the posterior musculature, therefore there is no counteracting moment to that produced by the weight of the trunk. **D:** After loss of the posterior column (−P). (Reproduced with permission from Haher TR, Bergman M, O'Brien M, et al. The effect of the three columns of the spine on the instantaneous axis of rotation in flexion and extension. *Spine* 1991;16:S312–S318.)

ing in clinical problems such as excessive kyphosis or occlusion of the spinal canal. A spinal implant therefore restores (or even reduces) the neutral zone range of motion.

Typical neutral zone plots are shown for three common types of thoracolumbar injuries in Figure 56. The plot shows the boundaries of the flexion/extension and lateral bending ranges plotted as a two dimensional map for comparative purposes. It was constructed by applying a load to an injured motion segment, in a cadaver experiment, then releasing it and recording the final position of the vertebra. As Figure 56 shows, a compressive (non bursting) injury with ligaments intact results in no difference in the neutral zone compared

with the intact spine, except in torsional loading. With a burst fracture, the flexion and lateral ranges are increased, while a flexion distraction injury results in a large increase in the flexion range only. It is interesting to note that although the neutral zone is enlarged in fracture, the intact and injured spine have similar flexion load-displacement behavior once the vertebra moves to a position where it can support load (116). This is due to the ability of the remaining uninjured structures to support the applied loads.

Certainly fractures with comminuted vertebral bodies and fractured endplates can be considered highly unstable (117). However, even in less severe injuries, it has been observed

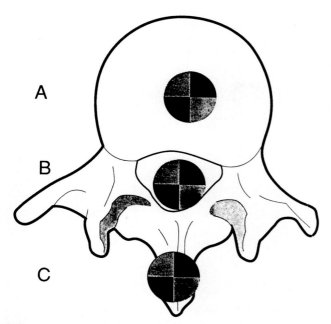

FIG. 54. Coronal plane view of a lumbar vertebra showing the locations of the axes of axial rotation of the spine, due to axial torsion. **A:** Facet joints injured. **B:** Intact spine. **C:** Facet joints and annulus injured. (Reproduced with permission from Haher TR, Bergman M, O'Brien M, et al. Instantaneous axis of rotation as a function of the three columns of the spine. *Spine* 1992;17:S149–S154.)

the flexion distraction injury to the lumbar spine, Neumann, et al. (118) proposed that instability be defined by lumbar kyphosis greater than 12 degrees, or a relative increase in interspinous process distance greater than 20 mm.

Fixation Biomechanics

Effect of Spinal Fixation

The function of a spinal implant is to restore lost mechanical stability to the spine and to minimize motion sufficiently to allow healing across the affected area. The implant usually is considered a temporary device in that once bone healing occurs it would have a lesser role in load transmission, the greater role being assumed by the healed bone. Several studies clearly demonstrate the necessity of stabilization by spinal fixation. For example, Gurr et al. (119) showed, in a model of posterior and anterior column disruption, that spinal segments were considerably more rigid in torsion with bone graft and posterior instrumentation than with either bone graft alone, or with no bone graft or implant. These conclusions were confirmed by Johnson et al. (120). Issues relate to the relative stiffness of the implant, which if too flexible may inhibit healing and if too stiff may induce stress shielding. Nagel et al. (121) found, in a sheep model of lumbar and lumbosacral nonunion, that 10% strain (interlaminar motion on x-ray film) defined a level below which a high certainty of fusion resulted. Evidence of device-related osteoporosis has been found in spines with rigid fixation; however, the overall properties of the fused segment are not at increased risk of fracture because of the greater cross-sectional area of the vertebra and incorporated fusion mass (122). With more rigid fixation, such as the use of transpedicular screws, the implant may continue to have a load-bearing role

that the decrease in height of the vertebral body is a potential indicator of residual stability of the injured spine, because a greater decrease from normal height implies greater laxity of the remaining intact ligaments. Although the specific relationship between height loss and increase in vertebral laxity has not been established for axial compression fractures, for

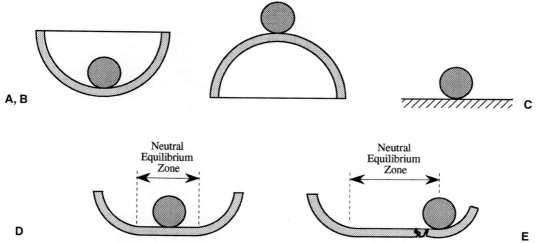

FIG. 55. Conceptual model of stability with reference to the injured spine. Concepts of stability. **A:** Stable equilibrium. **B:** Unstable equilibrium. **C:** Neutral equilibrium. **D:** The intact spinal motion segment, like a ball within a dish, allows a normal range of mobility but if this is exceeded, the soft tissue stabilizers return the vertebra to its neutral zone position. **E:** In the case of a fracture, the neutral zone is enlarged because the soft tissue stabilizers have been injured. (Reproduced with permission from Ching RP, Tencer AF, Anderson PA, Daly CH. A comparison of residual stability in thoracolumbar spine fractures using neutral zone measurements. *J Orthop Res* 1995;13:533–541.)

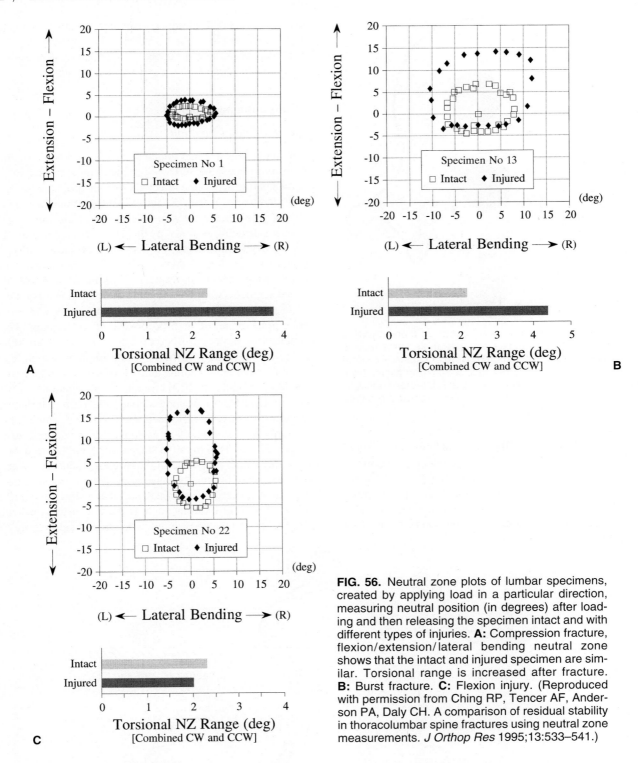

FIG. 56. Neutral zone plots of lumbar specimens, created by applying load in a particular direction, measuring neutral position (in degrees) after loading and then releasing the specimen intact and with different types of injuries. **A:** Compression fracture, flexion/extension/lateral bending neutral zone shows that the intact and injured specimen are similar. Torsional range is increased after fracture. **B:** Burst fracture. **C:** Flexion injury. (Reproduced with permission from Ching RP, Tencer AF, Anderson PA, Daly CH. A comparison of residual stability in thoracolumbar spine fractures using neutral zone measurements. *J Orthop Res* 1995;13:533–541.)

even after solid fusion is achieved. Kotani et al. (122) estimated, in their model of lumbar fusion using transpedicular screws, that the fixator supported about 27% of the total load, with reduction in volumetric density of surrounding bone. On the other hand, excessively rigid devices can have deleterious effects on posterolateral fusion. Craven et al. (123) showed that when pedicular screws were linked by 4.76-mm rods (in dog spines), stiffer fusions were achieved

than when 6.35-mm rods were used. They estimated that the 6.35-mm rods used in humans were similar in load-sharing ability and stiffness to the 4.76-mm rods used in their model.

Apart from the effect of the fixation on the strength of the fusion, concern has been expressed about how a fused segment affects the free segments around it. Quinnell and Stockdale (124) found that when a segment of the lumbar spine was fused, the motion was taken up by adjacent motion segments, most likely the segment just below the fused one. This may induce hypermobility or further degeneration of adjacent discs and should be a consideration because it may cause an asymptomatic disc to become symptomatic at a later date. Further, loss of lordosis with posterior instrumentation has significant effects. The residual hypolordosis of the operated region results in a compensatory hyperlordosis in proximal motion segments. Load across the fixation increases, putting it at greater risk for loosening during extension loading, and loading increases in the posterior column of the motion segment above the instrumentation, placing the facet joints at risk (125).

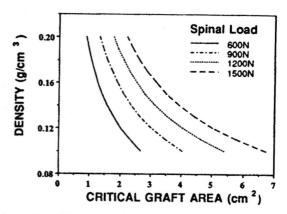

FIG. 57. Relationship of support area of trabecular bone under the graft and bone graft load capacity. (Reproduced with permission from Closkey RF, Lee CK, Parsons JR, Blaksin MF. Mechanics of interbody spinal fusion: analysis of critical bone graft area. Transactions of the 39th Annual Meeting of the Orthopedic Research Society, 1993:65.)

Properties of Iliac Grafts and Threaded Fusion Cages

The iliac corticol graft is an important component of the reconstruction procedure in spine trauma because it helps to reestablish at least the compressive load-carrying capacity of the anterior and middle columns of the injured vertebra and works in conjunction with the implant to resist forward flexion. Wolfinbarger et al. (126) tested a variety of prepared iliac grafts in compression. The results indicated that freeze-dried but nonrehydrated graft wedges have the lowest compressive strength compared to frozen and thawed grafts, or rehydrated grafts, and that, if used, they should be rehydrated *in vacuo* for at least 1 hour before being used. All grafts, however, supported very high compressive loads, averaging 5,438 N (greater than seven times body weight). Another important point related to graft use should be appreciated. The trabecular bone bed under the graft is as likely, or possibly more likely, to fail under load bearing than the graft itself, which is cortical bone, compared to the trabecular bone bed it lies on. The area required to support the graft within the range of physiologic loads must be larger as bone density decreases. As shown in Fig. 57, to support a load of two times body weight (definitely within the physiologic range in walking) requires a trabecular bone support area of 3 cm^2 under the graft for bone of 0.20 g/cm^2 density, and about 7 cm^2 if the bone density decreases to about 10 g/cm^2 (127).

In addition to the loads applied to the graft physiologically, precompressing the graft is important to assure that it does not displace and to encourage fusion. Krodel (128) pointed out the importance of slight kyphotic positioning of the fixation to enhance compression of the graft as opposed to lordotic positioning, which tends to unload the graft.

Threaded fusion cages are being used as substitutes for bone graft. Their performance has been investigated, although not in biomechanical models involving trauma. To provide stability, the threaded insert relies on intact tissues between the vertebrae to be fused, because the superior and inferior parts of the thread that the cage engages are in different bones (the two vertebrae). Greater distraction of tissues with placement of the threaded fusion cage will result in a reduced neutral zone (motion of the vertebrae with very little load applied) and greater stiffness. These devices, when placed into vertebrae with intact discs (except for the threaded insert drill hole) and ligaments, significantly reduce neutral zone motion and increase stiffness. As with bone grafts, the limitation on compressive load bearing is due to the trabecular bed that the fusion cage rests on, with a typical load-bearing capacity of close to 3,000 N. Also, the insertion site (lateral, posterolateral, or posterior) has no effect on stabilization, except in torsion where posterior placement damaged facets or lamina, thus increasing motion (129).

Mechanics of Indirect Reduction of Bone in the Canal

Biomechanical consideration should be given to the mechanism by which bone in the canal can be indirectly reduced during surgical placement of spinal implants. There are several mechanisms of posterior vertebral bone fragment reduction, because the fragments typically are hinged at the junction of the superior endplate and disc. The PLL, if intact, certainly acts to displace bone fragments anteriorly (out of the canal) if it is tensioned. Because it is important to restore vertebral body height along with lordosis (in the lumbar spine), the most effective way to use the PLL for indirect bone fragment reduction is to distract first (130), then place the vertebra in lordosis or kyphosis maintaining distraction, because lordosis will inherently slacken the PLL (Fig. 58) (131). However, even when the PLL is damaged, reduction can occur simply by restoring a space for the bone fragments to displace into, especially if the fragments are still connected to the superior disc or endplate (132). As Zou et al. (133) pointed out, it is important that the function of the instrumentation be considered when restoring vertebral height and lordosis and reducing the bone in the canal. They indicated that instrumentation that can provide independent control of lordosis and distraction best restores anatomic alignment and canal decompression. Techniques for accomplishing distraction and

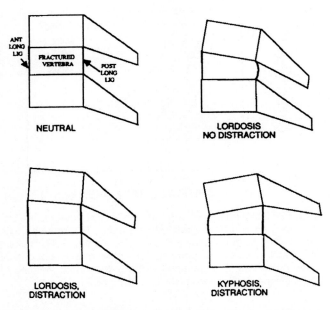

FIG. 58. Schematic demonstration of the tensions in the anterior and posterior longitudinal ligaments in an anterior and middle column injured lumbar motion segment due to positioning the vertebrae in different sequences with posterior instrumentation. (Reproduced with permission from Harrington RM, Budorick T, Hoyt J, Anderson PA, Tencer AF. Biomechanics of indirect reduction of bone retropulsed into the spinal canal in vertebral fracture. *Spine* 1993;18:692–699.)

lordosis with different instrumentation systems are shown in Fig. 59.

Bone–Implant Interface

The ability of an implant to transfer load depends on the strength of the bone–implant interface. With posterior instrumentation, the lamina, transverse process, or, in the case of pedicle screw attachment, the vertebral body bone, are the sites at which load is transferred. Pullout or direct posterior loading is considered to be a primary mechanism by which failure can occur in some instrumentation systems. This is due to the flexion moment acting on the spine (Fig. 60). In general, pullout strength increases in more distal spinal vertebrae and is greater for hooks compared to wires because they can spread the load (135). The lamina is the strongest purchase site in the posterior thoracolumbar spine and, significantly, is less affected by osteoporotic bone loss than the trabecular bone within the pedicle and vertebral body, the site of pedicle screw attachment (136). The hook–lamina interface is a connection that transfers load only in compression between the bone and hook material (Fig. 61). This provides resistance to posterior pull and axial compression or distraction forces. Pivoting occurs between the hook and lamina, so flexion rotation of the verte-

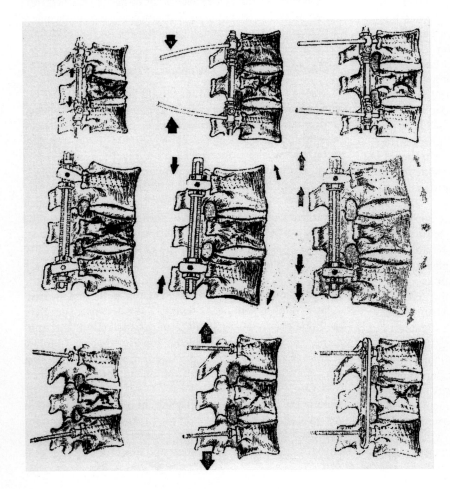

FIG. 59. Comparison of three techniques (left to right) for gaining distraction and lordosis along with indirect reduction of bone in the canal for different instrumentation systems. **Top:** AO fixateur interne uses posterior distraction and application of an extension moment to regain lordosis. **Middle:** Restoration of lordosis followed by distraction. **Bottom:** Steffee plate and manual positioning of vertebra followed by locking into position. (Reproduced with permission from Zou D, Yoo JU, Edwards WT, et al. Mechanics of anatomic reduction of thoracolumbar burst fractures. Comparison of distraction versus distraction plus lordosis in the anatomic reduction of the thoracolumbar burst fracture. *Spine* 1993; 18:195–203.)

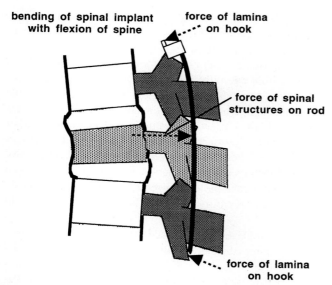

FIG. 60. Schematic diagram showing the flexion moment acting on the spine and the resulting three-point bending on a posterior fixation implant. Pullout forces result at hook fixation attachment sites.

bra is not directly controlled by the hook. However, interaction of the rod with the lamina does block flexion rotation (Fig. 62). Sublaminar wiring is not effective in transmitting axial load to the rods, and slippage of wire on the rod can result during lateral bending, flexion, and compression loading. Improvement in interface mechanics can be accomplished by combining implants, an example being the use of

offset laminar hooks with pedicle screws. Laminar hooks reduce bending moments applied to screws and resulting angular displacement (in testing from a mean of 8.1 to 1.9 degrees), and improve pullout strength, especially with screws having partially stripped holes, where pullout strength increased from a mean of 93 N without a supplemental hook to 290 N with a hook (137).

The pedicle screw presents an alternative to fixation by hooks or wires. This type of implant permits the transmission of moments in all directions, except about the axis of the screw, along with the ability to resist loads transverse to and along the axis of the screw. The pullout strength of pedicle screws, as with other bone screws, depends on several parameters (9). A most important controllable parameter is the diameter of the screw, because the bending stiffness (138), cyclic fatigue strength (139) (Fig. 63), and pullout strength (140,141) increase significantly with increasing diameter. A number of studies have documented the minimum sagittal and transverse widths of the pedicles to permit appropriate sizing of screws. Figure 64 shows a comparison of the results of several investigations. In general, the minimum pedicle diameter ranges from about 5 to 7 mm in the thoracic spine, but increases rapidly toward the distal end of the lumbar spine to between 15 and 18 mm at L-5 (141–144).

A second important parameter in determining the pullout strength of pedicle screws is the shear strength of the material into which they are embedded, that is, the shear strength of cancellous bone (139). Pedicle screw purchase in the spine has been correlated to shear strength, which is related to bone mineral density (Fig. 65B) (145–147) and the torque

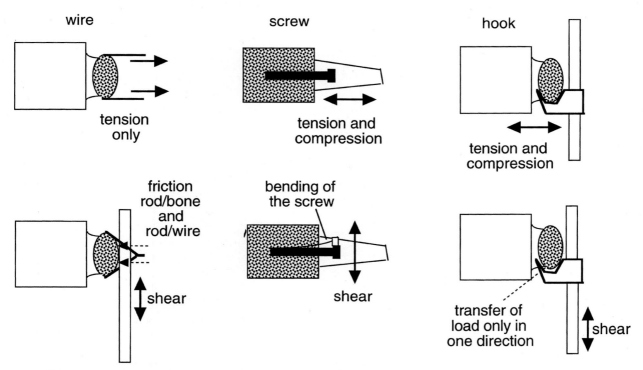

FIG. 61. A Methods of transferring load between two surfaces with wire, a screw, or a hook. **Top:** Tension and compression. **Bottom:** Shear parallel to the long axis of the spine.

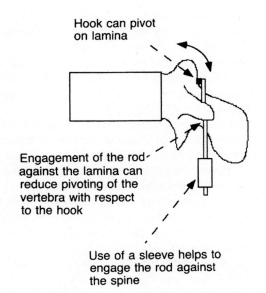

Hook can pivot on lamina

Engagement of the rod against the lamina can reduce pivoting of the vertebra with respect to the hook

Use of a sleeve helps to engage the rod against the spine

FIG. 62. Using a hook to couple the instrumentation to bone allows rotation at the hook–lamina interface, reducing control of flexion/extension motion. If the rod engages the posterior laminar wall of the vertebra or if a sleeve is used, rotation can be reduced.

applied during screw insertion (148). As well, bone density varies within the vertebra itself, being greatest near the endplates and cortical shell and least in the midplane. Wu et al. (149) showed that pedicle screws placed close to the endplates provide the greatest overall stability.

The contributions of some other factors to the mechanical performance of the pedicle screw have been studied. Altering hole preparation technique (3-mm K-wire probe vs. 4-mm drill bit) (139,150), screw thread shape (V or buttress, shallow or deep thread) (139,141,146), or depth of insertion into the vertebral body (50% of vertebral diameter vs. to anterior cortex) (143) produces little or no gain in screw pullout strength. However, screw depth of penetration (80% of vertebral diameter vs. 50%) does increase the moment required to cut the screw laterally through the vertebral wall (141). Also, screws pulled out at a mean load of 903 N when positioned near the anterior vertebral cortex and 1,186 N when they engaged the anterior cortex (143). In addition, tapered or conical shaped screws have been shown to increase the torque required for insertion but do not have greater pullout strengths than straight profile screws (151).

When pedicle screws are loaded in a caudocephalad direction (i.e., transverse to their long axis), a "toggle" type of displacement can result (143,152). This occurs because the narrowest part of the pedicle is its base (Fig. 66). The screw is sized to fit the base of the pedicle, which becomes a fulcrum about which it can rotate when load is applied transverse to the axis of the screw (152). Wittenberg et al. (146) showed that if a controlled displacement of ±2 mm is applied to the end of a screw in a caudocephalad direction, the initial load drops from about 200 N to less than half that value in fewer than 10,000 load cycles. The "butterfly" pattern of widening of the pedicle screw hole due to this type of loading is clearly seen in Fig. 67 and can be reduced by, for example, capturing the head of the screw so that it cannot displace, i.e., by locking it to the plate. With this method, the potential for rotation of the screw is eliminated by adding a second point of fixation. Alternatively, applying screws so they are not parallel and then cross linking them can reduce this toggle effect.

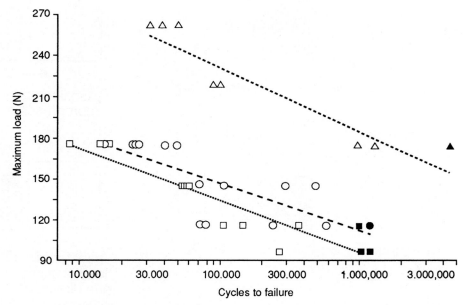

FIG. 63. Number of cycles to failure for 5.5- and 7.0-mm diameter lumbar pedicle screws loaded in bending. (Reproduced with permission from Moran JM, Berg WS, Berry JL, Geiger JM, Steffe AD. Transpedicular screw fixation. *J Orthop Res* 1989;7:107–114.)

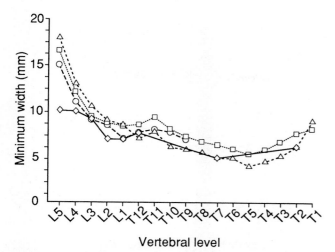

FIG. 64. Comparison of mean minimum pedicle diameters at different vertebral levels as reported in several studies. (Reproduced with permission from Moran JM, Berg WS, Berry JL, Geiger JM, Steffe AD. Transpedicular screw fixation. *J Orthop Res* 1989;7:107–114.)

Another area of concern with pedicle screws is fracture of the pedicle during insertion. Hasegawa et al. (153) showed that the bone mineral density of the pedicle was consistently lower in all regions of the cross sections of the pedicles of osteoporotic vertebrae. For example, the outermost region of the pedicle cortex (75% to 100% of the cross-sectional diameter) was only half as dense in osteoporotic vertebrae as in normal vertebrae. The risk for fracture of the pedicle was increased when bone mineral density of the pedicle was below about 0.7 mg/cm^2 and fill of the pedicle by the screw was beyond 70% (153).

Ashman et al. (154) described an event that can result in breakage of the screw instead of loosening, especially when adequate screw purchase is obtained in bone. If the instrumentation is applied posteriorly and there is little resistance to flexion in the stabilized spine (i.e., no graft is used to buttress the spine against flexion anteriorly), then the screws are loaded in bending (Fig. 68). Under these conditions, the tensile stresses (caused by the cantilever bending) at the base of the screw can exceed the endurance limit tensile stress for stainless steel at axial load levels below 150 N, which is well below the expected physiologic load (Fig. 69). If the endurance limit stress magnitude is exceeded, the implant is potentially liable to fail by fatigue. Protection against fatigue failure requires reducing the load experienced by the implant or increasing the minor diameter of the screw. Screws also can be unloaded by eliminating the rigid plate-screw connection (which reduces the bending moment on the screw), distributing the load among a greater number of screws, ensuring that an anterior vertebral body graft is well located to minimize flexion moments and protecting the surgical site against excessive repetitive stresses. Note, however, that eliminating the rigid screw-plate connection increases the potential for toggling as discussed previously. Therefore, ensuring an appropriately located graft able to support compression is probably the best way to guard against screw damage.

The resistance to lateral forces (perpendicular to the axis of the screw) of anterior vertebral body screws have been studied. As expected, the ability of the screw to resist load was correlated to vertebral body mineral density. The greatest resistance to lateral force was produced when the screw was placed bicortically along with a staple (155) or when placed in a superior oblique position (Fig. 70) (156).

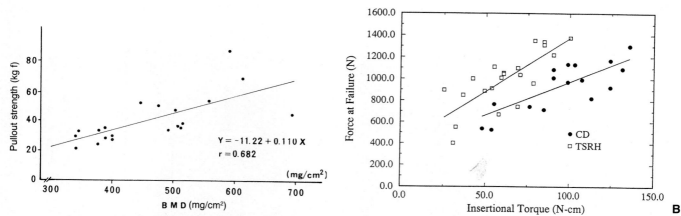

FIG. 65. A: Correlation between vertebral bone mineral density (BMD) and the pullout strength of AO 6.5-mm cancellous pedicle screws. (Reproduced with permission from Yamagata M, Kitahara H, Minami S, et al. Mechanical stability of the pedicle screw fixation systems for the lumbar spine. *Spine* 1992;17:S51–S54.) **B:** Relationship of the torque required for screw insertion and the measured pullout strength for two different types of screws. (Reproduced with permission from Myers BS, Belmont PJ, Richardson WJ, Yu JR, Harper KD, Nightingale RW. The role of imaging and in situ biomechanical testing in assessing pedicle screw pullout strength. *Spine* 1996;17:1962–1968.)

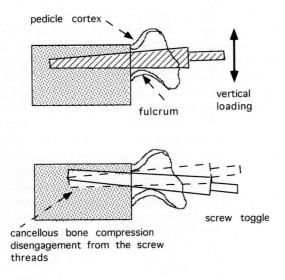

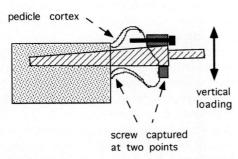

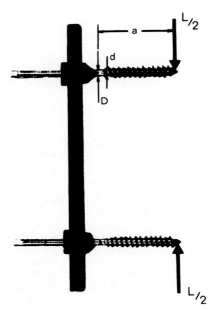

FIG. 66. Top: Mechanism by which the pedicle screw can toggle and ultimately loosen with caudocephalad loading. **Middle:** In this system, the base of the pedicle, being the most rigid region (there is the least cancellous bone for the screw to engage), becomes the fulcrum and the screw can toggle and loosen. **Bottom:** If the head of the screw is prevented from moving, this toggle is greatly diminished. (Reproduced with permission from Law M, Tencer AF, Anderson PA. Mechanism of loosening of pedicle screws. *Spine* 1993;18:2438–2443.

FIG. 68. Forces acing on a pedicle screw fixation system with the screws rigidly attached to the plate. The loads (L/2) applied to the screws through engagement with vertebral body bone bend the screws and plate. The screw acts as a cantilever beam, with the maximum stresses occurring at its base (the junction with the plate). The stresses are concentrated at this region because of the change in diameter from (d) to (D) in this region. (Reproduced with permission from Ashman RB, Galpin RD, Corin JD, Johnston CE. Biomechanical analysis of pedicle screw instrumentation in a corpectomy model. *Spine* 1989;14:1398–1405.)

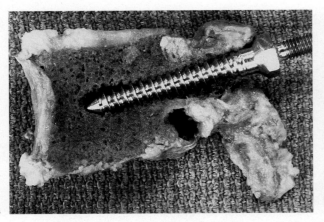

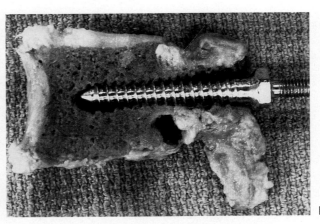

FIG. 67. Positions of a pedicle screw in maximum caudal position under load **(A)** and maximum cephalad position **(B)** demonstrating that cancellous bone has been crushed during vertical cyclic loading, causing the screw to loosen. (Reproduced with permission from Law M, Tencer AF, Anderson PA. Mechanism of loosening of pedicle screws. *Spine* 1993;18:2438–2443.)

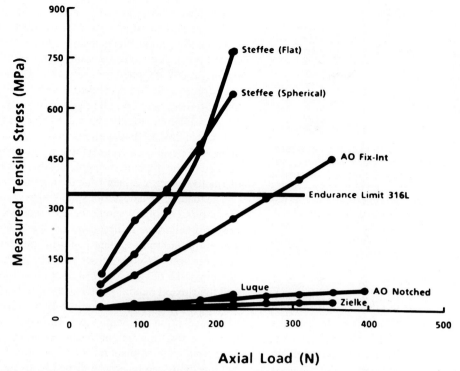

FIG. 69. Tensile stress measured from strain gauges located at the bases of various pedicle screws as a function of the axial load applied to the implant. Note that in some implants these stresses exceed the endurance limit of stainless steel, which indicates a potential for fatigue failure. (Reproduced with permission from Ashman RB, Galpin RD, Corin JD, Johnston CE. Biomechanical analysis of pedicle screw instrumentation in a corpectomy model. *Spine* 1989;14:1398–1405.)

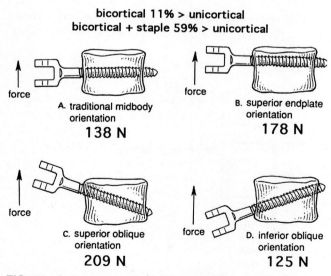

FIG. 70. Comparison of resistance to lateral forces of anterior body screws placed through one or two cortices, along with either a washer or staple (155) and the effect of screw orientation. (Adapted from Horton WC, Blackstock SF, Norman JT, Hill CS, Feiertag MA, Hutton WC. Strength of fixation of anterior body screws. *Spine* 1996;21:439–444.)

General Mechanical Principles of Fixation

Krag (157) outlined some important considerations when applying spinal constructs. In general, because of the location of the center of gravity of the torso anterior to the lower lumbar spine, flexion is a predominant mode of loading, along with compression, even when activities of daily living are restricted to sitting and standing. For the same applied moment, a construct in which the rod is applied over a larger number of spinal motion segments will produce smaller forces in the rod hooks or screws, because the larger moment arm of the rod reduces the magnitude of forces required at the rod–implant interface to generate a moment able to resist an externally applied flexion moment (Fig. 71).

The mechanical function of an anterior graft is illustrated in Fig. 72. With fixation to the vertebra above the injured one in a fracture when the anterior column is compromised, the moment generated by a short segment pedicle screw implant to counteract the externally applied flexion moment is equal to the force in the screw times the length of the moment arm (distance from the axis of the screw to the fulcrum of the system). Screw forces can be reduced by increasing the length of the moment arm, distributing the forces over a greater

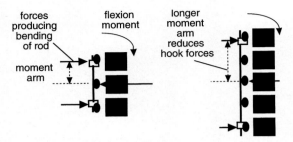

FIG. 71. Biomechanical comparison of long and short posterior rodding of the spine. **Left:** For the same externally applied flexion moment, the short rodded segment produces a resisting bending moment in the rod equal to the force at the hook site times the distance of the force to the center of the rod. **Right:** If the rod is longer, the center of the rod to hook site distance is greater; therefore, to counteract the same moment, the hook site force will be smaller. (Adapted from Krag MH. Biomechanics of thoracolumbar spinal fixation. A review. *Spine* 1991;16:S85–S98.)

number of screws, and/or using an anterior strut graft. The compressive force from a well-fitted anterior graft, times its distance from the fulcrum of the system, results in an additional moment to counteract the external flexion moment, thereby reducing forces in the implant. Given the previous discussion of the strength and preloading of grafts, it is important to ensure an adequate load-bearing surface area for the graft on the vertebral body and to precompress it, but not excessively.

A distraction type of instrumentation, such as one with hooks on the lamina of vertebrae above and below the injury site, applies axial tension (distraction) to the immobilized segment to regain height in the injured area, reduce retropulsed bone, and maintain the positions of the hooks on the lamina. Distraction also tensions remaining ligaments, which enhances stability of the injured motion segment. With this type of instrumentation, viscoelastic creep of the

soft tissues of the spine will decrease the distractive force over a period of time, resulting in lower hook purchase forces at the lamina. Nachemson and Elfstrom (158) demonstrated this using *in vivo* measurements of the axial force in Harrington rods applied for scoliosis. As shown in Fig. 6, the axial force in the rod decreased sharply after initial application of the implants and more gradually thereafter, so that by 18 days postoperatively the axial force of distraction was only about 25% of that applied initially. It is important when using soft tissue as a counterforce mechanism to distraction applied by the implant, to appreciate this effect and check the distractive force at a later time during the procedure.

The loading on a posterior spinal instrumentation with different types of injury should be distinguished. In the case of posterior element injury (loss of the posterior column), where the motion segment can still maintain resistance to compression through intact discs (anterior and middle columns), the flexion center of rotation has shifted anteriorly and the flexion neutral zone has enlarged, as discussed previously. Distractive force applied by the implant adds to the external flexion moment (Fig. 73). For the implant to contribute to resisting flexion of the spine, the distraction load produced by the implant must be converted to bending of the implant. This can be accomplished by using a sleeve placed between the implant and the lamina, which results in bending of the implant when resisting flexion and compression against the spinal lamina.

If the anterior column is disrupted, the flexion/extension center of rotation moves posteriorly and is located close to the facets and the posteriorly placed implant. The moment arm (distance from axis of rotation to axis of implant rod), and hence the resulting moment generated by the implant in resisting the forces applied to it, is small because it is close to the flexion/extension center (Fig. 74). In this situation, bending of the implant is a primary mechanism for resisting flexion deformity, as opposed to compressive force gener-

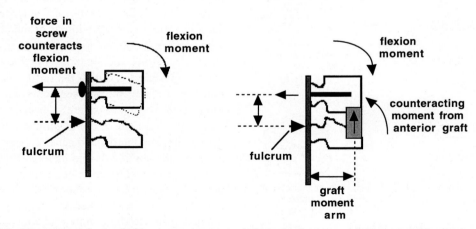

FIG. 72. The mechanical role of an anterior strut graft. **Left:** A moment is generated in the implant by screw forces due to the external flexion moment. The large force may cause screw toggle within the vertebra or high stresses in the screw without the support provided by an anterior strut graft. **Right:** An anterior graft produces a moment counteracting the external flexion moment, reducing force in the implant. (Adapted from Krag MH. Biomechanics of thoracolumbar spinal fixation. A review. *Spine* 1991;16: S85–S98.)

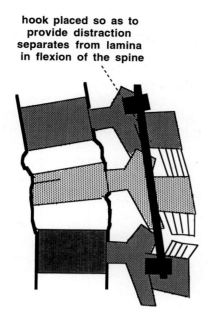

hook placed so as to
provide distraction
separates from lamina
in flexion of the spine

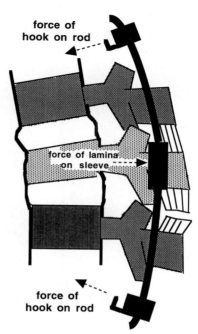

force of
hook on rod

force of lamina
on sleeve

force of
hook on rod

FIG. 73. Left: In the case of posterior element disruption, the flexion/extension axis shifts anteriorly. Distraction instrumentation contributes to the external flexion moment applied to the spine instead of resisting it, unless spinal flexion is converted into bending in the rod. **Right:** Placing a sleeve between the lamina and the implant produces bending in the implant when a flexion moment is applied, enhancing the ability of distraction instrumentation to resist flexion.

ated through the hooks. If both the anterior and middle columns are disrupted, the center of flexion/extension moves posterior to the facets. With the center of rotation in this position, a distractive force from the implant now opposes the

flexion
moment

compressive
force of hook
on lamina

moment
arm

anterior
column
injury

flexion
center of
rotation

FIG. 74. With anterior column disruption, the flexion/extension center of rotation shifts posteriorly and is located near the axis of a posteriorly positioned implant, decreasing its moment arm. Therefore, compressive force in the implant contributes little to opposing the external flexion moment.

external flexion moment applied to the spine (Fig. 75), in contrast to the case of posterior column disruption. However, the implant must be able to support direct compressive forces as well as bend in this very unstable situation.

A bursting injury with disruption of the facets is unstable in lateral bending and torsion. If an implant is applied that has separate rods or plates as the longitudinal members, fixed by screws (Fig. 76), the system can act as a four-bar mechanism, which allows the injured motion segment to displace laterally, providing little resistance to torsion and lateral bending (159). A coupler bar that connects the rods, making an H configuration. is a very effective method for increasing lateral bending and torsional stability.

Implant Performance in Posterior Column Injuries

A large number of studies have appeared comparing the stability offered by different forms of spinal constructs. It should be emphasized that the type and degree of injury play a large part in determining the stabilizing potential of various devices (160). Therefore, direct comparisons of the mechanical performance of various types of devices is given in the context of the type of injury that the implant is required to stabilize. This discussion is limited to studies that simulate a realistic bone–implant interface.

Before comparing implant performance, it is instructive to appreciate the positions that create the highest loads on an implant and the magnitudes of those loads. Rohlmann et al. (161) placed strain gauges on a posterior implant placed into

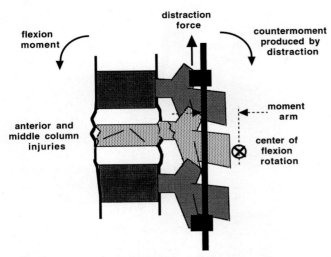

FIG. 75. When both the anterior and middle columns are disrupted, the flexion/extension center of rotation of the motion segment shifts posterior to the implant, so that distractive force from the implant also counteracts flexion.

the lumbar spine of a patient with degenerative instability. They found that load on the fixation was small for lying in a relaxed supine, lateral, or prone position. In walking, the force reached only about 170 N, and 2.7 Nm in flexion, whereas the torsional moment was below 1.2 Nm. The greatest loads occurred when the patient turned from a supine to a lateral position with the support of her hands. After a second procedure for anterior stabilization and once the patient became mobile, loads supported by the implant increased significantly, with bending moments between 5 and 8 Nm and axial forces close to 400 N (Fig. 77). The load magnitudes were measured 40 days after stabilization. These reported load magnitudes should be considered as the performance of various implants is discussed in the following paragraphs.

Fixation of Posterior Column (Flexion-Distraction) Injuries

With a posterior column injury (posterior ligaments disrupted), which can still support compression, lateral bending

and axial rotation, but is unstable in flexion, and where the center of rotation in flexion has moved anteriorly, posterior fixation should be considered. Shea et al. (162) compared several configurations of three types of instrumentation systems and found them all to provide considerable stiffness in compression and flexion. The only real difference occurred when using longer instrumentation, which increased flexion stiffness considerably (from about 100% of intact to 265% of intact). This demonstrates that the biomechanical advantage of applying a longer implant overshadows individual differences between most modern devices in posterior column injuries.

Fixation of Posterior Middle Column Injuries

This injury disrupts the posterior elements and the posterior half of the disc. The injured spine is unstable to loads in flexion, compression, lateral bending, and rotation and, therefore, places high demands on the instrumentation. The axis of flexion/extension rotation is anterior to its normal location; therefore, devices placed posteriorly and able to resist separation of the posterior part of the motion segment (i.e., spreading of the lamina) have the greatest resistance to flexion and lateral bending loads.

Panjabi et al. (163) compared the biomechanical properties of a number of constructs applied in this injury pattern, including the anterolaterally placed Dunn device, Harrington rods placed in distraction, compression, combined distraction and compression, or distraction with Edwards sleeves, and Luque rods, rectangle or short rectangle fixed with sublaminar wires. In flexion, most of the posterior constructs permitted only 52% to 23% of the motion of the intact spine, thereby enhancing stability. The anterior construct allowed greater than 250% of the angular motion of the intact spine, clearly indicating the ineffectiveness of applying anterior instrumentation to prevent flexion motions in this type of injury. In lateral bending, the least effective fixation was the Luque short rectangle (181% of intact spinal motion), and the most stabilizing were the Dunn device and Luque rod (72% of intact). Devices with distraction hooks cannot pre-

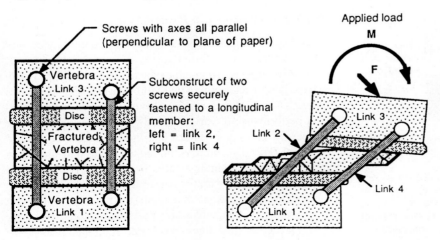

FIG. 76. Left: A fixation system arranged with parallel bars and parallel pedicle screws allows the fixation to act as a four-bar linkage resulting in lateral displacement of one vertebra, which makes the construct less rigid in lateral bending and torsion. **Right:** Addition of a coupler bar between the rods, creating an H configuration, prevents this motion. (Reproduced with permission from Gaines RW, Carson WL, Satterlee CC, Groh GI. Experimental evaluation of seven different fracture internal fixation devices using non failure stability testing. *Spine* 1991;16:902–909.)

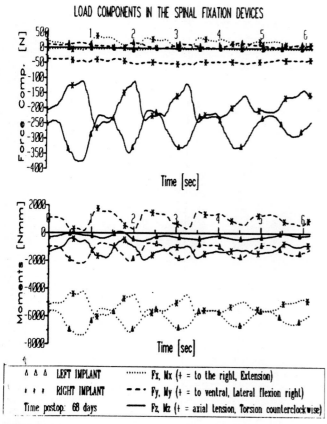

FIG. 77. Loads in six directions (three forces and three moments) in a posterior internal fixation device measured *in vivo* in a patient 40 days after posterior fixation and anterior grafting for spinal degeneration, during ambulation. (Reproduced with permission from Rohlmann A, Bergmann G, Graichen F, Mayer H-M. Telemeterized load measurement using instrumented spinal internal fixators in a patient with degenerative instability. *Spine* 1995;20:2683–2689.)

vent the lamina on the side away from the direction of bending from lifting off the hook. In extension, the Dunn device was least stable, and the Harrington distraction rods with and without sleeves were the most stable constructs. Because the spine lamina directly load the distraction hooks in extension, the superiority of distraction instrumentation in this loading mode is not unexpected. In torsion no construct was able to reproduce the stiffness of the intact motion. The main problem with the constructs tested in that experiment was the lack of a central coupler bar to prevent the implant from acting like a linkage, as discussed previously.

Fixation of Anterior Middle Column (Bursting) Injuries

An anterior/middle column injury shifts the flexion/extension center of rotation posterior to the instrumentation itself and is highly unstable to compression, flexion, lateral bending, and torsion loading. Gurr et al. (164) compared the Kaneda device (applied anteriorly) and posterior fixation devices including Harrington distraction rods, Cotrel-Dubousset instrumentation with 5-mm pedicle screws, Steffee plates

and screws, and the Luque rectangle. All the posterior devices were fixed between the first and fifth levels, with an anterior strut graft to replace the damaged vertebra. The results demonstrated the need for rigid fixation with either pedicle or vertebral screws in addition to the anterior strut graft to control the displacement produced by compressive force in this injury pattern. In flexion, the three implants with screw attachments were most effective in limiting angulation, although the most stiff constructs had displacements that were still nearly the same as that of the intact spine. This result shows the difficulty in controlling flexion when the middle column is injured. Also of note is that the strut graft alone does little by itself to control flexion angulation. Its function as a buttress is important, but possibly only at larger loads. In torsion, the implants fixed with screws were again able to produce constructs with stiffnesses greater than that of the intact spine. Similar observations have been made by others (165,166).

A survey of currently available devices shows how both anterior and posterior instrumentation can restore stability to the injured spine. Anterior devices with strut grafting installed on lumbar spines with burst fractures produce considerable decreases in motion, having the least effect in axial torsion (Fig. 78) (167). A promising enhancement to the pedicle screw instrumentation is the addition of supplemental hooks. Addition of the hooks increased the stiffness of short segment pedicle instrumentation in these injuries considerably, greater than 200% in some loading directions (Fig. 79) (168).

One aspect that has received less attention is the performance of these implants under cyclic stress below failure level. In a study of five posterior instrumentations, fatigue

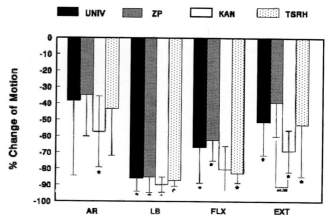

FIG. 78. Percent decreases in motion in four loading directions using anterior devices with an interbody graft in an anterior-middle column injury (burst fracture) of the lumbar spine. UNIV, University plate; ZP, Z plate; KAN, Kaneda device; TSRH, Texas Scottish Rite Hospital device; AR, axial rotation; LB, lateral bending; FLX, flexion; EXT, extension. (Reproduced with permission from An HS, Lim T-H, You J-W, Hong JH, Eck J, McGrady L. Biomechanical evaluation of anterior thoracolumbar spinal instrumentation. *Spine* 1995; 20:1979–1983.)

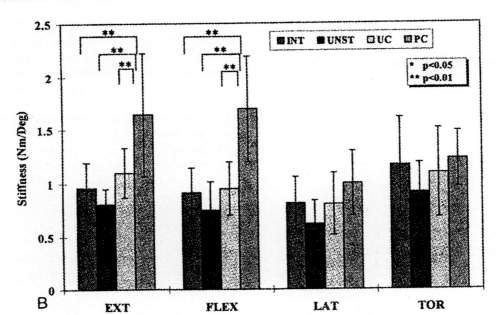

FIG. 79. Effect of a supplemental hook on the stiffness of lumbar spine burst fractures fixed with short segment pedicle screws. Mean stiffness for the different constructs in each of four loading direction: INT, intact; UNST, unstable; UC, pedicle screw construct without supplemental hook; PC, pedicle screw with supplementary hook. EXT = extension; FLEX = flexion; LAT = lateral bending; TOR = torsion. (Reproduced with permission from Chiba M, Mclain RF, Yerby SA, Moseley TA, Smith TS, Benson DR. Short-segment pedicle instrumentation. Biomechanical analysis of supplemental hook fixation. *Spine* 1996;21:288–294.)

failure of the implant was induced in three of six upper screws with the AO fixateur interne, five of six upper screws with the Steffee plate, and four of five rods with the Kluger fixateur interne. These failures occurred between 12,000 and 90,000 load cycles. In all cases, failure of the device occurred at a change in diameter along the screw or rod (169). It should be appreciated that these tests simulate a worst case situation where no healing or load transfer to bone occurs; however, it does point out the temporary nature of these implants in terms of their load-bearing function. One way to potentially reduce implant stresses as well as stimulating healing is by transfer of load to bone by dynamization of the implant, a common strategy in long bone fracture healing. Goel et al. (170) reported on the mechanical function of an implant that allows controlled axial collapse. Stability (motion less than that of the intact spine) was demonstrated in all loading directions except for axial rotation.

Fixation Systems for Anterior Middle Posterior Column Injuries

This type of injury is the most severe with all structures damaged and the spine unable to support any load at all. Ferguson et al. (160) compared posterior spine fracture constructs using Harrington rods with sublaminar wires, C rods (crossed segmentally wired C-shaped rods), Jacobs rods, the Vermont fixator, and Roy Camille plates fixed with pedicle screws at multiple levels. The multiple level screw fixation of the Roy Camille plate gave the greatest fixation stability in all loading directions, exceeding the stiffness of the intact spine.

The effectiveness of pedicle screw fixation systems in

producing rigid constructs in severe spinal injuries also was shown in the study by Gaines et al. (159), who ranked constructs produced by various instrumentation systems by their ability to limit angular and linear displacements in various directions. The Steffee plate produced the highest rank construct, and the Harrington rods alone the lowest. An extensive survey of 12 pedicular screw devices by Cunningham et al. (171) showed that the rank order of implant failure was similar in static and cyclic loading. This probably occurs because more flexible implants also usually have greater component internal stresses due to larger deformations of components. They also found that implants using interlocking rods could withstand more cycles to failure than those using plates. A summary of the cyclic fatigue characteristics of various spinal implants is shown in Fig. 80.

Lumbosacral Fixation: General Concepts

Fixation of the lumbosacral spine presents probably a greater challenge in some respects than thoracolumbar fixation. Although the degree of injury to the spine may be less severe, the lumbosacral junction will experience loads equivalent to those in the lumbar spine as well as greater shear forces because of the greater angulation of the L5–S1 junction. However, the most difficult aspect of fixation in this region is obtaining good screw purchase in the sacrum. A major difficulty with sacral screw placement is locating sites with adequate purchase that are clinically safe. As shown by Licht et al. (172), placement of sacral screws oblique to the ala puts the L-5 nerve root at risk, whereas locating them directly posterior to anterior may result in penetration of the iliac

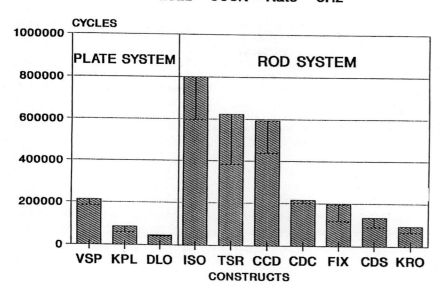

Load = 600N   Rate = 5Hz

FIG. 80. Number of cycles to failure at a peak load of 600 N for 12 different pedicle screw implant systems. VSP, Steffee plate; DLO, Dyna-lok plate; KPL, Kirschner plate; SIM, Simmons plate; ISO, Isola rod; TSR, Texas Scottish Rite Hospital rod; CCD, compact Cotrel-Dubousset rod; CDC, cold rolled rod; CDS, Cotrel-Dubousset standard rod; FIX, AO fixateur interne; KRO, Kirschner rod; ROG, Rogozinski rod. (Reproduced with permission from Cunningham BW, Sefter JC, Shono Y, McAfee PC. Static and cyclical biomechanical analysis of pedicle screw spinal constructs. *Spine* 1993;18:1677–1688.)

veins or the sympathetic chain, and at S-2 or S-3, the rectum. A safe zone for screw placement was defined in the midline of the sacrum, which limits the mechanical options for enhancing screw purchase.

Zindrick et al. (140) showed that the pullout strengths of screws located in the S-2 pedicle were considerably lower than those of screws located at the S-1 level. Also, the strengths of screws placed from posterior to anteromedial versus posterior to anterolateral have been compared. Screws placed posterior to anteromedial, through the promontory, have greater maximum load capacity that those located anterolaterally (Fig. 81) (140,173). In addition, when the screw is constrained against sagittal plane rotation (extension), greater force of failure can be developed (Fig. 81).

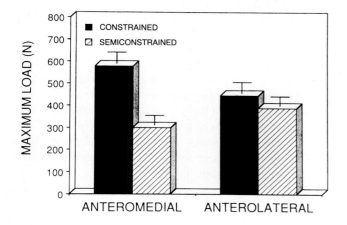

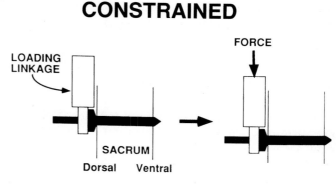

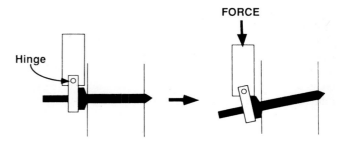

FIG. 81. Maximum vertical load (transverse to the axis of the screw) sustained by sacral screws placed from posterior to anteromedially into the promontory of the sacrum as opposed to anterolaterally into the ala, at S-1. Vertical (along the long axis of the spine) loading of a screw either "constrained" and "semiconstrained." The semiconstrained screw can rotate in the sagittal plane. (Reproduced with permission from Carlson GD, Abitbol JJ, Anderson DR, et al. Screw fixation in the human sacrum. *Spine* 1992;17: S194–S203.)

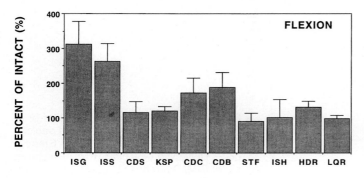

FIG. 82. Comparison of the rigidity of various constructs in flexion loading compared to the intact lumbosacral joint. ISG, ISOLA Galveston; ISS, ISOLA iliac screw; KSP, Kirschner sacral plate; CDC, Cotrel-Dubousset Chopin block; CDB, Cotrel-Dubousset butterfly plate; STF, Steffee plate; ISH, ISOLA sacral hook; HDR, Harrington distraction rods with sacral hooks; LQR, Luque rods with sublaminar wires. (Data adapted from McCord DH, Cunningham BW, Shono Y, Meyers JJ, McAfee PC: Biomechanical analysis of lumbosacral fixation. *Spine* 1992;17:S235–S243.

This is because, in the semiconstrained condition, a component of the applied load acts along the axis of the screw to produce pullout as the screw rotates. The maximum load capacity of sacral screws increases significantly with increasing bone density (a mean of 2 N for every 1 mg/cc increase in bone density), as with other screws. Also, there is only a 5% gain in strength with placement of screws bicortically (174). Therefore, the optimum location of sacral screws, for strength of purchase and safety, is medially toward the promontory at the S-1 level, but without penetrating the anterior cortex of S-1.

Comparison of Sacral Fixation Constructs

As with thoracolumbar spinal instrumentation, the number of alternative methods for fixing lumbosacral spinal injuries has increased significantly recently. McCord et al. (175) recently studied the performance of ten different methods of fixation in the lumbosacral joint in flexion to failure. This study provided a comparison between five fundamentally different methods of load transfer between the sacrum and the implant: sacral wiring, sacral screws, sacral hooks, iliac screws, and rods embedded into the ilium. The specific implants studied were the Galveston technique (rods embedded into the ilia), the ISOLA system using ¼-inch diameter rods, the ISOLA system with iliac screws, Cotrel-Dubousset rods with iliosacral screws, Kirschner sacral plates, Cotrel-Dubousset butterfly plates, Cotrel-Dubousset Chopin block, ISOLA hooks, Harrington distraction rods, Luque rods, and Steffee plates. The results of the flexion testing demonstrate that fixation into the ilia provides a clear advantage over other methods in developing a construct resistant to flexion loading (Fig. 82). Further, the constructs using iliac rod fixation failed at significantly greater loads than those with plate and screw fixation. The greater rigidity of fixation to the ilium can be attributed to the longer lever arm of the anchoring mechanism of the iliac rod compared with the sacral screw. The lumbosacral fixation acts as a complex lever. With flexion loading, rotation in the fixation system may occur at the screw or rod and bone interface, at the screw–rod or screw–plate junction, and by bending of the rod or plate. The longer lever arm of the iliac fixation reduces bone–implant motion.

The previous study compared fixations only in flexion loading at the lumbosacral junction; however, this region must resist loads in other planes. Puno et al. (176) compared several techniques, including Galveston fixation, Luque segmentally wired ring fixation, and Steffee plates with and without fixation to S-2, in several loading directions, in otherwise intact specimens. In compression, all implants produced constructs with stiffnesses similar to intact, except for the Galveston-Luque technique. In torsion and lateral bending, the Steffee plate constructs were most rigid, whereas extension loading produced almost identical results regardless of instrumentation. It is interesting to note the contribution of the S-2 screw, which improves fixation stiffness moderately in most loading modes, but significantly in flexion (82% without to 129% with the S-2 screw). Although the S-2 purchase site is weak (140), the gain in moment arm length between the S-1 and S-2 screws is such that a considerable additional resisting moment to flexion is generated in the instrumentation with the S-2 screw in place.

Similar observations were made by McCord et al. (177), who summarized the concepts involved in obtaining sacral purchase as extending the sacral purchase through the anterior sacral cortex, achieving more inferior purchase by extending fixation down to the S-2 pedicle, and obtaining purchase between the iliac cortices down to the superior acetabular bone. It is also possible to combine posterior fixation with anteriorly placed threaded fusion cages to obtain constructs of greater rigidity (178).

REFERENCES

1. Oxland TR, Panjabi MM. The onset and progression of spinal injury: A demonstration of neutral zone sensitivity. *J Biomech* 1992;25:1165–1172.
2. Panjabi MM, Duranceau J, Goel V, Oxland T, Takata K. Cervical human vertebrae. Quantitative three dimensional anatomy of the middle and lower regions. *Spine* 1991;16:861–869.
3. Panjabi MM, Goel V, Oxland T, Takata K, et al. Quantitative three dimensional anatomy. *Spine* 1992;17:299–306.
4. Bell GH, Dunbar O, Beck JS, Gibb A. Variation in strength of vertebrae with age and their relation to osteoporosis. *Calcif Tissue Res* 1967;1:75–86.
5. Young WC. *Roark's Formulas for Stress and Strain*, 6th edition. New York: McGraw-Hill, 1989:667–700.

6. McBroom RJ, Hayes WC, Edwards WT, Goldberg RP, White AA III. Prediction of vertebral body compressive fracture strength using quantitative computed tomography. *J Bone Joint Surg* 1985;67: 1206–1214.

7. Mosekilde L, Bentzen SM, Ortoft G, Jorgensen J. The predictive value of quantitative computed tomography for vertebral compressive strength and ash density. *Bone* 1989;10:465–470.

8. Keller T. Regional variations in the compressive properties of lumbar vertebral trabeculae: effects of disc degeneration. *Spine* 1989; 14:1012–1019.

9. Chapman JR, Harrington RM, Lee KM, Anderson PA, Tencer AF, Kowalski D. Factors affecting the pullout strength of cancellous bone screws. *J Biomech Eng* 1996;118:391–398.

10. Tran NT, Watson NA, Tencer AF, Ching RP, Anderson PA. Mechanism of the burst fracture in the thoracolumbar spine: the effect of loading rate. *Spine* 1994;20:1984–1988.

11. Nachemson AL. Disc pressure measurements. *Spine* 1981;6:93–97.

12. Doherty BJ, Heggeness MH. Vertebral body endplates deform under physiological axial loading. Transactions of the 39th Annual Meeting of the Orthopedic Research Society, 1993;88.

13. Brinckmann P, Frobin W, Hierholzer E, Horst M. Deformation of the vertebral end-plate under axial loading of the spine. *Spine* 1983; 8:851–856.

14. Holmes AD, Hukins DWL, Freemont AJ. End plate displacement during compression of lumbar vertebra-disc-vertebra segments and the mechanism of failure. *Spine* 1993;18:128–135.

15. Acaroglu ER, Iatridis JC, Setton LA, Foster RJ, Mow VC, Weidenbaum M. Degeneration and aging affect the tensile behavior of human lumbar annulus fibrosus. *Spine* 1995;20:2690–2701.

16. Adams MA, Green TP, Dolan P. The strength in anterior bending of lumbar intervertebral discs. *Spine* 1994;19:2197–2203.

17. Goel VK, Winterbottom JM, Weinstein JN, Kim YE. Load sharing among spinal elements of a motion segment in extension and lateral bending. *J Biomech Eng* 1987;109:291–297.

18. Haher TR, O'Brien M, Dryer JW, Nucci R, Zipnick R, Leone DJ. The role of the lumbar facet joints in spinal stability. *Spine* 1994; 19:2667–2671.

19. Miller JAA, Haderspeck KA, Schultz AB. Posterior element loads in lumbar motion segments. *Spine* 1983;8:331–337.

20. Lorenz M, Patwardhan A, Vanderby R. Load bearing characterisitcs of lumbar facets in normal and surgically altered spinal segments. *Spine* 1983;8:122–130.

21. Asano S, Kaneda K, Umehara S, Tadano S. The mechanical properties of the human L4-5 functional spinal unit during cyclic loading. *Spine* 1992;17:1343–1352.

22. Skipor AF, Miller JAA, Spencer DA, Schultz AB. Stiffness properties and geometry of lumbar spine posterior elements. *J Biomech* 1985;18:821–830.

23. Tencer AF, Ahmed AM, Burke DL. Some static mechanical properties of the lumbar intervertebral joint, intact and injured. *J Biomech Eng* 1982;104:193–201.

24. Tencer AF, Mayer TG. Soft tissue strain and facet face interaction in the lumbar intervertebral joint: part II. Calculated results and comparison with experimental data. *J Biomech Eng* 1983;105:210–215.

25. Panjabi MM, Goel VK, Takata K. Physiological strains in the lumbar spinal ligaments. *Spine* 1982;7:192–203.

26. Waters RL, Morris JM. An in vitro study of normal and scoliotic interspinous ligaments. *J Biomech* 1973;6:343–348.

27. Nachemson AL, Evans JH. Some mechanical properties of the third human lumbar interlaminar ligament (ligamentum flavum). *J Biomech* 1968;1:211–220.

28. Neumann P, Keller TS, Ekstrom L, Hansson T. Effect of strain rate and bone mineral content on the structural properties of the human anterior longitudinal ligament. *Spine* 1994;19:205–211.

29. Dumas GA, Beaudoin L, Drouin G. In situ mechanical behavior of posterior spinal ligaments in the lumbar region. An in vitro study. *J Biomech* 1987;20:301–310.

30. Yoganandan N, Pintar F, Butler J, Reinartz J, Sances A, Larson SJ. *Spine* 1989;14:1102–1110.

31. Fielding JW, Cochran GVB, Lawsing JF III, Hohl M. Tears of the transverse ligament of the atlas. *J Bone Joint Surg* 1974;56A: 1683–1691.

32. Ommaya AK. Mechanical properties of tissues of the nervous system. *J Biomech* 1968;1:127–138.

33. Tencer AF, Ferguson RL, Allen BL Jr. A biomechanical study of thoracolumbar spine fractures with bone in the canal: part III. Mechanical properties of the dura and its tethering ligaments. *Spine* 1985; 10:741–747.

34. Panjabi MM, Dvorak J, Duranceau J, et al. Three dimensional movements of the upper cervical spine. *Spine* 1988;13:726–731.

35. Fielding JW, Cochran GVB, Lawsing JF III, Hohl M. Tears of the transverse ligament of the atlas. *J Bone Joint Surg* 1974;56A: 1683–1691.

36. Crisco JJ III, Oda T, Panjabi MM, Bueff HU, Dvorak J, Grob D. Transections of the C1-C2 capsular ligaments in the cervical spine. *Spine* 1991;16:S474–S479.

37. Anderson LD, D'Alonzo RT. Fractures of the odontoid process of the axis. *J Bone Joint Surg* 1974;56A:1663–1674.

38. Mouradian WH, Fietti VG Jr, Cochran GVB, Fielding JW, Young J. Fractures of the odontoid: a laboratory and clinical study of the mechanisms. *Orthop Clin North Am* 1987;9:985–1001.

39. Doherty BJ, Heggeness MH, Esses SI. A biomechanical study of odontoid fractures and fracture fixation. *Spine* 1993;18:178–184.

40. Heggeness MH, Doherty BJ. The trabecular anatomy of the axis. *Spine* 1993;18:1945–1949.

41. Oda T, Panjabi MM, Crisco JJ III, Oxland TR. Multidirectional instabilities of experimental burst fractures of the atlas. *Spine* 1992; 17:1285–1290.

42. Panjabi MM, Oda T, Crisco JJ III, Oxland TR, Katz L, Nolte LP. Experimental study of atlas injuries. Biomechanical analysis of their mechanisms and fracture patterns. *Spine* 1991;16:S460–S465.

43. Sasso R, Doherty BJ, Crawford MJ, Heggeness MH. Biomechanics of odontoid fracture fixation. *Spine* 1993;18:1950–1953.

44. Gallie WE. Fractures and dislocation of the cervical spine. *Am J Surg* 1939;46:495–499.

45. Brooks AL, Jenkins EB. Atlanto-axial arthrodesis by the wedge compression method. *J Bone Joint Surg* 1978;60A:279–284.

46. Grob D, Magerl F. Dorsale Spondylodese der Halswirbelsaule mit der Hakenplatte. *Orthopade* 1987;16:55–61.

47. Magerl F. Spondylodesen an der oberen halswirbelsaule. *Acta Chir Aust Suppl* 1986;43:69–71.

48. Tucker HH. Technical report: method of fixation of subluxed or dislocated cervical spine below C1-C2. *Can J Neurol Sci* 1975; 2:381–382.

49. Grob D, Crisco JJ III, Panjabi MM, Wang P, Dvorak J. Biomechanical evaluation of four different posterior atlantoaxial fixation techniques. *Spine* 1992;17:480–490.

50. Hajek PD, Lipka J, Hartline P, Saha S, Albright JA. Biomechanical study of C1-C2 posterior arthrodesis techniques. *Spine* 1993;18:173–177.

51. van Mameren H, Sanches H, Beursgens J, Drukker J. Cervical spine motion in the sagittal plane: II. Position of segmental averaged instantaneous centers of rotation, a cineradiographic study. *Spine* 1992; 17:467–474.

52. Joffe MH, White AA, Panjabi MM. Clinically relevant kinematics of the cervical spine. In: Sherk HH (ed). *The Cervical Spine.* The Cervical Spine Research Society. Philadelphia: JB Lippincott, 1989: 57–82.

53. Conley MS, Meyer RA, Bloomberg JJ, Feeback DL, Dudley GA. Noninvasive analysis of human neck muscle function. *Spine* 1995; 20:2506–2512.

54. Pintar FA, Yoganandan N, Pesigan M, Reinartz J, Sances A Jr, Cusick JF. Cervical vertebral strain measurements under axial and eccentric loading. *J Biomech Eng* 1995;117:474–478.

55. Clasen JD, Goel VJ, Traynelis VC. Investigation of the role of the uncinate process and Luschka's joints using finite element analysis. Transactions of the 43rd Annual Meeting of the Orthopedic Research Society, 1997;22:359.

56. Zdeblick TA, Abitbol JJ, Kunz DN, McCabe RP, Garfin S. Cervical stability after sequential capsule resection. *Spine* 1993;18:2005–2008.

57. Panjabi MM, White AA III, Johnson RM. Cervical spine mechanics as a function of transection of components. *J Biomech* 1975;8:327–336.

58. McElhaney J, Snyder RG, States JD, Gabrielsen MA. Biomechanical analysis of swimming pool neck injuries. Transactions of the Society of Automotive Engineers, Paper 790137, 1979.

59. Yoganandan N, Haffner M, Maiman DJ, et al. Epidemiology and injury biomechanics of motor vehicle related trauma to the human spine.

Transactions of the Society of Automotive Engineers, Paper 892438, 1989.

60. Carter JW, Ching RP, Tencer AF, Mirza S. Transient changes in cervical spinal canal geometry during wedge compression fracture. Proceedings of the 6th Injury Prevention through Biomechanics Symposium, Detroit, Michigan, 1996:39–46.

61. James R, Nasmyth-Jones R. The occurrence of cervical fractures in victims of judicial hanging. *Forensic Sci Int* 1992;54:81–91.

62. Huelke DF, Mackay GM, Morris A, Bradford M. A review of cervical fractures and fracture dislocations without head impacts sustained by restrained drivers. *Accid Anal Prev* 1993;26:731–743.

63. States J. Soft tissue injuries of the neck. Transactions of the Society of Automotive Engineers, Paper 790135, 1979.

64. Kornhauser M. Delta-V thresholds for cervical spine injury. Transactions of the Society of Automotive Engineers, Paper 960093, 1996.

65. Myers BS, Winkelstein BA. Epidemiology, classification, mechanism, and tolerance of human cervical spine injuries. *Crit Rev Biomed Eng* 1995;23:307–409.

66. McElhaney JH, Diherty BJ, Paver JG, Myers BS, Gray L. Combined bending and axial loading responses of the human cervical spine. Transactions of the Society of Automotive Engineers, Paper 881709, 1988.

67. Pintar FA, Yoganandan N, Sances A Jr, Reinartz J, Harris G, Larson SJ. Kinematic and anatomical analysis of the human cervical spinal column under axial loading. Transactions of the Society of Automotive Engineers, Paper 892436, 1989.

68. Nightingale RW, Richardson WJ, Myers BS. The effects of padded surfaces on the risk for cervical spine injury. *Spine* 1997 (in review).

69. Ching RP, Watson NA, Tencer AF. Effect of post injury position on occlusion of the cervical spinal canal. *Spine* 1997;22:2380–2387.

70. Panjabi MM, Lydon C, Vasavada A, Grob D, Crisco JJ III, Dvorak J. On the understanding of clinical instability. *Spine* 1994;19:2642–2650.

71. Panjabi MM, Duranceau JS, Oxland TR, Bowen CE. Multidirectional instabilities of traumatic cervical spine injuries in a porcine model. *Spine* 1989;14:1111–1115.

72. Podolsky S, Baraff LJ, Simon RR, Hoffman JR, Larmon B, Ablon W. Efficacy of cervical spine immobilization methods. *J Trauma* 1983;23:461–464.

73. Wolf JW Jr, Johnson RM. Cervical orthoses. In: *The Cervical Spine. The Cervical Spine Research Society.* Philadelphia: JB Lippincott, 1990:33–103.

74. Lind B, Sihlbom H, Nordwall A. Forces and motions across the neck in patients treated with halo-vest. *Spine* 1988;13:162–167.

75. Anderson PA, Budorick TE, Easton KB, Henley MB, Salciccioli GG. Failure of the halo vest to prevent in vivo motion in patients with injured cervical spines. *Spine* 1991;16:S501–S505.

76. Whitehill R, Richman JA, Glaser JA. Failure of immobilization of the cervical spine by the halo vest. *J Bone Joint Surg* 1986;68A:326–332.

77. Walker PS, Lamser D, Hussey RW, Rossier AB, Farberov A, Dietz J. Forces in the halo vest apparatus. *Spine* 1984;9:773–777.

78. Krag MH, Beynnon BD. A new halo-vest: rationale, design and biomechanical comparison to standard halo-vest designs. *Spine* 1988;13:228–235.

79. Wang GJ, Moskal JT, Albert T, Pritts C, Schuch CM, Stamp WG. The effect of halo-vest length on stability of the cervical spine. *J Bone Joint Surg* 1988;70A:357–360.

80. Mirza S, Moquin RP, Anderson PA, Tencer AF, Steinmann J, Oamau D. Stabilizing properties of the halo apparatus. *Spine* 1997;22:727–733.

81. Kerwin GA, Chou KL, White DB, Shen KL, Salciccioli GG, Yang KH. Investigation of how different halo influence pin forces. *Spine* 1994;19:1078–1081.

82. Whitesides TE, Mehserle WL, Hutton WC. The force exerted by the halo pin. A study comparing different halo systems. *Spine* 192;17:S413–S417.

83. Amevo B, Aprill C, Bogduk N. Abnormal instantaneous axes of rotation in patients with neck pain. *Spine* 1992;17:748–756.

84. Pelker RR, Duranceau JS, Panjabi MM. Cervical spine stabilization. A three dimensional biomechanical evaluation of rotational stability, strength, and failure mechanisms. *Spine* 1991;16:117–122.

85. Rogers WA. Fractures and dislocations of the cervical spine: an end result study. *J Bone Joint Surg* 1957;39A:341–376.

86. Callahan RA, Johnson RM, Margolis RN, Keggi KJ, Albright JA, Southwick WO. Cervical facet fusion for control of instability following laminectomy. *J Bone Joint Surg* 1977;59A:991–1002.

87. Fairbank TJ. Spinal fusion after laminectomy for cervical myelopathy. *Proc R Soc Med* 1971;64:634–636.

88. Orozco Delclos R, Llovet Tapies R. Osteosintesis en las lesiones traumaticas y degeneratives de la columna vertebral. *Rev Traumatol Cirurg Rehabil* 1971;1:45–52.

89. Magerl F, Grob D, Seeman P. Stable dorsal fusion of the cervical spine (C2–T1) using hook plates. In: Kehr P, Weidner A (eds). *Cervical Spine I.* Berlin: Springer-Verlag, 1987:217–221.

90. Ulrich C, Woersdoerfer O, Kalff R, Claes L, Wilke H-J. Biomechanics of fixation systems to the cervical spine. *Spine* 1991;16:S4–S9.

91. Kotani Y, Cunningham BW, Abumi K, McAfee PC. Biomechanical analysis of cervical stabilization systems. An assessment of transpedicular screw fixation in the cervical spine. *Spine* 1994;19:2529–2539.

92. Richman JD, Daniel TE, Anderson DD, Miller PL, Douglas RA. Biomechanical evaluation of cervical spine stabilization using a porcine model. *Spine* 1995;20:2192–2197.

93. Grubb MR, Currier BL, Bonin V, Grabowski JJ. Biomechanical evaluation of anterior cervical spine stabilization in a porcine model. Transactions of the 39th Annual Meeting of the Orthopedic Research Society, 1993:8.

94. Choueka J, Spivak JM, Kummer FJ, Steger T. Flexion failure of posterior cervical lateral mass screws. *Spine* 1996;21:462–468.

95. Brantley AGU, Oxland TR, Koeneman JB. Effects of the BAK interbody implant system on cervical spine flexibility. Transactions of the 41st Annual Meeting of the Orthopedic Research Society, p 662, 1993.

96. Dvorak J, Panjabi MM, Chang DG, Theiler R, Grob D. Functional radiographic diagnosis of the lumbar spine. Flexion-extension and lateral bending. *Spine* 1991;16:562–571.

97. Dvorak J, Panjabi MM, Novotny JE, Chang DG, Grob D. Clinical validation of functional flexion-extension roentgenograms of the lumbar spine. *Spine* 1991;16:943–950.

98. McGregor AH, McCarthy ID, Hughes SP. Motion characteristics of the lumbar spine in the normal population. *Spine* 1995;20:2421–2428.

99. White AA III, Panjabi MM. *Clinical Biomechanics of the Spine,* 2nd edition. Philadelphia: JB Lippincott, 1990.

100. Lavender SA, Tsuang YH, Andersson GBJ, Hafezi A, Shin CC. Trunk muscle cocontraction: the effects of moment direction and moment magnitude. *J Orthop Res* 1992;10:691–700.

101. Tveit P, Daggfeld T, Hetland S, Thortensseon A. Erector spinae lever arm length variations with changes in spinal curvature. *Spine* 1994;19:199–204.

102. Schultz A, Andersson G, Ortengren R, Haderspeck K, Nachemson A. Loads on the lumbar spine. Validation of a biomechanical analysis by measurements of intradiscal pressures and myoelectric signals. *J Bone Joint Surg* 1982;64A:713–720.

103. Smith TJ, Fernie GR. Functional biomechanics of the spine. *Spine* 1991;16:1197–1203.

104. Posner I, White AA III, Edwards WT, Hayes WC. A biomechanical analysis of the clinical stability of the lumbar and lumbosacral spine. *Spine* 1982;7:374–388.

105. Holdsworth F. Fractures, dislocations, and fracture-dislocations of the spine. *J Bone Joint Surg* 1970;52A:1534–1551.

106. Ferguson RL, Allen BL Jr. A mechanistic classification of thoracolumbar spine fractures. *Clin Orthop* 1984;189:77–87.

107. Anderson PA, Rivara FP, Maier RV, Drake C. The epidemiology of seatbelt-associated injuries. *J Trauma* 1991;31:60–67.

108. Roaf R. A study of the mechanics of spinal injuries. *J Bone Joint Surg* 1960;42B:810–823.

109. Burkhardt R, Kettner G, Bohm W, et al. Changes in trabecular bone, hematopoiesis and bone marrow vessels in aplastic anemia, primary osteoporosis, and old age: a comparative histomorphometric study. *Bone* 1987;8:157–164.

110. Kazarian L, Graves GA. Compressive strength characteristics of human vertebral centrum. *Spine* 1977;2:1–14.

111. Denis F. The three column spine and its significance in the classification of acute thoracolumbar injuries. *Spine* 1983;8:817–831.

112. Panjabi MM, Oxland TR, Kifune M, Arand M, Wen L, Chen A. Validity of the three-column theory of thoracolumbar fractures: a biomechanic investigation. *Spine* 1995;20:1122–1127.

113. Haher TR, Bergman M, O'Brien M, et al. The effect of the three columns of the spine on the instantaneous axis of rotation in flexion and extension. *Spine* 1991;16:S312–S318.

114. Haher TR, Bergman M, O'Brien M, et al. Instantaneous axis of rotation as a function of the three columns of the spine. *Spine* 1992; 17:S149–S154.

115. Ching RP, Tencer AF, Anderson PA, Daly CH. A comparison of residual stability in thoracolumbar spine fractures using neutral zone measurements. *J Orthop Res* 1995;13:533–541.

116. Slosar PJ Jr, Patwardhan A, Lorenz M, et al. The three dimensional instability patterns of the thoracolumbar burst fracture. Transactions of the 38th Annual Meeting of the Orthopedic Research Society, 1992; 17:67.

117. Willen J, Lindahl S, Irstam L, Aldman B, Nordwall A. The thoracolumbar crush fracture, An experimental study on instant axial dynamic loading: The resulting fracture type and its stability. *Spine* 1984;9:624–631.

118. Neumann P, Nordwall A, Osvalder A-L. Traumatic instability of the lumbar spine. A dynamic in vitro study of flexion-distraction injury. *Spine* 1995;20:1111–1121.

119. Gurr KR, McAfee PC, Warden KE, Shih C-M. Roentgenographic and biomechanical analysis of lumbar fusions: a canine model. *J Orthop Res* 1989;7:838–848.

120. Johnson CE II, Welch RD, Baker KJ, Ashman RB. Effect of spinal construct stiffness on short segment fusion mass incorporation. *Spine* 1995;20:2400–2407.

121. Nagel DA, Kramerss PC, Rahn BA, Cordey J, Perren SM. A paradigm of delayed union and nonunion in the lumbosacral joint. A study of motion and bone grafting of the lumbosacral spine in sheep. *Spine* 1991;16:553–559.

122. Kotani Y, Cunningham BW, Cappuccino A, Kaneda K, McAfee PA. The role of spinal instrumentation in augmenting lumbar posterolateral fusion. *Spine* 1996;21:278–285.

123. Craven TG, Carson WL, Asher MA, Robinson RG. The effects of implant stiffness on the bypassed bone mineral density and facet fusion stiffness of the canine spine. *Spine* 1994;19:1664–1673.

124. Quinnel RC, Stockdale HR. Some experimental observations on the influence of a single lumbar floating fusion on the remaining lumbar spine. *Spine* 1981;6:263–267.

125. Umehara S, Zindrick MR, Patwardhan AG, Vrbos L, Havey RM, Lorenz M. Postoperative sagittal malalignment in instrumented lumbar fusion causes abnormal loading of the adjacent segment. Transactions of the 43rd Annual Meeting of the Orthopedic Research Society, 1997:360.

126. Wolfinbarger L, Zhang Y, Adam B-LT, Sutherland V, Gates K, Brame B. A comprehensive study of physical parameters, biomechanical properties and statistical correlations of iliac crest bone wedges used in spinal fusion surgery, III. Multivariate regression analysis and practical formulas for strength prediction. *Spine* 1994;19:284–295.

127. Closkey RF, Lee CK, Parsons JR, Blaksin MF. Mechanics of interbody spinal fusion: analysis of critical bone graft area. Transactions of the 39th Annual Meeting of the Orthopedic Research Society, 1993:65.

128. Krodel A. Mechanical principles of compressive interbody fusion. *Spine* 1996;21:821–826.

129. Tencer AF, Hampton D, Eddy S. Biomechanical properties of threaded inserts for lumbar interbody spinal fusion. *Spine* 1995; 20:2408–2414.

130. Fredrickson BE, Mann KA, Yuan HA, Lubicky JP. Reduction of the intracranial fragment in experimental burst fractures. *Spine* 1988;13:267–271.

131. Harrington RM, Budorick T, Hoyt J, Anderson PA, Tencer AF. Biomechanics of indirect reduction of bone retropulsed into the spinal canal in vertebral fracture. *Spine* 1993;18:692–699.

132. Cain JE, DeJong JT, Dinenberg AS, Stefko RM, Platenburg RC, Lauerman WC. Pathomechanical analysis of thoracolumbar burst fracture reduction. *Spine* 1993;18:1647–1654.

133. Zou D, Yoo JU, Edwards WT, et al. Mechanics of anatomic reduction of thoracolumbar burst fractures. Comparison of distraction versus distraction plus lordosis in the anatomic reduction of the thoracolumbar burst fracture. *Spine* 1993;18:195–203.

134. Butler TE, Asher MA, Jayaraman G, Nunley PD, Robinson RG. The strength and stiffness of thoracic implant anchors in osteoporotic spines. *Spine* 1994;19:1956–1962.

135. Tencer AF, Self J, Allen BL Jr, Drummond D. Design and evaluation of a posterior laminar clamp spinal fixation system. *Spine* 1991; 16:910–918.

136. Coe JD, Herzig MA, Warden KE, McAfee PC. Load to failure of spinal implants in osteoporotic spines. A comparison study of pedicle screws, laminar hooks, and spinous process wires. Transactions of the 35th Annual Meeting of the Orthopedic Research Society, 1989;14:71.

137. Hilibrand AS, Moore DC, Graziano GP. The role of pediculolaminar fixation in compromised pedicle bone. *Spine* 1996;21:445–453.

138. Brantley AGU, Mayfield JK, Koeneman JB, Clark KR. The effects of pedicle screw fit. An in vitro study. *Spine* 1994;19:1752–1758.

139. Moran JM, Berg WS, Berry JL, Geiger JM, Steffe AD. Transpedicular screw fixation. *J Orthop Res* 1989;7:107–114.

140. Zindrick MR, Wiltse LL, Widell EH, et al. A biomechanical study of intrapeduncular screw fixation in the lumbosacral spine. *Clin Orthop* 1986;203:99–112.

141. Krag MH, Beynnan BD, Pope MH, et al. An internal fixator for posterior application to short segments of the thoracic, lumbar or lumbosacral spine. Design and testing. *Clin Orthop* 1986;203:75–98.

142. Olsewski JM, Simmons EH, Kallen FC, Mendel FC, Severin CM, Berens DL. Morphometry of the lumbar spine: anatomical perspectives related to transpedicular fixation. *J Bone Joint Surg* 1990; 72A:541–549.

143. Zindrick MR, Wiltse LL, Doornik A, et al. Analysis of the morphometric characteristics of the thoracic and lumbar pedicles. *Spine* 1987;12:160–166.

144. Misenhimer GR, Peek RD, Wiltse LL, Rothman SLG, Widel EH Jr. Anatomic analysis of pedicle canal and cancellous diameter related to screw size. *Spine* 1989;14:367–372.

145. Yamagata M, Kitahara H, Minami S, et al. Mechanical stability of the pedicle screw fixation systems for the lumbar spine. *Spine* 1992; 17:S51–S54.

146. Wittenberg RH, Shea M, Swartz DE, Lee KS, White AA III, Hayes WC. Importance of bone mineral density in instrumented spinal fusions. *Spine* 1991;16:647–652.

147. Halvorson TL, Kelley LA, Thomas KA, Whitecloud TS III, Cook SD. Effects of bone mineral density on pedicle screw fixation. *Spine* 1994;19:2415–2420.

148. Myers BS, Belmont PJ, Richardson WJ, Yu JR, Harper KD, Nightingale RW. The role of imaging and in situ biomechanical testing in assessing pedicle screw pullout strength. *Spine* 1996;17:1962–1968.

149. Wu S-S, Edwards WT, Zou D, Ordway NR, Fay LA, Yuan HA. Transpedicular vertebral screws in human vertebrae: effect on screw-vertebra interface stiffness. Transactions of the 38th Annual Meeting of the Orthopedic Research Society, 1992;17:459.

150. George DC, Krag MH, Johnson CC, van Hal ME, Haugh LD, Grobler LJ. Hole preparation techniques for transpedicle fixation. Effects on pullout strength from human cadaveric vertebrae. *Spine* 1991; 16:181–184.

151. Kwok AWL, Finkelstein JA, Woodside T, Hearn TC, Hu RW. Insertional torque and pull-out strengths of conical and cylinderical pedicle screws in cadaveric bone. *Spine* 1996;21:2429–2434.

152. Law M, Tencer AF, Anderson PA. Mechanism of loosening of pedicle screws. *Spine* 1993;18:2438–2443.

153. Hasegawa HT, Takahashi HE, Washio T, et al. Structural changes in the pedicle and its fracture risk by pedicle screwing in osteoporotic spine. Transactions of the 43rd Annual Meeting of the Orthopedic Research Society, 1997:372.

154. Ashman RB, Galpin RD, Corin JD, Johnston CE. Biomechanical analysis of pedicle screw instrumentation in a corpectomy model. *Spine* 1989;14:1398–1405.

155. Snyder BD, Zaltz I, Hall JE, Emans JB. Predicting the integrity of vertebral bone screw fixation in anterior spinal instrumentation. *Spine* 1995;20:1568–1574.

156. Horton WC, Blackstock SF, Norman JT, Hill CS, Feiertag MA, Hutton WC. Strength of fixation of anterior body screws. *Spine* 1996;21:439–444.

157. Krag MH. Biomechanics of thoracolumbar spinal fixation. A review. *Spine* 1991;16:S85–S98.

158. Nachemsen A, Elfstrom G. Intravital wireless telemetry of axial forces in Harrington distraction rods in patients with idiopathic scoliosis. *J Bone Joint Surg* 1971;53A:445–465.

159. Gaines RW, Carson WL, Satterlee CC, Groh GI. Experimental evaluation of seven different fracture internal fixation devices using non failure stability testing. *Spine* 1991;16:902–909.

160. Ferguson RL, Tencer AF, Woodard PL, Allen BL Jr. Biomechanical comparisons of spinal fracture models and the stabilizing effects of posterior instrumentations. *Spine* 1988;13:453–460.

161. Rohlmann A, Bergmann G, Graichen F, Mayer H-M. Telemeterized load measurement using instrumented spinal internal fixators in a patient with degenerative instability. *Spine* 1995;20:2683–2689.

162. Shea M, Edwards WT, Clothiaux PL, et al. Three dimensional load displacement properties of posterior lumbar fixation. *J Orthop Trauma* 1991;5:420–427.

163. Panjabi MM, Abumi K, Duranceau J, Crisco JJ. Biomechanical evaluation of spinal fixation devices: II. Stability provided by eight internal fixation devices. *Spine* 1988;13:1135–1140.

164. Gurr KR, McAfee PC, Shih C-M. Biomechanical analysis of anterior and posterior instrumentation systems after corpectomy. *J Bone Joint Surg* 1988;70A:1182–1191.

165. Gurwitz GG, Dawson JM, McNamara MJ, Federspeil CF, Spengler DM. Biomechanical analysis of three surgical approaches for lumbar burst fractures using short segment instrumentation. *Spine* 1993; 18:977–982.

166. Slosar PJ, Patwardhan AG, Lorenz M, Havey R, Sartori M. Instability of the lumbar burst fracture and limitations of transpedicular instrumentation. *Spine* 1995;20:1452–1461.

167. An HS, Lim T-H, You J-W, Hong JH, Eck J, McGrady L. Biomechanical evaluation of anterior thoracolumbar spinal instrumentation. *Spine* 1995;20:1979–1983.

168. Chiba M, Mclain RF, Yerby SA, Moseley TA, Smith TS, Benson DR. Short-segment pedicle instrumentation. Biomechanical analysis of supplemental hook fixation. *Spine* 1996;21:288–294.

169. Wittenberg RH, Shea M, Edwards WT, Swartz DE, White AA III, Hayes WC. A biomechanical study of the fatigue characteristics of thoracolumbar fixation implants in a calf spine model. *Spine* 1992;17:S121–S128.

170. Goel VK, Hitchon PW, Grosland NM, Rogge TN, Sairyo K, Serhan HA. Comparative kinematics of a collapsible and rigid anterior devices. Transactions of the 43rd Annual Meeting of the Orthopedic Research Society, 1997:382.

171. Cunningham BW, Sefter JC, Shono Y, McAfee PC. Static and cyclical biomechanical analysis of pedicle screw spinal constructs. *Spine* 1993;18:1677–1688.

172. Licht NJ, Rowe DE, Ross LM. Pitfalls of pedicle screw fixation in the sacrum. *Spine* 1992;17:892–896.

173. Carlson GD, Abitbol JJ, Anderson DR, et al. Screw fixation in the human sacrum. *Spine* 1992;17:S194–S203.

174. Smith SA, Abitbol JJ, Anderson DR, Carlson GD, Taggart KW, Garfin SR. The effects of depth of penetration, screw orientation, and bone density on sacral screw fixation. Transactions of the 38th Annual Meeting of the Orthopedic Research Society, 1992;17:462.

175. McCord DH, Cunningham BW, Shono Y, Myers JJ, McAfee PC. Biomechanical analysis of lumbosacral fixation. *Spine* 1992; 17:S235–S242.

176. Puno RM, Bechtold JE, Byrd JA III, Winter RB, Ogilvie JW, Bradford DS. Biomechanical analysis of transpedicular rod systems. A preliminary report. *Spine* 1991;16:973–980.

177. McCord DH, Cunningham BW, Shono Y, Myers JJ, McAfee PC. Biomechanical analysis of lumbosacral fixation. *Spine* 1992; 17:S235–S243.

178. Glazer PA, Colliou O, Lotz JC, Bradford DS. Biomechanical analysis of lumbosacral fixation. *Spine* 1996;21:1211–1222.

179. Mow VC, Hayes WC. *Basic Orthopedic Biomechanics.* New York: Raven Press, 1991.

180. Adams MA, Hutton WC. The mechanical function of the lumbar apophyseal joints. *Spine* 1983;8:327–330.

181. Woo SL-Y, An K-N, Arnoczky SP, Wayne JS, Fithian DC, Myers BS. Anatomy, biology anf biomechanics of tendon, ligament, and meniscus. In: Simon SR (ed). *Orthopedic Basic Science.* Chicago: American Academy of Orthopedic Surgeons, 1994;45:87.

182. McElhaney JH, Myers BS. Biomechanical aspects of cervical trauma. In: Nahum AM, Melvin JW (eds). *Accidental Injury.* New York: Springer Verlag, 1993;311–361.

183. Shono Y, McAfee PC, Cunningham BW. The pathomechanics of compression injuries in the cervical spine. *Spine* 1993;18: 2009–2019.

184. Evans DC. Biomechanics of spinal injury. In: Gonza ER, Harrington IJ (eds). *Biomechanics of Musculoskeletal Injury.* Baltimore: Williams & Wilkins, 1982:31–86.

Surgery of Spinal Trauma,
edited by J.M. Cotler, J.M. Simpson, H.S. An, and C.P. Silveri.
Lippincott Williams & Wilkins, Philadelphia © 2000.

CHAPTER 4

Initial Evaluation and Management of the Spinal Injured Patient

Douglas C. Sutton, Christopher P. Silveri, and Jerome M. Cotler

Spinal trauma and spinal cord injuries are a major cause of disability in today's society. The goals of management of acute spinal trauma include (i) preservation of life, (ii) preservation of intact neurologic function, (iii) restoration of spinal stability and prevention of spinal deformity, (iv) treatment of associated injuries and prevention of complications, (v) enhancement of neurologic recovery, and (vi) facilitational of functional recovery. This chapter presents an overview of the protocols used for the evaluation and treatment of spinal trauma based on principles derived from our senior author's (JMC) many years of experience with the Regional Spinal Cord Injury Center of Delaware Valley (RSCICDV) and represents the knowledge accumulated during the treatment of more than 3,000 patients. Because spinal cord injury is not a reportable condition, the true incidence is unknown. It is estimated that the incidence of spinal cord injury is between 30 and 40 per million of population (1). Falls continue to be the leading cause of spinal cord injury in the population served by the RSCICDV (1). Gunshot wounds have increased steadily through the last number of years and now equal automobile accidents as the second leading cause of injury (1). Spinal cord injuries most commonly occur in persons in the age range between 15 and 30 years (1). However, the aging trends of our population has been associated with a concomitant increase in

the percentage of patients older than 60 years of age admitted with spinal cord injuries. Data obtained from the RSCICDV suggests that persons with spinal cord injury have a better opportunity for decreasing the associated morbidity and mortality if referred to a comprehensive spinal cord injury center within 72 hours of injury (1). A review from the RSCICDV during the period between 1990 and 1994 demonstrated the average length of stay for patients admitted within 72 hours of injury was 82.8 days versus 120.6 days for persons who were admitted after 72 hours. This was associated with earlier return to the community, with estimated cost savings of approximately $74,000 for such patients. The mortality rate during the initial acute care and rehabilitation period at the RSCICDV is approximately 5.5%. The mortality is age related, with approximate rates of 22.7% in patients older than 60 years of age compared with 1.3% in patients 30 years or younger (1).

EMERGENCY EVALUATION

Evaluation and management of known or suspected spinal injury comprises a staged process. Proper management of unstable spine injuries begins with the evaluation and treatment of patients by emergency personnel in the field and continues with proper patient immobilization and transport to the emergency center. Maintaining a high index of suspicion is the key to prevention of further neurologic injury during transport. All patients with head or high energy trauma, neurologic deficit, or complaints of neck or back pain must be assumed to have a spine injury until proven otherwise. Particular attention must be given to the unconscious patient or patient who is obtunded from substance abuse who may

D.C. Sutton: 486 Golden Gate Drive, Richboro, Pennsylvania 18954.
    C.P. Silveri: Fair Oaks Orthopaedic Associates, Fairfax, Virginia 22033.
    J.M. Cotler: Department of Orthopaedic Surgery, Thomas Jefferson University Hospital, Philadelphia, Pennsylvania 19107.

lack protective reflex muscle tone, as 5% to 10% of these patients may have a significant spine injury (2). The most effective method of immobilization for transport is through supine positioning of the patient on a spine board combined with use of a hard cervical collar and sandbags taped to either side of the head and torso to prevent rotation (3). A hard collar alone provides adequate control of flexion and extension, but fails to control cervical rotation. A Philadelphia collar has been demonstrated to be significantly better at preventing sagittal and translational rotation when compared to other semirigid orthoses and is an excellent choice for the acute stabilization and transport of patients with suspected cervical spine injuries (4). If possible, the cervical collar should have an anterior opening if an emergent cricothyroidotomy is necessary for establishment or maintenance of an airway (5). The patient should be secured to the board by taping or strapping of the forehead, chest, and extremities. Sandbags are helpful in controlling rotation of the head and trunk. Patients usually are placed with the occiput resting on the spine board. The exception to this is children under 6 years of age in whom the head is disproportionately larger compared to the trunk and, therefore, placing a young child on this board would inappropriately flex the cervical spine. In this scenario, the spine board should have a cutout to allow recession of the occipital region, thereby placing the cervical spine in a more neutral alignment. If this type of board is unavailable, then placing a pad behind the child's shoulders and upper back should help align the cervical spine in a more neutral alignment (6). Conversely, occipital padding may be necessary in adults with larger trunks to prevent undue hyperextension. The general principle is to keep the cervical spine neutrally aligned with the body while the Philadelphia collar is placed. In general, patients should be positioned as outlined above as long as it does not cause any increase in pain or change in neurologic function (7). The key to successful and safe transport is centered on having a high index of suspicion for potential injury. When feasible, a neurologic examination is advisable before moving any patient suspected of having a cervical injury. Once the examination is completed, a cervical collar is placed on the patient. Log rolling is the preferred method of patient mobilization onto the spine board, during which care is taken to maintain the head and neck in line with the body. The patient should be prevented from further movement of the spine until evaluation by a physician and radiographs are obtained in the emergency room (8,9).

Advanced trauma life support guidelines mandate an awareness of potential spine injury during primary and secondary resuscitative measures. During the primary patient survey, which is completed in the field, any manipulation of patient's airway must be accompanied by inline manual traction to prevent inadvertent motion of the spine. Patients with high cervical spinal cord injury may require a ventilator and/or circulatory support. Although a detailed, exhaustive neurologic exam is delayed until the secondary survey, an initial general neurologic assessment should be included in the primary survey. Prompt and accurate diagnosis of spinal injuries in the emergency room is essential. Frequently, spinal injuries are missed during trauma resuscitation because attention is focused on more obvious or life-threatening injuries. In a review of 300 cervical spine injuries, Bohlman (10) reported that 100 injuries were initially missed in the emergency room. The most common cause of missed cervical spine injuries in the emergency room include multiple trauma, multiple noncontiguous fractures, and altered consciousness (coma, intoxication). Diagnostic delay ranged from 1 day to more than 1 year. As many as 3% to 16% of patients with evidence of cervical fracture also will have a noncontiguous spine fracture, the most common cervical pattern being a fracture of the C1–2 complex and a second remote subaxial cervical spine fracture (11–13). In an analogous fashion, those patients who present for evaluation with known or obvious spine injuries require a thorough screening for associated injuries (14). Almost 50% of patients with acute spinal cord injury have other significant skeletal or visceral injuries (15–19).

Soderstrom et al. (18) reviewed records of 288 patients sustaining blunt cervical spine injuries and found that 4.2% had sustained significant intraabdominal injuries. All of these abdominal injuries were occult and detected by peritoneal lavage, which is a diagnostic aide that is especially useful in patients whose physical examination is difficult. Peritoneal lavage is highly sensitive, and detecting injuries can be done quickly and has a low morbidity (18). Computed tomography (CT), which may be used in evaluation of the cervical spine, is less sensitive than peritoneal lavage in determination of intraabdominal injury. Thoracolumbar and lumbar spine injuries in pediatric patients also require special attention. Retroperitoneal injuries have been reported in 30% to 50% of patients in this population (20,21). In addition, it has been reported that 25% to 50% of pediatric spinal cord injuries may present with concomitant head trauma (22,23). Significant mortality rates also are noted in severe spinal cord injuries. Up to 40% of individuals sustaining traumatic quadriplegia may die within the first year (7). The elderly are especially prone to fatal outcomes, with preexisting medical factors and poor response to recumbency contributing to a 23% mortality rate in one study (24). Pneumonia, cardiovascular disease, and septicemia are leading causes of death (25).

In the emergency treatment, advanced trauma life support protocols prevail (26). Airway management remains the first priority in the care of these patients. If intubation is required, a lateral radiograph of the cervical spine is first recommended. However, initial imaging is not always feasible depending on the patient's status. If no radiograph is available, nasotracheal intubation with the head and neck stabilized in a neutral position is recommended. If a contraindication to nasotracheal intubation exists, a cricothyroidotomy should be performed. Fiberoptic intubation may be a helpful technique in these situations and may minimize the need for cervical manipulation.

Assessment of the patient's circulatory status then follows. Sites of obvious hemorrhage must be identified and controlled, while secondary assessment for occult blood loss is completed. Hemodynamic data may be difficult to interpret, especially in the presence of spinal shock with the resultant neurogenic hypotension. Cervical and upper thoracic cord lesions may compromise the descending sympathetic nervous system, resulting in significant hypotension. Loss of peripheral vascular tone directly reduces systemic vascular resistance, increases venous stasis in the extremities, and decreases the return of blood to the heart. The body's ability to react to the hemodynamic changes is absent and so too is the typical reflex increase in cardiac output. The patient remains hypotensive with associated bradycardia and often hypothermia as well (2,27). Hypotension due to hypovolemia or traumatic hemorrhage is accompanied by tachycardia and often responds to aggressive volume resuscitation. In neurogenic shock, however, fluid resuscitation must proceed with caution so as to avoid overload and congestive heart failure. If occult sites of hemorrhage are ruled out, then gentle fluid administration is accompanied by atropine for its vagolytic properties and dopamine and other cardiovascular pressors to increase systemic vascular resistance and directly increase cardiac output. Trendelenburg positioning will augment venous return to the heart, and central venous monitoring and Foley catheterization will facilitate the resuscitation process. Supplemental oxygen is recommended to provide adequate oxygenation and prevent tissue hypoxemia, which may be a cause of secondary neuronal injury (27).

Throughout the emergency room process, these patients are best managed through a team approach. The resuscitation is supervised by a member of the trauma service, where evaluation and treatment of any spine injury are carried out by a three-member spinal cord team composed of members of the orthopedic, neurosurgical, and physical medicine rehabilitation services. Each member of this team is responsible for evaluating the patient. Precise neurologic examination is critical in the initial and follow-up assessment of the patient's status, with accurate documentation being essential. Serial examination should be performed by one or more physicians with motor and sensory evaluation and level of function determined in a standardized fashion. The most popular established guidelines are those of the American Spinal Injury Association (ASIA) (28). The presence or absence of distal motor function cannot be determined accurately until spinal shock has been reversed, and this is heralded by the return of the bulbocavernosus reflex.

The primary survey in the emergency room should include notation of certain neurologic criteria. The patient's level of consciousness is important to appreciate in the first instance because, with concomitant head and spinal injuries, there may be subtle deterioration in the patient. Alertness, orientation, patient cooperation, and the ability to follow simple commands, as well as the ability to communicate, are all descriptors that require notation. The Glasgow Coma Scale is also a standard by which the level of consciousness can be assessed (Table 1). At the same time, brain stem function needs assessment, in addition to general motor function to determine the presence of any gross neurologic deficits. Pupil reaction, response to painful stimuli, posturing, flaccid extremities, signs of incontinence, and priapism need to be documented. Perianal neurologic examination is most important in the evaluation of trauma patient and is important for the determination of the existing level of injury, completeness of neurologic damage, and subsequent potential return of function. The presence of perianal sensation, proprioception, and/or function indicates an incomplete lesion with function below the level of injury. Continued neurologic recovery, although possible, can only be estimated. Contraction of the bulbocavernosus reflex, which heralds the resolution of spinal shock, itself has no prognostic value. It is believed that the return of the bulbocavernosus reflex imparts a favorable prognostic indicator, as it may represent activity of the sacral myelomere and potential for neurologic improvement more cephalad. The exception to this is in a thoracolumbar injury at the level of the conus medullaris. Direct injury to the sacral cell bodies within the cord may not allow for the return of this reflex arc.

A careful neurologic exam in the emergency room is required, and additional confirmatory examination should be performed by consulting services. The lowest functioning neurologic level must be documented and any change or loss in neurologic function observed by other physicians or nursing staff reported immediately. Once the initial surveys have been completed, the patient then may be log rolled and each region of the spine palpated for interspinous ligament tenderness, spinous process tenderness, paraspinal muscle tenderness, ecchymosis, abrasions, or other signs of both obvious or occult trauma.

TABLE 1. *Glasgow Coma Scale*

	Response	Score
Eyes open	Spontaneous	4
	To sound	3
	To pain	2
	Never	1
Verbal response	Oriented	5
	Confused conversation	4
	Inappropriate words	3
	Incomprehensible words	2
	None	1
Motor response	Obeys commands	6
	Localizes pain	5
	Flexion withdrawal	4
	Abnormal	3
	Extension	2
	None	1

Adapted from Teasdale G, Jennett B. Assessment and prognosis of coma after head injury. *Acta Neurochineg* 1976; 34:45. Reproduced with permission from HS An, JM Simpson (eds). *Surgery of the Cervical Spine.* United Kingdom: Martin Dunitz Limited, 1994:104.

After the initial resuscitative measures, a complete history of the mechanism of injury should be obtained. If the patient is unresponsive, a detailed history must be obtained from family, friends, witnesses, emergency medical services, or police personnel. Reconstruction of the events leading up to the incident can provide the appropriate details needed to understand the forces involved and the mechanism of injury, both of which will allow the physicians to anticipate possible instability and jeopardy to the spinal cord.

Information gathered from the observations of the emergency medical service personnel at the scene also adds to the history. Position of the patient when found, the level of consciousness, victim's initial complaints, and degree of motor function contribute to the history of the event. Occasionally, the patient may have transient paraplegia or paralysis secondary to concussion of the spinal cord, which recovers before arriving at the emergency room. If the patient is conscious, a detailed history of the incident should precede further evaluation. This should include type of injury, blunt versus deceleration injury, level of consciousness, short- and long-term memory loss, dizziness, location of pain, numbness, paresthesia, or fasciculation at or since the time of the incident. If sudden flexion/extension forces were involved, the patient should recount experience of acute sensory or motor symptoms in the extremities or an "electric" shock sensation at the time of the accident.

Past medical history that is significant for preexisting cervical spinal pathology, such as ankylosing spondylitis or predisposing kyphosis, is important to note. Cervical spondylosis with congenital or rheumatologic causes of instability are important factors in predisposing the spinal cord to immediate injury with subsequent low tolerance for further motion as a result of the decreased space available for the cord. With the space available for the cord already compromised, sudden angular or translational movements may cause cord contusion with varying neurologic sequelae.

Inspection is critical in the initial management of the acutely injured patient. Although the patient may be unconscious, much can be derived from the general posture of the patient. The presence of maxillofacial trauma, lacerations, or other injury above the level of the clavicle, as well as ventilation difficulties, should lend suspicion to potential spine injury.

Neurologic examination is again performed with careful attention for accurate measurements of both motor and sensory levels. Muscle strength is graded as follows: 0 for paralysis, 1 for palpable visible contractions, 2 for range of motion in a gravity eliminated fashion, 3 for active range of motion against gravity without resistance, 4 for active range of motion with some resistance, and 5 for against range of motion with full resistance. Sensory evaluation is done to both sharp-dull discrimination as well as light touch. Proprioception also can be helpful when looking at dorsal columns. Patients then can be given a motor index score according to the ASIA scale, which provides a numerical grading system to document improvement or deterioration of function (26).

Motor score is graded bilaterally for the cervical C5–8 roots, T1, and lumbar L2–5 roots, and a total score based on individual ratings from 0 to 5 can be followed. The ASIA impairment scale places clinical presentation of spinal cord injury into one of five broad categories (29). An ASIA A stands for complete spinal cord injury with no sensory or motor function distal to the level of injury; B represents an incomplete spinal cord injury with preservation of sensation, but no motor function distal to the level of injury; C represents an incomplete spinal cord injury with motor function present below the level of injury with a motor grade of three or less; D represents an incomplete spinal cord injury with motor preservation greater than grade III below the level of injury; and E represents a normal neurologic evaluation. There are essentially two types of spinal cord injury: complete and incomplete. With complete injuries, little or no neurologic return is expected. No injury may be considered complete until spinal shock has resolved. The bulbocavernosus reflex, which is elicited by genital stimulation and produces anal contraction, is used to determine the absence of spinal shock. If no motor or sensory function is present in the absence of spinal shock, the injury is considered complete. The determination of complete injury usually can be made within the first 24 to 72 hours after injury.

Incomplete spinal cord syndromes are characterized by the presence of some function below the level of injury. Classically, these have been divided into four syndromes: the anterior cord syndrome, central cord syndrome, posterior cord syndrome, and the Brown-Séquard syndrome. Some patients will present with isolated nerve root dysfunction.

The anterior cord syndrome is usually the result of compression and/or flexion injuries to the spine. This syndrome is characterized by injury to the anterior horn cells opposite the area of the spinal injury with alteration of anterolateral white matter column function controlling pain and temperature sensation. The posterior columns and posterior horn areas of the gray matter are variously spared, controlling deep pressure and posterior sensation. This syndrome carries the poorest prognosis, with return to motor function being rare.

The central cord syndrome is common and typically involves an extension injury in an older patient with underlying spondylitic changes. A central hematomyelia results producing cord injury in the central gray matter where the motor horn cells for the upper extremities are housed. At this level, motor and sensory impulses in the sacral segments of the spinal cord are in the peripheral white matter and may be preserved, thus providing sacral sensation. Upper extremity weakness is more pronounced than lower extremity weakness. Patients with this syndrome will experience variable return to function, but some degree of spasticity is likely.

The Brown-Séquard syndrome has the best prognosis of all incomplete syndromes. This syndrome is caused by transverse hemisection of the cord and results in weakness and proprioceptive sensory loss on the side of injury, with pain and temperature loss on the contralateral side. Stab wounds and other penetrating trauma are the most common cause.

TABLE 2. *Incomplete spinal cord injuries*

Syndrome	Physical findings	Prognosis
Anterior cord	Motor loss Pain and temperature loss	Poor
Central cord	Weakness in upper extremities, lower extremities Perianal sensation preserved	Variable return
Brown-Séquard	Ipsilateral paralysis Contralateral pain and temperature loss	Good
Posterior cord	Motor function usually preserved Sensory function lost	Unknown

Reproduced with permission from HS An, JM Simpson (eds). *Surgery of the Cervical Spine.* United Kingdom: Martin Dunitz Limited, 1994:163.

Brown-Séquard syndrome caused by blunt trauma has a favorable prognosis for neurologic recovery.

The posterior cord syndrome is rare. With this injury, the posterior column sustains the brunt of the injury, preserving motor function, but there is associated loss of sensation below the level of injury. The prognosis for this injury is uncertain (Table 2).

RADIOGRAPHIC EVALUATION

The initial radiographic assessment of the spine consists of a mandatory cross-table lateral radiograph demonstrating the base of the skull, all seven cervical vertebrae, and the superior endplate of T-1. Anteroposterior and lateral radiographs also are obtained of the cervical, thoracic, and lumbar spine. Although the cross-table lateral radiograph is an excellent screening tool that, by itself, will diagnose 70% to 79% of all cervical spine injuries, a full cervical spine series is indicated in all patients suspected of cervical injury (30). A complete cervical spine series consists of lateral, trauma views or obliques, anteroposterior, and open-mouth views, which will diagnose 90% to 95% of all cervical spine injuries (31–34). In patients with large shoulders and/or short necks, it often is difficult to visualize the C7–T1 junction on a lateral film, and it may be necessary either to apply traction through the arms or to obtain a swimmer's view (35–37). Unconscious or uncooperative patients, and those with upper extremity fractures, may require computed or conventional tomography to evaluate fully the cervicothoracic junction.

In evaluating the lateral radiograph, four lines are drawn or visualized to ensure normal anatomic relationships, including the anterior spinal line, the posterior spinal line, the spinal laminar line, and the basilar line of Wackenheim (Fig. 1) (38). The anterior and posterior spinal lines course along the anterior and posterior margins of the vertebral bodies, respectively, forming continuous smooth lines. The overall contour should be a gently sloping lordosis in the cervical spine, kyphosis in the thoracic spine, and lordosis in the lumbar spine. The spinolaminar line is drawn, connecting the posterior aspect of the foramen magnum to the anterior cortex of each spinous process, and it also should be a smooth lordotic curve. There is one normal variation in this line, of which the interpreter must be aware. The spinolaminar line of C-2 may lie 2 to 3 mm posterior to that of C-3, but this is normal. The basilar line of Wackenheim lies along the posterior surface of the clivus and is at a tangent to the posterior cortex of the odontoid tip. This relationship is important in evaluating cranial vertebral relationships.

Additionally, lateral radiographic evaluation should include scrutiny of vertebral body height, articular pillars, alignment of the articular facets, interspinous widening, and spinous process fracture. The articular pillars are rhomboid in shape in the cervical spine, and the two pillars of any one vertebra should be superimposed on a true lateral view. With an absence of this normal relationship, the observer should be alert to the possibility of fracture or facet dislocation. The interspinous distance below the level of C-3 should be almost equal. An increased distance usually indicates posterior ligamentous injury. Translation greater than 3.5 mm and angulation greater than 11 degrees are regarded as unstable (39).

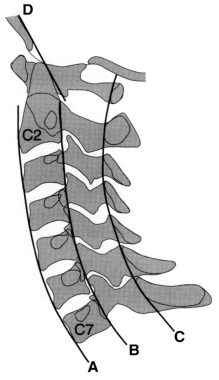

FIG. 1. Schematic view of the lateral cervical spine and its normal bony relationships. Line A, anterior spinal line. Line B, posterior spinal line. Line C, spinolaminar line, which connects the foramen magnum with the anterior aspect of each spinous process. Line D, basilar line of Wackenheim, which lies along the posterior clivus tangent to the posterior odontoid and defines craniocervical relationships.

The prevertebral (retropharyngeal) soft tissue should be evaluated on the lateral radiograph. A prevertebral soft tissue space measuring between 7 and 10 mm at C-2 indicates a possible abnormality, and additional studies should be considered. When this soft tissue space is larger than 10 mm, the patient must be considered to have a cervical injury and further workup is required (40).

The role of flexion/extension lateral radiographs in an emergency room setting remains controversial. Active motion flexion and extension radiographs may be useful in the alert, cooperative patient without neurologic deficit who complains of neck pain. In this setting, a positive flexion/extension study has obvious clinical implications, but a negative film does not rule out an acute injury. Patients with acute cervical spine injury may have muscle spasm that masks cervical instability for up to 2 to 3 weeks (41). Therefore, despite a negative study, for any patient in whom the index of suspicion is sufficiently high to obtain flexion/extension films, immobilization in a rigid cervical orthosis is recommended, and follow-up films are taken in 2 to 3 weeks.

The spinous processes also may be viewed on the anteroposterior radiograph for evidence of rotation or interspinous widening. An abrupt shift in position of any one spinous process may indicate a fracture of the articular pillar or dislocation of the associated facet joint. A widened interspinous distance 1.5 times that above or below the questionably injured segment indicates an anterior dislocation (42). The lateral border of the spine normally has an uninterrupted, wavy appearance. The facet joints themselves should not be seen on an anteroposterior projection. If a space is identified on this view, fracture of the pedicle or articular mass with subsequent rotation must be suspected. Open-mouth views are used in evaluation of the upper cervical spine. Characteristic abnormalities are detailed further in Chapter 7.

Computed tomography is an excellent method of evaluation in patients with spine injuries. Its advantages include speed, availability, supine position, axial imaging, and excellent cortical detail. As a result of the cost and relatively high dose of radiation, however, it should not be used as a screening modality. Rather, use of CT should be reserved to delineate the bony anatomy of fracture seen or suspected on plain radiographs, and for cases in which spinal anatomy cannot be adequately visualized. Scanning should consist of 2- to 3-mm consecutive images and include at least one vertebra above and below the suspected level of injury. In patients with neurologic deficit and no obvious fracture on plain radiographs, CT scanning can be used and should include one level above or below the level of neurologic deficit. Conventional tomography, for the most part, has been replaced by computerized scanning for the diagnosis of spinal fractures. However, plain tomography is used for the diagnosis of minimally displaced horizontal fractures. Horizontal fracture of the odontoid or facets may be missed on axial oriented computer tomograms and sagittal reconstructions, but are often well delineated on anteroposterior and lateral tomograms. Tomograms also are useful in the evaluation of the cervicothoracic junction and in the postoperative evaluation of graft placement and healing. Again, the usefulness of conventional tomography is becoming less frequent with the further improvements in axial reconstructions on CT.

Magnetic resonance imaging has become a popular modality in evaluating spine trauma and the spinal cord injury patient. In many ways it has revolutionized our ability to determine the extent of cervical spine and spinal cord injury (38,43,44). It generally has replaced myelography as a diagnostic tool in spine trauma. Advantages of magnetic resonance imaging (MRI) include lack of ionizing radiation, direct multiplane image capabilities, ability to detect noncontiguous fractures, and, most importantly, the ability to determine the degree of soft tissue injury, including the intervertebral disc, spinal cord, and ligamentous structures. Recent studies have demonstrated the incidents of disc injury complicating cervical spine trauma significantly higher than initially thought, and as more than 50% in some injury patterns (45–48). Magnetic resonance imaging is not only capable of accurately depicting the presence of injury to these structures, but it is able to quantitate the degree of injury to these structures as well (49–52). T2-weighted images are best for visualizing the spinal cord (50–52). Imaging signals, consisting of intramedullary hematoma and/or spinal cord contusion associated with edema, encompassing more than one spinal segment, has been shown to be associated with more severe neurologic deficits (50–52). Less severe injuries have been correlated with normal spinal cord signal and edema encompassing one segment or less (52). Whether this will be a useful modality to establish long-term prognosis remains uncertain. Magnetic resonance imaging is indicated in the following cases: (i) all patients with complete or incomplete neurologic deficits to search for and quantify the degree of spinal cord compression; (ii) any patient in whom the neurologic status deteriorates; and (iii) cases in which there is suspicion of posterior ligamentous injury despite negative plain radiographs. Currently, CT provides greater detail of bony anatomy; therefore, patients may require both computed tomograms and MRI scans. In the future, MRI may provide cortical detail equivalent to CT and, therefore, obviate the need for a second study. The disadvantages of MRI include relatively long acquisition time, limited availability in some institutions, and contraindications. Magnetic resonance imaging is contraindicated in patients with pacemakers, aneurysm clips, metallic fragments in the eye or spinal cord, and severe claustrophobia. Furthermore, ventilator support and cardiac monitoring of patients during MRI scanning must be accomplished with nonferromagnetic equipment.

EARLY MANAGEMENT CONSIDERATIONS IN CERVICAL SPINE INJURIES

There are many aspects of patient care that require early consideration in spinal injury. Once the patient's medical status is secured and diagnostic radiographic studies obtained, the stability or instability of the spine must be recognized, deformity and subluxation reduced and immobilized, and complications associated with spinal injury averted. The understanding of these topics is imperative to proper and successful management.

STABILITY

The concept of spinal stability, in many respects, is vague. Radiographic measurements of translation and angulatory abnormalities are helpful, but they are limited in the ability to recognize potential for neurologic injury in many fracture patterns. Spinal stability has been defined as "the ability of the spine under physiologic loads to maintain the relationship between vertebrae in such a way that there is neither initial nor subsequent damage to the spinal cord or nerve roots." Based on multifactorial considerations that determine stability, White et al. (39) suggested that a checklist of dynamic and static radiographic criteria and neurologic findings be used (Table 3). These criteria are particularly helpful in equivocal cases of instability, but they are not required in the vast majority of presenting spinal injuries. In brief, any of the following situations must be considered to represent an unstable injury of the spine: anterior and posterior column injury; any structural injury with injury to the spinal cord; and

TABLE 3. *Checklist for the diagnosis of clinical instability in the middle and lower cervical spine*

Element	Point value
Anterior elements destroyed or unable to function	2
Posterior elements destroyed or unable to function	2
Positive stretch test	2
Radiographic criteria	4
A. Flexion extension radiographs	
1. Sagittal plane translation >3.5 mm or 20% (2 pts)	
2. Sagittal plane rotation >20 degrees (2 pts)	
or	
B. Resting radiographs	
1. Sagittal plane displacement >3.5 mm or 20% (2 pts)	
2. Relative sagittal plane angulation >11 degrees (2 pts)	
Abnormal disc narrowing	1
Developmentally narrow spinal canal	1
1. Sagittal diameter <13 mm	
or	
2. Pavlov's ratio <0.8	
Spinal cord damage	2
Nerve root damage	1
Dangerous loading anticipated	1
Total of 5 or more = unstable	

Reproduced with permission from AA White, MM Panjabi. The problem of clinical instability in the human spine: a systematic approach. In: *Clinical Biomechanics of the Spine.* Philadelphia: JB Lippincott, 1987:314.

gross deformity of the spine with or without neurologic involvement. The classification schemes described by Holdsworth (53), Allen et al. (54), and Denis (55) help us to determine the applied forces responsible for injury and the extent of structural damage to the spine. These classifications may help the clinician in determining stability and treatment options.

REDUCTION AND IMMOBILIZATION OF CERVICAL INJURY

Cervical immobilization is required for any patient suspected of being injured. A rigid cervical orthosis is required while diagnostic studies are completed. When radiographs reveal significant osseous or ligamentous injury, it is preferable to immobilize the cervical spine by application of cervical traction. For most injuries, the authors prefer application of MRI-compatible Gardner-Wells tongs (Zimmer, Inc., Warsau, IN) with pins placed neutral or 1 cm behind the external auditory canal, and just above the pinna. Pins placed in front of this point will exert an extension moment on the spine whereas those placed behind will impart a flexion moment. In the emergency room, patients are placed on a manual turning frame (Stryker Corp., Kalamazoo, MI) and on admission to the intensive care unit are transferred to an automatic rotating bed. Positioning on a rotating bed allows for weight transfer and prevention of pressure points in areas at risk for skin breakdown. The rotating beds also allow for posterior hatches for examination of each region of the spine that can be opened sequentially for skin care without risking instability. It also allows for care of the peroneal region through removal of the sacral hatches. The weight required for immobilization of cervical spine injuries must be tailored to the individual injury, but, in most cases, 10–15 lbs of weight is sufficient. The posttraction alignment of the spine should always be checked after application of weight with plain radiographs as well as by neuromuscular assessment. In those cases where timing or logistics of the trauma resuscitation precludes thorough evaluation or application of traction, the patient should be maintained in this rigid cervical orthosis. Spinal deformity resulting from spinal injury is not only capable of causing the initial spinal cord injury, but also may be responsible for ongoing neurologic compromise via the destructive cycle of vascular compromise and edema.

Therefore, attempt at closed reduction is indicated in all cases of cervical spine injury demonstrating shortening, angulation, and/or translation. The goal of closed reduction is restoration of normal spinal alignment, which may result in decompression of the spinal canal, enhance neurologic recovery, restore the stability of intact bony elements, and prevent further neurologic injury. Many animal and several recent clinical studies demonstrated that the extent of neurologic recovery is influenced by the duration and length of neurologic compression (56–62).

Closed reduction should be attempted as rapidly as possible on admission to the hospital. Closed reduction must always be attempted in a closely supervised setting, with vigilant radiographic and neurologic monitoring. Patients should be awake, alert, and cooperative during an attempt at closed reduction to provide feedback during the procedure. Reduction is accomplished via a combination of skeletal traction, patient positioning, and postural bumps and wedges. The patient should be placed on a Stryker frame and Gardner-Wells tongs applied as previously described. Reduction begins with 10 lbs of applied traction and is increased by 4.5 kg in a sequential fashion at 10- to 20-minute intervals until an acceptable reduction is achieved. Evaluation of vertebral distraction is performed after each incremental change in the traction weight (Fig. 2). A lateral cervical spine radiograph is taken 5 to 10 minutes after the weight change. The patient's neurologic status is evaluated after each weight change through either the patient's ability to perform an established motor function or a change in sensory level. After reduction is achieved, the weight is reduced to 4.5 to 9.0 kg, and repeat lateral radiographs are obtained to confirm maintenance of reduction. Use of MRI-compatible tongs is preferred, unless a high weight reduction (approximately 30 kg or 70 lb) reduction is anticipated. Stronger stainless steel tip pins should then be used, as the MRI-compatible pins will undergo plastic deformation. The role of manipulation during closed reduction is controversial. It should be reserved for those familiar with its indications and techniques and should be utilized when the facets are perched and will not reduce. The weight required for reduction of an individual cervical spine injury is highly variable, and the maximum amount of weight that can be applied safely is not known (12). Attempt at closed reduction should be discontinued when (i) the spine is reduced; (ii) more than 1 cm of distraction occurs at the zone of injury and/or another location, or if the tip to tip position of the dislocated facets have fully been distracted; (iii) the patient's neurologic status deteriorates; or (iv) the physician believes additional attempts have little or no chance of success. Closed reduction has been achieved successfully in up to 90% to 95% of cases (63). Following successful closed reduction, preoperative alignment of the spine usually can be maintained with 4.5 to 6.7 kg of axial traction, but dictates that the patient remain in a supine position. In selected injury patterns, preoperative immobilization of unstable fractures in a halo vest is a safe and effective technique in maintaining reduction while facilitating patient mobilization, nursing care, and pulmonary toilet. However, close patient monitoring with serial radiographs is necessary to recognize any recurrent displacement (64). An MRI-compatible halo vest orthosis allows for further diagnostic intervention that may be required. Open reduction is indicated if acceptable vertebral alignment cannot be achieved closed (Figs. 2 and 3) and in most cases requires anterior and posterior decompression.

HALO APPLICATION

A halo fixation device has been used for cervical spine immobilization since it was first introduced by Perry and Nickel in 1959 to immobilize patients paralyzed by poliomyelitis (65,66). Today, the halo is mainly used to provide immobilization in conditions of spinal trauma or following a reconstructive procedure of the cervical spine. Compared with conventional orthoses, the halo has been shown to be more effective in restricting cervical motion and maintaining cervical alignment. In addition, numerous attachments to the support structure in custom vest designs allow rigid immobilization in more complex deformity patterns. However, up to 30% of normal cervical spine motion has been reported even after stabilization with the halo device (67). Therefore, careful attention to detail is necessary to reduce excess motion and complications and to maximize results. The advantages of using a halo in patients requiring cervical spine immobilization include the physical and psychological benefits of early mobilization, avoidance of complications associated with prolonged bed rest, shorter hospitalization and rehabilitation stays, and less interference with mandibular motion and eating. The halo also has the advantage of allowing the patient to be able to position the neck more precisely in the preferred alignment to counteract the forces of any instability present.

Our indications for halo use include unstable injuries of the upper cervical spine such as odontoid fractures, hangman's fractures and Jefferson fractures. Use of the halo for lower cervical spine injuries is not as well defined. Our preference has been to use the halo for unstable injury patterns whether the injuries are being treated operatively or nonoperatively. It cannot be overemphasized that nonsurgical management of cervical spine injuries and instability requires careful follow-up, because failure rates may range from 10% to 40% depending on the specific injury pattern (68–70).

Successful halo application is dependent on many factors to minimize complications. A thorough understanding of the desired final head and neck position is necessary to minimize any potential deforming forces that may result in loss of alignment. The head and neck position should be dictated by

FIG. 2. Serial reduction of a unilateral facet dislocation. **A:** Lateral radiograph of C4–5 unilateral facet dislocation. Note the posterior position of the traction tongs to allow for a flexion moment during reduction. **B:** Weights are added beginning with 10 lb, in 5- to 10-lb increments, to achieve reduction. In this case, 35 lb provides only disc space distraction. **C:** At 60 lb, reduction is achieved. Although distraction is significant as indicated by the spinous process widening, gross overdistraction of the disc space did not occur. The addition of weights in a serial judicious fashion will allow the practitioner to monitor the degree of distraction. **D:** Once reduction is achieved, the weights are lowered slowly while placing an extension moment on the cervical spine (best achieved by raising the patient's thoracic cavity). Immediate halo placement can occur or traction maintained.

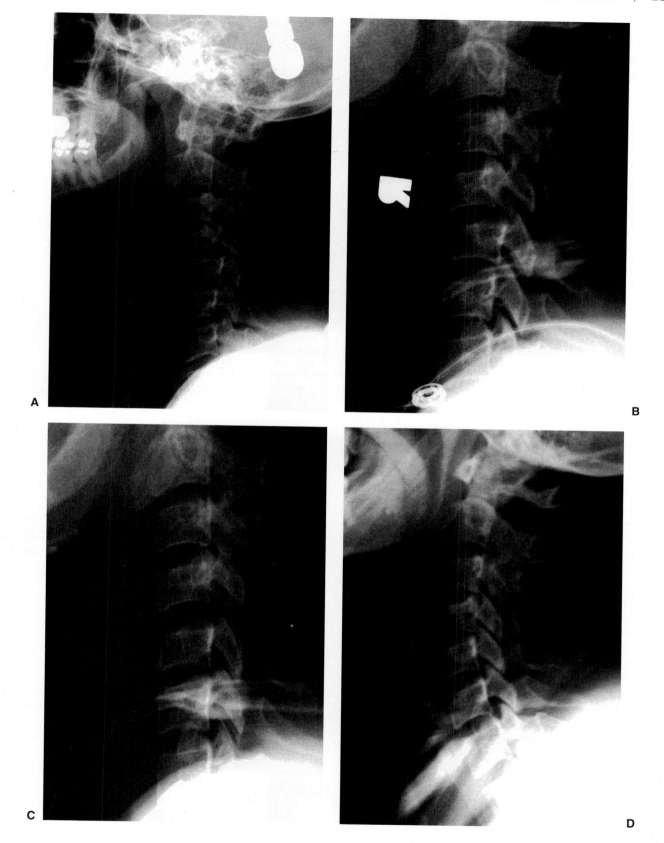

A

B

C

D

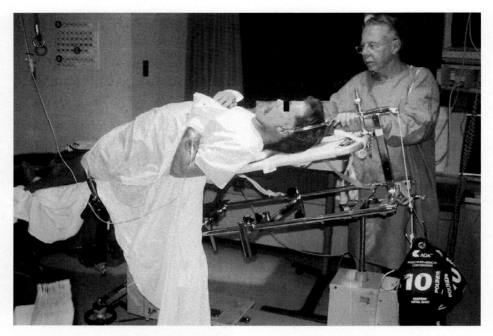

FIG. 3. Patient positioning for conscious closed reduction. The patient is alert, supine on the Stryker frame in reverse Trendelenburg position to utilize the weight of the body to counteract the distraction force of the weights. Our senior author (JMC) is seen here monitoring each incremental weight increase, with serial neurologic examinations, and inspection of pin integrity and position.

the particular instability pattern and deformity present; therefore, achieving an acceptable final position can be obtained more reliably if the necessary help is available. Several devices are available to aid in supporting the head and neck (i.e., a narrow board) during the application process. Our preference has been to use a minimum of three individuals: one to support the head, neck, and halo ring and two additional assistants to apply the pins and vest. When possible, patients are premeasured for an appropriate vest size before application, and a full complement of ring sizes should be available at the time of application. The decision to use a closed or open posterior ring must be made, with an open ring being preferred if there is any potential for high posterior cervical or occipital cervical surgical intervention. Informed consent and discussion of the risks and benefits is conducted before each application. Generally, patients are awake during the application, except when applied intraoperatively following surgical reconstructive procedures. Patients should be placed in a bed that will allow access to the posterior occipital region. Our preference has been to use a Stryker frame or a rotating-type bed because of the ease of access to the posterior occipital region. In addition, these types of beds allow assistants supporting the head and ring to support their forearms on the bed frame, thereby minimizing fatigue during the application. The halo ring and pins should be sterilized. Standard sterile techniques are used during the application. The ring size is chosen to allow clearance of the ears while placing the ring "below the equator" or positioning the ring below the greatest circumference of the patient's skull so that any pressure will be directed up into bone and

not out of position, avoiding the "French beret." Temporary positioning pins may be used to help with provisional placement of the ring. Once the ring is positioned properly, the insertion sites are prepared with povidone iodide (Betadine) and the posterior occipital region is shaved of any excess hair. A 25-gauge needle is used to inject 1% lidocaine into the skin, subcutaneous tissues, and periosteum under the selected entry holes of the ring. Intramuscular intravenous narcotics may be used to supplement the local anesthesia. The pins are inserted percutaneously and are designed with a sharp point and a broad shoulder to avoid penetration of the skull. The anterior pins should be inserted as inferiorly as possible and close to the lateral supraorbital ridge to achieve the most perpendicular angle of insertion (71). The pins should enter the lateral two thirds "safe zone" (Fig. 4) over the eyebrow, avoiding the medial one third and thereby reducing the risk of injury to the supraorbital and supratrochlear nerves (72). Anterior pins should not be placed over the temporalis fossa to avoid impaling the temporalis muscle and possible injury to the temporal artery. As the anterior pins are being tightened, the patient's upper eyelids should be kept closed to avoid tension at the insertion site. Following insertion, the patient should demonstrate eye opening and closing to be certain that the skin of the forehead is not preventing the eyes from opening and closing. The posterior pins are placed in the occipital bone, allowing sufficient clearance for the ears. Excessive inferior placement of the posterior pins may impale the mastoid bone and upper cervical musculature, causing increased pin site pain and soft tissue complications. Once provisional fixation is achieved, the final tightening is performed by simultaneously tightening opposite pin sites, i.e., left anterior and right posterior, and right anterior and left posterior. The pins then are tightened to the final tension in this alternate fashion. A recent prospective randomized study found that the halo pin insertion torque had no significant effect on halo pin complications when comparing 6 versus 8 in.lb. Our current protocol therefore utilizes insertion of pins with 6 in.lb of torque (73). After initial application, the pins should be routinely retorqued 24 to 48 hours after insertion. Once the ring is secured, it can be attached to the vest, which preferably should be placed beneath the patient before ring attachment. If this is not possible, then the patient is carefully log rolled and a posterior vest and uprights are placed beneath the patient. The patient's alignment is maintained carefully during this maneuver. The anterior half then can be applied after the four uprights are connected to the ring and torqued to 28 to 32 in.lb. The connections of the uprights to the ring and the vest vary considerably among manufacturers; therefore, familiarization with these connections is mandatory before application of the halo. Likewise, several companies have attachments that permit additional anterior or posterior translation and greater flexion and extension moments through accessory attachments, allowing for a wider range of positioning of complex cervical deformities. Careful attention must be taken to protect and pad areas of bony prominence to avoid skin breakdown, especially in the elderly and in patients with

regions of insensate skin secondary to neurologic compromise. Typically, gel pads are applied anteriorly over the flare of the anteroinferior costal margin and posteriorly over the spine of the scapula. Finally, careful adjustments and attention to the fit of the vest are essential to reduce any excess motion. A lateral radiograph should be obtained to verify that there has been no change in alignment during the application process. Early application has been proven to be an effective method of temporarily immobilizing unstable segments and preventing further neurologic compromise while waiting for surgical stabilization in spinal fracture patients. Patients may be immediately mobilized and safely transferred and transported for additional imaging studies and other patient care services. Routine periodic radiographs should be performed in nonsurgical cases to confirm maintenance of alignment. Most halo orthoses have traction bails available for use. Traction can be used to help facilitate reduction of traumatic injuries. The ring is applied, as outlined previously, followed by attaching the traction bail at the site of the outrigger or wing attachment. Halo traction can be useful intraoperatively to maintain reductions of unstable injury patterns and provide distraction over cervical segments in cases of anterior interbody fusions or anterior structural grafting after following single or multiple corpectomies. The halo ring allows for three to four points of added fixation that may be helpful in traumatic cervical spine injuries with concomitant skull fractures requiring cervical traction. Finally,

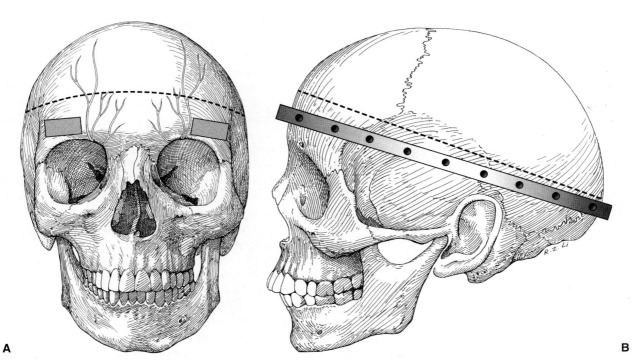

A   **B**

FIG. 4. A: Frontal view of skull. Anterior halo pins must be placed in the lateral two thirds of the supraorbital ridge or safe zone to avoid injury to the supraorbital and supratrochlear nerves. **B:** Lateral view of skull. Halo ring placement should remain below the equatorial ridge or line of greatest cranial circumference. Ideal placement is one finger breadth above the pinna of the ear with the posterior pins low in the occiput.

halo traction has been used successfully in a bivector fashion to reduce deformities requiring excessive flexion vectors, i.e., posterior displaced odontoid fractures or patients with ankylosing spondylitis or diffuse idiopathic skeletal hyperostosis with traumatic subluxations and dislocations in both the cervical and cervicothoracic regions.

Numerous investigators have reported on the complications of halo use, the most common of which are related to the pins (67,72,74,75). A thorough review of the complications is presented by Garfin et al. (72), who identified the following complications: pin loosening, pin site infection, pressure sores, nerve injury, dural penetration, dysphasia, disfiguring scars, and severe pin discomfort. Several recent studies have examined the effective insertion torque on these complications. Botte et al. (76) reported prospectively using 8 in.lb and noted loosening and infection rates at 7% and 2%, respectively. They also noted pressures up to 10 in.lb did not lead to penetration of the inner table and cadaver bone. Rizzolo et al. (77) in a randomized prospective study compared 6 and 8 in.lb and found loosening and infection rates of 5% and 13%, respectively, in the 6 in.lb group. There was no significant difference of halo pin loosening, infection, pain, or scarring between the torque protocols, but they did find a trend toward higher complications in the 8 in.lb of insertion pin torque group.

Several other studies have shown that both the angle and location of pin insertion sites can favorably affect the biomechanical strength of the halo (71,73). Pin insertion inferior position along the supraorbital ridge and perpendicular to the bone helps to maximize the pullout strength. Keeping the pins and the ring "below the equator" allows for fixation via a wedging effect and not by fixation from the individual pins. Our current belief is that 6 in.lb yields acceptable complication rates. Pins should be retorqued within 24 to 48 hours of insertion. Patients and family are both educated in the techniques of proper tract care before discharge from the hospital. This care consists of daily cleaning with soapy water or hydrogen peroxide followed by sterile saline. If a pin subsequently becomes loose, attempts at retorquing should be performed only if resistance is met during retorquing (within one full turn). If no resistance is met, than an alternative pin site should be chosen. A mildly erythematous pin or indolent infection should be retorqued if resistance is encountered, followed by orally administered antibiotics. A grossly infected pin with purulent drainage should be exchanged for another site and treated with oral or parenteral antibiotics.

PREVENTION OF PERIOPERATIVE COMPLICATIONS

Patient immobilization, which is required for many spinal injuries, predisposes the patient to a host of medical complications before surgical stabilization. These include pulmonary dysfunction, peptic ulcer disease, deep venous thrombosis, and skin breakdown. As indicated with most trauma patients, complication rates are most effectively reduced through rapid intervention and mobilization. In addition, prophylactic measures initiated on admission minimize patient risk. Prophylaxis of pulmonary complications includes prevention of aspiration and aggressive pulmonary toilet.

Gastrointestinal bleeding, usually the result of developing peptic ulcer disease, is reported to occur in 9% to 40% of patients and is most common 10 to 14 days after injury (10,78–80). The risk of ulceration may be aggravated by the use of steroids and can be combatted through the use of H2 receptor blockers and early enteral feeding. The incidence of deep vein thrombosis in spinal cord injury patients has been reported to be as high as 25% to 95% and is clinically relevant in 25% to 35% of patients (81,82). Although ongoing research continues, the current prophylaxis protocol calls for adjusted low-dose heparin and compression boots. Skin breakdown is best treated through prevention with vigilant nursing care and the use of rotating beds. Established skin ulcers must be treated aggressively with debridement, local wound care, and pressure release.

CORTICOSTEROIDS

The theoretical benefit of steroids in patients with acute spinal cord injury is to decrease inflammation and minimize neural tissue damage and dysfunction at the cellular level. The theoretical disadvantages are the undesirable systemic consequences of steroids, including, but not limited to, immunosuppression and gastrointestinal bleeding. Initial studies, using relatively low doses of steroids administered over a course of several weeks, resulted in significant increases in infection and gastrointestinal bleeding rates, with little or no improvement in neurologic function (83–85). In a recent multicenter randomized study, Bracken et al. (84) evaluated the safety and efficacy of large doses of methylprednisolone started within 8 hours of admission and administered over the first 24 hours. The authors reported a significant improvement in motor scores in patients with motor incomplete lesions who were treated with methylprednisolone as opposed to a placebo or naloxone. Infection rates of 7.9% versus 3.6%, and gastrointestinal bleeding rates of 4.5% versus 3%, were noted in the steroid and placebo groups, respectively. The shortcomings of this study include a lack of control over subsequent operative intervention between the study groups as well as no mention of the degree of functional motor improvement associated with increased motor scores. It must be reiterated that the study included only those patients treated within 8 hours of blunt spinal cord injury and did not include penetrating spinal cord injuries. The ultimate role of steroids in acute treatment of spinal cord injury thus remains unclear. Based on a relatively modest increase in complication rate noted in the more recent studies, the recommended bolus of methylprednisolone 30 mg/kg body weight is administered by the authors to all patients with acute (less than 8 hours) blunt spinal cord injury, followed by an infusion of 5.4 mg/kg/h over 23 hours. This represents the data collected from the National Acute Spinal

Cord Injury Study (NASCIS II). A subsequent NASCIS III study recently was reported (83). This study was done to evaluate the potential advantage of prolonging the administration of methylprednisolone if the initial bolus was given within 3 hours of injury. There was, however, no discernable advantage to prolonging the administration if the initial bolus was given within 3 hours. However, there did appear to be evidence of improved motor function with 48 hours of methylprednisolone infusion in the 3- to 8-hour window. This may lead to future changes in the previously mentioned protocol. However, the associated increased risks of sepsis and pneumonia must be taken into account when prolonging the steroid infusion.

CONCLUSION

The successful management of the patient sustaining spinal trauma and/or spinal cord injury is multifactorial. It requires a careful collaborative effort among all participating medical disciplines and ancillary services. A high index of suspicion for initial injuries as well as index of suspicion for potential complications associated with treatment is imperative. Early recognition and immobilization of the injured segment is imperative to maintaining and maximizing neurologic stability and spinal alignment with hopeful restoration of function.

REFERENCES

1. Fact sheet published by the Regional Spinal Cord Injury Center of Delaware Valley, Thomas Jefferson University, Philadelphia, PA. Supported in part by Grant H133N00027 from the National Institute on Disability and Rehabilitation Research, U.S. Department of Education, Washington, D.C.
2. McGuire RA, Degnan G, Amundson GM. Evaluation of current extrication orthoses in immobilization of the unstable cervical spine. *Spine* 1990;15:1064–1067.
3. Cohen M. Initial resuscitation of the patient with spinal cord injury. *Trauma Q* 1993;9:38–43.
4. Heckman JD (ed). *Emergency Care and Transportation of the Sick and Injured,* 5th edition. Chicago: American Academy of Orthopaedic Surgeons, 1992:334–349.
5. Ramzy AL, Parry JM, Greenberg J. Head and spinal injury: prehospital care. In: Greenberg J (ed). *Handbook of Head and Spine Trauma.* New York: Marcel Dekker, 1993:29–44.
6. Fielding JW. Fractures of the spine: part I. Injuries of the cervical spine. In: Rockwood CA Jr, Wilkins KE, King RE (eds). *Fractures in Children.* Philadelphia: JB Lippincott, 1984:683–705.
7. Green BA, Eismont FJ, O'Heir JT. Spinal cord injury: a systems approach. Prevention, emergency medical services, and emergency room management. *Crit Care Clin* 1987;3:471–493.
8. Raflin G, Jenneret B, Mageri F. Tetraplegia following cervical spine fusion. Presented at the Annual Meeting of the Cervical Spine Research Society, European Section, St. Gallen, Switzerland, 1989.
9. Saul TG, Ducker TB. The spine and spinal cord. In: Watt J, et al. (eds). *American College of Surgeons: Early Care of the Injured Patient,* 3rd edition. Philadelphia: WB Saunders, 1982:196–205.
10. Bohlman HH. Acute fractures and dislocations of the cervical spine: an analysis of 300 hospitalized patients and review of the literature. *J Bone Joint Surg Am* 1979;61:1119–1142.
11. Keenen TL, Anthony J, Benson DR. Non-contiguous spinal fractures. *J Trauma* 1990;30:489–491.
12. Miller LS, Cotler HB, DeLucia FA, Cotler JM, Hume EL. Biomechanical analysis of cervical distraction. *Spine* 1987;12:831–837.
13. Vaccaro AR, An HS, Lin SS, Sun S, Balderston RA, Cotler JM. Non-contiguous injuries of the spine. *J Spinal Disord* 1992;5:320–329.
14. Saboe LA, Reid DC, David LA, Warren SA, Grace MG. Spine trauma and associated injuries. *J Trauma* 1991;31:43–48.
15. Bohlman HH, Freehafer A, Dejak J. The results of treatment of acute injury of the upper thoracic spine with paralysis. *J Bone Joint Surg Am* 1985;67:360–369.
16. Kauffer H, Hayes JT. Lumbar fracture-dislocations: a study of 21 cases. *J Bone Joint Surg Am* 1966;48:712–730.
17. Meyer PR. *Surgery of Spina Trauma.* New York: Churchill Livingstone, 1989.
18. Soderstrom CA, McArdle DQ, Ducker TB, Militello PR. The diagnosis of intra-abdominal injury in patients with cervical cord trauma. *J Trauma* 1983;23:1061–1065.
19. Streitweiser DR, Knopp R, Wales LR, et al. Accuracy of standard radiographic views in detecting cervical spine fractures. *Ann Emerg Med* 1983;12:538.
20. Glassman SD, Johnson JR, Holt RT. Seatbelt injuries in children. *J Trauma* 1992;33:882–886.
21. Rumball K, Jarvis J. Seat-belt injuries of the spine in young children. *J Bone Joint Surg* 1992;74B:571–574.
22. Desmond J. Paraplegia: problems confronting the anaesthesiologist. *Can Anaesth Soc J* 1970;17:435–451.
23. Nand S, Goldschmidt JW. Hypercalcemia and hyperuricemia in young patients with spinal cord injury. *Arch Phys Med Rehabil* 1976;57:553(abst).
24. Flanders A, Andreychik DA, Stauffer ES. Early outcome in cervical spinal cord injury in patients greater than 50 years of age. *Spine* 1994;19:2299–2301.
25. Sonntag VKH, Douglas RA. Management of spinal cord trauma. *Neurosurg Clin North Am* 1990;1:729–750.
26. *Advanced Trauma Life Support Course by Committee on Trauma,* 3rd edition. Philadelphia: American College of Surgeons, 1991:9–24.
27. Slucky AV, Eismont FJ. Treatment of acute injury of the cervical spine. *J Bone Joint Surg* 1994;76A:1882–1896.
28. American Spinal Injury Association. *Standard for Neurologic and Functional Class of Spinal Cord Injury.* Chicago: American Spinal Injury Association, 1992.
29. American Spinal Injury Association. *Standards for Neurological and Functional Classification of Spinal Cord Injury.* Chicago: American Spinal Injury Association. 1992.
30. Daffner RH, Deeb ZL, Rothfus WE. The posterior vertebral body line: importance in the detection of burst fractures. *AJR Am J Roentgenol* 1987;148:93–96.
31. Galli RL, Spaite DW, Simmon RR. The cervical spine. In: *Emergency Orthopaedics.* East Norwalk, CT: Appleton & Lange, 1989:96–99.
32. Lahd WH. Efficacy of the post-traumatic cross table lateral view of the cervical spine. *Emerg Med* 1986;2:243.
33. More SE. Emergency evaluation of cervical spine injuries: CT versus radiographs. *Ann Emerg Med* 1985;14:973.
34. Stover SC. *Spinal Cord Injury: The Facts and Figures.* Birmingham, AL: University of Alabama, 1986.
35. Gisbert VL, Hollerman JJ, Ney AL, et al. Incidence and diagnosis of C7-T1 fractures and subluxations in multiple trauma patients: evaluation of the advanced trauma life support guidelines. *Surgery* 1989; 106:702–709.
36. Lodge T, Higgenbottom E. Fractures and dislocations of the cervical spine. *X-Ray Focus* 1966;7:2.
37. Scher A, Vambeck V. An approach to radiological examination of the cervicodorsal junction following injury. *Clin Radiol* 1977;28:24–43.
38. Kulkami MV, McArdle CB, Kopanicky D, et al. Acute spinal cord injury: MR imaging at 1.5 T. *Radiology* 1987;164:837.
39. White AA, Southwick WO, Panjabi MM. Clinical instability in the lower cervical spine. A review of past and current concepts. *Spine* 1970;1:15–27.
40. Templeton PA, Young JWR, Mirvis SE, Buddemeyer EV. The value of retropharyngeal soft tissue measurement in trauma of the adult cervical spine. *Skeletal Radiol* 1987;16:98–104.
41. Herkowitz HR, Rothman RH. Subacute instability of the cervical spine. *Spine* 1984;9:348–352.
42. Naidich JB, Naidich TP, Garein C, et al. Interspinous distance: a useful sign of anterior cervical dislocation in the spinal frontal projection. *Radiology* 1977;123:113–116.
43. Chakeres DW, Flickinger F, Bresnahan JC, et al. MR imaging of acute spinal cord trauma. *Am J Neurol Res* 1987;8:5.

44. Goldberg AL, Rothfus WE, Deeb ZL, et al. The impact of magnetic resonance on the diagnostic evaluation of acute cervicothoracic spinal trauma. *Skeletal Radiol* 1988;17:89.
45. Harrington JF, Likavel MJ, Smith AS. Disc herniation in cervical fracture subluxation. *Neurosurgery* 1991;29:374–379.
46. Pratt ES, Green DA, Spengler DM. Herniated intervertebral discs associated with unstable spinal injuries. *Spine* 1990;15:662–665.
47. Raynor RB. Cervical cord compression secondary to acute disc protrusion in trauma. *Spine* 1977;2:39–43.
48. Rizzolo SJ, Plazza MR, Cotler JM, Balderston RA, Schaefer D, Flanders A. Intervertebral disc injury complicating cervical spine trauma. *Spine* 1991;16[Suppl]:S187–S189.
49. Beers JG, Raque GH, Wagner GG, et al. MR imaging in acute cervical spine trauma. *J Comput Assist Tomogr* 1988;12:755–761.
50. Cotler HG, Kulkami MV, Bondurant FJ. Magnetic resonance imaging of acute spinal cord trauma: preliminary report. *J Orthop Trauma* 1988;2:1–4.
51. Kalfas I, Wilberger J, Goldberg A, Prostko R. Magnetic resonance imaging in acute spinal cord trauma. *Neurosurgery* 1988;23:295–299.
52. Schaefer DM, Flanders A, Northrup BE, Doan HT, Osterholm JL. Magnetic resonance imaging of acute cervical spine trauma: correlation with severity of neurologic injury. *Spine* 1989;14:1090–1095.
53. Holdsworth FW. Fractures, dislocations, and fracture-dislocation of the spine. *J Bone Joint Surg Am* 1970;52:1534–1551.
54. Allen BL, Ferguson RL, Lehmann TR, O'Brien RP. A mechanistic classification of closed, indirect fractures and dislocations of the lower cervical spine. *Spine* 1982;7:1–27.
55. Denis F. The three column spine and its significance in the classification of acute thoracolumbar spinal injuries. *Spine* 1983;8:817–831.
56. Aebi M, Mohler J, Zach GA, Morscher E. Indication, surgical technique and results of 100 surgically treated fractures and fracture-dislocations of the cervical spine. *Clin Orthop* 1980;203:244–257.
57. Burke DC, Berryman D. The place of closed manipulation in the management of flexion-rotation dislocations of the cervical spine. *J Bone Joint Surg Am* 1971;53:165–182.
58. Cotler JM, Nasuti J, Ditunno JF, An HS. Improvement of motor index score after rapid closed reduction of traumatic cervical spine dislocation using traction weights up to 130 pounds. Presented at the Annual Meeting of American Spinal Injury Association, Toronto, Ontario, Canada, 1992.
59. Dolan EJ, Tator CH, Endrenyi L. The value of decompression for acute experimental spinal cord injury. *J Neurosurg* 1980;53:749–755.
60. Levi L, Wolf A, Rigamonti D, Regheb J, Mirvis S, Robinson WL. Anterior decompression of cervical spine trauma. Does timing of surgery affect outcome? *Neurosurgery* 1987;29:216–222.
61. Rorabeck CH, Rock GM, Hawkins RL, Bourne RB. Unilateral facet dislocation of the cervical spine. An analysis of results in 26 patients. *Spine* 1987;12:23–27.
62. Tartov IM. Spinal cord compression studies. Time limits for recovery after gradual compression in dogs. *Arch Neurol Neurosurg Psychol* 1954;71:588–597.
63. Star AM, Jones AA, Cotler JM, Balderston RA, Sinha R. Immediate closed reduction of cervical spine dislocations using traction. *Spine* 1990;15:1068–1072.
64. Ramsey M, Rizzolo SJ, Cotler JM, Balderston RA, Solit R. Temporary immobilization of unstable cervical spine injuries in the halo-vest orthosis. Presented at the Annual Meeting of the Cervical Spine Research Society, Palm Desert, California, December 1992.
65. Perry J. The halo in spinal abnormalities: practical factors and avoidance of complications. *Orthop Clin North Am* 1972;3:69–80.
66. Perry J, Nickel VL. Total cervical spine fusion for neck paralysis. *J Bone Joint Surg Am* 1959;41:37–60.
67. Koch RA, Nickel VL. The halo vest: an evaluation of notion and forces across the neck. *Spine* 1978;3:103–107.
68. Bucci MN, Dauser RC, Maynard FA, et al. Management of post traumatic cervical spine instability: operative fusion versus halo vest immobilization. Analysis of 49 cases. *J Trauma* 1988;28:1001–1006.
69. Bucholz RD, Cheung KC. Halo vest versus spinal fusion for cervical injury: evidence from an outcome study. *J Neurosurg* 1989;70:884–892.
70. Cooper PR, Maravilla KR, Sklar FH, et al. Halo immobilization of cervical fractures: indications and results. *J Neurosurg* 1979;50:603–610.
71. Ballock RT, Thay QI, Triggs KT, et al. The effect of pin location on the rigidity of the halo pin bone interface. *Neurosurgery* 1990;26:238–241.
72. Garfin SR, Botte MJ, Waters RL, et al. Complications in the use of the halo fixation device. *J Bone Joint Surg Am* 1986;68:320–325.
73. Triggs KT, Ballock RT, Lee TQ, et al. The effect of angled insertion on halo pin fixation. *Spine* 1989;14:781–783.
74. Johnson RM, Hart DL, Simmons EF, et al. Cervical orthosis. *J Bone Joint Surg Am* 1977;59:332–339.
75. Kostuik J. Indications for use of halo immobilization. *Clin Orthop* 1980;154:46–50.
76. Botte MJ, Byrne TP, Garfin SR. Application of the halo device for immobilization of the cervical spine utilizing an increased torque pressure. *J Bone Joint Surg Am* 1987;69:750-752.
77. Rizzolo SJ, Piazza MR, Cotler JM, et al. The effect of torque pressure on halo pin complications: a randomized prospective study. *Spine* 1993;18:2163–2166.
78. Albert TJ, Levine MJ, Balderston RA, Cotler JM. GI complications in spinal cord injury. *Spine* 1991;16[Suppl]:5522–5525.
79. Bohlman HH, Zdeblick TA. Complications of treatment of fractures and dislocations of the cervical spine. In: Epps C (ed). *Complications of Orthopaedic Surgery*. Philadelphia: JB Lippincott, 1985:897–918.
80. Leramo OB, Tator CH, Hudson AR. Massive gastroduodenal hemorrhage and perforation in acute spinal cord injury. *Surg Neurol* 1982;17:186–190.
81. Green D, Lee MY, Ito V, et al. Fixed versus adjusted dose heparin in prophylaxis of thromboembolism in spinal cord injury. *JAMA* 1988;260:1255–1258.
82. Merli GJ, Herbison GJ, Ditunno JF, et al. Deep venous thrombosis prophylaxis in acute spinal cord injury patients. *Arch Phys Med Rehabil* 1988;69:661–664.
83. Bracken MB, Collins WF, Frieman DF, et al. Efficacy of methylprednisolone in acute spinal cord injury. *JAMA* 1984;25:45–52.
84. Bracken MB, Shephard MJ, Collins WF, et al. A randomized controlled trial of methylprednisolone or naloxone in the treatment of acute spinal cord injury. Results of the second national acute spinal cord injury study. *N Engl J Med* 1990;322:1405–1444.
85. Bracken MB, Shepard MJ, Hefenbrand KG, et al. Methylprednisolone and neurologic function of year post spinal cord injury. *J Neurosurg* 1985;63:704–713.
86. Bracken MB, et al., for the National Acute Spinal Cord Injury study. Administration of methylprednisolone for 24 or 48 hours or tirilazad mesylate for 48 hours in the treatment of acute spinal cord injury. Results of the Third National Acute Spinal Cord Injury Randomized Controlled Trial. *JAMA* 1997;277:1597.

Surgery of Spinal Trauma,
edited by J.M. Cotler, J.M. Simpson, H.S. An, and C.P. Silveri.
Lippincott Williams & Wilkins, Philadelphia © 2000.

CHAPTER 5

Radiographic Evaluation of Spinal Injuries

Evelyn M.L. Sklar, Armando Ruiz, and Steven Falcone

Spine trauma is one of the most serious disorders affecting humans, constituting one of the leading causes of disability. In the last 2 decades, important imaging developments have taken place that have improved diagnosis and have paralleled the development of better clinical and more aggressive surgical management of spinal injuries. In choosing a particular radiographic protocol, numerous factors should be taken into account. These include the neurologic status of the patient, the level of injury, the age of the lesion, and the potential benefit that might be derived from each of the different imaging modalities.

IMAGING MODALITIES USED IN THE EVALUATION OF SPINAL TRAUMA

Plain Radiographs

Plain films remain indispensable in the evaluation of bony imaging and are the foundation on which the initial evaluation of spinal injuries is based. The anteroposterior and lateral views must be evaluated for fracture lines, endplate discontinuity, subluxation, abnormal orientation or separation of facets, pedicles or spinous processes, loss of height of vertebral bodies and intervertebral discs, and signs indicative of abnormalities of the surrounding soft tissues and adjacent bony structures. The main disadvantage of plain films is their

inability to provide information about injuries to the neural elements of the spine.

Computed Tomography

Computed tomography (CT) is one of the fundamental tools used in the evaluation of patients with spinal trauma. It has largely replaced conventional tomography in the evaluation of bony injuries to the spine; however, the latter retains some utility in cases where nondisplaced horizontal fractures are suspected. Computed tomography has the ability not only to detect fractures of the spine, but also to determine the presence of displaced bone fragments, degree of compromise of the spinal canal, and disruption of the posterior elements (Fig. 1), and to evaluate the paravertebral soft tissues. Computed tomography is a nonreplaceable modality in the evaluation of spinal trauma because of its high resolution in evaluation of osseous anatomy and fractures.

Computed tomography traditionally has been a diagnostic imaging modality where cross-sectional axial scans are acquired one slice at a time. The patient is stationary while each image is obtained. The couch moves between scans to cover the area of interest. With the new technology of spiral CT, the patient couch moves through the scan plane in a fluid motion rather than incremental steps while the x-ray tube rotates continuously, creating a ribbon or helix of data. The pitch is the distance the table travels per revolution of scan frame and depends on couch speed and the number of seconds per revolution. In a standard helix, the slice thickness equals the distance the table travels per revolution. An extended helix covers 50% more anatomic area per revolution than a standard helix. Images can be reconstructed anywhere

E.M.L. Sklar and S. Falcone: Department of Radiology, University of Miami School of Medicine, Miami, Florida 33136.
A. Ruiz: Department of Radiology (R-308), Neuro Radiology Section, MRI Center, Miami, Florida 33136.

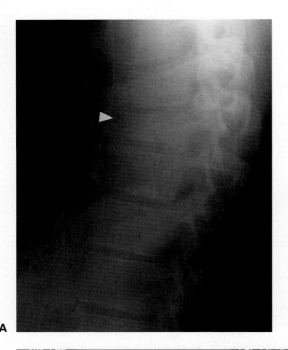

FIG. 1. Male patient involved in a motor vehicle accident **A:** Lateral thoracic spine plain film demonstrates anterior wedging deformity of T-7 *(arrowhead)*. The visualized portion of the posterior elements is limited. **B,C:** Two contiguous axial cuts (bone and soft tissue windows, respectively) through T-7 showing severe nature of the fracture seen in **A**. The burst fracture is associated with fracture of the posterior arch and costotransverse process *(arrowhead)*. The canal is severely compromised by retropulsed bone *(open arrow)*. The patient was paraplegic, due to severe cord damage. (Reproduced with permission from Ruiz A, Post MJD, Sklar EML. Traumatic thoracic and lumbar fractures. *Appl Radiol* October 1996: 49–57.)

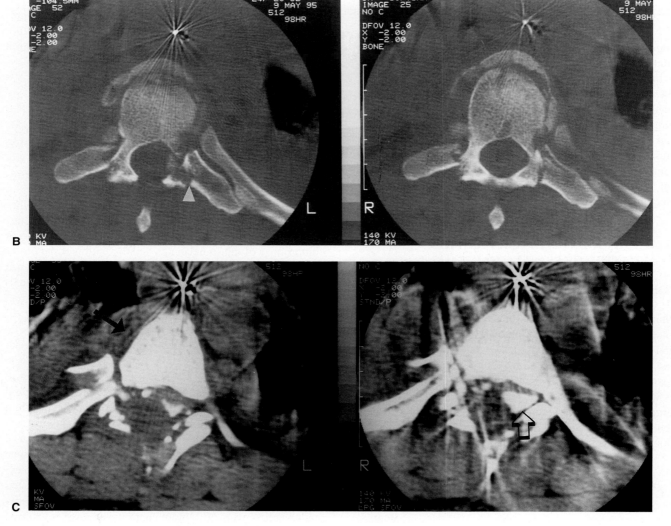

along the volume of data without rescanning the patient. Reconstructions also may be obtained in different planes, which is very helpful in the detection of horizontally oriented fractures that may be missed on axial CT. Another major advantage of spinal CT is the capability to scan rapidly, which is extremely useful in patients who have to be scanned quickly, such as unstable patients in the setting of trauma.

Many fractures are missed or incompletely shown at radiography, mainly because of suboptimal studies obtained in obtunded uncooperative trauma patients. At our institution, Nunez et al. (1) compared radiographs and helical CT in 88 patients. Thirty-two of these patients had cervical spine fractures that were not revealed or were incompletely demonstrated at radiography but were depicted by helical CT. Most missed fractures occurred at the C1–2 and C6–7 levels, and most involved the transverse processes and posterolateral elements of the vertebrae. One third of the patients with missed fractures had either clinically significant or unstable injuries.

The reconstructions obtained with spiral CT are extremely helpful in the management of trauma patients. For example, posterior transarticular screw fixation of the C1–2 complex has become an accepted method of rigid internal fixation for patients requiring posterior C1–2 fusion. The main limitation of this procedure is the location of the vertebral artery. Paramore et al. (2) used reconstructions from spiral CT to visualize the potential path of a transarticular screw (see section on odontoid fractures). On the basis of their data, they postulate that 18% to 23% of patients may not be suitable candidates for posterior C1–2 transarticular screw fixation on at least one side.

Computed tomography also assesses the paraspinal and intraspinal soft tissues. Acute intraspinal hemorrhage (epidural hematomas, intradural blood), herniated disc material, and pseudomeningoceles often can be demonstrated with CT (Fig. 2).

For those patients in whom magnetic resonance imaging (MRI) evaluation is not possible because of metallic foreign bodies (Fig. 3), claustrophobia, or MRI-incompatible life support systems, CT myelography allows for indirect visualization of the cord and nerve roots. Extradural defects and cord or nerve root compression can be appreciated easily. Computed tomographic myelography also is useful in diagnosing dural tears (Fig. 4), nerve root avulsion (especially small avulsions that may not be detected with other modalities), and cord cysts. The main disadvantage of CT myelography is that it is an invasive procedure that requires the placement of intrathecal iodinated material with its intrinsic risks. In addition, acutely injured spinal cord patients often are immobilized, necessitating cervical puncture rather than lumbar puncture. Also, coexistent brain injury with mass effect may preclude performance of a spinal puncture. Patient positioning during the performance of a cervical puncture may be difficult in patients who are in traction or who have orthopedic devices. Visualization of the intrinsic spinal cord is not possible with myelography, which is of particular importance in patients with progressive posttraumatic myelopathy.

Magnetic Resonance Imaging

Magnetic resonance imaging is a proven tool in the evaluation of both the acutely injured spinal cord patient and the patient who develops late sequelae from spinal cord trauma. Prior to MRI, CT myelography was the most accurate method in the evaluation of the spine and its contents. The

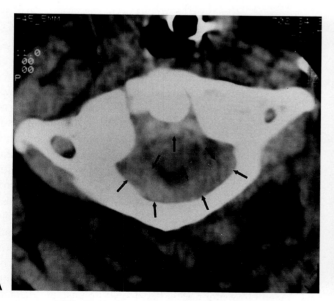 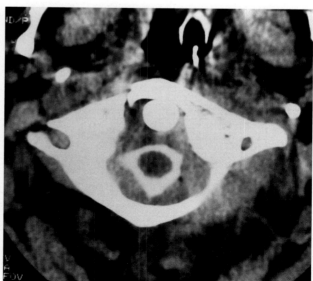

A   B

FIG. 2. Patient with fracture of anterior arch of C-1. **A:** Noncontrast computed tomography shows high density in epidural space *(arrows)* consistent with epidural hemorrhage. **B:** Computed tomographic myelogram demonstrates circumferential narrowing of contrast-filled thecal sac by epidural hemorrhage.

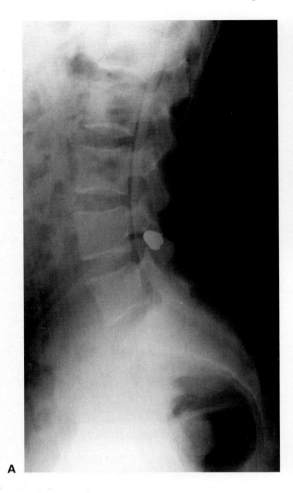

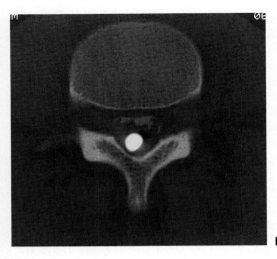

FIG. 3. Male patient with a history of gunshot wound to the lumbar spine and a clinical concern for dural leak. Postmyelogram lateral plain film **(A)** and axial computed tomographic view **(B)** of the lumbar spine showing the intraspinal extradural location of the bullet fragment. There was no active leak of contrast. (Reproduced with permission from Ruiz A, Post MJD, Sklar EML. Traumatic thoracic and lumbar fractures. *Appl Radiol* 1996: 49–57.)

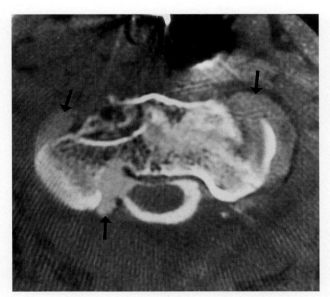

FIG. 4. Dural tear. Fracture of the body of C-2 produced a dural tear in this patient. Computed tomographic myelogram shows extravasation of contrast *(arrows).*

necessity of a spinal puncture and the inability to adequately evaluate the spinal cord parenchyma are major inherent limitations of myelography. Myelography has several other disadvantages compared to MRI. Acutely injured spinal cord patients often are immobilized and/or on a backboard, requiring a more risky cervical puncture rather than lumbar puncture. Coexistent brain injury with mass effect may preclude performance of a spinal puncture. Myelography frequently requires meticulous patient positioning, which may be difficult or impossible in patients who are in traction or who have concomitant orthopedic injuries. Magnetic resonance imaging, however, is noninvasive and has the ability to better image the spinal cord parenchyma. The major advantages of MRI include superior contrast resolution, multiplanar capability, ability to directly visualize the spinal cord, lack of ionizing radiation, and its noninvasive nature. These benefits have resulted in the replacement of CT myelography by MRI in the evaluation of both the acutely injured spinal cord patient and the patient who develops late sequelae form spinal cord trauma. Magnetic resonance imaging may not be the procedure of choice in all patients, as in those patients who need close monitoring because of an unstable medical condition, in those conditions in which ferromagnetic material cannot be eliminated, or in those patients who have absolute/relative contraindication to MRI such as the presence of aneurysm clips, pacemaker, heart valve, etc. When feasible, MRI is preferred over myelography in the evaluation of both the acutely injured spinal cord patient and patients who develop late sequelae of spinal cord trauma.

Plain radiographs and a CT scan should be the first radiographic examination obtained in the evaluation of the acutely injured spinal cord patient. Magnetic resonance imaging is reserved for those acutely injured spinal cord patients when neurologic deficits are not explained by plain film or CT findings, to evaluate the degree of canal compromise or cord compression in the presence of displaced fractures, and before operative stabilization to exclude the presence of a disc herniation (3). The primary role of MRI is in the detection of surgically correctable lesions that can go undiagnosed by plain radiography and CT. This includes the evaluation for epidural hematomas, traumatic disc herniations, and ligamentous injuries. Magnetic resonance imaging also can be used as a prognostic tool, as patients with spinal cord hemorrhage do not fair as well as those who do not exhibit cord hemorrhage (4–8). There is no indication for MRI in the routine workup of patients with acute whiplash injury when plain radiography shows no signs of fracture or subluxation (9).

Magnetic resonance imaging is the imaging procedure of choice in patients who develop delayed or progressive neurologic deficits months to years after acute spinal injury (10,11). The primary role of MRI is in the detection of spinal cord cysts, spinal cord tethering/myelomalacia, and spinal cord compression related to bony deformities or disc herniations. The identification of treatable causes for progressive neurologic deficits is crucial in the quadriplegic or paraplegic patient, because preservation of any remaining neurologic function may result in major differences in their rehabilitation and daily activity or comfort.

The acutely injured spinal cord patient requires special considerations before entering the MRI environment. Performing MRI on these patients requires a team approach. The participation of a technologist, respiratory therapist, nurse, and spine surgeon often is necessary, as these patients are imaged on a backboard, in tongs, with a halo, and may be ventilator dependent.

When possible, surface coils are used to obtain the highest quality images. A flat linear surface coil can be placed underneath the patient if there is supervision by the spine surgeon. A volume neck coil can be used if a cervical collar is not in place. A body coil provides sufficient images to evaluate the cervical spine if the patient cannot be moved. Backboards free of ferromagnetic material will allow the generation of diagnostic images. Imaging of the patient in tongs (made of titanium) is a challenging but easily accomplished task. Performing MRI on these patients is accomplished by attaching water bottles of appropriate weight to the end of a rope, which is attached to the head holder. After the patient is transferred to the scanner, the rope is dangled over the edge of the magnet with the water bottles suspended at the end of the rope. Magnetic resonance imaging-compatible ha-

los with special geometric designs are widely available and routinely utilized. Ventilator-dependent patients can be imaged safely, provided appropriate personnel are present and monitoring equipment is used. Although MRI-compatible ventilators are commercially available, we choose to manually ventilate the patient. An MRI-compatible pulse oximeter is utilized to monitor the patient's heart rate and oxygen saturation. The patient's blood pressure can be monitored with an automated MRI-compatible sphygmomanometer.

We use both T1-weighted (T1W) and T2-weighted (T2W) imaging sequences in the axial and sagittal planes to evaluate the acutely injured spinal cord patient. Coronal images may be helpful in the evaluation of nerve root avulsions. Gradient-echo T2* sequences are preferred to conventional T2W spin-echo sequences because T2W spin-echo sequences are less sensitive to deoxyhemoglobin. Fast spin-echo T2W sequences are even less sensitive to deoxyhemoglobin when compared to T2W sequences due to the repetitive application of the 180-degree pulse. In the acutely injured spinal cord patient, we recommend acquiring T2* gradient-echo images in both the axial and sagittal planes.

Imaging of the chronically injured spinal cord patient can be challenging. These patients may be ventilator dependent or may suffer from uncontrollable muscle spasms. Diagnostic images cannot be obtained when significant spasms are experienced during image acquisition, because the images will be degraded by motion. Magnetic resonance imaging can be performed successfully in patients with muscle spasms if sufficient medical therapy is instituted.

Routine imaging of the chronically injured spinal cord patient includes both T1W and T2W sequences in both the axial and sagittal planes. A T2*W sequence is not as useful as in the acute setting, because the detection of blood products is not a prime concern. We strongly encourage the use of conventional dual-echo spin-echo sagittal sequences, because analysis of the first and second echoes may be critical in the distinction between a confluent spinal cord cyst and myelomalacia. If the patient has undergone prior operative stabilization with metallic hardware, a T2W fast spin-echo sequence is utilized. The fast spin-echo sequence is less susceptible to metallic artifacts compared to a routine spin-echo sequence. A sequence we commonly use in the chronically injured spinal cord patient is a gradient-echo cerebrospinal fluid (CSF) flow study. A CSF flow study is useful for the confirmation and diagnosis of posttraumatic spinal cord tethering. Spinal cord cyst pulsatility also can be assessed with a CSF flow study (12).

CERVICAL SPINE TRAUMA

Acute Spinal Injury

Ligamentous Injury

The only imaging modality that can give direct evidence for ligamentous injury is MRI (13–15). The presence of ligamentous injury can be inferred by plain radiography when significant bony displacement or soft tissue swelling is present. The absence of vertebral column malalignment or soft tissue swelling does not exclude the presence of a ligamentous injury. Flexion/extension radiographs, which may be useful in the evaluation of instability and ligamentous injury, are contraindicated in patients with acute focal neurologic deficits and patients with an alteration of mental status. The integrity of the anterior longitudinal ligament (ALL), posterior longitudinal ligament (PLL), interspinous ligaments, ligamentum nuchae, ligaments of the craniovertebral junction, and ligaments about the dens can be assessed with MRI. Kulkarni et al. (15) detected ligamentous injury in 78% of patients suffering acute cervical injury using MRI.

The MRI findings of ligamentous injury depend on the ligament in question. Indirect signs of ligamentous injury, such as prevertebral soft tissue swelling with or without hemorrhage (ALL) and flaring of the spinous processes (interspinous ligaments), can be evaluated accurately with MRI. Direct evidence of a damaged ligament includes interruption of a continuous low signal intensity of the ligament in question (Fig. 5) and associated intermediate or high signal intensity on T1W or T2W images within or around the ligaments (7,13–16). An interrupted continuous low signal can be particularly evident with ALL, PLL, and transverse ligament disruption. Both T1W and T2W images may reveal discontinuity of the low signal intensity of a ligament. Dickman et al. (16) showed MRI to be useful in the management of patients with injury to the transverse atlantal ligament. Dickman et al. (16) used thin-section (2 to 3 mm) high-resolution T2W axial MRI through the transverse ligament to classify patients into two groups. Type 1 injuries involved the midportion or periosteal insertion of the ligament and required early surgery with internal fixation. Type II injuries involved an associated comminuted fracture of the lateral mass of C-1 or an avulsed tubercle of the lateral mass of C-1 that healed with nonoperative external immobilization in nearly 75% of cases. Interspinous ligament injury usually is manifest by increased signal between the spinous processes.

Fractures

Flexion Injuries

Bilateral Interfacetal Dislocation. Bilateral interfacetal dislocation is dislocation of both interfacetal joints at the same level. Interlocking of the articular facets begins with the movement of the inferior articular facets of one vertebra forward over the articular facets of the underlying vertebra. This causes the laminae and spinous processes to distract and the vertebral bodies to sublux.

Radiographically, this is characterized by anterior displacement of the dislocated segment. The inferior facets of the dislocated vertebra lie anterior to the superior facets of the adjacent segment. Often this injury is referred to as "double locked" vertebra. This lesion is acutely unstable due to its skeletal and soft tissue disruption at the level of injury.

Unilateral Interfacetal Dislocation. Unilateral interfacetal dislocation results from simultaneous flexion and rotation (Fig. 6). The posterior ligament complex and the capsule of the dislocated facetal joint are disrupted. The ALL, PLL, and the disk are disrupted.

The interfacetal joint on the side of the direction of rotation acts as the pivotal point while the contralateral side including its inferior facet rides upward and forward over the tip of the superior facet of the inferior vertebra. The dislocated facet is locked and fixed. The contiguous facets are no longer in apposition and are uncovered, or exposed, "naked" facets. There may be fractures of either of the articular facets with tiny fragments having no clinical significance but large fractures rendering the interfacetal dislocation unstable.

In the anteroposterior radiograph, unilateral interfacetal dislocation is evidenced by rotation of the spinous processes from the level of the dislocation upward off the midline in the direction of the side of the dislocated interfacetal joint.

In the lateral view, there is forward displacement of the dislocated vertebra. While the vertebrae below are in the true lateral projection, the vertebrae above are seen obliquely because of the rotational component of the mechanism of injury. This results in a "bowtie" appearance of the articular pillars of the dislocated vertebra. In the anteroposterior projection the spinous processes are displaced from the midline toward the side of the dislocated interfacetal joint at the level of the dislocation and above. Fractures of the vertebral spinous processes may be associated with injuries that cause dislocation of the articular facets.

Simple Wedge (Compression) Fracture. Simple wedge (compression) fracture is characterized by impaction of the superior endplate and the anterior cortical margin of the body.

Clay Shoveler's Fracture. Clay shoveler's fracture is an avulsion of the spinous process of C-6, C-7, or T1 (Fig. 7).

Flexion Teardrop Fracture. The flexion teardrop fracture is composed of complete disruption of all the ligaments and the intervertebral disc, disruption of the interfacetal joints, and a large triangular fragment consisting of the anterior inferior aspect of the involved vertebral body.

Extension Injuries

Extension Teardrop Fracture of the Axis. Extension teardrop fracture of the axis shows a triangular fragment with its vertical height equal to or greater than its transverse width. This fragment represents the anteroinferior corner of the C-2 body, which is avulsed by the intact ALL during hyperextension.

Hangman's Fracture. Usually, hangman's fracture represents bilateral fractures of the pars interarticularis of the axis (Fig. 8). Less commonly, one or both fractures may involve the superior articulating facet or may be more anteriorly located at the junction of the posterior arch and posterior aspect of the body of C-2.

Laminar Fracture. Isolated laminar fractures involve that portion of the posterior arch of the lower cervical vertebrae

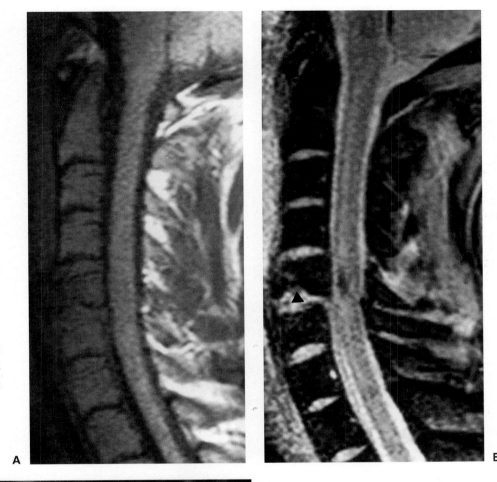

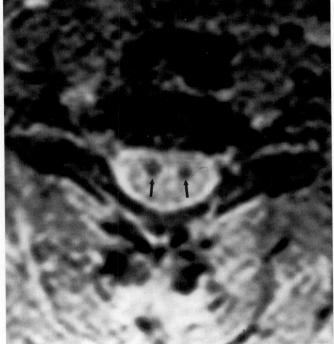

FIG. 5. Vertebral body fracture, spinal cord hemorrhage, and anterior longitudinal ligament (ALL) rupture. **A:** T1-weighted sagittal image. **B:** T2-weighted gradient-echo sagittal image. **C:** T2-weighted gradient-echo axial at C-5. Acute quadriparesis status post motor vehicle accident. Evaluation of the sagittal images from ventral to dorsal reveals discontinuity of the *black line* of the ALL at C4–5 to C5–6 *(arrows)*. The signal of the ventral aspect of the C-5 body is abnormal, with decreased signal on the T1-weighted images. Note also the disruption of the inferior cortical line of the C-5 body and upward herniation of C5–6 disc material *(arrowhead)*. Deoxyhemoglobin is also present in the C5–6 disc space. There is mild subluxation at C5–6, with ventral compression of the subarachnoid space. Abnormal T2 signal in the ventral horns at C-5 (best seen on axial image) *(arrows)* is consistent with deoxyhemoglobin.

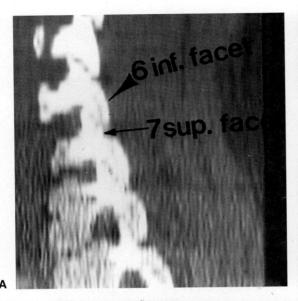

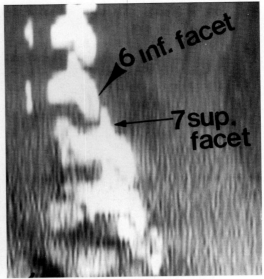

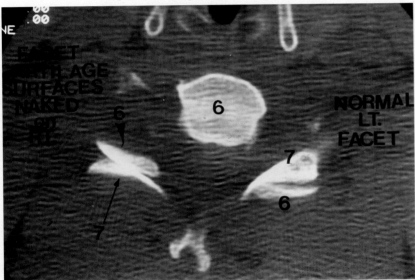

FIG. 6. Unilateral interfacetal dislocation. Sagittal reformatted images of computed tomography (CT) show normal left side **(A)** and dislocated right inferior facet of C-6 *(arrowhead)* anterior to the contiguous superior facet of C-7 *(straight arrow)* **(B). C:** Axial CT shows the dislocated articular mass of C-6 *(arrowhead)* anterior to its subjacent counterpart, the superior facet of C-7, which is "naked."

between the articular mass and the spinous process. It is an uncommon fracture that occurs in older patients with cervical spondylosis. Radiographically, these fractures are subtle and are characterized by disruption of the laminae on the lateral projection but are best identified by CT (Fig. 9).

Diverse or Poorly Understood Mechanisms

Acute Traumatic Rotatory Atlantoaxial Dislocation. Acute traumatic rotatory atlantoaxial dislocation is a rare injury (17–21) in which there is partial or complete derangement of the lateral atlantoaxial articulations. The lateral masses of the atlas are displaced, one anteriorly and one posteriorly with respect to the articular masses of C-2. The distances between the atlas and the dens become asymmetric (Fig. 10). In the lateral projection, there is prevertebral soft tissue swelling. The rotation of the atlas about the dens

causes the anterior arch of C-1 to lose its normal configuration. In addition, the atlantoaxial interval on the lateral projection becomes indistinct. Axial CT scans through C1–2 in patients with clinically diagnosed atlantoaxial rotatory fixation demonstrate the rotated position of C-1 on C-2 (22–24). The CT appearance of the atlantoaxial complex in a patient with torticollis is identical (25). To differentiate these groups, Kowalski et al. (25) suggested a functional scan through C1–2 in which patients are scanned initially as they present with their heads fixed in lateral rotation. Subsequent scans are obtained with their heads turned to the maximum contralateral rotation. Computed tomographic scans of patients with atlantoaxial rotatory fixation demonstrate no motion at C1–2 in this maneuver, but those patients with transient torticollis show a reduction or reversal of the rotation of C-1 on C-2.

Torticollis. Torticollis or atlantoaxial rotatory displace-

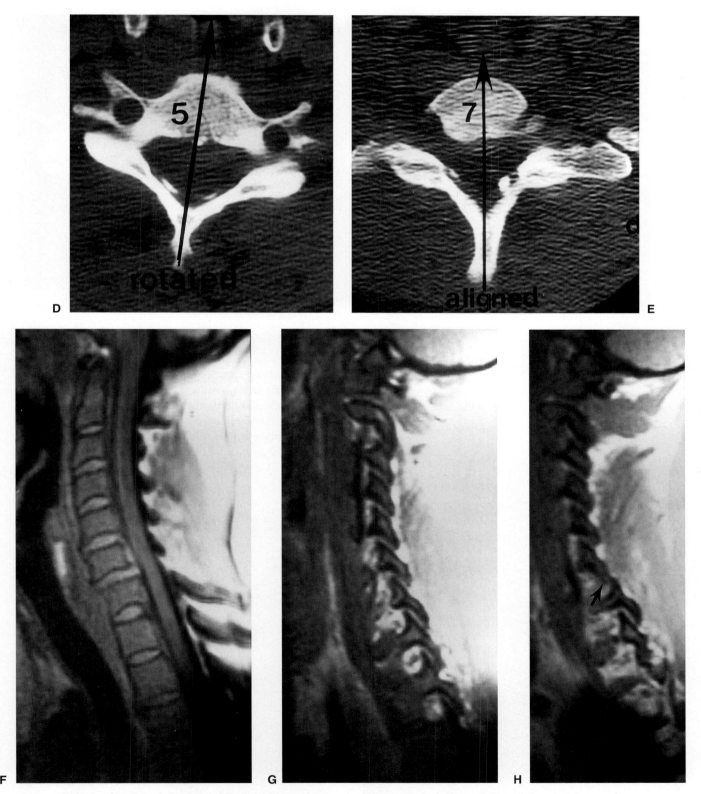

FIG. 6. *Continued.* **D:** Axial CT scan above the level of dislocation shows rotation of the vertebra and spinous process. **E:** Axial CT scan below the level of dislocation shows no rotation. **F:** Sagittal magnetic resonance imaging scan through the midline shows anterior translation of C-6 on C-7. Sagittal T1-weighted image shows normal left facets **(G)** and dislocated inferior facet of C-6 *(arrow)* anterior to the contiguous superior facet of C-7 *(curved arrow)* **(H).**

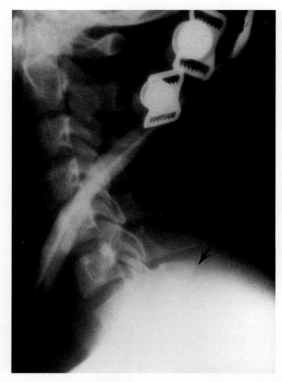

FIG. 7. Clay shoveler's fracture of the spinous process of C-7 *(arrow)*. Note the teardrop fracture of the axis.

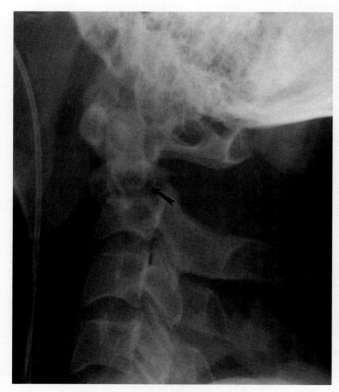

FIG. 8. Hangman's fracture. Fracture through the pars interarticularis *(arrow)*.

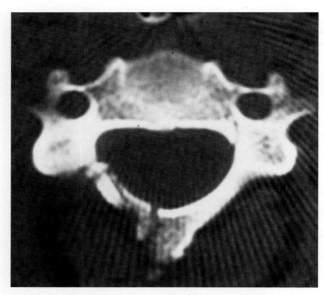

FIG. 9. Laminar fracture of C-3 seen by axial computed tomography.

ment is not associated with a pathologic injury as opposed to acute traumatic rotatory atlantoaxial dislocation (described earlier) (26). In this entity, the relationship of the atlas to the axis is a position normally attained during physiologic rotation (27). Fielding and Hawkins (28) used the term "rotational displacement" to describe the physical changes at the atlantoaxial articulation. This term has no implication of abnormality. Torticollis is a clinical condition of unknown eti-

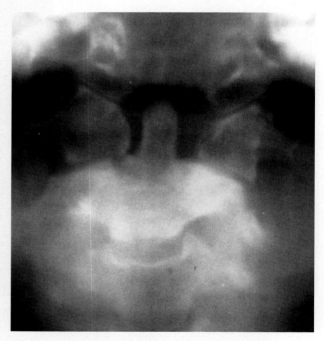

FIG. 10. Acute traumatic rotatory atlantoaxial dislocation. On this tomogram, the distances between the atlas and the dens are asymmetric.

ology that is seen frequently in childhood and early adolescence. It usually occurs spontaneously but may follow minor trauma or be associated with acute infections. The deformity usually reverses spontaneously.

In the radiographic evaluation of a patient with torticollis, no attempt should be made to straighten the head and neck to obtain a good anteroposterior radiograph. The lateral tilt and rotation of the head that occurs in torticollis result in physiologic movement of the atlas and axis. Lateral tilt of C-1 causes unilateral displacement of its articular masses with respect to the dens and those of C-2, which results in asymmetry of the spaces between the dens and the articular masses of the atlas, asymmetry of the lateral margins of the lateral atlantoaxial joints, increase in the transverse diameter of the anteriorly rotated articular masses of the atlas, and displacement of the spinous process of C-2 from the midline in the direction opposite that of the torticollis deformity.

Vertical Compression

Jefferson Bursting Fracture. The original description of this lesion was that of bilateral fractures of both the anterior and posterior arches of C-1. The Jefferson fracture, however, may result from a single break in each ring.

On plain films, in the frontal projection, there is bilateral displacement of the articular masses of C-1. In the lateral projection, the anterior arch fracture is seen rarely but the posterior arch fracture is noted frequently. On the lateral projection, the Jefferson fracture cannot be distinguished from an isolated hyperextension fracture of the posterior arch of the atlas. These fractures can be demonstrated on CT and less well on MRI (Fig. 11).

Burst Fracture. The burst fracture of the lower cervical spine is a comminution fracture of the vertebral body with retropulsion of bone into the spinal canal. Computed tomog-

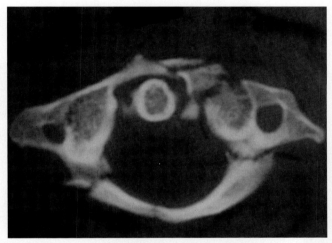

A

FIG. 11. Jefferson fracture. A: Axial computed tomography shows multiple fractures through C-1. B: Magnetic resonance imaging at the same level demonstrates the difficulty frequently encountered in diagnosing fractures with magnetic resonance imaging. C: Coronal T1 images shows bilateral displacement of the articular masses of C-1 (arrows).

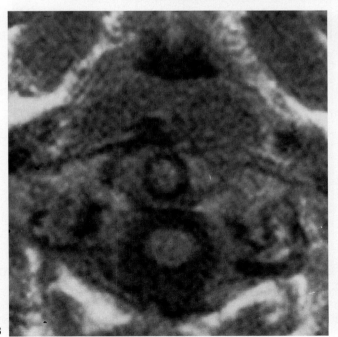

B

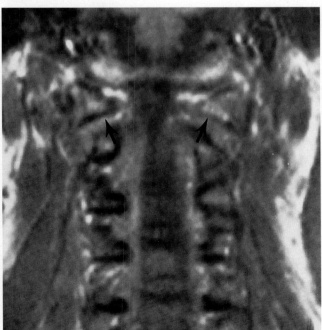

C

raphy has demonstrated that a posterior arch fracture usually is present. On a lateral radiograph, there is comminution of the vertebral body with retropulsion of the posterior body fragments. The alignment of the posterior elements is normal. A vertical fracture of the vertebral body is seen on the frontal projection, but the posterior arch fracture is only seen on CT.

Odontoid Fractures

Fractures of the dens can occur with either forced hyperflexion or forced hyperextension of the head or the neck. Hyperflexion injuries cause the dens to be displaced anteriorly, and there is forward subluxation of C-1 on C-2. Hyperextension injuries cause the dens to be displaced posteriorly, and there is posterior subluxation of C-1 on C-2. The dens moves with C-1 unless there is rupture of the transverse ligament. Fractures of the dens also can occur without subluxation of C-1 on C-2. Fractures of the dens without displacement of C-1 on C-2 can be most difficult to recognize. Polytomography of the dens may be helpful in detecting these fractures.

Odontoid fractures have been classified by Anderson and D'Alonzo (29) into three types. Type I is an avulsion fracture of the top of the dens, which is rare. Type II is a transverse fracture of the dens above the body of the axis. Type II fracture has a propensity to develop nonunion. Type III is a fracture of the superior portion of the axis body that involves one or both articulating facets (Fig. 12). This type of fracture is not really a fracture of the dens but is actually a fracture of the superior portion of the axis body. Because it involves an area of cancellous bone, it heals more readily.

Although MRI is not the imaging modality of choice for fracture detection, most bony injuries can be identified by MRI (Fig. 13). This is particularly true of vertebral body fractures (13). Nondisplaced fractures involving the posterior elements are not detected as easily (14). The importance of plain radiographs and CT for fracture detection cannot be overstated. Magnetic resonance imaging is not a substitute for CT. The ability of MRI to determine if displaced bone fragments compress vital structures such as the spinal cord, however, makes it an invaluable tool in pa-

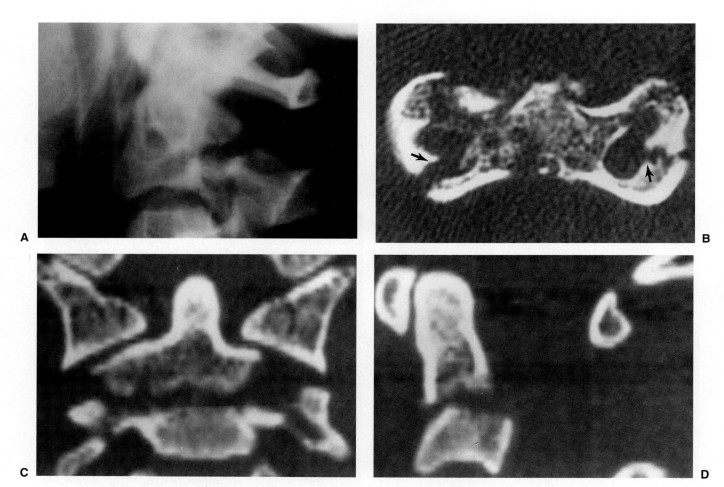

FIG. 12. Type III odontoid fracture. **A:** Lateral plain film. Note the anterior translation and displacement of the dens. **B:** Axial computed tomographic scan through the axis body shows fracture lines that traverse both transverse foramina *(arrows)*. **C:** Coronal reconstructed image shows fracture through the axis body. **D:** Sagittal reconstruction through the midline shows the anterior displacement of the dens.

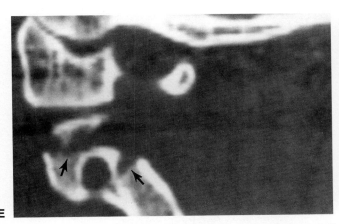

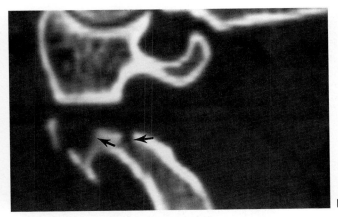

FIG. 12. *Continued.* **E,F:** Right and left parasagittal reconstructed images, respectively, show fractures extending through both transverse foramina and therefore do not allow posterior transarticular screw fixation *(arrows).*

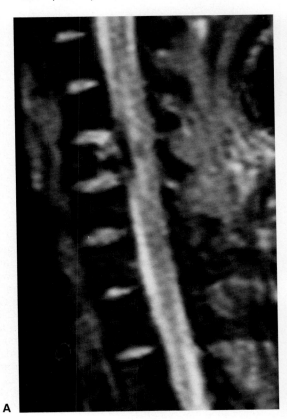

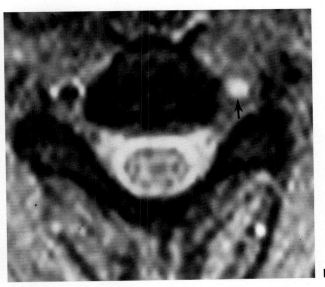

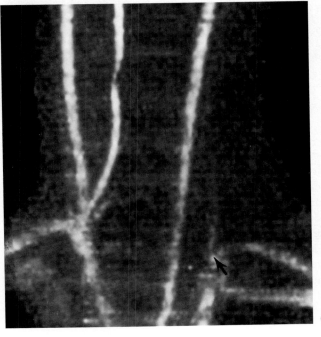

FIG. 13. Burst fracture of C-5. Vertebral artery injury. **A:** T2-weighted gradient-echo sagittal image. **B:** T2-weighted gradient axial image. **C:** Coronal maximum intensity projection from a two-dimensional time-of-flight angiogram. **A:** C-5 burst fracture is present with cord hemorrhage and edema. Axial image **(B)** reveals asymmetric signal in the vertebral arteries. The right vertebral artery demonstrates low signal, whereas the left is bright *(arrow).* Magnetic resonance angiography **(C)** reveals lack of time-of-flight enhancement in the left vertebral artery just distal to its origin from the subclavian artery *(arrow).* At the level of injury, the right vertebral artery is narrowed.

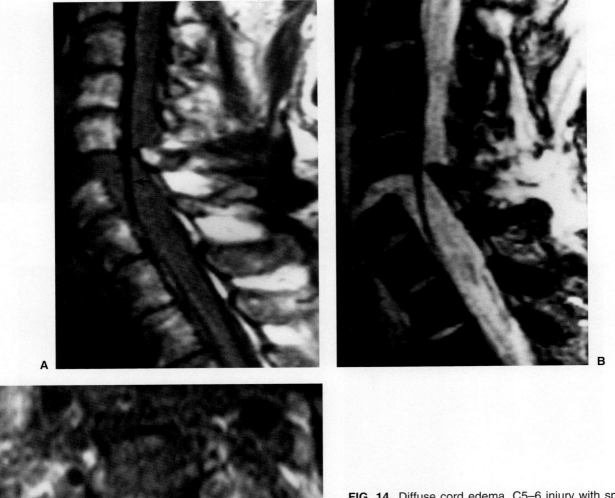

FIG. 14. Diffuse cord edema, C5–6 injury with spinal column disruption, bony spinal cord compression, and subligamentous edema versus hematoma. **A:** T1-weighted sagittal image. **B:** Gradient-echo sagittal image. **C:** T1-weighted axial image. There is distraction at the C5–6 intervertebral disc space, with subluxation of the C-5 vertebral body. The posterior elements of C-6 relative to those above have slipped forward. Resultant severe cord compression is present. Although the posterior longitudinal ligament (PLL) appears to be intact, it is lifted away from the C-6 vertebral body *(arrow)*. Just anterior to the PLL is soft tissue that is isointense to the spinal cord, most likely edema. The cord signal is diffusely abnormal, which is compatible with extensive edema.

tients with displaced fractures (Fig. 14). In addition, the detection of associated soft tissue abnormalities, such as herniated discs, ligamentous injury, and epidural hematomas, is unrivaled.

Several MRI signs exist that indicate the presence of a spine fracture. The T2W and T2* images are best suited for the detection of cortical interruptions (6). Although we do not routinely use fat saturation sequences, they may be helpful in the detection of marrow edema (30). Interruption of the dark signal of cortical bone, the presence of a fracture line

that is isointense to hypointense signal on T1W images and hyperintense signal on T2W images, identification of abnormal marrow signal (relative decreased signal intensity on T1W images and relative increased signal intensity on T2W images) secondary to edema or marrow hemorrhage (13,15,31), or loss of vertebral body height are all direct signs of a spine fracture. Parasagittal images are particularly suited in the evaluation of facet subluxations/dislocations (Fig. 15) (13), whereas midline sagittal images are useful in the evaluation of vertebral body subluxations.

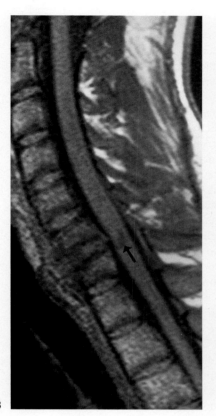 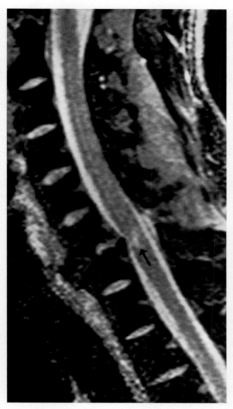 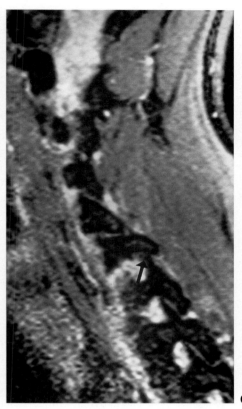

A,B   C

FIG. 15. Cord contusion, facet subluxation, and facet cord subluxation contusion. **A,B:** T1-weighted and T2-weighted gradient-echo sagittal images. **C:** Right parasagittal T2-weighted gradient-echo image. Significant acute injury has occurred at the C6–7 level. After partial reduction, the patient underwent magnetic resonance imaging, which demonstrated a focal cord contusion at C6–7 *(arrows)*. There is minimal residual bony cord compression. Parasagittal image reveals that the inferior facet of C-6 is nearly perched on the superior facet of C-7 *(arrow)*. Incidentally seen is acute hemorrhage in the C6–7 disc space, with ventral herniation of disc material.

Extradural Lesions

The identification of extradural compressive lesions is the prime consideration in the MRI evaluation of the acutely traumatized spine. Accurate identification and localization of these extradural compressive lesions is important so that the surgeon can relieve the mass effect on the spinal cord. The benefit of rapid decompression of an acutely compressed spinal cord is based on experimental evidence that the degree of permanent neurologic deficit is related to the duration of cord compression (32–34). Early decompression of the traumatized spinal cord can improve neurologic outcome.

The information that MRI provides concerning the nature of posttraumatic extradural lesions is crucial in the preoperative evaluation. Meticulous description of lesion location and lesion extent is important in the determination of the surgical approach (35). Both T1W and T2W sequences along with CT correlation are necessary for accurate characterization of posttraumatic extradural lesions.

It has been shown that extradural soft tissue masses are more easily diagnosed by MRI compared to CT myelogra-

phy (7,14). The common posttraumatic lesions include epidural hematomas, disc herniations, and bone fragments. Bone fragments are detected easily with CT, but direct visualization of spinal cord compression by displaced bone fragments can only be achieved with myelography/CT myelography or MRI (Fig. 14).

One problem encountered when interpreting magnetic resonance image in the first 72 hours after injury is distinguishing small focal epidural hematomas from subligamentous edema, engorged epidural veins, or herniated discs. In this hyperacute to acute period, a sufficient amount of methemoglobin may not be present, resulting in a "watery" appearance of the hematoma. Instead of hyperintense T1 signal, isointense signal is present on T1W images and hyperintense signal on T2W or T2* images (13). In this early period of epidural hematoma formation, T2* images may provide the only clue to the etiology of the extradural lesion as areas of hypointense signal may be identified. Note, however, that this hypointense signal, which represents deoxyhemoglobin in an acute hematoma, also could be secondary to hemorrhage in a traumatic disc herniation or be confused with a bone fragment. Tarr et al. (14) reported a case of an epidural hematoma that demonstrated hyperintense T1 signal within 24 hours of injury. The distinction between extensive epidural hematomas and other posttraumatic extradural lesions is not as problematic as small focal epidural hematomas.

Magnetic resonance imaging is superior to CT myelography in the detection of posttraumatic disc herniations (7). In some series, posttraumatic disc herniations were seen in up to 100% of cases using MRI (31). Except for the presence of acute intradiscal blood, MRI cannot reliably distinguish a traumatic from a nontraumatic disc herniation. The signal within a traumatic disc herniation may parallel the signal of the parent intervertebral disc space or reflect the presence of edema and/or blood products. Disc space narrowing may or may not be present.

Spinal Cord

The information that MRI can provide regarding the acutely injured spinal cord is unrivaled (Fig. 14). Magnetic resonance imaging has been found to be superior in the detection of spinal cord parenchymal abnormalities compared to myelography/CT myelography (6,7,13,14). Magnetic resonance imaging is the only imaging study that can directly image the spinal cord parenchyma with sufficient contrast resolution and demonstrate intrinsic signal abnormality even in the absence of cord enlargement. Myelography and CT myelography can only provide information regarding spinal cord size or spinal cord compression. Magnetic resonance imaging can reliably determine if acute posttraumatic cord enlargement is related to edema or hemorrhage and identify hemorrhage or contusive change in a nonenlarged cord.

Kulkarni et al. (15) were one of the first to report signal cord parenchymal changes in the acutely injured spinal cord utilizing a 1.5-T magnet. Three types of MRI signal patterns in patients imaged 1 day to 6 weeks after injury were reported by Kulkarni et al. (15). In 19 patients who demonstrated MRI evidence of cord injury, 5 had evidence of cord hemorrhage with decreased T2 signal within 72 hours of injury. A peripheral T2 hyperintense rim with persistence of central T2 hypointensity images was seen up to 7 days after injury. In a second group of 12 patients, only cord edema was appreciated (Fig. 14). This cord edema, which manifested with increased T2 signal, showed evidence of some resolution from 7 days to 3 weeks after injury. A mixture of hemorrhage and edema with central hypointensity surrounded by a rim of hyperintensity on T2W images was identified as a third pattern of cord injury in two patients. Resolution of cord lesion with blood products was slower than those cord lesions that were nonhemorrhagic. In the early period after injury, T1W images were only useful in demonstrating cord swelling and failed to reveal significant signal change in the cord parenchyma.

Many authors have tried to correlate parenchymal MRI signal changes and the degree of neurologic impairment in the acute setting (4,5,8,15). Flanders et al. (6) studied 104 patients with acute cervical injury using MRI. In this comprehensive report, Flanders et al. (6) related the degree of motor recovery with the extent of cervical spinal cord damage as seen by MRI within 72 hours of injury. In this series of patients, the authors concluded that the presence of intramedullary hemorrhage or an extensive segment of spinal cord edema was predictive of worse motor recovery 1 year after injury in comparison to patients with smaller nonhemorrhagic lesions. Flanders et al. (5) showed that 91% of their patients with complete neurologic injury demonstrated evidence of parenchymal edema involving more than 1 cm of the cord. Significant neurologic improvement can be anticipated if the initial magnetic resonance image reveals no parenchymal abnormality.

The T2W images are most important in the detection of intramedullary spinal cord damage. Studies have shown that T1W images demonstrate spinal cord enlargement and offer less information about parenchymal signal abnormalities (4,7,15,33,36–38). Various authors also reported that spin-echo T2W images are best for demonstrating cord edema (Fig. 14), whereas T2* images are superior for demonstrating blood products (4,5,37). T2* images may not depict edema as well as T2 spin-echo sequences (37).

Significant evidence exists that the presence of intramedullary cord hemorrhage and extensive cord edema are poor prognostic indicators of neurologic recovery. What is the best sequence for hemorrhage detection in the acute period after injury? T2* images are the most sensitive sequence in the acute phase. Deoxyhemoglobin results in signal loss on T2* images (Fig. 16). The development of methemoglobin is somewhat delayed in intramedullary spinal cord hematomas when compared to brain hematomas and may not be present for at least 7 days or more after injury (5). This delay may be the result of a relatively ischemic environment within the spinal cord.

Progressive Posttraumatic Myelopathy

Spinal Cord Cysts

Posttraumatic myelopathy can occur in up to 32% of chronically injured spinal cord patients (39). Posttraumatic myelopathy may present as early as 2 months after injury or as late as 36 years after injury (39). Progressive posttraumatic myelopathy may be related to several etiologies. One of the more common treatable parenchymal abnormalities is a spinal cord cyst (Fig. 17) (22). Progressive myelopathy also can be seen in the presence of myelomalacia and cord tethering (Figs. 18 and 19) (40). Cord tethering likely plays a significant role in the development of both myelomalacia and spinal cord cysts. There also is evidence that myelomalacia and spinal cord cysts are part of a continuum (10,22,40–44). Imaging plays a key role in the differentiation between spinal cord cyst and myelomalacia, because there is a lack of clinical distinction (10,40,41,42,45). Magnetic resonance imaging is the imaging modality of choice in

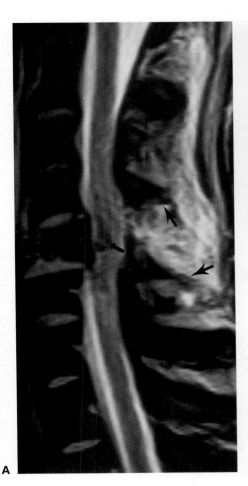

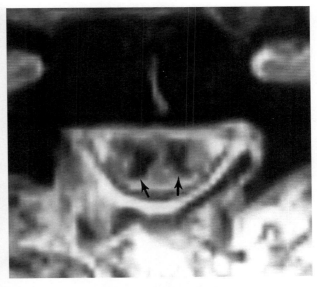

FIG. 16. Acute spinal cord hemorrhage, interspinous ligamentous injury, and burst fracture. This young man suffered an automobile accident several hours prior to this scan. T2-weighted gradient-echo sagittal **(A)** and T2-weighted gradient-echo axial image through C-5 **(B)**. **A:** Burst fracture of the C-5 vertebral body is present. Note the associated decrease in ventral subarachnoid space and mild cord compression. Underneath this injury there is decreased signal intensity predominantly involving the central gray matter of the spinal cord *(arrows)*. This is most consistent with acute hemorrhage (deoxyhemoglobin). The C4–5 interspinous ligaments are disrupted with splaying of the spinous processes *(arrows)*, fracture of the C-5 spinous process, and increased T2 signal in the intervening soft tissues.

the evaluation of patients with progressive posttraumatic myelopathy (11). Less common causes of posttraumatic myelopathy that also are detectable by MRI include cord compression from malalignment, herniated disc, or osteophytes, arachnoid cysts, and cord atrophy.

Quencer et al. (11) first demonstrated the benefit of MRI compared to immediate and delayed CT myelography in differentiating spinal cord cysts from myelomalacia. In addition to the obvious drawbacks of myelography, both false-positive and false-negative cases of spinal cord cysts were found with myelography. Spinal cord cysts can best be evaluated with axial and sagittal T1W MRI images.

Spinal cord cysts almost always follow CSF signal intensity on MRI (Fig. 17) (11). Cerebrospinal fluid pulsation-induced signal loss or flow-related enhancement that may be seen in large pulsatile cysts can alter the MRI appearance (46). Although the cyst contents may contain an elevated protein content compared to CSF and theoretically shorten T1 and T2 relaxation, this is rarely a problem. A well-defined border usually can be traced around the cyst, although when a cyst develops in a region of severely damaged spinal cord tissue, the entire border may not be well defined (11). Posttraumatic spinal cord cysts may be single cavities or contain septations and may occur above, below, or at the site of initial injury. Cine images may be helpful in the determi-

nation of cyst pulsatility (12). Postoperative cine evaluation may help determine if shunting of the cyst was successful.

Myelomalacia

Closed spinal cord trauma is a common mechanism leading to a myelomalacic or soft cord. Histologically, myelomalacia is characterized by microcysts, reactive astrocytosis, and thickening of the pia-arachnoid (20). Intraoperative observations at our institution have always revealed associated cord tethering (Figs. 18 and 19). The cord is tethered by arachnoid fibrous adhesions associated with thickening of the overlying dura. Recognition of posttraumatic myelomalacia may be important, because recent observations implicate myelomalacia as a cause of progressive myelopathy. Untethering of the spinal cord may lead to clinical improvement (40).

On MRI (Figs. 18 and 19), a myelomalacic cord typically reveals abnormal hypointense signal that is greater in intensity than the CSF on T1W images. T2W images reveal corresponding hyperintensity within the spinal cord. The proton density or spin density sequence may be helpful when there is difficulty distinguishing between myelomalacia and a spinal cord cyst. Myelo-

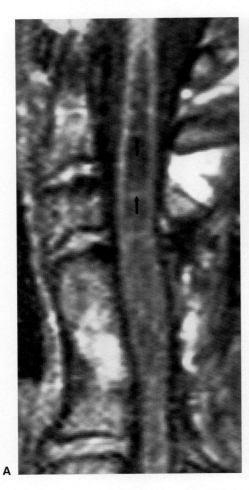

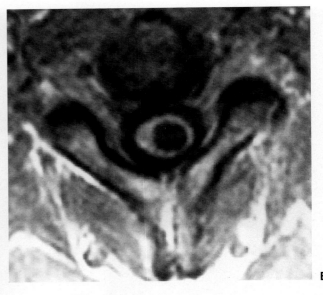

FIG. 17. Traumatic spinal cord cyst. T1-weighted sagittal image **(A)** and axial image **(B)**. This patient underwent prior an anterior corpectomy discectomy and fusion (ACDF). for spinal fracture he suffered many years ago. He is an incomplete quadriplegic who is experiencing an ascending myelopathy. The spinal cord signal is abnormal from C1–C7, with expansion of the cord from C3–C6. Axial image through C2–C3 best demonstrates the nature of the signal abnormality, with a well-defined and marginated eccentric spinal cord cyst. Note the septations within the cyst on the sagittal view *(arrows)*.

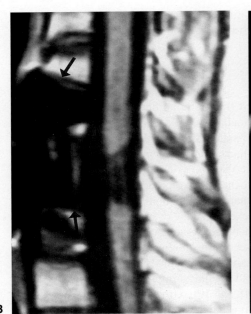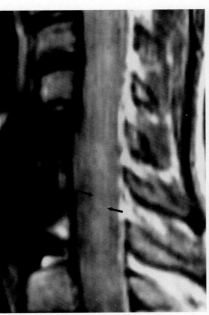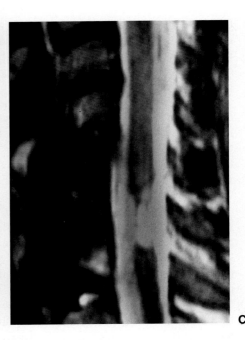

FIG. 18. Microcystic myelomalacia, cord atrophy, cord tethering, and wallerian degeneration. A 16-year-old boy who suffered acute traumatic quadriparesis several years ago now presents with worsening neurologic deficit. **A:** T1-weighted sagittal image. **B:** Proton density (PD) sagittal image. **C:** T2-weighted sagittal image.

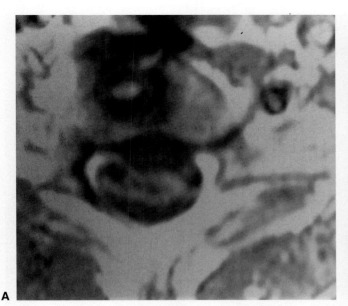

A

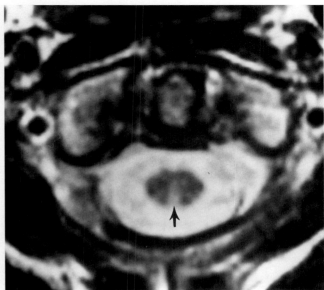

B

FIG. 18. *Continued.* **D:** T1-weighted axial image at C5–6. **E:** T2-weighted axial image at C-1. Metallic artifact from ACDF is present from C5–C7 *(arrows)*. The spinal cord is small below the level of injury, which is indicative of spinal cord atrophy. At the level of injury, a focal signal abnormality is present within the spinal cord, which does not follow CSF signal on PD image *(arrows)*. The cord is also deformed at this level and tethered to the right **(D)**. **E:** Hyperintense signal in the dorsal columns is compatible with wallerian degeneration *(arrows)*.

malacia will not parallel CSF and reveals isointense to hyperintense signal change relative to normal spinal cord on spin density images (40). The margins of a myelomalacic cord usually are irregular and ill defined. A myelomalacic cord may be normal in size, atrophic, or expanded.

Cord tethering is usually a coexistent feature of myelomalacia. Tethering manifests on MRI as an asymmetric loss of the subarachnoid space. Loss of the subarachnoid space most commonly occurs dorsally. This presumably results from the prolonged recumbency of these patients, although ventral tethering also has been appreciated. Cord expansion, which may be associated with myelomalacia, results from a "pulling apart" of the spinal cord by fibrous adhesions. These adhesions may be visualized on MRI (40). We have found that gradient-echo cine MRI may be useful in the confirmation and detection of cord tethering. Loss of normal CSF flow patterns are seen in patients with a tethered cord. Flow studies are useful after untethering, because these studies will demonstrate reestablishment of flow in areas of previous tethering (unpublished data).

Wallerian Degeneration

Once the neuronal cell body has been damaged and loses its axonal connection, disintegration of the axon and its myelin sheath ensues (47). This process results in damage to tissue remote from the primary site of injury. Little is known about the clinical significance to the identification of these lesions. Recognition is important so that other etiologies are not ascribed to the signal alterations that occur with these lesions.

Terae et al. (48) described 6 patients in whom high signal was observed on long TR images in the posterior columns cephalad to the primary site without corresponding abnormality on T1W images. These signal alterations were seen 10 weeks to 12 months after injury. Magnetic resonance imaging with histologic correlation from postmortem spinal cords of patients who suffered traumatic spinal cord injury demonstrated that wallerian degeneration occurred at an injury to death interval greater than 7 weeks (24). Becerra et al. (24) also showed that wallerian degeneration occurred below the primary injury site within the corticospinal tracts. Areas of wallerian degeneration are best appreciated on axial T2 images (Fig. 18) (24,48).

THORACOLUMBAR SPINE TRAUMA

Fractures of the thoracolumbar spine follow in frequency fractures of the cervical spine. Thoracolumbar spine fractures represent one third of the spinal fractures (49,50). Sixty to seventy percent of the thoracic and lumbar spine fractures occur at the thoracolumbar junction (T12–L2), and about 40% of these fractures are associated with different degrees of neurologic deficits (51).

Important Anatomic Features of the Thoracic and Lumbar Spine

Twelve vertebrae compose the thoracic spine. The vertebral body is the load-bearing portion, whereas the posterior neural arch, which consists of the paired pedicles, laminas, ar-

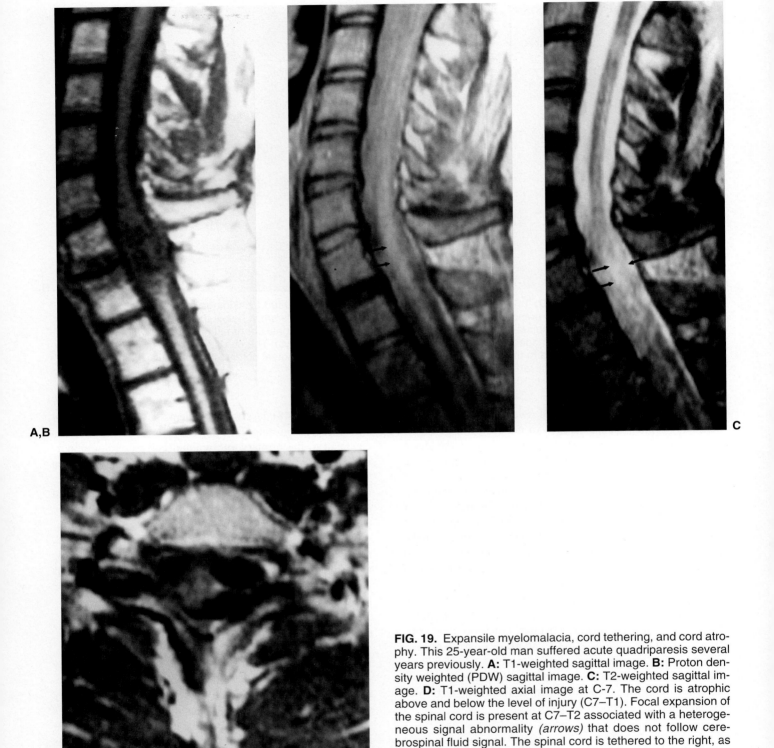

FIG. 19. Expansile myelomalacia, cord tethering, and cord atrophy. This 25-year-old man suffered acute quadriparesis several years previously. **A:** T1-weighted sagittal image. **B:** Proton density weighted (PDW) sagittal image. **C:** T2-weighted sagittal image. **D:** T1-weighted axial image at C-7. The cord is atrophic above and below the level of injury (C7–T1). Focal expansion of the spinal cord is present at C7–T2 associated with a heterogeneous signal abnormality *(arrows)* that does not follow cerebrospinal fluid signal. The spinal cord is tethered to the right, as demonstrated on the axial image.

ticulating facets, and transverse processes, deals with tensional forces.

The height of the thoracic vertebral bodies is 2 to 3 mm less anteriorly than posteriorly, which accounts for the mild kyphosis that characterizes the thoracic spine. From T-1 to T-12 the anteroposterior and transverse diameters of the thoracic spine increase progressively. A coronal orientation of the thoracic spine articulating facets is the anatomic and biomechanical landmark of this segment of the spine.

The coronal orientation of the articulating facets provides stability in the anteroposterior plane by limiting any significant motion in this direction. Another stabilizing factor that enhances the strength and shock-absorbing capabilities of the thoracic spine in situations of trauma is provided by articulating facets for the ribs at the costotransverse articulation and the vertebral body itself. This articulation occurs by way of demifacets above and below the disc space.

As opposed to the cervical and lumbar spine, the thoracic spine has the smallest concentric canal diameter. The intervertebral discs are smaller but have thicker anuli fibrosis. The thoracic spine ligamentous apparatus is similar to the rest of the spine and is composed of the ALL, PLL, ligamentum flavum, interspinous, supraspinous, and capsular ligaments (52).

In the absence of a transitional segment, the lumbar spine is composed of five vertebrae. The lumbar spine lacks articulating processes of ribs. The rest of the bony elements of the lumbar spine are similar to those of the rest of the spine.

The spinal canal increases in concentric diameter from the thoracolumbar junction to the lumbosacral junction. In the lumbar spine, the facet joints, instead of being oriented coronally, are oriented in the sagittal plane. This anatomic configuration is helpful to resist rotational biomechanical forces.

Because the thoracic spine and chest cage act as a single unit with limited range of motion, the thoracolumbar junction becomes a fulcrum for spinal motion, allowing abnormal forces to cause fractures and/or subluxations with increased frequency in this area.

Spinal Injury and Associated Osseous Abnormalities

Fractures of the Upper Thoracic Spine

Fractures of the upper thoracic spine (T1–10) are different from other levels of spinal fractures because they are relatively stable as a result of the presence of the rib cage and the strong attaching costovertebral ligaments that limit the degree of motion of this segment of the spine. An axial orientation of the facet joints limits rotational forces in the axial plane.

The injuries that usually affect the upper thoracic spine occur in flexion or extension. Upper thoracic spine injuries not uncommonly are associated to injuries of the head, cervical spine, and chest.

The most common type of fracture that occurs in the upper thoracic spine is the compression or axial loading fracture, which leads to different degrees of anterior wedging of

the vertebral body being affected. When neurologic deficit occurs, it usually is due to cord compression secondary to the presence of retropulsed bone within the spinal canal. Alternatively, the cord may be compressed by herniated nucleus pulposus or epidural hematomas. Posttraumatic thoracic disc herniations are an uncommon event. Nevertheless, when the disc herniates, it usually protrudes through a torn PLL.

In addition to the anterior wedging fractures, the upper thoracic spine may be affected by burst fractures usually secondary to a severe axial loading force applied to the vertebra. Burst fractures of the upper thoracic spine may have associated fractures of the posterior neural arch (Fig. 1). Any comminuted retropulsed bone fragment can cause cord compression or cord maceration, a finding that is well demonstrated on MRI.

A third type of posttraumatic upper thoracic spine fracture is the sagittal slice fracture. In this type of fracture, the vertebra above telescopes into the vertebra below, with secondary lateral displacement of the latter. Severe cord damage usually supervenes with this type of fracture. If, in addition to the vertebral fracture, anterolisthesis or retrolisthesis is present, this should be considered a sign of likely rupture of the ALL or PLL. Severe dislocations usually are accompanied by ligamental disruption and facet dislocation, findings that frequently are associated with severe cord injury. Seventeen percent of upper thoracic spine fractures are associated with a second, noncontiguous spinal fracture. This second site of fracture often will be located in the upper cervical spine and/or the thoracolumbar junction. Therefore, investigation of these areas with plain films, CT, or MRI may be warranted in patients in whom the clinical symptoms and neurologic findings are not easily explained by the thoracolumbar spine fracture.

More than half of patients with injury to the upper thoracic spine may present with radiographic findings of mediastinal widening, pleural fluid, and apical cap, findings that are seen in patients with traumatic aortic transection. If a fracture of the upper thoracic spine is detected in a patient with mediastinal widening and an apical pleural cap, aortic rupture becomes a less likely diagnosis only if the clinical symptoms and signs do not support this diagnosis. Nevertheless, it is necessary to keep in mind that aortic rupture and acute spinal fractures can be present with signs of paraparesis or paraplegia, the former by impairing the cord vascular supply leading to ischemia and infarct; the latter by compressing the cord.

Trauma to the upper thoracic spine may be associated with a fracture of the sternum, with posterior displacement of the upper sternal fragment. The sternal fracture usually results from a spinal fracture and/or spinal dislocation, with forces transmitted to the sternum through the ribs.

Although most of the upper thoracic spine fractures are stable, instability needing surgical correction is seen in instances of complete dislocations, kyphosis greater than 40 degrees, progressing kyphosis, persistent pain, and progressive neurologic deficits. Another indication for surgical intervention in patients with upper thoracic fractures is given by the MRI demonstration of disruption of the spinal supporting ligaments. In the setting of acute trauma, radiographic findings suggestive of spinal instability include vertebral subluxation, widening of the interspinous or interlaminar distance, disruption of the posterior body line, and vertebral wedging greater than 40% (52).

Fractures of the Thoracolumbar Junction

The thoracolumbar junction (T11–L2) is one of the areas most commonly affected during spinal trauma. Most of the thoracolumbar injuries occur between T12–L2, which represents the area of transition between a stiff and a more mobile segment of the spine. In addition, a changing orientation of the facet joints, absence of adjacent supporting structures, and a greater range of motion of the spine favor an increased incidence of neurologic deficit, which has an incidence as high as 40% in patients with this type of fracture (53).

Ferguson and Allen (54), McAfee et al. (55), and Dennis (56) have created a mechanistic classification for the thoracolumbar fractures. In this classification, the "three column" concept divides the vertebra into three main regions: the anterior column, middle column, and posterior column. The anterior column is composed of the ALL, the anterior anulus fibrosus, and the anterior vertebral body. The middle column is represented by the posterior vertebral body margin, the PLL, and the posterior anulus fibrosus. The posterior column is represented by all the structures behind the PLL (neural arch). The main purpose of this classification is to predict the stability and neurologic sequela of the fractures of the thoracolumbar region. Thus, an intact middle column equals spinal stability and vice versa. Fractures of the anterior column rarely will be associated with neurologic deficit (56).

From the studies of McAfee et al. (55), three basic types of forces act to injure the middle column: axial compression, axial distraction, and lateral translation. These vectors of force are applied in the x, y, or z axis of the spine and produce the following types of injuries:

Hyperflexion Injuries

This is the most common type of injury affecting the thoracolumbar spine. The anterior column is compressed while the posterior elements are distracted. There are several types of hyperflexion injuries.

Hyperflexion Compression Fractures. This type of fracture commonly affects T-12, L-1 and L-2 (Fig. 20). The compression force can occur anteriorly or laterally, which becomes manifest on x-ray or MRI by loss of height of the vertebral body anteriorly or laterally, focal kyphosis/scoliosis, and/or fracture, usually of the anterosuperior endplate or the presence of a paraspinal hematoma. The CT analysis requires careful review of the scout or pilot view, which would show the loss of height of the vertebral body injured. The disc space may or may not be narrow. A prever-

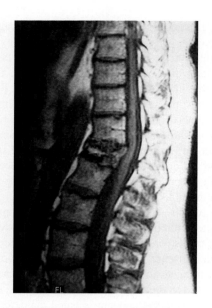

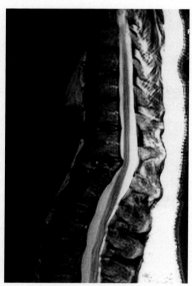

FIG. 20. Chronic hyperflexion compression fracture of T-12. Sagittal T1-weighted and T2-weighted images. There is severe loss of height of the T-12 body anteriorly, with associated endplate disruption. Note the focal kyphos deformity indenting the sac and the cord. (Reproduced with permission from Ruiz A, Post MJD, Sklar EML. Traumatic thoracic and lumbar fractures. *Appl Radiol* October 1996: 49–57.)

tebral/paraspinal hematoma usually is present. If the axial force applied to the vertebral body is large enough, the posterior column may disrupt and distract, leading to dislocation and instability (49).

Flexion/distraction Injury. This type of injury more often occurs from L1–3 and may occur in two different ways. In one instance, the middle and posterior columns may be disrupted by the tensional forces applied with secondary rupture of the anulus fibrosus and secondary subluxation. A second way for this type of spinal injury is when hyperflexion occurs around an axis anterior to the ALL. When this occurs,

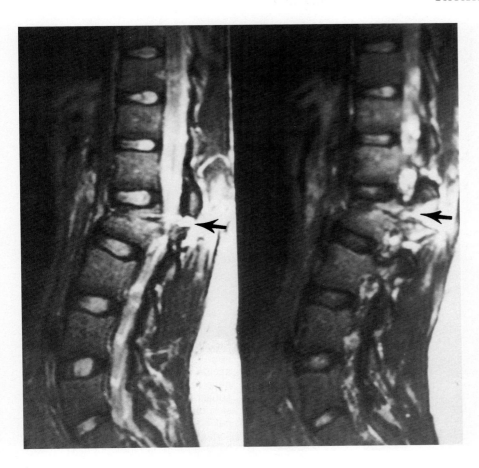

FIG. 21. Chance fracture. Female adolescent involved in a motor vehicle accident while wearing a lap seat belt. The patient sustained a flexion/distraction injury. Contiguous sagittal T2-weighted images demonstrate a split fracture through the posterior elements and posterior L-2 body. There is injury to the posterior spinal ligaments (*black arrows*). (Reproduced with permission from Ruiz A, Post MJD, Sklar EML. Traumatic thoracic and lumbar fractures. *Appl Radiol* October 1996: 49–57.)

the entire vertebra is pulled apart or distracted by a tensile force. This type of spinal injury leads to what is known as a Chance fracture or seat belt injury (Fig. 21).

Radiographically, a split fracture through the spinous processes, pedicles, and lamina is demonstrated. The fracture line extends upward to involve the vertebral endplate anterior to the neural foramen. There is also severe disruption of the spinal ligaments and distraction of the intervertebral disc and facet joints. The fracture is unstable and usually is associated with severe abdominal injuries (57,58). Two thirds of the thoracolumbar spine flexion/distraction injuries are associated with some degree of neurologic deficit. In the case of the Chance fracture, the neurologic compromise reaches up to 20%.

Flexion/rotation Injuries. Flexion/rotation injury is an unusual and very unstable injury that frequently is associated with severe neurologic damage/sequela such as paraplegia (Fig. 22). The anterior column is compressed undergoing rotation, whereas the middle and posterior columns are disrupted by tensional forces. Subluxation and dislocation are frequent imaging findings as well as widening of the interspinous distance and fractures of the laminae/transverse processes, facets, and adjacent ribs. Facet dislocation, when present, gives the finding of a "naked facet" on CT (59,60). This CT sign is the appearance in the transverse plane of the vertically distracted articular process.

Shearing Fracture-dislocation. In shearing fracture-dislocation, all three columns are damaged secondary to an impacting force applied in the horizontal plane from posterior to anterior or vice versa, thereby producing anterior and posterior dislocation with secondary facet fracture and/or dislocation.

Hyperextension Injury

Hyperextension injury is a rare type of injury that occurs when a patient falls and hyperextends over an object. Radiographically, there is widening of the disc space anteriorly, posterior subluxation, avulsion fracture of the anterosuperior corner of the vertebra, and fracture of the posterior neural arch.

Axial Compression Fractures

The characteristic fracture in this group is the burst fracture (Fig. 23). An axial loading force pushes the intervertebral disc through the endplate inferiorly (vertical disc herniation), with secondary comminution of the vertebral body. Ninety percent of burst fractures occur from T9–L5. A second burst fracture is present in less than 10% of cases. Radiographic findings characteristic of this fracture are severe anterior vertebral body wedging, bone retropulsion with different de-

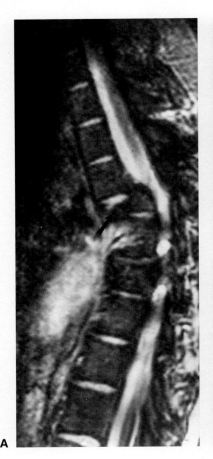
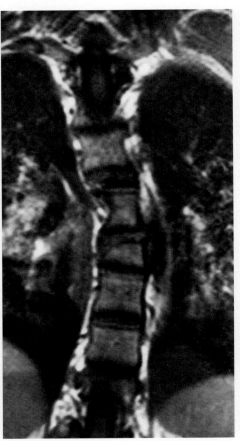

FIG. 22. Flexion/rotation injury in a 45-year-old woman involved in a boating accident. **A:** Sagittal T2-weighted magnetic resonance image shows marked subluxation of T-3 on T-4 with compression deformity of T-4 *(arrow).* **B:** Coronal T1-weighted image shows the rotational component of this injury. The T-3 body is rotated to the right of T-4.

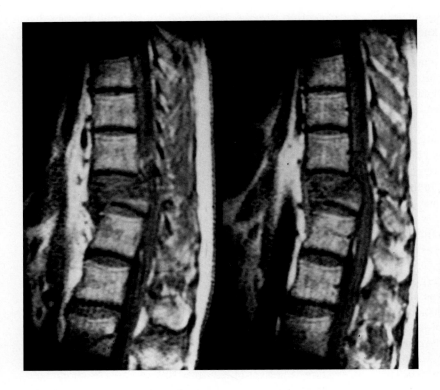

FIG. 23. Axial compression fracture of T-12. Sagittal T1-weighted images demonstrate superior endplate fracture, wedging deformity, and retropulsion of T-12, severely compressing the cord. The decreased signal of T-12 vertebra is due to marrow edema. (Reproduced with permission from Ruiz A, Post MJD, Sklar EML. Traumatic thoracic and lumbar fractures. *Appl Radiol* October 1996: 49–57.)

grees of neural canal narrowing, neural element compression, increased interpediculate distance, and vertical fracture through the vertebral body, pedicle, or laminae. Depending on the degree of bone retropulsion and level of injury, different degrees of cord, conus, and cauda equina damage may be present (61,62). This injury is an unstable one. Computed tomography and MRI are the best modalities to evaluate this injury. Computed tomography former will demonstrate the degree of bony canal narrowing, whereas MRI provides superb information about the relationship between the retropulsed bone and spinal neural elements, including the level and degree of neural damage. Magnetic resonance imaging also gives information about the status of the disc and ligamental apparatus.

Sacrococcygeal Injuries

Fractures that involve the sacrum and coccyx do not occur frequently because of the immobility of this segment and because of the protection given by the pelvis. When they are fractured, the trauma usually is quite severe and the pelvis is fractured as well. In these cases, the plain films often are inadequate due to the overlying soft tissue and bowel shadows (29). Computed tomography is ideal for diagnosing sacrococcygeal spinal fractures and for detecting bony fragments in the spinal canal. Computed tomography also detects associated pelvic fractures and hematomas (Fig. 24).

Other Thoracolumbar Spine Fractures

Fractures of the Transverse Process

Fractures of the transverse process may occur as an isolated injury or as part of other spinal fractures. In the lumbar spine, this type of fracture usually results from a direct blow to the flank or strenuous contraction of the quadratus lumborum and/or psoas muscles. One of the several transverse processes may fracture. The fracture may be unilateral or bilateral. Distraction of the fracture fragments usually is seen. The clinical evaluation of patients with this type of fracture must include a careful search for associated neural or aortic injuries. The neurologic evaluation must be oriented to exclude injury to the lumbar plexus, which may be present in transverse process fractures affecting the L-3, L-4, or L-5 vertebrae.

Fractures of the Lower Lumbar Spine

Fractures of the lower lumbar spine are uncommon. The mechanism of injury usually is a severe axial loading force and hyperflexion at the L-4 or L-5 level. Bone retropulsion may be present. If the retropulsed bone occupies more than 60% of the spinal canal diameter and there is neurologic deficit, surgical stabilization is advocated (63).

Delayed Posttraumatic Vertebral Collapse (Kummell's Disease)

Delayed vertebral collapse usually occurs in the thoracic and thoracolumbar regions. It is believed that minor trauma without any overt fracture leads to this entity. The pathophysiology of this injury is thought to be related to avascular necrosis (a significant number of patients suffering from this phenomenon have been receiving steroids for long periods of time). The theory of avascular necrosis has been supported by angiographic and pathologic studies. In addition to vertebral body collapse, intravertebral and intradiscal vacuum phenomena often are demonstrated radiographically (64).

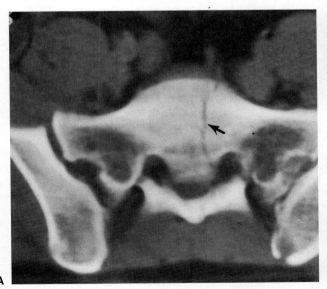
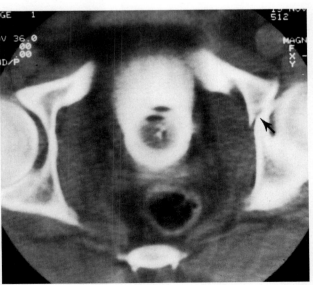

FIG. 24. Patient who sustained multiple pelvic and sacrococcygeal fractures. **A,B:** Computed tomographic axial images show fractures of the body of S-1 and of the left acetabulum *(arrows)*.

Nonosseous Posttraumatic Thoracolumbar Abnormalities

Extradural Lesions

Traumatic disc herniations occur at the cervical, thoracic, and lumbosacral levels. In one series, the cervical spine was the most frequent site of involvement (65). The thoracic spine is not affected frequently because the rib cage and thoracic muscles provide protection to this part of the spine. Herniated discs may be unrecognized if CT or MRI is not used. In patients with fracture-dislocations who are to undergo stabilization, the discovery of one associated herniated disc may indicate the need for a prompt surgical intervention, specifically a decompression discectomy and fusion.

Spinal epidural hematomas may produce spinal cord and/or cauda equina compression. The clinical presentation is that of sudden acute back or neck pain followed by sensory and motor deficits, with progression to paraplegia or quadriplegia. Although epidural hemorrhage in the spinal canal has been regarded in the literature as uncommon, with the availability of MRI this diagnosis is being made more often. These hematomas may show some compression of the thecal sac as well as compression of the spinal cord (Fig. 25). They show variable signal intensity. Magnetic resonance imaging is an excellent modality for diagnosing spinal epidural hematomas. Broad regions of the spine can be surveyed for abnormality and the full extent of the hematoma determined. The degree of compression of the thecal sac and cord can be quantified.

Avulsion of Nerve Root and Pseudomeningoceles

Trauma may cause damage to the nerve root sheath, the nerve roots themselves, or both (Fig. 26). When laceration of a nerve root and adjacent dura and arachnoid occurs, the nerve root stump retracts distally, producing a cavity that fills with CSF. Avulsions of the lumbosacral roots are not as frequent as those of the cervical roots, partly because of the stability and relative immobility of the pelvis and because of the deep location of the lumbosacral plexus. Typically, young adults who have avulsions of the lumbosacral roots have pelvic fractures and sacrococcygeal involvement. Myelography has been used to diagnose avulsions of nerve roots shown by irregular shaggy collections of contrast material, pseudomeningoceles, that extend beyond the normal confines of the nerve root sheath in the neural foramen. Computed tomographic myelography localizes the sites of these dural disruptions, demonstrates their intraspinal and extraspinal extension, and is the procedure of choice for small tears, although larger tears may be seen on T2W MRI.

Pseudomeningoceles may be caused by avulsed nerve roots or by an unintentional tear of the dura during surgery. If the tear heals, then communication with the subarachnoid space is lost and myelography may not show the communication (66,67). One then may see displacement of the contrast-filled true subarachnoid spaces, which indicates the presence of an extradural lesion, the pseudomeningocele. If large, the extradural location of the lesion is indicated on MRI by splaying of fat in the epidural space.

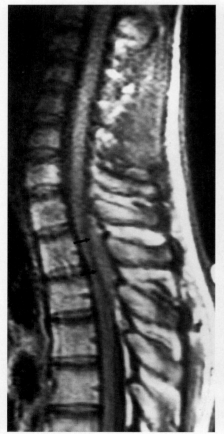
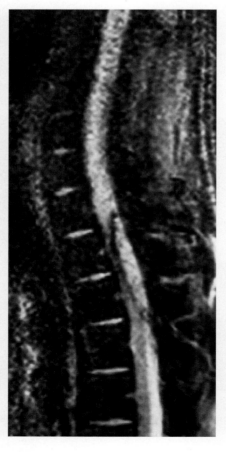

A,B

FIG. 25. Epidural hematoma. **A:** T1-weighted sagittal image shows an acute epidural hematoma *(arrows)* that is isointense relative to cord displacing the sac anteriorly. **B:** On gradient-echo image, the lesion becomes hyperintense. (Reproduced with permission from Sklar EML, Ruiz A, Whiteman MLH, Post MJD, Lebwohl NH. Vertebral and paravertebral abnormalities. In: Edelman RR, Hesselink JR, Zlatkin MB. *Clinical Magnetic Resonance Imaging,* 2nd edition. Philadelphia: WB Saunders, 1996;1278–1301.)

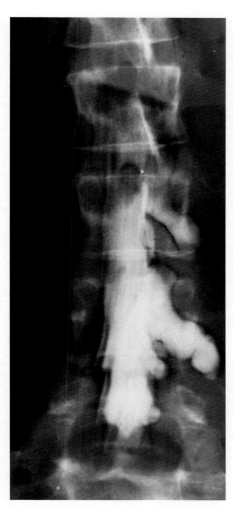

FIG. 26. A 25-year-old woman was involved in a motorcycle accident. After decreased strength in the left lower extremity was noted, a myelogram was performed. There are pools of contrast in the spaces left by the L-3, L-4 and L-5 nerve roots on the left. These indicate the nerve roots have been overruled at these levels. (Reproduced with permission from Sklar EML, Ruiz A, Whiteman MLH, Post MJD, Lebwohl NH. Imaging of thoracolumbar trauma. *Semin Spine Surg* 1992;4;111–125.)

Chronic Sequelae of Trauma

Posttraumatic spinal cord cysts and myelomalacia also occur in the thoracic spine. These lesions were described in the section on cervical spine trauma.

Subarachnoid cysts may occur as the sequelae of trauma (66). The definitive radiologic diagnosis of spinal subarachnoid cysts is difficult. In the past, radiologic evaluation has included plain films and computed tomography-myelography. Plain films may show only associated bony abnormalities, and myelography may be nondiagnostic if the cysts do not fill with contrast. Also, if a CSF block is present, diagnosis may not be possible.

From our experience, MRI appears to be the most efficient way to diagnose and characterize acquired subarachnoid cysts and associated abnormalities (66). T1-weighted images demonstrate a subarachnoid cyst as a low-intensity signal collection that becomes higher in intensity on T2W images

(Fig. 27), paralleled by CSF intensity. These collections usually produce mass effect on the cord, with indentations of the cord. These cysts seem to behave variably. In some, the subarachnoid cyst may be loculated and not in direct communi-

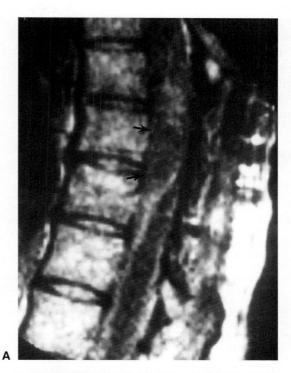

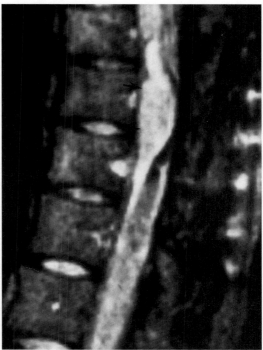

FIG. 27. Subarachnoid cyst. T1-weighted magnetic resonance image **(A)** shows focal area of low-intensity signal that becomes hyperintense on T2-weighted image **(B)** at T-9 and T-10. (Reproduced with permission from Sklar EML, Quencer RM, Green BA, et al. Acquired subarachnoic cysts: evaluation with MR, CT, myelography and intraoperative sonography. *AJNR Am J Neuroradiol* 1989;10:1097–1104.)

cation with the subarachnoid space. In this case, the cyst fluid is hyperintense relative to CSF on routine MRI studies. This is because the fluid within the cyst is loculated and not receiving enough pulsation to cause spin dephasing. In other cases, the cysts freely communicate with the rest of the subarachnoid space and the signal is lower or more heterogeneous.

Intraoperative sonography may be used to confirm the presence of a posttraumatic cyst either within the cord or within the subarachnoid spac, and at the same time provide a reliable means to confirm adequate decompression at surgery.

REFERENCES

1. Nunez DB, Zuluaga A, Fuentes Bernardo DA, Rivas LA, Becerra JL. Cervical spine trauma: how much more do we learn by routinely using helical CT? *Radiographics* 1996;16:1307–1318.
2. Paramore CG, Dickson CA, Sonntag VKH. The anatomical suitability of the C1-2 complex for transarticular screw fixation. *J Neurosurg* 1996;185:221–224.
3. Cornelius RS, Leach JL. Imaging evaluation of cervical spine trauma. *Neuroimaging Clin North Am* 1995;5:451–463.
4. Mascalchi M, Dal Posso G, Dini C, et al. Acute spinal trauma: prognostic value of MRI appearance at 0.5T. *Clin Radiol* 1993;48:100–108.
5. Flanders AE, Schaefer DM, Doan HT, Mishkin MM, Gonzalez CF, Northrup BE. Acute cervical spine trauma: correlation of MR findings with degree of neurologic deficit. *Radiology* 1990;177:25–33.
6. Flanders AE, Spettell CM, Tartaglino LM, Friedman DP, Herbison GJ. Forecasting motor recovery after cervical spinal cord injury: value of MR imaging. *Radiology* 1996;201:649–655.
7. Mirvis SE, Geisler FH, Jelinek JJ, Joslyn JN, Gellad F. Acute cervical spine trauma: evaluation with 1.5T MR imaging. *Radiology* 1988;166:807–816.
8. Yamashita Y, Takahashi M, Matsuno Y, et al. Chronic injuries of the spinal cord assessment with MR imaging. *Radiology* 1990;175:849–854.
9. Ronnen HR, de Korte PJ, Bring PRG, van der Bijl HJ, Tonino AJ, Franke CL. Acute whiplash injury: is there a role for MR imaging? A prospective study of 100 patients. *Radiology* 1996;201:93–96.
10. Gebarski JS, Maynard FW, Gabrielsen TO, Knoke JE, Latack JT, Hoff JT. Posttraumatic progressive myelopathy. *Radiology* 1985;157:379–385.
11. Quencer RM, Sheldon JJ, Post MJD, et al. Magnetic resonance imaging of the chronically injured cervical spinal cord. *AJNR Am J Neuroradiol* 1986;7:457–464.
12. Post MJD, Quencer RM, Green BA, Hink RS, Horen M, Labus J. The role of cine-MR in the evaluation of the pulsatile characteristics of posttraumatic spinal and subarachnoid cord cyst. *AJNR Am J Neuroradiol* 1988;9:1001–1002.
13. McArdle CB, Crofford MJ, Mirfakhree M, Amparo EG, Calhoun JS. Surface coil MR of spinal trauma: preliminary experience. *AJNR Am J Neuroradiol* 1986;7:885–893.
14. Tarr RW, Drolshagen LF, Kerner TC, Allen JH, Partain CL, James Ce. MR imaging of recent spinal trauma. *J Comput Assist Tomogr* 1987;11:412–417.
15. Kulkarni MV, McArdle CB, Kopanicky D, et al. Acute spinal cord injury: MR imaging at 1.5T. *Radiology* 1987;164:837–843.
16. Dickman CA, Greene KA, Sonntag VKH. Injuries involving the transverse atlantal ligament: classification and treatment guidelines based upon experience with 39 injuries. *Neurosurgery* 1996;38:44–50.
17. Corner EM. Rotatory dislocations of the atlas. *Ann Surg* 1907;45:9–26.
18. El Khoury GY, Clark CR, Gnaveth AW. Acute traumatic rotatory atlantoaxial dislocation in three children. *J Bone Joint Surg* 1984;66A:774–777.
19. Greeley PW. Bilateral (ninety degrees) rotatory dislocation of the atlas upon the axis. *J Bone Surg* 1930;12:958–962.
20. Jacobson C, Alden DC. An evaluation of lateral atlantoaxial displacement in injuries of the cervical spine. *Radiology* 1953;61:355–362.
21. Jacobson C, Alden DC. Examination of the atlantoaxial joint following injury with particular emphasis on rotational subluxation. *AJR Am J Roentgenol* 1956;76:1081–1094.
22. Barnett HJM, Jousse T, Ball MJ. Pathology and pathogenesis of progressive cystic myelopathy as a late sequel to spinal cord injury. In: Walton JN (ed). *Major Problems in Neurology*. London: WB Saunders, 1973:179–219.
23. Baumgarten M, Mouradian W, Boges D, Watkins R. Computed axial tomography in C1-C2 trauma. *Spine* 1985;10:187–192.
24. Becerra JL, Puckett WR, Hiester ED, et al. MR-pathologic comparisons of Wallerian degeneration in spinal cord injury. *AJNR Am J Neuroradiol* 1995;16:125–133.
25. Kowalski HM, Cohen WA, Cooper P, Wisoff JH. Pitfalls in the CT diagnosis of atlantoaxial rotary subluxation. *AJNR Am J Neuroradiol* 1987;8:697–702.
26. Harris HR Jr, Eideken-Monroe B. Diverse or poorly understood mechanisms. In: Grayson T (ed). *The Radiology of Acute Cervical Trauma*. Philadelphia: Williams & Wilkins, 1987:220–255.
27. Wortzman C, Dewar FP. Rotatory affixation of the atlantoaxial joint: rotational atlantoaxial subluxation. *Radiology* 1986;90:479–487.
28. Fielding JW, Stillwell WT, Chynn KY, Syropoulos EC. Use of computed tomography for the diagnosis of atlantoaxial fixation. *J Bone Joint Surg Ann.* 1978;60:1102–1104.
29. Anderson CD, D'Alonzo RT. Fractures of the odontoid process of the axis. *J Bone Joint Surg Am* 1974;56:1663–1674.
30. Enzmann DR, DeLaPaz RL. Trauma. In: Enzmann DR, DeLaPaz RL, Robin JB (eds). St. Louis: CV Mosby 1990;237–259.
31. Beers GJ, Raque GH, Wagner GG, et al. MR imaging in acute cervical spine trauma. *J Comput Assist Tomogr* 1988;12:755–761.
32. Marshall LF, Knowlton S, Gartin SR, et al. Deterioration following spinal cord injury: a multicenter study. *J Neurosurg* 1987;66:400–404.
33. Dolan EJ, Tator CH, Endernyi L. The value of decompression for acute experimental spinal cord compression injury. *J Neurosurg* 1980;53:749–755.
34. Tarlov IM. Spinal cord compression studies: III. Time limits for recovery after gradual compression in dogs. *Arch Neurol Psychiatr* 1954;71:588–597.
35. Hall A, Wagle V, Raycroft J, et al. Magnetic resonance imaging in cervical trauma. *J Trauma* 1993;34:21–26.
36. Kalfas I, Wilberger J, Goldberg A, Prostko ER. Magnetic resonance imaging in acute spinal cord trauma. *Neurosurgery* 1988;23:295–299.
37. Manelfe C. Magnetic resonance imaging of the spinal cord. *Diagn Intervent Radiol* 1989;1:3–4.
38. Kadoya S, Nakamura R, Kobayashi S, Yamamato I. Magnetic resonance imaging of acute spinal cord injury. *Neuroradiology* 1987;29:252–255.
39. Umbach I, Heilport A. Review article: post spinal cord injury syringomyelia. *Paraplegia* 1991;29:219–221.
40. Falcone S, Quencer RM, Green BA, Patchen SJ, Post MJD. Progressive posttraumatic myelomalacic myelopathy: imaging and clinical features. *AJNR Am J Neuroradiol* 1994;15:747–754.
41. MacDonald RL, Findlay JM, Tator CM. Microcystic spinal cord degeneration causing post traumatic myelopathy. Report of two cases. *J Neurosurg* 1988;68:466–471.
42. Fox JL, Wener L, Drennan DL, Manz HJ, Won DJ, Al-Mefty O. Central spinal cord injury: magnetic resonance imaging confirmation and operative considerations. *Neurosurgery* 1988;22:340–347.
43. McLean DR, Miller JDR, Allen PBR, Ezzedin SA. Post traumatic syringomyelias. *J Neurosurg* 1973;39:485–492.
44. Seibert Ce, Dreisbach JN, Swanson WB, Edgar RE, Williams P, Hahn H. Progressive post traumatic cystic myelopathy. *AJNR Am J Neuroradiol* 1981;2:115–119.
45. Stevens JM, Olney JS, Kendall BE. Post traumatic cystic and non-cystic myelopathy. *Neuroradiology* 1985;24:48–56.
46. Enzmann DR, O'Donohue J, Rubin JB, et al. CSF pulsations within non-neoplastic spinal cord cysts. *AJNR Am J Neuroradiol* 1987;8:517–525.
47. Waller AV. Experiments on the section of the glossopharyngeal and hypoglossal nerve of a frog, and observations of the alterations produced thereby in the structure of their primitive fiber. *Philos Trans R Soc Lond Biol Soc* 1850;140:423–429.
48. Terae S, Taneichi H, Abumi K. MRI of Wallerian degeneration of the injured spinal cord. *J Comput Assist Tomogr* 1993;17:700–703.

49. Murphy MD, Batnitzky S, Bramble JH. Diagnostic imaging of spinal trauma. *Radiol Clin North Am* 1989;27:855–872.
50. Ruiz A, Post MJD, Sklar EML. Traumatic thoracic and lumbar fractures. *Appl Radiol* October 1996: 49–57.
51. Brant-Zawadzki M, Brooke JR Jr, Minagi H, et al. High resolution CT of thoracolumbar fractures. *AJR Am J Roentgenol* 1993;160:95–102.
52. El-Khoury GY, Whitten CG. Trauma to the thoracic spine: anatomy biomechanics and unique imaging features. *AJR Am J Roentgenol* 1993;160:99–102.
53. Pathnia MN, Petersilge CA. Spine trauma. *Radiol Clin North Am* 1991; 29:847–865.
54. Ferguson RL, Allen BL Jr. A mechanistic classification of thoracolumbar spine fractures. *Clin Orthop* 1984;189:77–88.
55. McAfee PC, Yuan HA, Frederickson BE, et al. The value of computed tomography in thoracolumbar fractures. An analysis of 100 consecutive cases and a new classification. *J Bone Joint Surg* 1983; 65A:461–473.
56. Denis I. The three column spine and its significance in the classification of acute thoracolumbar spinal injuries. *Spine* 1983;8:817–831.
57. Reid AB, Letts RM, Black GM. Pediatric chance fractures: association with intra-abdominal injuries and seat belt use. *Trauma* 1990;30: 384–391.
58. Smith WS, Karfer H. Patterns and mechanisms of lumbar injuries associated with lap seat belts. *J Bone Joint Surg* 1969;51A:239–254.
59. Manaster BJ, Osborn AG. CT patterns of facet fracture dislocations in the thoracolumbar region. *AJR Am J Roentgenol* 1987;143: 335–340.
60. O'Callaghan JP, Ullrich CG, Yuan HA, et al. CT of facet distractions in flexion injuries of the thoracolumbar spine: the "naked" facet. *AJR Am J Roentgenol* 1980;134:563–568.
61. Atlas SW, Rogenbogen V, Rogers LF, et al. The radiographic characterization of burst fractures of the spine. *AJR Am J Roentgenol* 1986;147:575–582.
62. Shumar WP, Rogers JV, Sickler ME, et al. Thoracolumbar burst fractures: CT dimensions of the spinal canal relative to post-surgical improvement. *AJR Am J Roentgenol* 1985;145:337–341.
63. Stouffer ES. Current concepts review: internal fixation of fractures of the thoracolumbar spine. *J Bone Joint Surg* 1984;66A:1136–1138.
64. Brower AC, Downer EF Jr. Kummell disease: report of case with serial radiographs. *Radiology* 1981;1141:363–364.
65. Post MJD, Green BA. The use of computed tomography in spinal trauma. *Radiol Clin North Am* 1983;21:327–375.
66. Sklar EML, Quencer RM, Green BA, et al. Acquired subarachnoic cysts: evaluation with MR, CT, myelography and intraoperative sonography. *AJNR Am J Neuroradiol* 1989;10:1097–1104.
67. Teplick JG, Peyster RH, Teplick SK, et al. CT identification of post laminectomy pseudomeningocele. *AJNR Am J Neuroradiol* 1983;4: 179–182.

Surgery of Spinal Trauma,
edited by J.M. Cotler, J.M. Simpson, H.S. An, and C.P. Silveri.
Lippincott Williams & Wilkins, Philadelphia © 2000.

CHAPTER 6

Medical Management and Rehabilitation of the Spinal Cord Injured Patient

David F. Apple

Management of spinal cord injury with paralysis has its roots in the antiquities where the ancient Egyptians had labeled it "an ailment not to be treated." Prior to World War II, that was almost true, as only 15% of those with spinal cord injuries survived. However, in 1944, Sir Ludwig Guttmann established a spinal cord injury treatment center in England that was devoted exclusively to management of paralysis. A similar categorical unit was first developed in the United States in Boston by Dr. Donald Monroe in the late 1940s and early 1950s. Around the same time, Drs. Herb Talbert, Estin Comarr, and Ernst Boer began developing spinal cord injury treatment centers through the Veterans Administration system to manage the large numbers of spinal cord injuries resulting from World War II. In 1964, the staff at Rancho Los Amigos Hospital diverted part of their resources from treating polio to setting up a spinal cord injury unit modeled after Sir Ludwig Guttmann's concepts. In 1968, the federal government of the United States became involved after a group of physicians treating spinal cord injury made the Congress aware of the needs of spinal

cord injury victims and the state of poor coordination of care. Through the Rehabilitation Services Administration, Congress funded the first spinal cord injury care system at Good Samaritan Hospital in Phoenix, Arizona. Subsequently, more centers have been recognized and presently there are 19 model centers across the United States (Fig. 1).

This initiative started by the Rehabilitation Services Administration and continued by the Department of Education through the National Institution of Rehabilitation and Research had two requirements for becoming a model center. One was to have a system of care, and second there would be a national statistical database. For a spinal cord injury center to develop, there were two critical ingredients. One, there must be a sufficient patient population to support a center. That number has been determined to be somewhere between 12 and 16 patients. This figure was derived from the necessary staffing required to develop the expertise to maintain the unit with an average length of stay of 90 days. There would need to be at least four new patients per bed, which means about 80 to 100 admissions per year. In recent years, the average length of stay has been reduced to 45 days; thus, the number of required admissions has doubled.

D.F. Apple: Emory University School of Medicine, Shepard Center, Atlanta, Georgia 30309.

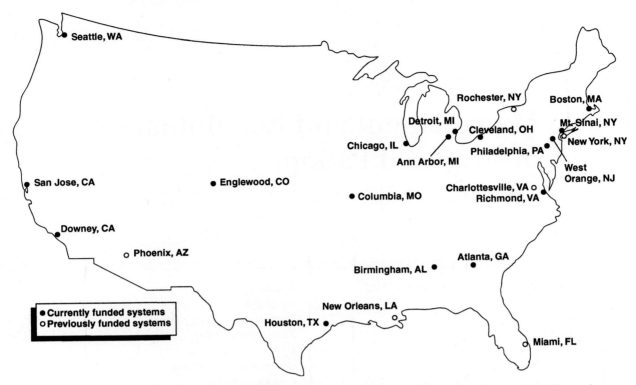

FIG. 1. Spinal cord injury centers that have been or are funded by the National Institute on Disability and Rehabilitation Research.

The second ingredient the center needs is a well-trained staff led by a knowledgeable physician who understands a system of care. Engineering defines a system as an assemblage of components operating within a prescribed boundary and united by some form of interaction or interdependence to form a coherent integrated whole. Applying that definition to the medical model for spinal cord injury means having a team of physician, nurse, physical therapist, occupational therapist, speech therapist, vocational therapist, recreational therapist, and psychological help as a minimum. This group of individuals needs to know how to work together in an interdisciplinary method. In such a method the physical therapist does not focus totally on the area of mobility, but must be able to interact on goals such as dressing, feeding, and, grooming, as well as wheelchair skills. For the team to function fully and provide a good result, education of the patient and family is mandatory.

As originally described, the system included the spinal cord injury center being involved with acute management, that is, from the time of injury into acute surgical management, to acute and long-term rehabilitation, psychological intervention, and community reintegration. With the onset of managed care, this model has been modified to meet imposed fiscal restraints. As an outgrowth, subacute hospitalization has occurred, which treats those patients who still require medical care but are not well enough to be in a full-scale rehabilitation program, defined as 3 hours of therapy on a daily basis.

Once the patient has moved through the subacute and into full-scale rehabilitation, there arises a time, particularly in those with paraplegia, when inpatient care is no longer critical. The treatment can be continued in a day hospital. Day hospital is defined as one where the patient and the significant other stay in a hotel or apartment situation close to the spinal injury center and come to the center for 8 hours, 5 days a week. As can be readily understood, this means the patient and the caregiver understand all the nursing issues, that is, skin, bowel, and bladder. Therefore, the focus of early rehabilitation has been changed so there is more emphasis on the nursing skills aspect as the patient goes through the acute and subacute phases. The idea is to get the patient into a day hospital or outpatient setting as quickly as possible. This alteration in the system has allowed the length of inpatient stay to be reduced over 50% but still allows the patient to achieve the same rehabilitation goal, which is to be as independent as possible consistent with the level of neurologic involvement.

EARLY CONSIDERATIONS IN MANAGEMENT OF SPINAL CORD INJURY

An insult to the spinal column of sufficient intensity will produce spinal cord injury that affects motor, sensory, and reflex functions of the cord. Depending on the intensity of the insult, a complete spinal cord injury may occur in which motor and sensory function below the bony level of injury is lost permanently. Less intense injury will produce an incomplete

TABLE 1. *Incomplete spinal cord injuries*

Syndrome	Physical findings	Prognosis
Anterior cord syndrome	Motor loss. Pain/temperature loss. Partial pain.	Poor for any functional return.
Central cord syndrome	Distal motor function better than proximal. Sensory function altered. Usually cervical.	Variable return of upper extremity function. Spasticity.
Brown-Sequard syndrome	Paresis or paralysis of ipsilateral side. Pain and temperature loss contralaterally.	Significant return usually occurs.
Posterior cord syndrome	Variable motor loss. Pain intact.	Unknown.
Conus medullaris	Injury at T11–L2. Loss of bowel and bladder control.	Usually not much improvement.
Cauda equina	Injury at L1–L5. Variable motor loss.	Usually some return of motor function.

spinal cord injury where there will be partial motor and/or sensory function below the bony level of injury. These incomplete syndromes are listed in the Table 1. Diagnostically, the degree of completeness can be ascertained within the first 24 hours by determining the presence or absence of the bulbocavernosus reflex. If this reflex is present, and it usually is within the first 4 to 24 hours, and there is no motor or sensory function below the bony level of injury, the injury is a complete one. If there is any function below the level of injury with concomitant partial sensation in the rectal area, the injury is incomplete. Table 2 outlines the American Spinal Injury Association classification (previously the Frankel classification), which has been accepted by the major orthopedic and neurosurgical groups managing spinal cord injury throughout the world.

The epidemiology has undergone changes over the past 20 years, as authenticated by the National Spinal Cord Injury database. This database is maintained at the University of Alabama as part of the collaborative efforts of the model spinal cord injury systems that are funded by the National Institute on Disability and Rehabilitation Research. The average has dropped from 61% of injuries occurring between the ages of 16 and 30 years to 58% in the last 10 years. Eighty-two percent of the injuries occurred in males, and the proportion of African-Americans has increased to almost 20% versus 12% in 1990. The primary etiology in 1990 was motor vehicle accidents at 48%; this has dropped to 44% in the most recent analysis. Acts of violence increased to 17% from

15%. July and August remain the most frequent months for injury, and Saturday and Sunday the most frequent days for injury.

One of the most important advances in the last 20 years in management of spinal cord injury has been the care that is given by the emergency medical service personnel at the scene of the injury. The improved care has resulted in more incomplete injuries. Immobilization of both the cervical and thoracic lumbar spine has been critical in this improvement. Safe removal of the patient from the emergency setting to the emergency room and awareness of potential for spinal cord injury, especially in the unconscious patient, has added to the improvement and potential outcome. Documentation of the mechanism of injury is important, as well as a good physical examination that must include a motor level, a sensory level, and examination of the rectal area, to ascertain sensation and reflex function (Fig. 2). At the completion of this examination, routine x-ray films should be obtained. For suspected cervical injury, the examining physician should have films that delineate the seven critical factors outlined in Table 3.

The x-rays films of the thoracic and lumbar area should be of sufficient integrity to allow for evaluation of the level of the injury, the width of the pedicles, the relationships of the facet joints, the vertebral body configuration, and the relationship of one vertebra to the other.

Medications that may be indicated would be high doses of prednisolone, which were introduced in May 1990 following a multicenter study that showed some enhanced neurologic

TABLE 2. *ASIA impairment scale*

Grade	Type	Description
A	Complete	No motor or sensory function in sacral segments S4–5.
B	Incomplete	Sensory but no motor function below the neurologic level. Extends through sacral segments S4–5.
C	Incomplete	Motor function below the neurologic level, and the majority of key muscles below the neurologic level have a muscle grade less than three.
D	Incomplete	Motor function is preserved below the neurologic level. Most key muscles below this level have a muscle grade greater than or equal to three.
E	Recovery	Motor and sensory function is normal.

ASIA, American Spinal Injury Association.

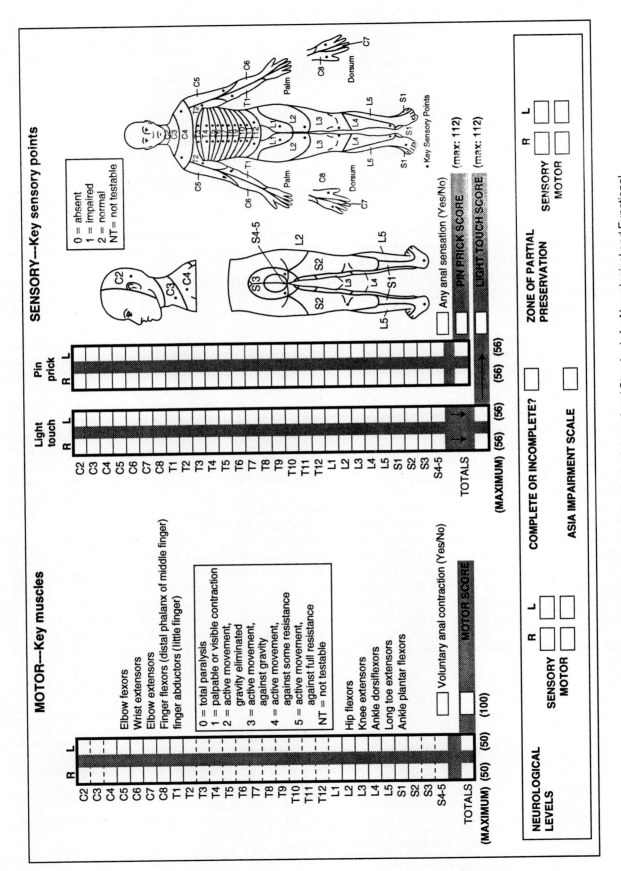

FIG. 2. Motor and sensory scoring tables for the International Standards for Neurological and Functional Classification of Spinal Cord Injury.

TABLE 3. *Cervical spine x-ray review*

1. Adequate film of C1–T1
2. Soft tissue swelling of the anterior inferior body of C-3, 5 mm or less
3. Cervical body configuration
4. Alignment of the posterior aspects of the bodies
5. Alignment of the facet joints
6. Spinous process integrity
7. Atlantoaxial relationship

improvement with the use of high doses of methylprednisolone on the following regimen: 30 mg/kg of body weight for the first hour and then 5.4 mg/kg over the next 24 hours. Studies are being conducted to ascertain the efficacy of using gangliosides alone or in combination with the methylprednisolone, but the results of this multicenter study are not available. Antiulcer prevention medication should be instituted and consideration should be given to anticoagulation, although this medication usually is started in the later postinjury period.

Following these initial evaluations, the treating surgeon may want to consider additional studies. If there is a question about bony integrity, computerized tomography is the diagnostic procedure of choice, and metrizamide myelography may be done concomitantly to gain more information about the soft tissues. However, it must be considered that, with myelography, the patient will need to be turned in the prone position, which may be contraindicated in case of an unstable cervical or thoracic lumbar fracture. The additional diagnostic study that may be indicated is magnetic resonance imaging (MRI), which is a more sensitive examination for soft tissue and would include evaluation of ligamentous injury and disc damage.

On completion of all the diagnostic studies, the treating surgeon should be able to make a reasonable judgment as to the stability of the spine and thus the cause for the paralysis. In the author's experience, and those of his colleagues at the center where he practices, very seldom is the offending agent a disc, but is more likely to be displacement of the bony elements of the spine through fracture or ligamentous disruption.

There have been numerous classification systems for spine fractures in the orthopedic literature, some of which are difficult to understand and others of which are cumbersome. With the sponsorship of the National Institute of Disability and Rehabilitation Research (NIDRR) and the support of the American Spinal Injury Association, a group of five physicians (P. Meyer et al.) (1), all doing traumatic spine surgery, have developed a classification system. The goals of the system were that it would be easy to use and understand, would allow physicians regardless of specialty to communicate about spine fractures, and would provide spine surgeons a standardized tool to track treatment methods versus outcomes.

The three fundamental components of the system are (i) number of columns injured, (ii) extent of translatory displacement, and (iii) anterior vertebral distortion resulting in angulation. Based on these parameters, the fracture is assigned as type A, B, or C. The system has demonstrated that it is applicable from cervical to lumbar spine, anatomically correct in all three dimensions, valid, reliable, and reproducible, and it correlates to outcome data (Fig. 3).

Physicians are able to use the new spine fracture classification system to suggest the extent of stability of the spine fracture, identify the relationship between canal compromise and neurologic injury, suggest the appropriate surgical approach based on the classification, and provide improved follow-up of management outcomes.

It is not within the scope of this chapter to discuss the operative management of the spinal column injury. However, there are some general statements that can be made referable to restoration of spinal stability and the course of rehabilitation. The overriding goal of the treating surgeon should be to establish spinal stability (2). This may be done nonoperatively with the use of a halo brace in the cervical spine and by postural realignment and recumbency in the thoracic lumbar spine. However, with the instrumentation available now, operative treatment utilizing plates, screws, wires, rods, or a combination either anteriorly, posteriorly, or both, has proven to be safe in experienced hands and allows quicker mobilization for the rehabilitation course (3–5).

The second goal of the treating surgeon should be to create no further neurologic damage (6). This is particularly true in the cervical spine, where loss of one nerve root has a significant bearing on the functional outcome and thus the rehabilitation course. In the thoracic spine, the loss of one nerve root is not as catastrophic, but in the lumbar spine, the loss of a nerve root may be the difference between ambulation and nonambulation. In these areas, wires under the lamina, screws that violate the cortex of the pedicle, and hooks that take up space within the canal need to be critically considered before utilization. The third goal of the operating surgeon should be to improve the possibility of neurologic return. This is particularly true in the cervical spine, where

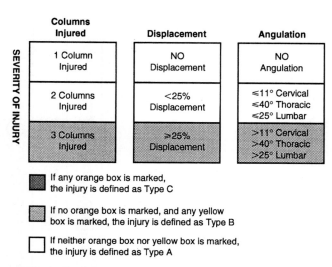

FIG. 3. Radiologic classification of spinal column injury.

improving the space for nerve root may enhance the return of that nerve root's function and thus improve the rehabilitation outcome. The final goal concerns those patients who are neurologically intact in whom any loss of function through a surgical procedure is a catastrophic happening. Thus, a surgical approach should be considered only if there is significant reason that a nonoperative approach will not produce a stable, painless outcome.

With the reestablishment of spinal stability, the patient's rehabilitation can proceed. Recent developments fostered by managed care have seen several concepts evolve. One is a clinical pathway that allows for more effective management of patients as they proceed through the rehabilitation course, leading them to achieve the function as depicted in Figure 4 and the goals as outlined in Figure 5. The pathway allows for the interdisciplinary rehabilitation team to proceed without significant interruption except when there are exceptions to progress as outlined on the pathway.

The second critical development is enhancement of the continuum of care. Prior to the early 1990s, rehabilitation was performed almost exclusively in an inpatient setting. However, this is a costly way to deliver care and different elements have been added. Two of these elements, subacute care and day hospital, were discussed earlier. The final treatment element is an enhanced outpatient setting where patients who have met nursing care goals and do not need a full therapy program can be maintained in a similar manner as the day hospital patient.

Finally, in a model system concept, the job is not completed until the patient has returned to the community and is functioning in that community on as high a level as possible. This means monitoring the patient for secondary complications with the goal of prevention. It also means having the patient involved in the community recreationally and vocationally. It has been established that if this system of care is provided, the total cost of lifetime care is reduced over other care models in which the commitment stops with the discharge of the patient from the inpatient rehabilitation program (7).

CLINICAL PATHWAY

A multidisciplinary model to provide care for patients is a long-standing tenet in rehabilitation. The next developmental step is to take an interdisciplinary approach and transform this approach into true collaborative care. This is accomplished through critical pathways and case management models (8). Critical pathways provide a framework for moving the patient toward positive measurable outcomes (Fig. 4,

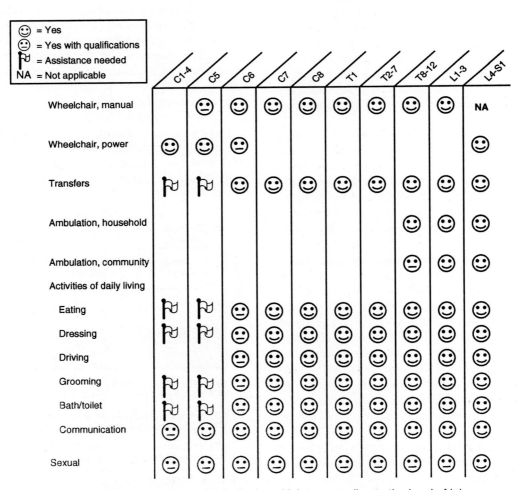

FIG. 4. Functional expectations in spinal cord injury according to the level of injury.

TABLE 4. *Cervical region: clinical presentation and goals by neurological level*

	Sensory	Motor	Test	Goals
C1–3	To the neck	Cervical flexors and extensors	Trapezius Shoulder shrug	Respiratory dependent Blink or head control wheelchair Environmental control unit Computer Mouth stick
C–4	Shoulder mantle	Deltoid Diaphragm	Shoulder abduction Breathing	Dependent Electric wheelchair with chin control
C–5	Lateral arm Thumb	Biceps	Elbow flexion	Partial Independence with adaptive equipment Electric wheelchair with arm control
C–6	Index, long fingers	Wrist extensors	Wrist extensors	Independent with equipment Driving hand controls Manual wheelchair with pegs
C–7	Long, index fingers	Triceps Wrist flexor Finger extensors	Elbow extension Finger extension	Independent transfers and ADLs Standard manual chair
C–8	Fifth finger	Finger flexors Interosseus	Flex fingers Spread fingers	Independent ADLs without splints Independent transfers

Tables 4 and Table 5). That rehabilitation medicine has always expressed its goals for patients in terms of measurable functional outcomes makes it compatible for the critical pathway model.

Outcome measurement is not the only benefit of a critical pathway. One advantage is an opportunity for process improvement. The critical pathway is embedded in the core of the medical record. Benefits are as follows:

1. The pathway becomes the center of all documentation and serves as the standard in which the staff may chart the patient's progress. Predetermined outcomes are clustered by diagnostic groups and specific to what the rehabilitation center has determined as reasonable as delineated from its own historical data.
2. The rehabilitation staff chart on pathways using a charting by exception model (9) that uses as little subjective narrative as possible. In the charting by exception model, staff document interdisciplinary care delivery and patient outcome achievements. Narrative notes are used to document variances from expected norms or outcomes.
3. Because the expected outcomes are predetermined, the staff has a concrete yardstick against which to measure performance (both the patients' and their own). This allows them to focus their energy and create new solutions for problems requiring individualization while ensuring that the core plan of the treatment is not forgotten.
4. All staff who give direct patient care document on the pathway.
5. The pathway is the plan of care for the patient and is the treatment record and therapy notes.
6. As an interdisciplinary document, the pathway facilitates communication between all disciplines and improves the internal case manager's ability to prepare a comprehensive report for external case managers. In most instances, the pathway document may serve as the team conference report.

TABLE 5. *Thoracolumbar region: clinical presentation and goals by neurological level*

	Sensory	Motor	Test	Goals
T1–10	Chest to umbilicus	Intercostals Spine extensors	Normal upper extremity	Independent in all skills for living
T11–12	Inguinal ligament	Rectus abdominis	Elevate trunk	Independent stand in long leg braces
L1–2	Anterior and medial thigh	Iliopsoas adductors	Hip flexion	Ambulation with long leg braces in household
L3–4	Medial calf	Quadriceps Hamstrings	Knee extension	Community ambulation with long leg (possibly short leg) braces
L4–5	Dorsum foot	Anterior tibial	Dorsiflexion of foot	Community ambulation with short leg braces
L5–S1	Lateral foot	Gastrocnemius Toe flexors	Plantar flexion of foot	Community ambulation with short leg braces
S2–5	Perianal region	Gluteus Sphincters	Hip extension Anal tone	Community ambulation, possibly without braces

7. The pathway system provides a mechanism for various tracking, examines individual outcomes, and tracks system problems within the institution.
8. Pathways are a visible interactive documentation system that uses standards of current practice. Because of the increased visibility, the pathway is a more fluid document than a policy book and can be adapted more quickly to change with the needs of the organization.

The second advantage of the critical pathway system is patient focused care. The pathways direct all documentation to focus on patient outcome measures. These pathways provide an all encompassing proactive plan that drives forward the care of the patient. With this care map, patients are encouraged to participate in their care and goal setting by use of patient versions of the pathways.

To best implement a system, the development team must consist of people who will actually be using the system and have hands-on experience in rehabilitation care. A critical pathway system will not function well if it is developed by consultants.

ACUTE COMPLICATIONS

Neurogenic Bladder Function

Spinal cord injury causes loss of control of the external urethral sphincter and thus the ability to control urination (10). Spinal cord injury may affect upper urinary tract function as well. Immediately after injury, the bladder is drained most effectively by an indwelling catheter that should remain in place for at least the first 24 hours or until the diaphoretic period has passed and cardiovascular stability has been achieved.

Following this initial period after injury, the type of voiding dysfunction can be ascertained. The history will include spinal cord injury either caused traumatically or otherwise induced. The physical examination should include assessment of the abdomen and genitalia as well as the rectum. The neurologic examination should check for perineural sensation and tone, presence of the bulbocavernosus reflex, and deep tendon reflexes. Urodynamic testing allows for specific qualification of the type of voiding dysfunction (11). Qualification of certain parameters such as bladder sensation, bladder capacity, and the ability of the detrusor muscle to maintain the bladder volume or expel urine during voiding can be obtained. Type and level of neurologic injury can be useful to predict the type of voiding dysfunction leading to the treatment options, but urodynamics allows for more specific delineation and more accurate diagnosis.

There are four main types of neurologic disorders.

1. Normal voiding with functional incontinence. These patients have normal capacity and compliance of the bladder with normal detrusor function. Because of cognitive deficits, however, such patients may experience incontinence. Treatment options for such patients include assisted and timed voiding with behavioral modification.

2. Detrusor hyperreflexia, i.e., the presence of uninhibited detrusor contractions. The ability of the patient's bladder to act as a reservoir is impaired by spasticity of the detrusor muscle. Urodynamics demonstrates basic increases in detrusor pressure that are involuntary. The treatment of these patients generally involves the administration of antispasmodic and anticholinergic medications that eliminate these contractions and allow for adequate bladder capacity. When medications are ineffective or poorly tolerated, surgical means to improve bladder capacity are indicated. Among the operations that are useful for this problem, augmentation enterocystoplasty is the most popular. This operative intervention involves increasing the capacity of the bladder by enlarging its diameter by means of the anastomosis of a patch of bowel to the bladder.

3. Detrusor areflexia. In this condition, the bladder muscle does not push in a reliable fashion to enable complete voiding. These patients commonly present in urinary retention. Treatment generally involves intermittent catheterization (12), which involves emptying the bladder. It is associated with a relatively low risk for urinary tract infection and lower urinary tract trauma. Other means would include intubation with an indwelling Foley catheter or suprapubic tube and urinary diversion with either incontinent diversion (i.e., ilioconduit) or continent diversion (i.e., kock or Indiana pouch).

4. Detrusor sphincter dyssynergia. This usually is associated with patients with cervical injuries. There is dyscoordination of detrusor contractility with external sphincter muscle contractility. Normally coordinated voiding occurs when the detrusor muscle contracts and the external sphincter relaxes simultaneously, therefore affecting low pressure voiding. In patients with detrusor sphincter dyssynergia, the bladder muscle contracts simultaneously with the external sphincter contraction. The result is high bladder pressures that can be associated with urinary tract infection, bladder trabeculation, and diverticula formation as well as vesicoureteral reflux and subsequent renal deterioration.

Patients may be symptomatic with autonomic dysreflexia, i.e., headaches and sweating when the patient reflex voids with these high pressures. This disorder can be diagnosed using urodynamic studies (13). The management of the disorder involves eliminating the detrusor contractions or the external sphincter contractions. As most patients with this disorder have high levels of injury, treatment of external sphincter spasm is usually the most practical, because such treatment will allow the patient to be a reflex voider. The traditional way to eliminate external sphincter spasm is sphincterotomy. Other means to ablate the activity of the spastic muscle include the prescription of alpha blockade (i.e., terazosin) (14), performance of sphincterotomy with laser, and insertion of an intraurethral stent to hold the sphincter muscle open (i.e., urolume prosthetic device by Mentor Corporation). All of these options are potentially less morbid than traditional sphincterotomy. Other treatment options include paralysis of the bladder muscle with medications with the addition of intermittent catheterization, as well as construction to allow for urinary diversion.

Upper urinary tract function can be adversely affected by high bladder pressures. Patients with detrusor sphincter dyssynergia (discussed earlier) are at high risk for this complication because of the high bladder pressures that can be transmitted to the kidneys. For this reason, the aggressive management of detrusor sphincter dyssynergia can prevent deterioration of renal function in patients with this condition. Monitoring of the upper tract on a regular basis is indicated in all patients with spinal cord injury. This monitoring can be performed with an intravenous pyelogram, ultrasound, and KUB or nuclear renal scan performed every 1 to 3 years. The choice of diagnostic modality is based on the patient's past urologic history, allergies, and age.

Bowel Function

The same control mechanisms that affect bladder function affect bowel management in patients with spinal cord injury. Bowel incontinence is one of the primary barriers to achieving independence. Constipation, fecal impaction, and non-functional prolonged evacuation affects success of the bowel management program. One study indicated that 19.7% of patients had bowel accidents monthly, and 18% to 49% had other significant gastrointestinal problems.

The extent of bowel control loss is determined by location and completeness of spinal cord injury. Left colonic motility is decreased in high cord lesions and increased in low cord lesions. Colonic transit time is increased as much as two times the rate prior to an injury (15). An injury to the spinal cord can result in two types of neurogenic bowel dysfunction. A cord injury to the upper motor neurons results in a reflex spastic bowel; a lower motor neuron results in an autonomous flaccid bowel. In either case, voluntary bowel function is lost. In both types of neurogenic bowel, principles of proper fluid and fiber management as well as the importance of a scheduled routine program are emphasized. The act of defecation is approached differently because the defecation reflex function is destroyed in those with a lower motor neuron injury. The neurogenic bowel assessment must include a history that identifies current elimination patterns, stool consistency, use of medications, diet, and lifestyle. In instances of intractable evacuation problems with interference of quality of life, transit time evaluation and rectal studies can be undertaken and elective colostomy considered.

Following assessment, appropriate treatment options can be designed to help an individual achieve continence. Bowel management programs are essential and are based on the premise of starting with a disimpacted bowel, instituting a high-fiber diet, establishing a regularly scheduled pattern, and choosing an appropriate mechanism of evacuation (digital stimulation or suppository). The first step in a bowel management program is to have a clean large colon. This can

be accomplished using a large-volume catheter flush enema or the pulsed enhanced bowel evacuation system (PIEE) designed to flush the large intestine. After the bowel is empty, bowel elimination is placed on a schedule and a high-fiber diet is instituted. All patients are recommended to ingest 25 to 30 g of fiber per day. Cereals high in fiber are the easiest ways to meet this high-fiber requirement and do not produce the abdominal bloating that some of the synthetic products cause. One cereal high in soluble fiber and low in calories is Fiber One by General Mills.

Adequate fluid intake is imperative with a high-fiber diet. Patients are instructed to drink 30 mL/kg of body weight per day. Establishing a scheduled time of day for the bowel management program is the next important component. It is determined from the premorbid history and from tracking the results of an everyday program. An a.m. or p.m. program should be maintained and, when this is achieved, most people can convert to an every other day pattern. Eating prior to the bowel program stimulates the gastrocolic reflex, which stimulates function. A final component of bowel management is establishing an evacuation mechanism. The patients with an upper motor neuron lesion and spastic bowel respond well to digital stimulation. The only contraindication to using this method is if the patient is unable to tolerate it due to hemorrhoids or sensation. If a suppository is indicated, as in a lower motor neuron lesion with a flaccid bowel, choose an appropriate suppository. Experience has shown that water-based disocodyl suppositories have the fastest and most complete results and should be the most tried. Alternative suppositories are available, and their mechanism of action should be evaluated before recommending them. Finally, stool softeners, laxatives, and enemas are best avoided for long-term use.

Skin

The skin of the insensitive areas of the body following a spinal cord injury are continuously at risk for breakdown. If the skin does not receive sufficient pressure relief to allow reoxygenation and clearing of the toxic byproducts of metabolism from the pressured area, the skin will break down, producing a decubitus ulcer or skin sore. To prevent this, meticulous attention must be paid to pressure relief by the nursing staff. This can be accomplished by frequent turns, usually on a 2-hour schedule, with appropriate padding of the commonly recognized pressure areas such as the greater trochanter, sacrum, and bony prominences around the upper torso.

When the patient is in a sitting position, it is necessary to relieve the pressure on the ischii by doing appropriate weight shifts. Initially the patient should shift weight every 15 minutes, relieving pressure for at least 1 minute. As skin tolerance improves, this could be lengthened to every 30 minutes. During the early phase after injury, management of the skin, both in the lying and sitting positions, is up to the nursing and therapy staff. However, as the patient progresses through the rehabilitation process, responsibility for skin management needs to be placed on the patient. Each patient's program will vary according to patient's weight, skin texture, and general health.

It should be the goal of the skin management program to increase the tolerance to pressure, maintain skin integrity, educate the family and the patient regarding the risk factors, and develop an effective discharge plan for skin maintenance, all the while enforcing the notion that to maintain the integrity of the skin, the patient must accept the responsibility. The experience in spinal cord injury centers is that the patient generally will remember this responsibility for about 2 years, but beyond that time the incidence of skin breakdown increases. Surprisingly, this is more true in paraplegics than in the quadriplegics. Breakdown of the skin leading to a grade IV decubitus ulcer is a very time-consuming, and thus costly, inpatient care problem. The best treatment is prevention.

Deep Venous Thrombosis and Pulmonary Embolus

Deep venous thrombosis (DVT, thrombophlebitis) remains a serious complication for the spinal cord injured patient with significant morbidity of recurrent disease, leg edema, and cost to prolonged hospitalization expensive therapy. The danger of life-threatening pulmonary embolus is a feared event. Depending on the type of testing, the incidence ranges from 100% with iodine 125 fibrinogen studies, to 14% by clinical examination. An excellent review of the subject was reported in 1992 by David Green (16). Shepherd Center institutional data suggests approximately 30% incidence of clinically significant (iliofemoral to popliteal) DVT. Diagnostic testing and prophylaxis have been improving over the last 10 years. A push to limit acute inpatient hospital days may change the risks and diagnosis of this disease. Surprisingly there is little uniformity as to the best approach. The risk is highest 1 to 3 weeks after injury, especially during the second week, decreases over the next 6 to 8 weeks, and approaches the risk to the general population by 4 to 6 months.

Pathogenesis of DVT is explained by Virchow's triad of blood flow changes, vessel wall damage, and increased coagulability. With immobility and traumatic injury, paralyzed patients are at higher risk. Testing for DVT involves high clinical suspicions because the risks are high. The tests for high-risk DVT include impedance plethysmography, Doppler ultrasound, and duplex study with good sensitivity and specificity. Rarely, contrast venography is used. Physical examination for DVT is not helpful, and suggestive findings such as swelling and redness occur late in the disease process. These findings also may be indicative of heterotopic ossification. Pain is not seen with sensory deficits. Frequently unexplained fever may be the only sign. Similarly, the usual signs and symptoms for pulmonary emboli may not be present. Chest pain or pressure, dyspnea, hemoptysis, cough, and fever may be noted as changing oxygen needs, unexplained infiltrate, or an abnormal electrocardiogram.

Hypercarbia as a presenting sign in a ventilated patient with fixed ventilation has been seen. With an acceptable level of suspicion, a radionuclide study or pulmonary angiogram can be performed.

Fatal pulmonary embolus is reported in 1% to 2% of all spinal cord injury deaths within the first 3 months of injury, with the highest risks within the first 3 weeks. Risks for pulmonary embolization in the spinal cord injured patient are increased by the absence of spasticity, obesity, age, and concomitant serious infections. In the later stages of injury, the presence of heterotopic ossification increases the risk of pulmonary embolization.

Because spinal cord injury patients are at high risk, "treatment" ideally should be prevention. Various regimens have been tried. The current approach is low molecular weight heparin associated with sequential compression, stockings, and early mobilization (17). Adjusted dose heparin also is good for treatment, but anticoagulation testing is required, thus raising costs. Unfortunately, low molecular weight dextran (low molecular weight heparin) is expensive. Ideal dosing and duration is not known. Older data suggest that the risks for DVT remain above normal for up to 3 months, but more recent pooled information suggests the highest risks are in the first month. Possibly earlier mobilization has decreased the frequency (18,19). Currently low molecular weight heparin is used only in the first month. Noninvasive flow studies are done at admission and prior to stopping low molecular weight heparin. Sequential stockings are discontinued after daily activities are started.

The treatment of DVT/pulmonary embolus is still standard heparin infusion with eventual warfarin (Coumadin) substitution. Future treatment probably will be use of high-dose low molecular weight heparin followed by warfarin. Currently the anticoagulation is continued for 3 months.

Cardiovascular

Spinal cord injury produces physiologic situations similar to a sympathectomy that occurs below the level of injury, especially if it is above the thoracic sympathetic outflow between T-6 and T-12. Two significant situations may develop because of this, one of which is bradycardia. Cervical cord injuries are at risk because of marked bradycardia during the acute phase of injury. The incidence approaches 100% the more cephalad the injury. Bradycardia may be seen with the initial injury, but it also may be induced by endotracheal suctioning or manipulation, or it may occur spontaneously. Bradycardia may be associated with hypoxia and has been called apneic bradycardia. Etiology is related to unopposed vagal tone with disruption of the infraspinal sympathetic nerves at the cervical level. It persists for approximately 3 to 6 weeks and generally resolves spontaneously.

In addition to the bradycardia, there may be associated vasodilatation similar to the mechanisms in the vasovagal reflex and syncope. This further exaggerates the hypotension due to the bradycardia and may hasten syncope or near syncope. Symptomatic bradycardia requires intervention. Avoidance of hypoxia and the symptomatic or prophylactic use of atrophine may be required. Long-term prevention with drugs such as propantheline has been reported. Temporary transvenous pacemakers may be required and can be left in place for several weeks as needed as long as absolute sterile technique during placement is observed. Permanent pacemakers usually are not required, as the bradycardia is self-limited and usually resolves 3 to 6 weeks after injury; however, there are reports of cases in which the recurrent bradycardia persisted and required permanent pacemakers.

Arrhythmias seen with spinal cord injury approach those seen with sinoatrial nodal dysfunction of the elderly. These include marked sinus bradycardia, sinus pauses, and sinus arrest with extremely slow junctional or ventricular escaped rhythm, or asystole that may be prolonged.

The second cardiovascular problem in addition to bradycardia that occurs is hypotension, which is not due to the bradycardia but may be orthostatic. In the acute injury, especially cervical cord levels, hypotension with or without bradycardia due to vasodilatation may be severe and require treatment with careful fluid and vasopressor therapy. Hypotension due to cord injury must be differentiated from hypovolemia caused by other trauma and blood loss.

Symptomatic orthostatic hypotension occurs almost universally in tetraplegic patients and less frequently in paraplegics. With time, symptomatic orthostasis decreases and usually resolves by 3 to 4 months, although significant postural hypotension may still be demonstrated. Initially these patients have lost sympathetic control of peripheral vasoregulatory mechanisms, which include tachycardia, increased cardiac output, and vasoconstriction response to the upright position. With time, some of these reflexes are regained, with recovery of spinal postural reflexes and perhaps changes in cerebral vasoregulation.

Treatment modalities of orthostatic hypotension include pressure gradient stockings, abdominal binding, and antigravity suits. Medications include mineralocorticoids, such as fludrocortisone, and vasoconstrictors, such as ergotamines and ephedrine. Clonidine has a paradoxical hypertensory response in spinal injury patients and has been reported as effective in orthostasis. However, as in the general population, effectiveness of all these modalities is limited.

Respiratory

Normal respiratory function depends on the interaction of four muscle groups that support the respiratory effort: the diaphragm, abdominal muscles, chest wall muscles, and accessory neck muscles. Respiratory complications are extremely common in the paralyzed patient (20), especially those with an injury above T-10. These respiratory problems become even more significant the more proximal the spinal cord lesion. Respiratory problems can be divided into two basic areas: (i) inadequate respiratory volume secondary to phrenic nerve damage, and (ii) inability to clear secretions with resultant infection and atelectasis (21).

Of the four muscle groups, the most important in respiration is the diaphragm, which is unique in that although it is anatomic at the T12–L1 level, it is innervated from the C3–5 cervical nerve roots. For this reason, patients injured at the C-5 level do not die from asphyxia with the initial injury and usually can be successfully weaned from ventilators. Injury between C-3 and C-5 levels produces varying respiratory disability. Frequently minimal innervation from an accessory pathway will be adequate for independent respiration. Patients can easily survive with one phrenic nerve intact. Complete spinal cord lesions above the C3–4 level can leave the patient without spontaneous respirations with an intact phrenic nerve. These patients are excellent candidates for phrenic pacing (22,23). Six months should elapse from injury to phrenic nerve pacing, because many patients will develop enough spontaneous recovery and thus not require phrenic pacing.

Interestingly, the diaphragm is an inspiratory muscle only. It contracts during respiration and is completely passive during expiration. Coughing requires closure of the glottis and forcible contracture of the abdominal muscles and, to some extent, the thoracic intercostal muscles. All quadriplegic patients and most paraplegic patients have significant problems clearing the secretions. The inability to cough promotes atelectasis and pneumonia. Those caring for paralyzed patients must be well trained in the technique of assisted or "quad" coughing.

Atelectasis in the acute quadriplegic is the most common respiratory complication and usually involves the left lower lobe (24). This is because suction catheters usually go straight into the right mainstem bronchus but do not reach the left. Left lower lobe atelectasis frequently can be missed on x-ray examination. Any patient with secretion problems, i.e., a history of tobacco abuse, vigorous treatment is indicated to prevent atelectasis and pneumonia. Vigorous pulmonary toilet with bronchodilators, physical therapy, postural drainage, and aggressive assistive coughing are indicated. The InExsufflator (25), which is a device that delivers a positive pressure followed by slightly higher negative pressure, gently facilitates secretion mobilization. Aerosol or intermittent positive pressure breathing treatments with acetylcysteine (Mucomyst) may liquefy secretions but must be used with caution because of the potential of severe bronchospasm. In patients with artificial airways, lavage with sodium bicarbonate will loosen secretions. Some patients will require frequent bronchoscopies for adequate secretion clearance.

Secretion problems in the quadriplegic do not subside rapidly; therefore, early tracheostomy is indicated in the patient with continuous secretion problems or a patient who is orally intubated. These patients who had an oral or nasal airway for 24 hours or more may have significant swallowing problems after removal. Extubating orally intubated patients in tongs or halos may be particularly dangerous and requires personnel expertly trained in intubation with fiberoptic laryngoscope or bronchoscope. Once the secretions of a patient with a tracheostomy have decreased to normal amounts, the tracheostomy tube can be replaced with an Olympic or Montgomery button. This keeps the stoma open by allowing more room in the airway to clear secretions. If the patient can go 3 to 7 days without suctioning through the button, the button can be removed and the stoma allowed to close. If the patient develops respiratory difficulty, suctioning can be done through the button, or the button can be removed and replaced with a tracheostomy tube.

Temperature Malfunction

Temperature is relatively tightly controlled by various autonomic, metabolic, and behavioral mechanisms. In response to a stimulus, regulatory counterresponses cause a return to a more physiologic state. In response to cold, sensory nerves carry information centrally to the hypothalamus. Local responses include vasoconstriction and shivering. Autonomic response involves decreased sweating, and behavioral response causes search for warmth and adding protective clothing. In response to heat, protective effects include increased sweating (the most effective), shedding of clothes, and moving to cooler air and vasodilatation. Conduction, radiation, and evaporation are used for heat loss.

With infection, a cascade mechanism starts with release of endogenous pyrogens including interleukin 1, tumor microsis factor, and interferons. There are perhaps other cytokines that stimulate the hypothalamus and brainstem (26). The central nervous system induces the appropriate temperature response. Spinal cord injury, with its loss of sensory input and autonomic nervous system, causes problems with temperature control (27). Associated loss of voluntary motor control may limit the ability to have an appropriate behavioral response.

Because sympathetic outflow occurs at the thoracic spine, cervical and high thoracic lesions lose the ability to respond to this pathway. Initially, acute spinal cord injury causes the person to become a "partial poikilotherm," which generally induces hypothermia and is seen in spinal shock. With time, an active and passive rewarming technique reestablishes a normal temperature. The injured patient continues to have fluctuations based on exogenous (environmental) and endogenous (infections, metabolic) stimuli. The physiologic response to the abnormal temperature can remain deranged. Fever remains a problem for the nonacutely injured patient. A recent study showed 85% of patients with injury above T-6 manifested fever during the rehabilitation stay, usually related to infection or inflammatory causes (28). These causes are familiar to those commonly treating spinal cord injured patients. Included are urinary tract infections, respiratory tract, both upper (bronchitis) and lower (pneumonia), infectious decubitus ulcer, certain diarrheas such as *Clostridium difficile,* colitis, sinusitis, and intravenous line infections. Less obvious sources of fever include prolonged ileus with translocation of bacterial products, drug fever, DVT with or without pulmonary emboli, heterotopic ossification, and autonomic dysreflexia.

The usual workup for fever includes history and physical examination with high index of suspicion for urinary and respiratory sources, intravenous access, nasogastric tubes, rectal tubes, and wounds. Laboratory examination includes complete blood count with differential, urinalysis, and culture, blood cultures if indicated, and chest x-ray film if indicated. Because examination of the extremities has limited usefulness for phlebitis, appropriate examination for either DVT or pulmonary embolus should be made. Review of the medications should be done if other sources are not found.

Therapy for fever should start with control of temperature because the ideal temperature is not known. Environmental manipulations with exposure of the skin to air, cooling with ice, and fans can be used to replace loss of sweat ability (evaporation). Antipyretics also can be used. Antibiotics are used if infection is suggested. The decision for antibiotics is based on apparent source of infection, presence of chills or fevers, elevated white blood cell count, or band forms. Response to antibiotics seem to be typical of nonspinal cord injured patients. If all of the tests are negative for an offending source, then one can make a diagnosis of fever of spinal cord injury. In such cases, the patients can be continued in the rehabilitation program, because even though they are running a high fever, they do not feel sick. If the fever persists, then the testing should be repeated within 2 weeks. If results of all the tests are within normal limits again, then the diagnosis of fever of spinal cord injury is reasonably confirmed. The elevated temperature usually will run its course over 6 to 8 weeks as the body temperature control mechanisms adjust to the newer circumstances.

Heterotopic Ossification

Heterotopic ossification is seen in 20% to 30% of patients with spinal cord injury. Heterotopic ossification is the development of calcification around a joint, most frequently the hip joint, it may involve the knee joint and shoulder joint, and infrequently it involves the elbow. The onset of heterotopic ossification may be seen as early as 3 to 4 weeks after injury but is usually later than that. In the able bodied person, the signs are similar to that of acute arthritis, but this is not reliable in the paralyzed because of the insensate joints. Usually the therapists are the first to notice a problem as the patient exhibits loss of range of motion, usually in the hip. Heterotopic ossification may show itself as a swollen limb; thus heterotopic ossification is part of the differential diagnosis of DVT.

Once the therapist or nurse notices either a decreased range of motion or swelling, then the diagnosis is confirmed by an elevated alkaline phosphatase level. The appearance of heterotopic ossification on x-ray film is a later phenomenon. Thus, treatment should be initiated when swelling or loss of range of motion and an elevated alkaline phosphatase level are present. The treatment of choice is disodium etidronate 20 mg/kg for the first 2 weeks and then 10 mg/kg for 2.5 months for a total treatment time of 3 months. This treatment will retard the process but will not cause dissolution of any heterotopic ossification that has already formed. It is effective in about 90% of patients.

In those patients in whom surgery is necessary either to debulk the joint or to provide motion in an almost alkalosed joint, it is necessary for the patient to receive 2 weeks of preoperative sodium etidronate and continue with the medication for 6 months to 1 year postoperatively. Surgery should not be undertaken until the alkaline phosphatase level has returned to normal and the calcium deposit looks mature on x-ray film. Heterotopic ossification has a fuzzy outline in the active stage that converts to a smooth border in the mature stage. The goal in surgery should be to obtain enough range of motion so that the patient can sit comfortably in a wheelchair without causing excessive pressure on the ischium and sacral area.

CHRONIC COMPLICATIONS ASSOCIATED WITH SPINAL CORD INJURY

Spasticity

Spasticity is a disorder characterized as increased muscle tone, abnormalities of muscle relaxation, and exaggerated deep tendon reflexes. Spasticity is a common problem in spinal cord injury. This disorder is regarded as clinically difficult and challenging. Several treatment modalities often are necessary to obtain reasonable control and include pharmacologic agents, physical rehabilitation, chemodenervation, and surgery with the intent of improving function and facilitating nursing care or patient hygiene (29). The physiology of spasticity includes a variety of upper motor neuron syndromes that result from disruption of descending inhibitory tracts, corticospinal and corticobulbar tracts, and sensory affects. The simplistic concept of overactive muscle spindles, or motor fibers, is no longer sufficient. Table 6 lists some of

TABLE 6. *Positive and negative phenomen associated with upper motor neuron syndromes*

Negative phenomenon	Positive phenomenon
Weakness	Velocity-dependent tone
Fatigability	increase
Slow initiation	Abnormal relaxation phase
Reduced motor recruitment	Clonus
Reduced dexterity	Rigidity
	Dystonia
	Flexor and extensor spasms
	Stretch hyperreflexia
	Cutaneous hyperreflexia
	Autonomic hyperreflexia
	Babinski reflex
	Triflexion reflex

the positive and negative phenomena associated with upper motor neuron syndromes.

It is well understood that spasticity is the imbalance of inhibition and excitation occurring at the motor neuron level of the spinal cord. The goals of management of spasticity are (i) to identify patients appropriate for specific types of therapy, and (ii) to establish treatments that take advantage of changes in the motor system, such as use of antispasticity medications, dorsal rhizotomy, botulinum toxin, and intrathecal baclofen therapy, to monitor changes in basic impairments (flexibility, strength, timing, and sequencing of contractions) and disabilities (gait, transfers, and activities of daily living after therapy).

Pharmacologic agents are an important component in the management of spasticity. The most commonly administered drugs include baclofen, diazepam, and dantrolene sodium. Newer adjunctive treatments include oral and transdermal forms of clonidine and tizanidine. Other investigational agents are presently underway. Botulism toxin A (botox) and intrathecal baclofen are important drugs now used for spasticity management.

Baclofen is an analog of γ-aminobutyric acid (GABA) binding to the GABA-B receptor. Baclofen inhibits monosynaptic and polysynaptic reflexes and depressor fusimotor activity. Baclofen decreases response to noxious peripheral stimuli. Gastrointestinal absorption is rapid, with peak plaza levels occurring 1 to 2 hours after administration with a half-life of approximately 2 to 6 hours. Baclofen is eliminated predominantly in the kidneys, although a small portion is metabolized in the liver. Baclofen is a potent antispasticity drug, has a wide therapeutic range, and generally has tolerable side effects; therefore, it has a primary role in spasticity control. Baclofen is particularly effective for the flexor and extensor spasms commonly seen in spinal cord injury patients. Baclofen may improve bladder control by decreasing hyperreflexic contractures of the external urethral sphincter. It has been shown to be safe and effective for long-term use. Doses in adults begins at approximately 5 mg given three times daily, and this is gradually titrated to produce an optimal clinical response. There is a wide variation of the response among individuals. The manufacturer's recommended dose is 80 mg/day, but most clinicians go as high as 120 mg/day and doses in the range from 200 mg/day are commonly used in Europe. Side effects, including confusion, sedation, ataxia, hypertonia, and hallucinations, are in low occurrence, but do increase with higher dosage and increased patient age. Sudden withdrawal of baclofen leads to seizures and hallucinations. Intrathecal administration of baclofen with an implanted pump has been approved in the United States for treatment of spasticity of spinal origin. Advantage of intrathecal baclofen administration lies in the ability to achieve higher therapeutic concentrations at potential sites of action within the spinal cord without incurring concomitant systemic toxicity.

Diazepam and the benzodiazepine class of drugs exert antispasmodic effects through facilitation of the postsynaptic effects of GABA, resulting in an increase in presynaptic inhibition at spinal and supraspinal sites within the central nervous system. Diazepam is effective in decreasing resistance to passive movement to deep tendon reflexes and painful spasms. It is absorbed in the gastrointestinal tract, undergoes transformation in the liver, and is excreted in the urine. It is highly lipid soluble and rapidly crosses the blood–brain barrier. Use of benzodiazepines for spasticity is most common among patients with spinal cord injury. This drug has a side effect profile that includes amnesia, sedation, and the potential for physiologic addiction, which has impeded its wider use for the treatment of spasticity. Withdrawal symptoms may appear if benzodiazepine is tapered too rapidly. Treatment with diazepam generally begins at doses of 2 mg given twice daily and may be slowly titrated in 2-mg increments to a maximum of 40 to 60 mg/day in divided doses.

Dantrolene sodium is the only drug in clinical use for spasticity that acts peripherally at the muscular level rather than at the reflex level. Its action is exerted on muscle fibers where it inhibits release of calcium from the sarcoplasmic reticulum. There is a decrease in the force produced by the exertion of contraction coupling. Effects of dantrolene are more evident in the fast twitch fibers than in slow muscle fibers. It reduces activities of phasic stretch reflexes. It is metabolized mostly in the liver and eliminated in the liver. Its half-life is approximately 8 hours. It is less likely to cause lethargy or cognitive impairment than baclofen or diazepam. Dantrolene reduces maximum voluntary power, and its effect on spastic hypertonia generally is observed without impairment of motor function. Weakness is a prominent side effect, however, especially in patients with marginal strength. Sedation is noted at higher doses. Malaise, nausea, vomiting, dizziness, and diarrhea have been reported. Significant hepatotoxicity may occur and has been reported in approximately 1% of patients. Therefore, hepatic function tests must be monitored periodically and the drug tapered or discontinued if hepatic enzyme elevations are noted. Doses range from 50 to 800 mg/day, although the manufacturer's recommended dose is 100 mg/day. Treatment is usually begun at 25 mg/day and slowly increased.

Clonidine acts centrally on α_2-adrenogenic receptor agonist whose mechanism of spasticity reduction has not been clearly elucidated. The α_2-adrenergic binding sites are in the substantia gelatinosa intermediolateral cell columns of the thoracic spinal cord. The suggested mechanism of action includes depression of spinal motor neurons as well as polysynaptic reflexes. Clonidine has assumed an adjunctive role in the management of spasticity. It is being used in conjunction with baclofen in patients with spinal cord injury. Some patients experience adverse effects with this drug, particularly orthostatic hypotension, dry mouth, and lethargy. There have been favorable results using transdermal clonidine in spinal cord injury patients. Side effects occasionally have resulted in discontinued use of the medication.

Tizanidine is a centrally acting α_2 agonist and imidazoline derivative and is structurally similar to clonidine (30). The antispasmodic activity of tizanidine is thought to result from the indirect depression of polysynaptic reflexes, probably through the facilitation of the action of glycine, an inhibitory neurotransmitter, and antagonizing excretory actions of spinal neurons. It reduces the tonic stretch reflexes and enhances presynaptic inhibition in animal studies. The greatest reduction in spasticity coincides with peak serum concentrations. Double-blind comparative studies indicated it is as effective as baclofen and diazepam in reducing tone and is as tolerable as these two drugs. Dosage typically begins at 2 mg given twice daily and can be increased in 4-mg increments every 4 to 7 days to a maximum of 37 mg/day in three or four divided doses. Side effects include drowsiness, dizziness, hypertension, and orthostatic hypotension. Side effects are dose related and often are resolved with decrease in the dose. Tizanidine was available outside the United States for 10 years but in December 1996 was approved by the Food and Drug Administration for use in the United States (31). Ketazolam, threonine, and orphenadrine citrate are three drugs currently under investigation for antispasmodic effects.

In summary, there are many treatment options for spasticity: (i) prevention by avoidance of noxious stimuli; (ii) physical therapy with passive or active range of motion exercises, strengthening, gait training, and splinting; (iii) occupational therapy with skilled training in tactile desensitization; (iv) surgery, which includes tendon lengthening, transfer, capsular release, rhizotomy, and dorsal root entry zone ablation; (v) medication; (vi) intrathecal medication, which includes the baclofen infusion pump; and (vii) chemodenervation with botulinum toxin (botox), which is a comparatively new agent for management of spasticity. It is useful for patients who are still in the recovery phase following spinal cord injury because its effects are short term, i.e., 2 to 3 months. There is no single correct dose of botox yet established. It can be injected without the use of electromyography and superficial palpation techniques. It is found to be safe but expensive.

Fractures

Fractures in both the upper and lower extremities occur frequently with spinal trauma. Modern concepts of fracture management recommend internal fixation whenever possible, and this is even more true when the long bone fractures are associated with paralysis secondary to spinal trauma, especially if the fractures occur in the limbs that are anesthetic. The paralyzed patient will be subjected to the possibility of skin sores if treated in traction or in a cast. It is the goal in rehabilitation to mobilize the patient as quickly as possible, and this is enhanced with internal fixation. Thus, aggressive treatment of fractures where feasible and safe is the management of choice in the acutely injured patient as well as the paralyzed patient during the first 3 to 6 months.

Beyond 3 to 6 months, the situation changes. The bones become osteoporotic, and obtaining adequate internal fixation either by screws and plates or rods is problematic.

Therefore, it is best to treat the fractures in the chronic spinal cord injured nonoperatively if at all possible. Treatment will include use of splints made of soft material, such as a pillow or well-padded removable splints, so the skin can be checked on a frequent basis. Such splinting does not completely immobilize the fracture site, but healing will occur almost universally except for those fractures of the femoral neck that must be internally fixed. One may be willing to accept a nonunion.

Fortunately, fractures in the chronically spinal cord injured patient heal more rapidly. For instance, a fractured femur will show significant callous in 3 to 4 weeks and be firmly healed usually in 6 to 8 weeks. Two aspects that the treating surgeon should keep in mind is that, when the treatment is completed for the fracture, the functional level is unchanged. The second aspect is that if the fracture has the possibility of causing skin problems, i.e., a large spike close to the skin, fracture repositioning must be carried out or attempts made at open reduction.

In summary, treatment of a fracture in an acutely injured paralyzed patient should be aggressive, utilizing internal fixation where possible. However, in the chronically paralyzed patient, nonoperative means should be pursued, utilizing soft splints to maintain satisfactory positioning (32,33).

Posttraumatic Syringomyelia

Posttraumatic syringomyelic syndrome was first described in 1898 by Harvey Cushing. Improved understanding of the clinical and pathologic features of posttraumatic syringomyelia did not occur until the antibiotic era and with prolonged survival of large numbers of spinal cord injured patients after World War II. Interest in widespread recognition of this syndrome arose from the monograph by Barnett and associates (34) in 1966. Syringomyelia continued to evolve as heightened clinical awareness and sophisticated neuroimaging techniques augmented experience with this devastating but treatable delayed complication of spinal cord injury.

Posttraumatic syringomyelia is characterized by the development of delayed progressive myelopathy away from the segment of the initial level of injury. The incidence varies from 1.3% to 51% of spinal cord injuries, and such variation may be related to the referral pattern of the particular institution. The mean latency from the injury to the development of new symptoms has been reported to be 4 to 9 years. The cyst may vary in size from a few millimeters to involving the entire length of the spinal cord. The presence of the cyst is not significant unless it is causing symptoms. The initial presenting symptom is often pain at or above the level of the original spinal cord injury and is usually localized to the chest or arms. The patients may notice increased spasticity, paresthesia, ascending level of numbness, and loss of motor strength in previously functioning muscles. Symptoms may be related to activities that cause increased pressure in the cyst, such as coughing or straining.

Examination reveals hypesthesia, especially to pain and temperature, extending cephalad to the spinal injury level. If the cyst extends into the lower brainstem, there may be associated dysphasia, atrophy of the tongue, and facial hypesthesia. Less frequent signs include Horner's syndrome, Charcot joints, and autonomic dysreflexia (causing increased sweating).

The natural history of this condition, although not well documented, generally causes gradual progression of neurologic deficits over months to years (35,36). The pathogenesis of posttraumatic syringomyelia is not completely defined. Cystic myelomalacia may follow clearance of chronic debris at the site of the spinal cord injury, as well as transduction of the fluid along paths of least resistance. Coughing and sneezing cause transmission of pressure from the abdomen, thoracolumbar epidural venous plexus, and, hence, to the cystic fluid, which usually migrates cephalad through the tissue planes that offer the least resistance.

Previously the diagnosis was made by performing a CT myelogram with water-soluble iodinated contrast material (Metrisamide) and taking delayed x-ray films 12 to 24 hours later. The contrast seeped from the subarachnoid space into the cystic cavity outlining the syrinx on the delayed 24-hour x-ray films. This has recently been superseded almost entirely by the MRI scan, which is so sensitive that it will readily outline very small cysts in the spinal cord. In a recent study by Backe and associates (37), 45 of 88 patients (51%) admitted to a rehabilitation unit had posttraumatic spinal cord cysts. Posttraumatic spinal cord cysts thus are much more frequently seen among spinal cord injured patients than as a clinical syndrome, and sound judgment has to be exercised on the need for surgical intervention based entirely on imaging. Surgical treatment is recommended in patients with documented neurologic deterioration accompanied by a positive MRI scan.

The surgical approach is to drain the cyst by performing a myelotomy of the dorsal spinal cord. Reaccumulation of the cyst and spontaneous closure of the myelotomy site are prevented by placement of a shunt. The most commonly recommended shunt is from the syrinx to the subarachnoid space (syringosubarachnoid shunt) (38–40). In the presence of significant subarachnoid scar tissue, the shunt can be diverted to the peritoneal cavity or pleural cavity. Cordectomy or terminal ventriculostomy with or without shunt has been effective in patients with complete spinal cord injury. Motor abnormalities are more likely than sensory deficits to improve following surgery, and drainage of the cyst is effective in pain control in carefully selected patients. Occasionally the treatment may not lead to significant functional recovery. Postoperative MRI scan may be helpful in detecting malfunctioning shunt and reaccumulation of the syrinx.

Sexual Functioning

Genital sensation and function are altered following spinal cord injury, but the emotional needs for continuation of sexual function remain intact. Sexual counseling has become a mainstay in the early rehabilitation of the patient (41). This issue is addressed early in the recovery phase. The centers that use the interdisciplinary approach to treatments are directed to both the physiologic needs of the patient as well as the cognitive behavioral strategy adapted to different lesion types.

In the last decade, there has been a rapid development regarding enhanced performance of the male with spinal cord injury (42). The vast majority of spinal cord injured males have the ability to have reflex erections, but these erections often are unpredictable and unsustained. During the 1970s and 1980s, implantation of prosthetic devices gained wide acceptance. However, enthusiasm has waned as long-term outcomes have shown an unacceptably high complication rate (43). These complications included infection, early and late erosion, as well as mechanical failure of the inflatable penile prosthesis. In addition, replacing the corporal bodies with a prosthetic device precluded the patient from using other options that have now become available.

Vacuum erection devices have gained wide acceptance among spinal cord injury males and offer the least invasive treatment for restoration of erectile function. Drawbacks to this treatment are related to the cumbersomeness of the device as well as the difficulty in manipulating them with an associated spinal cord injury. Newer devices such as the Osbon Esteem have allowed for easier use.

Intercavernous pharmacotherapy has gained wide acceptance among males. Pharmacologic agents that induce smooth muscle relaxation are injected into the corpora cavernosum (44). This allows for filling of the lacunar space with blood and subsequent compression of the emissary veins, producing a physiologic sustained erection. The initial agent used was papavarine, a cost-efficient smooth muscle relaxant. However, side effects such as corporal fibrosis, priapism, and nodularity were complications, but the manufacturer removed any indecision regarding its use by pulling the drug off the market. The most common agent used today is alprostadil (PGE1), which was approved by the Food and Drug Administration in 1996 (45). PGE1 causes less side effects than papavarine but is more expensive. Caution should be taken when using these compounds in the neurologically impaired patient because these agents are prone to cause priapism. Dosages should be generally lower than in the able bodied population. The institution of pharmacologic erection program must be a multidisciplinary approach involving the patient, partner, sexual counselor, and physician extender, who can thoroughly train the patient in proper injection techniques and educate him about prevention of complications.

The latest development for treatment of erectile dysfunction involves the administration of PGE1 to the distal urethra by proprietary drug delivery system. The PGE1 then is absorbed via the urethral mucosa to the erectile bodies (the corpora cavernosus and corpora spongiosus). This has particular appeal to the spinal cord injury patient who is accustomed to performing self-catheterization and has no urethral dysfunction.

Unfortunately, studies and research on physiologic changes of the female sexual response are sorely lacking (46). Although Comarr and Vigue (41) reported on women who could achieve organism through breast and genital stimulation, studies on the physiologic responses such as vaginal contractions and lubrication are limited. Despite these many new developments, return to sexual function must include the physical as well as psychosocial rehabilitation of the patient with spinal cord injury.

Pain

Recent studies have shown the incidence of severe pain following spinal cord injury to be 65% and the incidence of disabling pain to be in the range of 30% to 40%. Chronic pain is usually described as pain persisting 6 months or more following injury. There are three major categories of chronic pain related to spinal cord injury: (i) neuropathic or neurogenic pain, (ii) musculoskeletal pain secondary to spasticity, and (iii) musculoskeletal pain arising from abnormal use patterns of muscles and joints secondary to functional changes caused by the injury. Many patients will have more than one type of pain. It is important to differentiate and quantify the types of pain that are present for purposes of selecting optimal treatment.

Neuropathic pain syndromes are the type most commonly seen following spinal cord injury and are variously labeled neurogenic pain, phantom pain, causalgia, anesthesia dolorosa, and deafferentation pain. This type of pain is commonly described as a burning numbness that may be regional or dermatomal in distribution and is usually present continuously.

Treatment of neuropathic pain has been difficult and often case refractory. Current protocols for neuropathic pain management utilized a stepwise application of treatment modalities beginning with the optimization of medical management and proceeding to neuromodulation, intraspinal drug administration, and possibly neurodestructive procedures. A recent survey assessing the results of treatment algorithms of this type of pain showed satisfactory pain control in 60% of patients (47).

A serotonin reuptake inhibitor (amitriptyline, doxepin, sertaline, paroxetine) are the drugs utilized with medical management. To these drugs an analeptic drug such as clonazepam, carbamazepine, or gabapentin can be added. Mexiletine, an orally administered system of local anesthetic, has been used with some series. Dosages are gradually increased to maximum recommended levels until pain relief or side effects are noted. In general, it is best to add medications in a parallel fashion while continuing previously prescribed drugs, because may be synergistic or superadditive effects among the medications. If pain relief is obtained with certain combination medications, selective medication may be tapered as symptoms allow. There are no controlled prospective studies that demonstrate superior effectiveness of any one medical regimen.

When medical therapy alone is ineffective, neuromodulation techniques should be considered. These include transcutaneous electrical nerve stimulation and spinal cord stimulation. Transcutaneous electrical nerve stimulation unit trial is safe and inexpensive and should be considered for almost all patients. Studies involving the use of spinal cord stimulation for neuropathic pain in spinal cord injury showed this treatment is largely ineffective in cases of complete cord transection (48). Patients should be considered for spinal cord stimulation only if there is partial sensory sparing and the pain tends to follow a dermatomal or radicular pattern. Spinal cord stimulation also has been recently tried for control of chronic spasticity in spinal cord injury.

Patients with intractable symptoms should be considered for long-term subarachnoid administration through the use of an implantable infusion pump. Morphine sulfate, the most commonly used drug in subarachnoid infusions, was initially believed to be relatively ineffective for neuropathic pain. There are now studies that support the effectiveness of subarachnoid morphine alone or in combination with other drugs for control of neuropathic pain in spinal cord injury (49). Before considering long-term intrathecal drug therapy, trial injections of subarachnoid morphine should be performed to ascertain effectiveness and dose requirements. Intrathecal baclofen, which is currently used for control of spasticity, has been reported in one series to effectively relieve neuropathic pain (50). This is presumably due to the role played by GABA-B receptors of the dorsal horn in some neuropathic states. Other studies have shown that baclofen is not effective in reducing neuropathic pain but does relieve muscular pain associated with spasticity. At the present time, morphine and baclofen are the only two drugs approved in the United States for intrathecal infusion. Studies from other countries have shown that the α_2 agonist, clonidine, is effective in reducing neuropathic pain and intrathecal infusion, either alone or in combination with morphine.

Pain secondary to spasticity is described as aching or cramping. It is present intermittently and usually associated with visible muscle spasm. The severity of the pain does not always correlate with degree of spasticity. The treatment of musculoskeletal pain associated with spasticity in spinal cord injury is accomplished through control of the spasticity. As a first step, oral administration of baclofen, diazepam, or clonazepam may be tried. In cases refractory to oral medication, a trial of intrathecal baclofen is performed. Patients with a positive response may be managed with chronic intrathecal baclofen infusion through an implanted pump.

Musculoskeletal pain arising from structural or functional changes following spinal cord injury may have multiple causes. Myofascial pain syndromes are common and are caused by abnormal use patterns, especially in the postural muscles of the neck and shoulder girdle. These syndromes are characterized by pain on movement, restricted range of motion, and the presence of distinct trigger points within the affected muscle. Pressure on these trigger points reproduces the familiar pain pattern. Another form of muscular pain arises from the disuse of partially denervated muscles. This pain is characterized by diffuse muscle tenderness and stiffness. Last, there are pain syndromes that arise from overstress or dysfunctional joints. These problems include sacral iliac joint dysfunction, facet joint syndromes, and costochondritis.

Treatment of patients with musculoskeletal pain syndromes that arise from abnormal muscle use patterns should first be treated with appropriate physical measures for muscle strengthening, stretching, and conditioning. In refractory cases, trigger point injections may be used to give initial pain relief and relaxation for compliance with physical therapy. If symptoms recur, medical management with serotonin reuptake inhibitor and nonsteroidal antiinflammatory agents may be indicated. A percutaneous electrical neuromuscular stimulator may be helpful in refractive cases. Biofeedback therapy may be used for symptoms involving neck pain and muscle tension headache.

Painful conditions involving specific joints, such as sacroiliac joint syndrome, facet joint syndrome, or costochondritis, may be treated with nonsteroidal antiinflammatory drugs or injection of steroid into the affected joint or cartilage. In addition to yielding initial pain relief, these procedures provide a therapeutic window for more intensive therapy directed at reconditioning and mobilization (Table 7).

Autonomic Dysreflexia

Autonomic dysreflexia is a paroxysmal syndrome of hypertension, hypohydrosis above the level of injury, bradycardia, flushing, and headache in response to noxious visceral and other stimuli. It occurs in cervical cord injury and thoracic

TABLE 7. *Medications commonly used for neuropathic pain*

Tricyclic antidepressants	
Amitriptyline	25–150 mg/day
Doxepin	25–150 mg/day
Selective serotonin reuptake inhibitors	
Fluoxetine (Prozac)	20–40 mg/day
Paroxetine (Paxil)	10–40 mg/day
Sertraline (Zoloft)	50–300 mg/day
Analeptics	
Carbamazepine (Tegretol)	300–1600 mg/day
Gabapentin (Neurontin)	300–1800 mg/day
Clonazepam (Klonopin)	1–4 mg/day
Systemic Local Anesthetics	
Mexiletine	450–600 mg/day
GABA-B agonists	
Baclofen	20–80 mg/day

GABA, γ-amino butyric acid.

cord injury above the level of the sixth thoracic vertebra. Symptoms are those of sudden severe sympathetic discharge, although plasma catecholamines do not appear to rise. The exact pathophysiologic mechanism has not been delineated.

Autonomic dysreflexia is most commonly triggered by bladder distention with or without infection, and next most commonly by fecal impaction and rectal distention. Other potential participating events are muscle spasm, cutaneous stimulation, labor, surgery, electrical stimulation for semen collection, and pulmonary embolus. The dystrophy rarely occurs less than 2 months following injury and usually persists more than 6 months. Approximately 60% of patients with high cervical injury and 20% of those with high thoracic cord injuries will exhibit dysreflexia.

With those demonstrating dysreflexia, approximately 10% may show evidence of malignant hypertension with transient neurologic deficit, nausea, dyspnea, or chest pain. Untreated, the severe hypertension can lead to seizures, transient visual loss, aphasia, or intracranial hemorrhage. The precise risks are unknown in most cases. With most cases with proper management, the risks are low.

Treatment includes removal of the noxious stimuli, elevation of the patient, and antihypertensive drugs as needed. Rapidly acting antihypertensives such as parenteral hydralazine or intravenous nitroprusside may be used acutely. Long-term prevention has been effective with prazosin.

In the field of disabled sports, autonomic dysreflexia has taken on a new perspective. The disabled athletes, particularly those with paralysis, have learned that it may enhance their performance by "boosting." Boosting is accomplished by the athlete sitting on a sharp object, thus creating a noxious stimulus, or by occluding the catheter, both of which will cause an increase in the blood pressure and pulse rate and provide a potential enhancement of the athletic activity. Athletes who are doing this can usually be detected because of the sweating that usually accompanies the dysreflexic episode. The International Paralympic Medical Commission recently has taken taken a stand prohibiting boosting in athletic events.

Contractures

Contractures will develop in joints that are not used or in joints where preaxial muscles have more tone than the postaxial muscles. This is a frequent occurrence in patients with spinal cord injury. In the early postinjury period, the nursing staff will need to be attuned to this fact or else contractures will develop in the upper extremities which will interfere with becoming as functional as the paralyzed level will allow. In the upper extremities, this will affect dressing and the ability to do transfers. In the lower extremities, transfer also will be more difficult if contractures are present, and good positioning of a wheelchair will be made more difficult.

One of the options in nonoperative management is the use of the halo. Patients treated in this manner are particularly prone to having shoulder problems with decreased range of motion, i.e., contractures, and increased pain. Thus, it is especially necessary that both the therapists and the nurses perform daily range of motion exercise of the shoulders and the positioning at night at least have some time with the shoulders abducted.

The foot and ankle are prone to develop contractures. The reason for this is that either the supine or prone position favors plantar flexion. In the long term, the hips and knees are more likely to develop contractures because of the time spent sitting in wheelchairs. To counterbalance this, it is tantamount that the patient be taught to sleep prone, at least a portion of the night, to stretch out these two major joints.

On the positive side, in quadriplegics, particularly the C6s, tightness in the flexor muscles will enhance the tenodesis effect and, thus, some amount of contracture would be positive for improving function. On the negative side, the patients with contractures tend to be more prone to skin sores because of the positioning problems, not only increasing pressure on at-risk areas but also the difficulty of changing to a safer position. When skin sores occur and contractures are present, it often is necessary to relieve the contractures before being able to have a satisfactory skin repair outcome.

REHABILITATIVE CONSIDERATIONS IN POSTTRAUMATIC QUADRIPLEGIA AND PARAPLEGIA

Psychological Considerations for Spinal Cord Injury Patients

Spinal cord injury is a family disease that affects each member of the family in a different way. The average person has little knowledge of what it really means to have such an injury. Most people assume that only walking is affected. Some may realize that there may also be hand and arm involvement. Rarely, however, do people know the potential implications of other bodily functions, such as bowel, bladder, and sexual ability. Additionally, many people assume that spinal cord injuries can be "fixed" or "cured" due to the many miracles that are seen on television and the movies. Consequently, spinal cord injuries are devastating emotionally and physically. Patients have described spinal cord injury as impossible, my worst nightmare, hell on earth.

Adjustment to spinal cord injury is a lifelong process with no end point and different issues arising at different developmental phases of a person's life after injury. A variety of factors influence one's ability to adjust. Preinjury personality and coping skills have a dramatic effect. Additionally, the presence or absence of a good family support system, financial stability, age, and the ability to return to work or school play key roles in the adjustment process (51). Regardless of a patient's success in dealing with adversity prior to sustaining a spinal cord injury, all patients undergo major emotional challenges as a result of these newly imposed physical limitations.

TABLE 8. *Program type: C1–3 ventilator dependent complete tetraplegia expected L.O.S. 5 weeks (rehab phase)*

Day/Date Unit	Pre-Admission	Admission Day First 24° Day 1	48–72°	Acute Phase
HEALTH STATUS • Consults/Tests • Assessments: • Cognitive • Nutrition • Respiratory management • Medications • Skin integrity • Pain • Neurological level	• Obtain current medical record (H&P; D/C notes; Operative report), X-rays; films. (Adm.) • If pt is adolescent, request family to bring confirmation of immunication status.	• Urology; Int Med; Ed; PT; OT; TR; Voc; Nutrition; Counseling • Assessment of spinal stabilization and mobility orders (attending MD). • H&P; Labs; X-ray of injury level and fractures, CXR; Diet; Meds; pain control; Lovenox (resident) • C&S urine to be **done ONLY when** Urology orders • BFS, DVT prophylaxis • ABG's, add co-oximetry to ABG's if admitted within 48 hrs. of injury. FVC, Neg Ins. Force, Baseline, CXR, CBC, ALB, Pre- ALB, SMA 18, Sputum C&S, • order metabolic studies for pts on nutritional support (diet) • EKG • Artificial Airway • Leave on transfer vent settings until ABG done. Adjust accordingly • Aerosol or MDI • Add 10–15 cm pressure support if not already on any pressure support • Lavage with suctioning • Weigh patient (RN) • Assess BCR positive/Negative (RN) • Establish am, or pm bowel program (RN)	• Address any new health problems not addressed with Adm. (MD, RN) and all • Check IVP and urodynamics scheduling • FIM & ASIA complete (PT; OT) • Assessment complete Estab. goals & treatment plan (PT; OT, RN) • Evaluate for midline catheter • Check with Urology to D/C foley, begin IC q4h (RN) • If skin breakdown present, complete skin assessment weekly until resolved (RN) • Initiate speech screening: (i.e. communication swallowing & cognitive D (Speech)	• Re-evaluate pt motor & sensory 1 month post admission (OT/PT) • Repeat BFS 1 month after initial study to D/C Lovenox & Zantac • Metabolic studies completed for patients on nutritional support (diet) • Eval for portable vent (RC) • TR completes initial assessment and estab. goals and tx plan. ongoing _____ • Evaluate C-3 candidacy for vent weaning pathway (RC; RN; PT) • ABG pm • Wean from supplemental O2, DAP to prepare for port. vent, as tolerated (RC) • Evaluate to D/C telemetry if not already D/C'd. (MD, RN) • Establish pain management program as appropriate. (MD, RN) • IVP; renal scan (for adolescents) completed? (RN) • Urodynamics completed? (RN) • Monitor I.C. volumes when ≤ 500 cc q4° for 48° ↓ I.C.'s to q 6° (RN) • If reflex occurs, obtain urine C&S → treat if appropriate. • If reflex persists check with urologist re: videourodynamics (RN) • Referral made to speech therapy for evidence of CHI on H & P and/or questionable cognitive status (i.e., reduced alertness, ↓ recall; comprehension problems; confusion with unexplainable etiology)

Pathways are to be used as a guideline; they do not represent a standard of care. Individual plans of care may differ based on each patient's individual needs. Sheperd Center, Inc. Rehab Pathways, copyright 4/3/96.

Grieving is the primary goal in helping a spinal cord injury patient. The objects of grief relate to physical loss, resulting life changes, altered body image, and changed roles in various contexts. Whereas more people can relate to the loss of a loved one, few people can relate to personal physical loss and all of its implications. This can result in feelings of isolation and despair. The benefits of rehabilitation transcend the physical arena. Meeting other patients with similar struggles can relieve some of the loneliness. Seeing people in more advanced stages of rehabilitation provides hope and creates a picture of possibilities that far exceeds the explanation from an able bodied professional.

Professional intervention by a counselor and/or psychologist enhances the adjustment process. Unfortunately, patients do not have the luxury of putting their physical needs and rehabilitation goals on hold until they feel more able to cope with them. This is especially true with the advent of managed care and the resultant shortened length of inpatient stay. At a minimum, psychological help during the rehabilitation process consists of the identification of obstacles such as denial, anxiety, or depression that may interfere or obstruct the rehabilitation process. Psychotropic medications can be a tremendous asset in the care of some patients. Additionally, the identification of alcohol and drug issues, as well as cognitive issues, ensures that all the patient's needs are addressed (52). A psychologist and/or a counselor can help patients work through their initial shock and disbelief in a supportive environment. Understanding the normal and expected emotions that come with grieving can help a patient cope better with his or her feelings. Anticipating one's return to the world after rehabilitation allows a patient to have some coping strategies to use proactively, which maximizes long-term adjustment potential. Finally, many, if not most, patients require postdischarge professional help to smooth the patient's reentry into the community.

Leisure and Recreation

Leisure activities can be a problem for people with spinal cord injuries because their injuries may limit their participation in familiar activities. Having a spinal cord injury may result in dramatic changes in how an individual spends his or her spare time. A person with spinal cord injury typically does not return to work immediately and must adjust to sudden "forced" leisure. Many people, unsure about what to do with this additional free time, return to substance abuse and a sedentary lifestyle. Studies have shown that there is a direct relationship between leisure patterns and secondary medical complications. For example, the more passive a person is, the more medical complications increase and the less satisfied a person may become with his or her leisure time. A long-term goal of spinal cord injury rehabilitation is to help patients achieve community reintegration, regain their maximal functional ability, and return to an active preinjury lifestyle (53). For a person to achieve a meaningful life and not just physically survive functional gains and just more

than physical skill, activities of daily living must be achieved. Other skills such as leisure and creative recreation, negotiating community barriers (architectural and interpersonal), creative problem solving, and accessing community resources must be required (54). Therapeutic recreation is a vital part of the comprehensive rehabilitation program in that it helps persons with spinal cord injury establish goals and skills required for leading a productive leisure lifestyle. Therapeutic recreation also provides opportunities for patients to become aware of their leisure options, learn new skills, and/or become familiar with adaptive equipment with their leisure interests. A qualitative research project conducted at the Shepherd Center illustrated that individuals perceived that therapeutic recreation also benefited them by providing motivation and self-confidence by providing hope and a sense of future possibilities. A thorough assessment of a patient's leisure history and interests, leisure resources used, and his or her attitude toward recreation should be completed by a therapeutic recreation specialist. Based on the assessment, the leisure goals are established with input from the patient. These goals focus on areas such as community reintegration, leisure education, leisure skill development, mobility training, and advocacy.

As with other kinds of therapy, patients are seen throughout the day for their individual treatment time to provide counseling about returning to preinjury leisure interests, developing new leisure interests, and possible adaptations needed to pursue those interests. Patients are encouraged to identify benefits of their leisure time and to consider the important part leisure played in their lives before their injury. Leisure education classes may be provided to help patients discover their leisure values and assess their preinjury values. In addition, the information on leisure resources and access to these resources is discussed. Advocacy, assertiveness training, and problem solving are topics essential to help patients return to the community.

In addition to leisure education, community reintegration outings should be provided. On outings, patients are given the opportunity to improve barrier management and problem solving skills and to practice leisure skills. Patients can confront issues of body image, self-esteem, and self-advocacy, which helps adjustment to their injury. Often the community reintegration outing is the culminating event that proves to the patient that the skills learned in the therapy environment have been mastered. Such an outing is often the final key that opens the patient's eyes to the very broad world that is still available to them, despite their injury. This often assists a patient in making a more comfortable return to the community. Providing patients with the necessary skills to develop active lifestyles is often the first and most important step to their success and recovery and reintegration back to the community.

Vocational Counseling

Planning for a spinal cord injured patient to reenter the workforce has to start early. It is important for the vocational counselor to see patients as part of their initial rehabilitation. The vocational aspect of the rehabilitation process is a highly individualized endeavor. An interview by a vocational counselor should result in a profile that contains work and educational history as well as assessment of the role work and motivational goals play in the patient's life before injury. Ascertaining the importance of work to each patient early after injury is critical because the desire to return to work may be an important motivational factor for other therapies. Thus, the initial interview should take place when the patient is medically stable and beginning the rehabilitation process. The vocational counselor has several options that can be established after the initial assessment. The patient may be able to return to the preinjury employer in the same job or modified version of the job. Or the patient may return to a different job with the preinjury employer, which may require additional training and education. Finally, the patient may need to completely rethink the job and the employer. Vocational testing is a useful tool for both the individual and the counselor and for deciding which direction to follow. A thorough evaluation performed by an evaluator who is familiar with spinal cord injury and who is able to appropriately modify tests as needed can result in recommendations that provide the individual with options for course of study and career path directions. Recommendations should include information about community resources that will assist the individual in achieving these vocational goals.

As part of the assessment, particularly if the patient intends to return to his or her preinjury job, is a work site evaluation. Following this, the vocational counselor can make recommendations for modification as well as being established as a resource for the employer in returning a productive employee to work. Often other disciplines such as occupational therapy may need to participate in the work site visit.

The vocational counselor will be able to give the patient information on state vocational rehabilitation agencies, social security work incentive programs, and resources for students with disabilities in educational settings. Because individuals who are newly injured can be overwhelmed with information, it is best to provide verbal and written information that can be reviewed as needed. In getting the patient back to work, it often is necessary to provide a continuum of services that can be individualized to match the journey from injury to employment. This continuum should include the previously mentioned components of initial assessment, evaluation and testing, education, job and work site analysis, as well as resource coordination, career exploration, job development, and job placement assistance. Traditional services may need to be supplemented with innovative programs such as internships. In individuals who are not ready to actively pursue vocational goals, this continuum should be readily available on an outpatient basis. Individuals with spinal cord injuries should be provided with the necessary information to be informed consumers, to know what resources are available to assist them in identifying vocational goals, and, most important, to know that a productive lifestyle after spinal cord injury can be a reality. It is documented that individuals who return to productive activity will do better physically and emotionally (55). Access to vocational services on an inpatient and outpatient basis is an important element of rehabilitation for people with spinal cord injuries.

ACKNOWLEDGMENTS

Acknowledgments and thanks go to the following for their contributions to this chapter: Sally Atwell, M.S., Bruce G. Green, M.D., Tariq Javed, M.D., Tammy King, R.N., Jill Koval, Ph.D., Donald Peck Leslie, M.D., John David Mullins, M.D., James A. Settle, M.D., Robert L. Whipple, M.D., and Andrew D. Zadoff, M.D.

REFERENCES

1. Meyer P, Apple DF, Cotler J, Gupta P, Zigler J. The New Spine Fracture Classification, Instructional Course Presentation, American Spinal Injury Association Annual Meeting.
2. Donovan WH. Operative and nonoperative management of spinal cord injury. A review. *Paraplegia* 1994;32:375–388.
3. Collins WF. Surgery in the acute treatment of spinal cord injury: a review of the past forty years. *J Spinal Cord Med* 1995;18:3–8.
4. Duh MS, Shepherd MJ, Wilberger JE, Bracker MB. The effectiveness of surgery on the treatment of acute spinal cord injury and its relation to pharmacological treatments. *Neurosurgery* 1994;35:240–248.
5. Alho A. Operative treatment as a part of the comprehensive care for patients with injuries of the thoracolumbar spine. A review. *Paraplegia* 1994;32:509–516.
6. Carwell JE, Grady DJ. Complications of spinal surgery in acute spinal cord injury. *Paraplegia* 1994;36:389–395.
7. DeVivo M, Richards J. Community reintegration and quality of life following spinal cord injury. *Paraplegia* 1992;30:108–112.
8. Zander K. Collaborative care: two effective strategies for positive outcomes. In: Zander K (ed). *Managing Outcomes Through Collaborative Care: The Application of CareMapping and Case Management.* Chicago, IL: American Hospital Publishing, Inc., 1995;1–38.
9. Burke L, Murphy J. Cost-effective, quality documentation systems are exception-based. In: Burke L, Murphy J (eds). *Charting by Exception Applications: Making It Work in Clinical Settings.* Albany, NY: Delmar Publishers, 1995;3–11.
10. Green B, Foote J, Gray M. Urologic management during acute care and rehabilitation of the spinal cord injured patient. *Phys Med Rehab* 1993.
11. Chancellor M, Killholma P. Urodynamic evaluation of patients following spinal cord injury. *Semin Urol* 1992;10:83–94.
12. Gittman L, Frankel H. The value of intermittent catheterization in the early management of traumatic paraplegia and tetraplegia. *Paraplegia* 1966;4:63–84.
13. Kuhlemeier KV, Lloyd LK, Stover SL. Urological neurology and urodynamics: long term follow up of renal function after spinal cord injury. *J Urol* 1985;134:510–513.
14. Thomas DG, Philip NH, McDermott TED, et al. The use of urodynamic studies to assess the effects of pharmacologic agents with particular reference to alpha-adrenergic blockade. *Paraplegia* 1984;22:162–167.
15. Zejdlick CM. Reestablishing bowel control. *Management of Spinal Cord Injury,* Belmont, CA: Wadsworth Inc., 1992;397–417.
16. Green D (ed). Deep vein thrombosis in spinal cord injury. *Chest* 1992;102[Suppl]:633s–663s.
17. Weingarden SI. Deep venous thrombosis in spinal cord injury. Overview of the problem. *Chest* 1992;102:636s–639s.
18. Green D, Lee MY, Lim AC, Chmiel JS, Vetter M, Pang T, et al. Prevention of thromboembolism after spinal cord injury using low-molecular weight heparin. *Ann Intern Med* 1990;113:571–574.
19. Hull RD, Pineo GF. Low-molecular-weight heparin for the treatment of venous thromboembolism. *Semin Respir Crit Care Med* 1996;17:65–70.

20. Jackson AB, Groomes TE. Incidence of respiratory complications following spinal cord injury. *Arch Phys Med Rehabil* 1994;75:270–275.
21. Mansel JK, Norman JR. Respiratory complications and management of spinal cord injures. *Chest* 1990;97:1446–1451.
22. Bach JR, Smith WH, Michaels J, et al. Airway secretion clearance by mechanical exsufflation for post-poliomyelitis ventilator assisted individuals. *Arch Phys Med Rehabil* 1993;74:170–177.
23. Glenn WIWL, Hogan JF, Loke JSO, Ciesielski TE, Phelps ML, Rowedder R. Ventilatory support by pacing of the conditioned diaphragm in quadriplegia. *N Engl J Med* 1984;310:1150–1155.
24. Schmidt-Nowara WW, Altman AR. Atelectasis and neuromuscular respiratory failure. *Chest* 1984;85:792–796.
25. Bach JR, Smith WH, Michaels J, et al. Airway secretion clearance by mechanical exsufflation for post-poliomyelitis ventilator assisted individuals. *Arch Phys Med Rehabil* 1993;74:170–177.
26. Saper C, Breeder C. The neurologic basis of fever. *N Engl J Med* 1994;330:1880–1886.
27. Schmidt K, Chan C. Thermoregulation and fever in normal persons and in those with spinal cord injuries. *Mayo Clin Proc* 1992;67:469–475.
28. Colachis SC, Otis SM. Occurrence of fever associated with thermoregulatory dysfunction after acute traumatic spinal cord injury. *Am J Phys Med Rehabil* 1995;72:114–119.
29. Whyte J, Robinson KM. Pharmacologic Management. In: Glenn MB, White J (eds). *The Practical Management of Spasticity in Children and Adults.* Philadelphia: Lea & Febiger, 1990:201–226.
30. Yablon SA, Sipski ML. Effect of transdermal clonidine on spasticity: a case series. *Am J Phys Med Rehabil* 1993;72:154–157.
31. Nance PW, Bugaresti J, Shellenberger K, et al. North American Tizanidine Study Group. Efficacy and safety of tizanidine in the treatment of spasticity in patients with spinal cord injury. *Neurology* 1994; 44[Suppl]:44–52.
32. Freehafer AA. Limb fractures in patients with spinal cord injury. *Arch Phys Med Rehabil* 1995;76:823–827.
33. Cochran TP, Bayley JC, Smith M. Lower extremity fractures in paraplegics: pattern treatment and functional results. *J Spinal Disord* 1988;1:219–223.
34. Barnett HJM, Botterell EH, Jousse AT, Wynne Jones M. Progressive myelopathy as a sequel to traumatic paraplegia. *Med Serv J Can* 1966;22:631–650.
35. Edgar R, Quail P. Progressive posttraumatic cystic and noncystic myelopathy. *Br J Neurosurg* 1994;8:7–22.
36. Yarkony GM, Sheffler LR, Smith J, Chen D, Rayne SZ. Early onset posttraumatic cystic myelopathy complicating spinal cord injury. *Arch Phy Med Rehabil* 1994;75:102–105.
37. Backe HA, Betz RR, Mesgarzadeh M, et al. Posttraumatic spinal cord cysts evaluated by magnetic resonance imaging. *Paraplegia* 1991;29:607–612.
38. Anton HA, Schweigel JF. Posttraumatic syringomyelia: the British Columbia experience. *Spine* 1986;11:865–868.
39. Barnett HJM, Foster JB, Hudgson P. *Syringomyelia.* Toronto: WB Saunders Company, 1973.
40. Rossier AB, Foo D, Shillito J, Dyro FM. Posttraumatic cervical syringomyelia—incidence, clinical presentation, electrophysiological studies, syrinx protein and results of conservative and operative treatment. *Brain* 1985;108:439–461.
41. Comarr AE, Vigue M. Sexual counseling among male and female patients with spinal cord and/or cauda equina injury. *Am J Phys Med* 1978;57:215–229.
42. Courtois FJ, Charvier KF, Leriche A, Raymond DP, Eysette M. Clinical approach to erectile dysfunction in spinal cord injured men. A review of clinical and experimental data. *Paraplegia* 1995; 33:628–635.
43. Green BG, Killorin EW, Foote J, Bennett JK, Sloan S. Complications of penile implants in spinal cord injured patients. *Topics Spinal Cord Injury Rehabil* 1995;1:44–52.
44. Lloyd LK, Brown J, Black K. Intracorporeal injections for neurogenic impotence: five year follow up. *J Urol* 1994;151:454A.
45. Padma-Nathan H, Helstrom JG, Kaiser FE, Labranski F, et al. Treatment of men with erectile dysfunction with transurethral alprostadil. *N Engl J Med* 1997;336:1–7.
46. Sipski ML, Rosen R, Alexander C. Physiologic studies of sexual responses in spinal injured females. Paper presented at the 33rd Annual Scientific Meeting of the International Medical Society of Paraplegia, Kobe, Japan, June 1994.
47. Fenollosa P, Pallares J, et al. Chronic pain in the spinal cord injured: statistical approach and pharmacological treatment. *Paraplegia* 1993;31:722–729.
48. Cioni B, Meglio M, et al. Spinal cord stimulation in the treatment of paraplegia pain. *J Neurosurg* 1995;82:35–39.
49. Siddall P, Gray M, Cousins MJ. Intrathecal morphine and clonidine in the management of spinal cord injury pain: a case report. *Pain* 1994;59:147–148.
50. Loubser P, Nafiz M. Effects of intrathecal baclofen on chronic spinal cord injury pain. *J Pain Symptom Manage* 1996;2:241–247.
51. Krause JS, Crewe NM. Prediction of long term survival of persons with spinal cord injury: an 11 year prospective study. *Rehabil Psychol* 1988;32:205–213.
52. Miller TW, Carmona JJ, Bishop-Trent E. Substance abuse in clinical issues in the spinal cord injured person. *SCI Psychosocial Proc* 1996; 9:14–47.
53. Caldwell L, Dattilo J, Kleiber D, Lee Y. Perceptions of therapeutic recreation among people with spinal cord injury. *Annu Ther Recreation* 1994–1995;V:13–26.
54. DeVivo M, Richards J. Community reintegration and quality of life following spinal cord injury. *Paraplegia* 1992;30:108–112.
55. Whaley HK. Psychological and sociological theories concerning adjustment to traumatic spinal cord injury: the implications for rehabilitation. *Paraplegia* 1992;30:317–326.

Surgery of Spinal Trauma,
edited by J.M. Cotler, J.M. Simpson, H.S. An, and C.P. Silveri.
Lippincott Williams & Wilkins, Philadelphia © 2000.

CHAPTER 7

Traumatic Injuries of the Adult Upper Cervical Spine

Christopher P. Silveri, Mark C. Nelson, Alexander Vaccaro, and Jerome M. Cotler

The cervical spine is unlike any other structure in the musculoskeleton. Its fluid, tacit mobility is vital to our appreciation of various sensations, balance, coordination, communication, and virtually all components of human existence. Implicit in the grandeur of its form and function is its ability to provide complex three-dimensional range of motion, while at the same time protecting the most delicate of life's tissues—the neural elements. Contributing to its unique design is the lack of homogeneity regarding its overall structure. This results in a construct of connecting parts all working in unison to provide painless, coordinated range of motion while providing stability and control, despite segmental structural differences. Cranial vertebral, atlantoaxial, and subaxial relationships are biomechanically and anatomically distinct, and therefore these structures respond to yield stresses in a characteristically unique fashion.

This chapter reviews the anatomic differences of the up-

per cervical spine, the classifications used to describe traumatic injury, and their radiographic features as well as treatment alternatives, surgical techniques, and potential problems. (Injuries to the subaxial spine are discussed in Chapter 8.) By consensus, the upper cervical spine consists of the occiput, the occipitocervical junction, and the atlantoaxial complex. With respect to traumatic injuries to the cervical spine, this subdivision accounts for the majority of fatal cervical spinal injuries, due to the respiratory dysfunction associated with high spinal cord injury. Most commonly, fractures of the axis with severe displacement account for the majority of these cases (1). High-speed motor vehicle accidents or falls from a height are causes of these traumatic injuries. Given the degree of force imparted to the cervical spine, these patients typically present with other musculoskeletal or visceral injuries that also contribute to the their high degree of mortality. The significant space available for the cord at this region, when associated with less energy imparted to the spine, provides the potential for survival, and in many cases, those patients with upper cervical spine injuries who do survive will typically do so with minimal or no neurologic impairment or subtle cranial nerve abnormalities. Despite the lack of significant neurologic loss, appreciation of these injuries and their characteristic radiographic find-

C. P. Silveri: Fair Oaks Orthopaedics Associates, Fairfax, Virginia 22033.

M. C. Nelson: Department of Orthopaedic Surgery, George Washington University, Washington, D.C. 20037.

J. M. Cotler: Department of Orthopaedic Surgery, Thomas Jefferson University Hospital, Philadelphia, Pennsylvania 19107.

ings will heighten the physician's awareness, and therefore prevent further iatrogenic injury by appropriate immobilization and definitive stabilization.

OCCIPITAL CONDYLE FRACTURES

One of the most elusive causes of posttraumatic neck pain is the occipital condyle fracture. First described in 1817 by Sir Charles Bell, fewer than 60 cases have been reported in the literature. Its rarity has resulted in a low index of suspicion by practitioners, and thus it has become known as the "forgotten condyle" (2,3). In fact, little has been written regarding its impact on morbidity and mortality due to its infrequent diagnosis. As with all upper cervical spine fractures, there exists a high rate of mortality when injuries occur in this area. Bucholz and Burkhead (4) in 1979 reviewed 100 cases of postmortem motor vehicle accidents and noted an 8% incidence of occipital condyle fractures in patients with cervical spine injuries. Furthermore, in Goldstein et al.'s (5) study, occipital condyle fractures resulted in fatalities in 44% of cases. In patients who survive these injuries, the incidence of these fractures is still unknown because so many often go undiagnosed secondary to vague complaints of neck pain. Only more recently, with the advent of computed tomography (CT) scan evaluation of such patients, have the more subtle fractures been detected. This is most evident in the recent literature; 9 of 55 patients (16.4%) reported by Bloom et al. (6) had occipital condyle fractures detected on CT scans with nondiagnostic plain cervical radiographs. Quite commonly, patients with these injuries appear with neck pain; however, they are dismissed after negative cervical spine films are obtained. Unexplained prevertebral

swelling, cervical pain, impairment of skull mobility, disproportionate torticollis, and at times cranial nerve symptomatology have all been noted as defining features associated with occipital condyle fractures (7,8). Several authors have noted the association of occipital condyle fractures with lower cranial nerve palsies that occur either immediately following the injury, after a period of loss of consciousness, or in a delayed fashion as described in a case report of late glossopharyngeal and vagus nerve paralysis following an apparent closed head injury (9–11). The cranial nerves that are frequently injured are those that are in the closest proximity to the occipital condyle, namely the 9th, 10th, and 11th cranial nerves, which exit the jugular foramen lateral to the condyle, as well as the 12th cranial nerve, which exits the hypoglossal canal at the base of the occipital condyle. Delayed nerve injuries, as in Urculo et al.'s (10) report, result from less trauma to the nerve, and the subsequent prognosis is much more favorable. In all cases, however, routine CT scan of the head in such patients must include the cranial-vertebral junction, and ideally should involve the sagittal as well as coronal reconstructions to best view the occipitocervical junction.

Injuries to the occipital condyles and their clinical manifestations are best understood when one appreciates the local bony ligamentous and neural anatomic structures (Fig. 1). The convex occipital condyles project downward and laterally to meet the upward and inward facing, concave, superior articulations of the atlas. This cradle allows for a significant degree of flexion and extension. Despite this freedom of motion, which allows for 50% of upper cervical spine flexion and extension, several ligamentous restraints exist that maintain the stability of the articulation. Most important is the su-

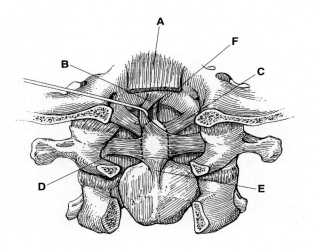

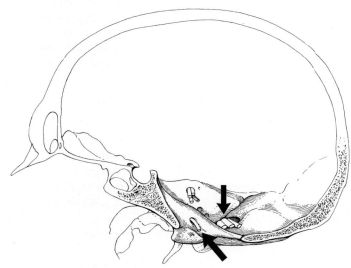

A

B

FIG. 1. A: Bony and ligamentous anatomy of the craniovertebral junction. *A*, tectorial membrane; *B*, rostral crus of the transverse atlantal ligament; *C*, alar ligaments; *D*, transverse atlantal ligament; *E*, caudal crus of the transverse atlantal ligament; *F*, apical ligament located anterior to the rostral crus from the tip of the dens to the clivus. **B:** Lateral view of the occipital condyle. Note the close proximity of the hypoglossal canal with exiting of the hypoglossal nerve *(large arrow)* and the jugular foramen with exiting 9th, 10th, and 11th cranial nerves *(small arrow)*.

perior extension of the posterior longitudinal ligament, known as the tectorial membrane, originating as a broad expansion from the posterior aspect of the bodies of C2 and C3, superiorly attaching to the anterior aspect of the occipital bone superior to the clivus. This membrane has a checkrein effect against distraction of the occipitocervical complex as well as anterior-posterior translation. Capsular attachments at the occipitoatlantal articulation as well as small contributions of the upper band or rostral crus of the transverse atlantal ligament gives some stability to the area; however, the second most important complex of ligaments are the alar ligaments, which are just anterior to the cruciate or transverse atlantal ligament and originate at the odontoid process and attach bilaterally to each occipital condyle. They have a significant effect on rotational stability as well as lateral flexion and extension of the occipitocervical junction. Injury at this

location typically produces an avulsion fracture of the condyle at their insertion. Finally, the apical ligament of the dens, which extends from the tip of the odontoid process to the clivus or anterior foramen magnum, acts to stabilize the odontoid to the anterior occiput.

Classification

Anderson and Montesano (12) described a classification system for occipital condyle fractures in terms of mechanism of injury, fracture morphology, and eventual treatment (Fig. 2). Type I injury occurs secondary to an axial load injury to the occipital condyle, resulting in comminution and impaction. Most importantly, the tectorial membrane and alar ligaments are weakened, but not ruptured, and overall anatomic stability is preserved. Type II injuries occur after blunt trauma to

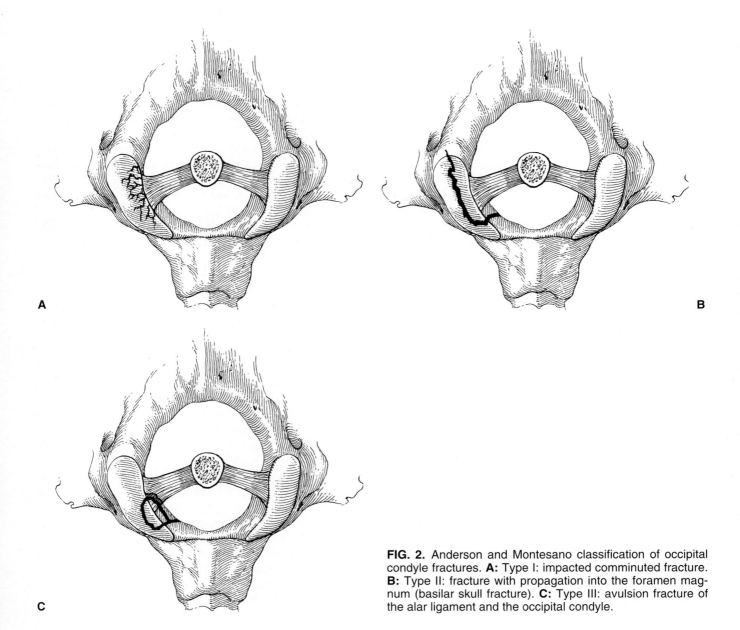

FIG. 2. Anderson and Montesano classification of occipital condyle fractures. **A:** Type I: impacted comminuted fracture. **B:** Type II: fracture with propagation into the foramen magnum (basilar skull fracture). **C:** Type III: avulsion fracture of the alar ligament and the occipital condyle.

the occiput with a fracture of the occipital condyle propagating into the foramen magnum. Such a basilar skull fracture may involve one or both occipital condyles and are typically stable due to an intact tectorial membrane and/or atlantal ligament. Finally, type III is an avulsion fracture involving the alar ligament. This is typically unilateral and is secondary to a mechanism of forced rotation with lateral bending. Because these injuries result from sheer or rotational forces, ligamentous injury is more likely and usually results in atlantooccipital dislocation, subluxation, or the potential for severe instability.

Treatment

The first principle in our overall treatment of these injuries is maintaining a high index of suspicion due to the rarity of their incidence and the subtlety in their presentation. Attention to detail will result in appropriate imaging with CT scan evaluation of the bony elements and magnetic resonance imaging (MRI) of the soft tissue structures, ligamentous integrity, and neural integrity. As mentioned earlier, axial load type I injuries rarely result in significant displacement and are typically stable and can be treated as such with a rigid cervical orthosis for 3 months' duration. In situations where patient compliance may be a problem, a halo orthosis can also be substituted and maintained for the same duration. A similar treatment protocol can be used for type II injuries, which occur without significant ligamentous instability. Type III injuries, however, which typically result in gross instability at the atlantooccipital junction, require halo immobilization in all cases for 3 months. At the conclusion of 3 months of immobilization for all three fracture types, dynamic radiographs in flexion and extension should be done to ensure that residual instability is not present; if it is, operative intervention may be necessary. In most instances, however, all three types of injuries can be treated successfully nonoperatively, except in cases with neurologic compromise or documented instability during immobilization. Surgical intervention is rarely noted in the literature. Only three reports have been identified, and their indications include brainstem compression, vertebral artery injury, or required stabilization due to concomitant suboccipital injuries (13, 14).

ATLANTOOCCIPITAL INJURIES

Known cases of traumatic instability of the occipitocervical junction are rare. As with many high-speed injuries, many patients with head and neck injuries are fatalities at the scene, and therefore are not counted in the absolute known incidence of this injury. Death occurs quickly secondary to the proximity of the respiratory center at this level of the spinal cord and lack of prompt respiratory assistance at the scene. Of the few patients who do survive transport to the hospital, the majority present as and remain pentaplegics. One of the largest studies in the literature was by Alker et al. (1), who examined, in postmortem, 312 traumatic fatalities and found 19 patients with atlantooccipital dislocations. A similar study by Bucholz and Burkhead (4) found nine cases of atlantooccipital injury in 112 victims examined. Both of these studies alluded to potential mechanisms of injury resulting in such disruption, although Alker et al. believed that a hyperflexion force was necessary to produce cranial cervical disruption. The Bucholz study associated the injury with more of a hyperextension and distraction force. In all likelihood, the vector of forces, either hyperflexion or hyperextension with or without rotational moments, could produce such an injury, and if severe enough, would likely result in either anterior or posterior translation of the occiput on the cervical spine. Regardless of the mechanism of injury, failure has to occur in both the ligamentous stabilization of the cranial cervical junction, namely the tectorial membrane, and the alar ligaments, along with injury through the atlantooccipital joint capsule and bony articulation.

A small subset of surviving victims of this injury may present with significant cranial cervical injury and preserved neurologic status. It is in this situation, as in many cervical spine injuries, that the nature and extent of the injuries may be overlooked if a high index of suspicion is not maintained. Bucholz and Burkhead (4) showed that atlantooccipital dislocation is more frequent in children than adults and postulated that this is due to their smaller and more horizontal occipitocervical articulations. The difficulty with evaluating children in the trauma setting as well as the reported incidence of a delayed or misdiagnosis in one-third of cases emphasize the need for attention to detail when evaluating these patients clinically and radiographically (15,16).

The clinical evaluation of such patients is similar to those who present with occipital condyle fractures and all upper cervical injuries. Survivors of atlantooccipital dislocations can present with a myriad of neurologic deficits with upper motor neuron long track findings, hemiparesis, and quadriplegia. Motor paralysis occurs due to compression of the medullary foraminal tracts as they descend from the cerebrum. If the compression is at the level of the pyramids proximal to their decussation, total spastic quadriplegia results. If compression occurs at the level of the decussation at an area where only upper extremity fibers are crossing, then only upper extremity paresis is noted.

An injury can be mistaken for a central cord syndrome if the foraminal tract injury occurs in the midline compressing primarily the upper extremity fibers as compared to the lower extremity ones. This was originally described by Bell and has been known as cruciate paralysis (15,16a,17). In the unconscious patient, much of the physical examination depends on the identification of these upper motor neuron findings, evaluation of their spontaneous respiratory function, and other indicators of central nervous system injury. Subtle cranial nerve abnormalities can be detected on examination as well as indirect cerebral injury secondary to trauma to the vascular structures in the neck. Significant distraction, flexion, extension, as well as lateral rotational trauma to the atlantooccipital articulation can cause significant neural complications; however, associated vascular complications are more subtle and difficult to appreciate. The vertebral artery's course moves cephalad through the foramina transversarium between C6 and C1. Superior to the arch of C1, the vertebral artery courses medially and superiorly through the atlantooccipital membrane and dura, and eventually into the skull through the foramen magnum.

Significant rotatory or angular displacements of any vertebral body can jeopardize the integrity of the vertebral artery, resulting in vasospasm, intimal tears, thromboses with eventual occlusion, dissection, or aneurysmal dilatation. Typically these injuries result in a neurologic deficit either acute in onset or delayed for minutes to several days and may appear with relatively normal appearing x-rays (18). In addition to vertebral artery injury, the internal carotid artery exists in proximity to the atlantooccipital complex, immediately anterolateral to the lateral mass of C1. Significant hyperrotation of this articulation potentially can impinge upon the artery and cause flow abnormalities (Fig. 3) (19). When vertebral artery injuries occur, they are associated with altered states of consciousness, nystagmus, swallowing difficulties, ataxia, diplopia, and dysarthria, all of which would not be normally associated with cervical spine trauma. An example of this is Wallenberg's syndrome, which presents as cerebellar ataxia, ipsilateral cranial nerve injuries involving

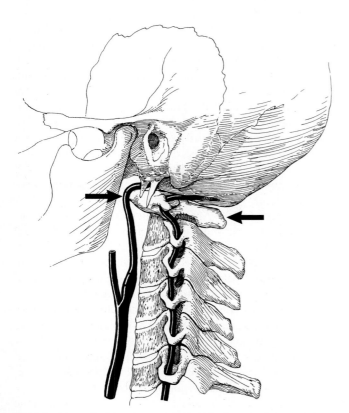

FIG. 3. Abnormalities in occipitocervical and atlantoaxial relationships can potentially impinge on the nearby vertebral and internal carotid arteries.

the 5th, 9th, 10th, and 11th nerves, contralateral loss of pain and temperature function, and an ipsilateral Horner's syndrome. The clinical picture is all the more confusing when initial evaluation in the emergency room is further complicated by direct head trauma, intraabdominal injury, hypotension, and cardiovascular collapse. Diagnosis can be made by arteriogram or magnetic resonance angiography. The latter technique, although limited in its ability to distinguish between spasm and other forms of occlusion, does identify vertebral artery injury and has been useful in prospective evaluation of cervical spine trauma patients, establishing an incidence of 19.7% in one study (20).

Radiographic Evaluation

The diagnosis of occipital cervical dislocation is difficult at times, clinically due to altered mental status, trauma, and compounding musculoskeletal or abdominal injuries. With improvements made in prehospital emergency care and transportation of these patients, survival has been more common with atlantooccipital injuries and the potential for iatrogenic neurologic deterioration needs to be minimized by careful evaluation of plain films. Although radiographic evaluation is not always clear, numerous parameters have been established to standardize the interpretation. Most of our clinical acumen relies on objective radiographic measurements based on initial roentgenographic surveys and secondary CT or MRI scans. As with any plain film evaluation of the cervical spine, one begins with the soft tissues. Significant trauma to the ligamentous or bony structures, in most cases, is evident by enlarged soft tissue plains with vertebral soft tissue dimensions anterior to the atlantoaxial complex measuring up to 7 mm (17,21). Any soft tissue swelling or retropharyngeal hematoma is a significant finding and warrants further evaluation of possible occipitocervical or upper cervical injury. Cadaver studies have shown retropharyngeal hematomas sufficiently large to cause obstruction of the airway, and laceration of the posterior pharynx with retropharyngeal gas has also been associated with these injuries secondary to a hyperextension mechanism of injury (4, 22).

The osseous structures of the atlantoaxial complex have also been well defined based on their radiographic appearance (Figs. 4 and 5). In normal subjects, a line constructed from the anterior aspect of the dens should be in line with the leading edge of the clivus or basion (23). In a similar fashion, the clivus baseline, also known as the basilar line of Wackenheim, is constructed from the posterior surface of the clivus extended inferiorly to be within the posterosuperior one-third of the dens or tangential to the posterior cortex of the odontoid process (24,25). This distance between the dens and the basion is typically between 8 and 10 mm in the adult and 4 and 5 mm in the child and is known as the basion-dental interval (15,26).

One of the most commonly referred to parameters for measuring atlantooccipital incongruity is known as the Pow-

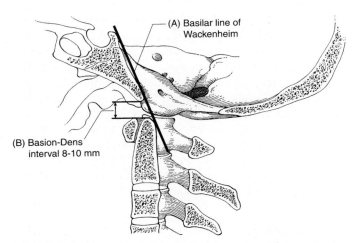

FIG. 4. Occipital cervical relationships. **A:** Basilar line of Wackenheim: a tangent from the clivus to the posterior superior aspect of the dens. **B:** Basion-dens interval, usually 8–10 mm in adults.

ers ratio (27). After studying the x-rays of 150 normal people, the ratio of the distance from the basion to the anterior aspect of the posterior arch of the atlas divided by the distance of the posterior aspect of the foramen magnum to the posterior aspect of the anterior arch of the atlas typically measured, on average, 0.77. When this ratio, BC/OA (see Fig. 5), was greater than 1, atlantooccipital incongruity existed representing a 2.6 standard deviation from the mean. The limitations to this ratio are that it was originally described for anterior translational abnormalities only, and its validity may be in question in the pediatric population as well as when significant distraction or posterior displacement is present (20).

Plain film evaluation has been well documented; however, it is not without question. Difficulties in visualization, radiographic techniques, and intraobserver and interobserver variability may diminish the reliability of any one technique

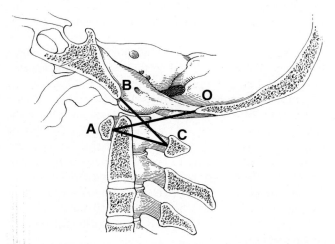

FIG. 5. Powers ratio—ratio of BC/OA measures on average 0.77. Anterior subluxation is noted with ratios greater than or equal to 1.

(28). Nevertheless, further evaluation with plain tomography or CT evaluation of the bony articulations is warranted in questionable cases. Furthermore, soft tissue ligamentous and neural tissues are well visualized on MRI, and its usefulness is also clear (29). Recent studies have also shown that both sagittal CT reconstructions and sagittal MRI allow for the diagnosis of infratentorial subarachnoid hemorrhage, which is associated with cranial cervical junction injuries, as well as late posttraumatic retropharyngeal pseudomeningocele, which can be delayed with neurologic deterioration from undiagnosed atlantooccipital dislocation (30,31).

Classification and Treatment

The classification system for occipital injuries is divided into three categories as proposed by Traynelis et al. (32). Type I injuries exhibit mainly longitudinal distraction without significant translation. Type II injuries are noted more commonly and result from anterior subluxation or translation of the atlantooccipital articulation. Type III injuries consist of posterior subluxation or dislocation.

The treatment of these injuries is based on the knowledge that severe ligamentous injury in the cervical and occipitocervical spine results in significant instability and poor healing potential. Diagnosis of the injury is followed immediately by provisional stabilization and reduction of alignment if need be to protect neurologic structures. Pure distraction injuries require immediate halo application and do not necessitate formal reduction. Occult occipitocervical dislocations associated with other cervical abnormalities are possible, and initial cervical traction in any instance should begin with careful, gradual application of up to 5 lb of traction with frequent radiographs to ensure that overdistraction does not occur through an injured segment. In type II and type III injuries where there is significant translation or dislocation, reduction should be achieved expediently, but with only light weights. It has been suggested that up to 1 to 2 kg of skeletal traction be used in graded increments (21,33). As with most ligamentous injuries of the cervical spine, nonoperative treatment rarely results in stability.

Persistent instability has been demonstrated as long as 5 months status postimmobilization in adults, and 3 to 4 months in pediatric cases of instability (17,34). Occipitocervical fusion has been the recommended treatment for these injuries. Various wiring techniques as well as plate fixation techniques have been used to secure rigid stabilization of the occipitocervical complex. Wertheim and Bohlman (35) have described the classic occipitocervical arthrodesis using iliac crest bone graft and wiring technique (Fig. 6). This posterior wiring technique is simple and provides excellent surface area for bone graft incorporation with minimal internal fixation while still providing excellent fixation; 16- or 18-gauge wires are placed through unicortical holes on each side of the inion with a trough made connecting these holes between the inner and outer tables of the occiput with a right-angle burr or towel clip. Bicortical holes may also be used, but with fur-

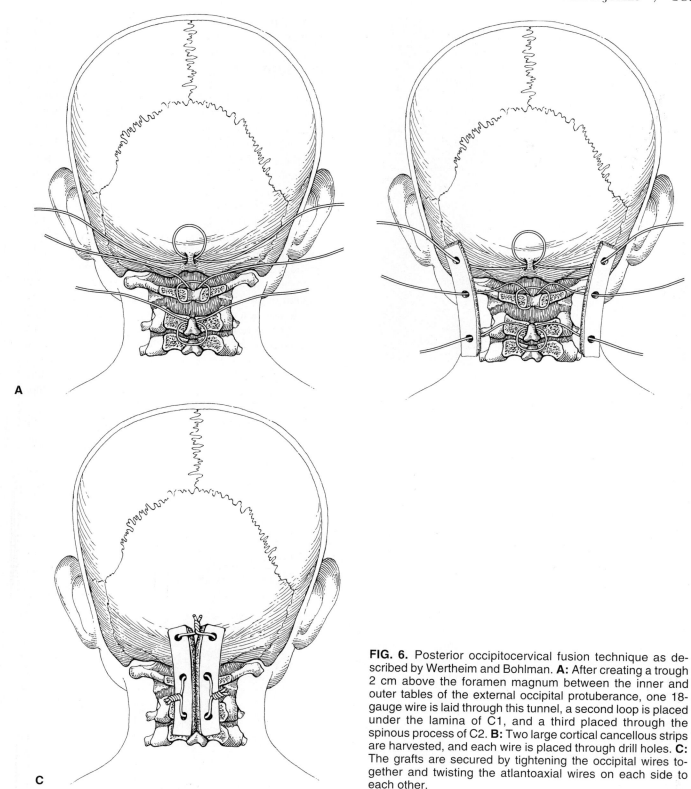

FIG. 6. Posterior occipitocervical fusion technique as described by Wertheim and Bohlman. **A:** After creating a trough 2 cm above the foramen magnum between the inner and outer tables of the external occipital protuberance, one 18-gauge wire is laid through this tunnel, a second loop is placed under the lamina of C1, and a third placed through the spinous process of C2. **B:** Two large cortical cancellous strips are harvested, and each wire is placed through drill holes. **C:** The grafts are secured by tightening the occipital wires together and twisting the atlantoaxial wires on each side to each other.

ther risks to epidural veins, large venous sinuses, and the dura. A second sublaminar wire is placed under the lamina of C1, and a third wire looped through or around the spinous process of C2 with all three pairs of wires opened up so each

arm is extended laterally to accept a cortical cancellous bone strut. Similar fixation has also been advocated using Luque rod constructs and onlay bone grafting (Fig. 7) (36). This technique also necessitates the presence of intact posterior

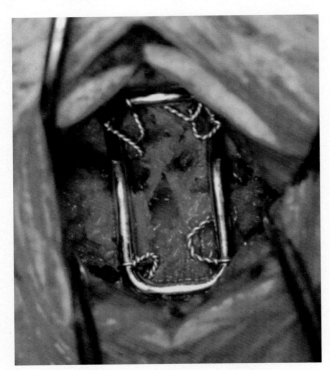

FIG. 7. Intraoperative photo of Luque ring and wire fixation of the craniocervical junction, occiput-C2. Uni- or bicortical holes are drilled in the occiput to accept wire passage and are accompanied by sublaminar wire fixation of C1 and C2.

above the superior nuchal line. The confluence of the transverse sinuses bilaterally and the sagittal sinus in the midline meets at a level just above or at the external occipital protuberance. Screw fixation, therefore, must remain below the superior nuchal line, and the thickness of the occiput increases from caudad to cephalad, with the thickest region being along the external occipital crest. Standard AO pelvic reconstruction plates can be used bilaterally in the occipitocervical junction and be contoured to allow for lateral mass and cervical C2 pedicle fixation and lateral to centrolateral fixation of the occiput bilaterally. Small or large reconstruction plates can be used depending on the size of the anatomy. Given the limited thickness of the inferior aspect of the occiput, 2.7-mm cortical screws may need to be used for the shorter screw lengths; however, 3.5-mm screws can be used if the distance between the inner and outer tables of the occiput is at least 10 mm. The surgeon's drill-tap technique needs to be done cautiously to avoid overpenetration and subsequent dural or venous sinus injury. Bone wax can be used with insertion of a screw to diminish the cerebrospinal fluid leakage or venous bleeding; however, if through-and-through sinus penetration occurs, fatal subdural hematoma may result. Experience with the anatomy and with occipitocervical plating will dictate whether a surgeon chooses unicortical versus bicortical screw fixation in a similar fashion as in the above wiring techniques.

Augmentation of occipitocervical fusion has been facili-

elements for purchase and fixation. There are, however, instances where laminar fractures or the need for intraoperative laminectomy would obviate the ability to use these wiring techniques. Rigid fixation has also been obtained using the Roy-Camille technique of occipitocervical fixation with contoured plates (Fig. 8) (37). In cases where laminar defects are present, this technique may be more advantageous, with strong purchase obtained in the occiput as with bilateral C2 pedicle screws and lower cervical lateral mass fixation (Fig. 9) (38).

Occipitocervical plate and screw instrumentation allows the physician to obtain rigid fixation in the occiput either with unicortical or bicortical screws. It is critical to understand the anatomy of the venous sinuses and neurologic structures within the occiput if bicortical screw fixation is attempted. Exposure of the occiput reveals bony landmarks that are useful markers for the underlying neurologic and vascular structures. After identification of the posterior rim of the foramen magnum, one must identify the inferior nuchal line and its parallel counterpart more cephalad—the superior nuchal line, which as prominent bony ridges serve as points of muscular attachment. Connecting these two in the midline is the external occipital crest, and the confluence of the superior nuchal line at this location forms the external occipital protuberance or inion. This is the most prominent aspect of the occipital bone during the surgical dissection.

Bicortical drill or screw placement must avoid the large transverse venous sinus, which is typically located at or

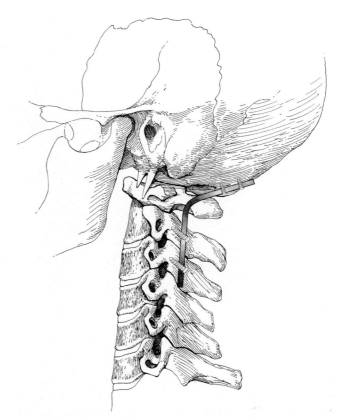

FIG. 8. Plate fixation of the occipitocervical junction.

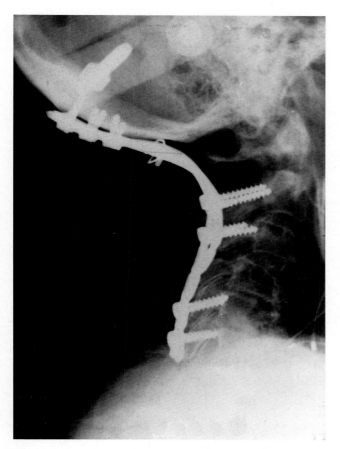

FIG. 9. Example of occipital cervical arthrodesis with plate fixation using bilateral C2 pedicle screws and lateral mass screws below.

tated by the use of cervical C2 pedicle or isthmus screw fixation. Exposure of the posterior elements of C2 as in the technique for transarticular screw fixation needs to involve subperiosteal dissection of the lamina and the medial aspect of the isthmus of C2 as it forms the lateral border of the spinal canal. Palpation of the isthmus or pedicle of C2 allows approximation of the screw direction and angulation, and evaluation of cortical penetration medially. Lateral mass fixation typically orients the screw in a superolateral direction; however, instrumentation of the C2 pedicle requires a medial deviation to avoid the vertebral artery, which is coursing from a medial to lateral direction as it enters the transverse foramina of C1. To avoid the lateral position of the vertebral artery at this location, the screw direction is initiated at a starting point in the superomedial quadrant of the C2 lateral mass and directed approximately 10 to 25 degrees medially and 15 to 25 degrees cranially (38,39). The medial direction is determined most accurately by intraoperative palpation of the medial border of the isthmus and appropriate alignment based on that structure. Drill-tap technique is used in the standard fashion; however, to diminish the risk of bony perforation and injury to arterial or venous structures, a 2-mm burr may be used to sound the C2 pedicle periodically check-

ing the cortical integrity of the medial and lateral walls. The posterior cortical entrance can then be tapped, and a 3.5-mm screw is inserted with sizes typically ranging from 14 to 18 mm in length. Preoperative CT scan evaluation is critical to determine the size of the C2 isthmus and whether or not it will accommodate a screw. Given the significant risk to vertebral artery and neural elements and the excellent purchase of the screw against the circumferential cortical margin of the pedicle, complete tapping of the screw path is not always warranted. Occipitocervical fusion with plate fixation can then be extended inferiorly as needed with lateral mass fixation in the subaxial spine as noted elsewhere in this text.

Occipitocervical fusion as the treatment of choice for these injuries has traditionally been extended to the level of C2 and beyond as needed for proper surface area for bone grafting and rigid fixation. Modifications of the posterior wiring technique have been made to allow for occipitocervical fusions to include only the ring of C1 with careful attention not to extend the dissection to the arch of C2. This has been used in treating children with occipitocervical dislocation; 18- or 20-gauge wire is used and passed through a trough made in the occiput and secured to sublaminar wires extending from the arch of C1 to stabilize iliac crest bone graft placement in this interval. Dissection is specifically avoided over the bony elements of C2 to prevent extension of the fusion, which commonly occurs in the pediatric population, and to maximize range of motion once healing has occurred (Fig. 10) (34,40).

ATLANTOAXIAL ROTATORY SUBLUXATION

Atlantoaxial rotatory subluxation and its related conditions have been termed in the literature atlantoaxial rotatory fixation, spontaneous hyperemic dislocation, rotation deformity, rotational subluxation, and unilateral atlantoaxial subluxation (41–43). Since its earliest review at the turn of the 20th century, its presence has continued to be an uncommon yet potential diagnosis of the adult and pediatric population (44).

Multiple etiologies have been associated with atlantoaxial rotatory subluxation including severe trauma, minor trauma, upper respiratory infections, tonsillitis, Down syndrome, tumor, ankylosing spondylitis, pharyngeal surgery, juvenile rheumatoid arthritis, rheumatoid arthritis, and tuberculosis (39,42,45–47). The majority of cases occur in children following retropharyngeal infections, commonly referred to as Grisel's syndrome (48). Lymphovenous connections of the retropharynx and upper cervical spine are thought to conduct pathogens that inflame, loosen, and disrupt the atlantoaxial joint (49). The resulting ligamentous laxity may allow subluxation to occur, and the inflamed synovial tissues may prevent spontaneous reduction (42). Bony abnormalities such as cervical anomalies, spondylosis, assimilation of the atlas to the occiput, basilar impression, odontoid abnormalities, and facet tropism are potential causes for a tilted or rotated torticollis (50). Clinical evaluation of a cervicothoracic scoliosis may also note an abnormality in head alignment.

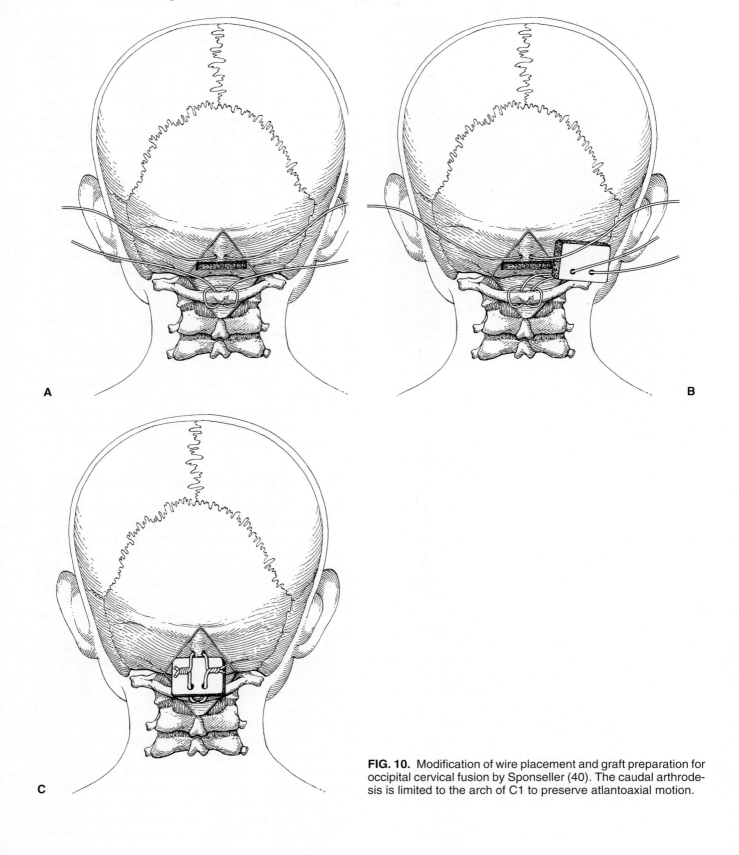

FIG. 10. Modification of wire placement and graft preparation for occipital cervical fusion by Sponseller (40). The caudal arthrodesis is limited to the arch of C1 to preserve atlantoaxial motion.

In many cases, however, atlantoaxial rotatory subluxation spontaneously corrects prior to seeking medical attention (51). It is incumbent on the physician, however, to correctly diagnose atlantoaxial rotatory subluxation as it can become recurrent or fixed with subsequent poor sequelae (42). Historically, atlantoaxial rotatory subluxation was associated with a delay in diagnosis. Its diagnosis can be often confused with torticollis or spasm (congenital muscular torticollis). A heightened degree of clinical suspicion and improved imaging techniques have shortened the time to diagnosis (52).

Classic physical findings should alert the clinician to the presence of atlantoaxial rotatory fixation. These include torticollis, cock robin position, ability to increase the rotation but not correct it, limited cervical extension, and facial flattening in long-standing cases (42). In contrast to congenital torticollis where the sternocleidomastoid on the side opposite the rotation is shortened, the ipsilateral sternocleidomastoid is observed to be in spasm as if attempting to correct the deformity (42). The so-called cock robin position is approximately 20 degrees of tilt to one side, 20 degrees of rotation to the opposite side, and slight flexion. This position has been likened to that of a robin listening for a worm (42,53). The anterior arch of the atlas and a step-off at C1-C2 may be palpable through an open mouth (52,54). Neurologic signs may or may not be present (42,52).

Atlantoaxial rotatory subluxation is primarily a ligamentous injury (52). Although commonly associated with local infection or inflammation with probable synovial capsular effusion, the true mechanical etiology for the irreducible nature of such subluxation is unknown. Fixed rotatory subluxation typically does not result in death and eventual postmortem examination. Injury, if present, is usually minor, disproportionate to the degree of deformity and pain that results. Past theories have suggested entrapped alar ligaments, or inflamed synovial fringes caught in the atlantoaxial articulation (17). Long-standing fixation can then lead to attenuation of supporting capsular and ligamentous structures, further dislocation, eventual contracture, and fibrosis of the local tissues, thereby preventing reduction.

The primary stabilizer against anterior subluxation of the atlas is the transverse ligament (55). When it is intact, the atlantodens interval (ADI) does not exceed 3 mm (56). Secondary stabilizers include the alar ligaments, facet joint capsules, the apical ligament, and accessory atlantoaxial ligaments (55). In the face of a force sufficient to disrupt the stout transverse ligament, the alar ligaments' ability to prevent anteroposterior (AP) translation has been questioned (55). Osseous congruity of the atlantoaxial articulation is shallow and more horizontal than the lower articular facets. This accounts for the added degree of rotation at this articulation. Approximately 50% of rotation in the cervical spine occurs here with only a few degrees of flexion/extension, lateral bend, or translation (57). Rotational stability is provided by the alar ligaments and facet joint capsules. The alar ligaments become taut at 45 degrees of rotation (47,58). Lateral flexion, however, relaxes the ipsilateral alar ligament and allows another 20 degrees of rotation (58). Bilateral facet dislocation occurs at 63 degrees of rotation (56). Approximately 64 degrees of rotation can occur before the space available to the cord is reduced to a centimeter (56). If anterior translation is present, the amount of rotation necessary to produce significant cord compression is significantly less. At 5 mm of anterior C1-C2 subluxation, rotatory dislocation occurs at only 45 degrees (42). The vertebral arteries are located in the transverse foramina of the atlantoaxial complex and are protected during normal range of motion. However, severe rotation can occlude, transect, or cause vasospasm in these arteries, resulting in cerebral ischemia and severe neurologic sequelae (59,60).

Classification

The classification of atlantoaxial rotatory fixation proposed by Fielding and Hawkins (42) is based on the functional anatomy of the C1-C2 articulation and is useful in prognosis and treatment algorithms (Fig. 11). It is a description based on the degree of atlantoaxial translation as well as concomitant rotation. Many cases of rotatory subluxation or fixation are known to occur within the range of normal physiologic rotation, and these cases make up type I. The ADI measurements remain less than 3 mm, which is consistent with an intact transverse ligament. This is the most common type, seen frequently in children. Such rotatory fixation without anterior displacement of the atlas is accompanied by the least amount of ligamentous/capsular injury.

Type II injuries are characterized by rotatory fixation with anterior displacement of the atlas 3 to 5 mm (ADI 3–5 mm). Disruption or injury to the transverse ligament allows for anterior displacement of the atlas with one lateral mass displaced anteriorly while the other remains located and acting as the pivot.

Type III fixation occurs with rotatory dislocation and anterior displacement of more than 5 mm (ADI >5 mm). Disruption of the transverse ligament and secondary ligamentous restraints (alar ligaments, lateral mass, and capsular ligaments) allows anterior displacement of the atlas with anterior displacement of both lateral masses. Severe compromise of the space available for the cord occurs with lateral radiographs revealing the accentuated atlantodens interval.

The last group, or type IV, is extremely rare and involves rotatory fixation with posterior displacement of the atlas. Deficient or absent dens allows posterior displacement of both lateral masses. Subsequent reports have documented traumatic type IV injuries in previously normal individuals (52). Severe hyperextension with rotation secondary to high-velocity trauma or motor vehicle accident can result in this posterior dislocation (61).

Radiologic Features

The key to diagnosis is demonstration of a fixed subluxation of the atlantoaxial joint. Useful imaging modalities include

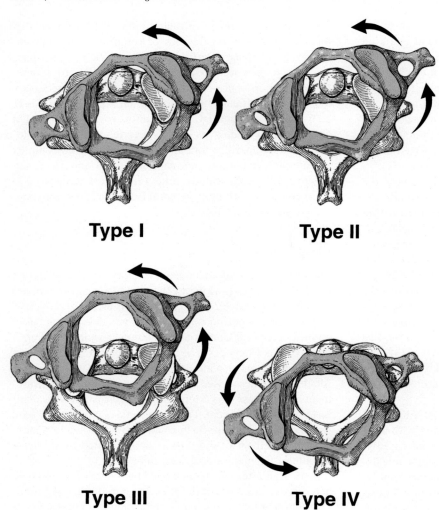

Type I

Type II

Type III

Type IV

FIG. 11. Classification of rotatory fixation as proposed by Fielding and Hawkins. **A:** Type I: rotatory fixation with no displacement with the odontoid acting as a pivot. **B:** Type II: rotatory fixation with 3 to 5 mm of anterior displacement pivoting about one lateral articular process. **C:** Type III: rotatory fixation with greater than 5 mm anterior displacement. **D:** Type IV: rotatory fixation with posterior displacement.

plain roentgenograms, cineroentgenography, tomography, CT, and MRI.

Difficulty in interpretation occurs with routine roentgenograms due to the tilt of the patient's head obscuring the AP view and causing poor positioning of the lateral view. The open-mouth anterior-posterior odontoid projection is the most useful view. Rotation of the atlas leaves one lateral mass anterior and superior to the opposite lateral mass. The anterior lateral mass appears wider, more superior and closer to the midline. The posterior lateral mass appears comparatively narrow and lateral. The "wink sign" occurs when posterior rotation of one C1 lateral mass obscures its radiographic joint space while that of the contralateral side remains well demonstrated (Fig. 12) (39,52). The joint space is not seen due to overlap with the ipsilateral superior articular facet of C2. Comparison open-mouth AP views at neutral and 15 degrees of left and right rotation may aid in diagnosis, if the atlantoaxial relationship does not change with rotation (53). However, these views are difficult to obtain and interpret and are inferior to CT and MRI. The AP view also demonstrates the position of the chin rotated in the same direction as the C1 rotatory fixation. Because the occiput and atlas move in unison, anterior rotatory fixation of a unilateral lateral mass causes the bifid spinous process of C2 to rotationally displace opposite to the rotational axis of C1 and lie on the same side of the midline as the chin. The midline deviation of the C2 spinous process occurs only when C1-C2 rotation exceeds 50% of normal. The lateral view is important for soft tissue evaluation, presence of edema, mass effect, assimilation of the arch of C1 to the occiput, and anterior position of a lateral mass of C1 with respect to the odontoid. Measurement of the ADI is crucial but may be difficult if one lateral mass is rotated far anterior and is also frequently better assessed on CT or MRI sections.

Cineroentgenography was the diagnostic procedure of choice prior to the advent of CT. Its use is currently limited because of its high radiation dose, the difficulty in obtaining an adequate exam, and the ready availability of CT (58). Such studies were able to show that unlike their normal independent motion, motion studies in patients with rotatory fixation demonstrate movement of C1 and C2 in unison.

Along the same lines, anteroposterior tomograms are capable of clearly demonstrating the lateral masses of the atlas

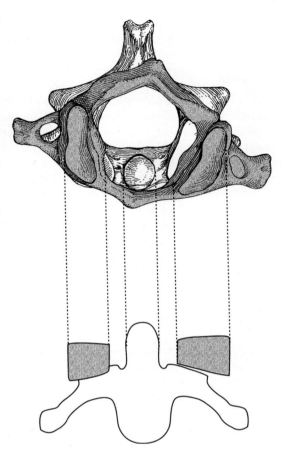

FIG. 12. Schematic representation of the "wink sign." Atlantoaxial fixation produces a characteristic feature on the AP odontoid view radiograph. The lateral mass rotating anteriorly will appear closer to the midline, larger and more cephalad as compared to the contralateral side. Severe cases cause the smaller more posterior lateral mass to fall below the anterior C2 superior articular process, obscuring the atlantoaxial articulation, known as the wink sign.

positioned in different planes (52). CT, however, has largely replaced standard tomography.

The advent of CT represents a quantum leap in the diagnosis of atlantoaxial rotatory subluxation (62). Dynamic CT scans are now the diagnostic gold standard (46,58). In this technique, 3-mm axial cuts are made from the occiput to C2 parallel to the ring of C1 (Fig. 13). Scanning is repeated with the head maximally rotated to each side. A positive scan shows no motion or limited asymmetrical motion between the atlas and axis (46). Three-dimensional (3D) reconstructions of CT scans are now available and can dramatically demonstrate atlantoaxial rotatory subluxation. Their value in the management of atlantoaxial rotatory subluxations, however, remains to be demonstrated. Similarly to CT, MRI has the ability to show sequential axial cuts. Its superior resolution of soft tissues is ideal for evaluating possible cord compression and may be advantageous in delineating ligamentous injuries and epidural or posterior pharyngeal collections.

Treatment

The goal of treatment is restoration of cervical motion and the prevention of deformity, recurrence, or neurologic compromise. As atlantoaxial rotatory subluxations are comparatively rare, well-controlled treatment protocols are not available. Prudence dictates that treatment plans be customized to each individual case with an eye on the complicating factors of each case.

Factors that influence treatment include duration of torticollis, amount of rotation, ligamentous integrity, and neurologic status (42,46,52). Fielding and Hawkins (42) also noted an average delay in diagnosis of 11.6 months, which contributes added difficulty in reduction. The majority of cases involve Fielding types I and II of recent onset without significant trauma and without neurologic deficit. Treatment alternatives, success of reduction, and time to reduction are related to the duration of torticollis before treatment (46):

Torticollis for 1 week or less: Many cases resolve spontaneously with a soft collar and bed rest for 1 week (58,63). Close follow-up is necessary. If spontaneous reduction does not occur hospitalization and cervical traction are indicated (46).

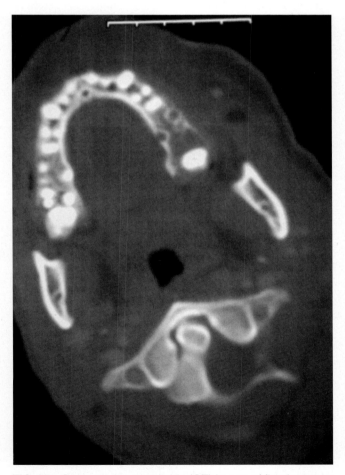

FIG. 13. Computed tomographic (CT) image of fixed rotatory subluxation of the atlantoaxial complex.

Torticollis for more than 1 week and less than 1 month: Hospitalization with cervical traction is indicated for torticollis present for more than 1 week (46). Traction may be either chin halter or skeletal traction dependent on the circumstances (58). Chin halter traction in children should begin at 1.35 to 2.3 kg (3–5 lb) depending on size. Oral analgesics and muscle relaxant sedatives may be administered as needed. Traction may be discontinued when active lateral rotation to each side is equal. Postreduction immobilization for 6 weeks is recommended in a cervical collar (58).

Torticollis for more than 1 month: Skeletal traction is indicated when rotatory subluxation has been present for more than 1 month or remains resistant to halter traction (42, 46). Traction weights in children should begin at approximately 3.2 kg and should be increased every 3 to 5 days by increments of 0.5 to 0.9 kg to a maximum of 6.8 kg (42). Initial weights in adults may be up to 6.8 kg with a maximum of 9.1 kg (42). Traction may be attempted for as long as 3 weeks and may not achieve complete reduction (42, 46). If the deformity is corrected, 3 months of immobilization should be completed after 2 to 3 weeks of continued traction. Minerva jacket or halo brace are typical forms of immobilization (39,42). However, as recurrence of deformity is common after long-standing subluxations and reduction is often incomplete despite prolonged traction, consideration should be given to fusion (46).

Most authors have advocated traction as the appropriate means to reduction, and have accepted some residual displacement rather than attempt direct manipulations (42). Others have questioned the efficacy of traction alone and have proposed alternative closed and open reduction techniques (52,64). Presence of the deformity for more than 1 month offers a poor prognosis for response to conservative treatment, and operative intervention is likely (42,58).

Surgical Techniques

Indications for surgery include atlantoaxial instability, recurrence of deformity after reduction, incomplete reduction, transverse ligament insufficiency, anterior displacement of the atlas, neurologic deficit, and deformity present for more than 3 months (42,52,58,63). Preoperative traction should be instituted to achieve as much reduction as possible (42). Most authors recommend atlantoaxial arthrodesis using various modified techniques of Gallie or Brooks (63,65). These techniques are discussed elsewhere in this chapter. However, some aspects of atlantoaxial arthrodesis unique to atlantoaxial rotatory subluxation warrant consideration.

Compensatory counter–occipital-atlantal subluxation may be present (66,67). Some authors have recommended in situ occiput-C2 fusion, reasoning that this condition represents an unstable occipital-atlantal joint (67). Others have opted to preserve occipital-atlantal motion by performing only atlantoaxial fusion and managing the occipital-atlantal subluxation with a halo vest postoperatively (66). Caution should

be exercised during reduction attempts as traction to reduce the atlantoaxial deformity may increase the occipital-atlantal subluxation, with potentially disastrous sequelae (67).

Few cases of posterior displacement or Fielding type IV injuries have been reported in the literature (68). Moskovich et al. (69) recommended a three-stage reduction maneuver with skeletal traction, and was summarized by Vaccaro and Cotler (39). Stage I consists of longitudinal skeletal traction with slight flexion needed to maintain the anterior arch of C1 in proximity to the posterior dens. This will prevent cord injury, maximize the space available for the cord, and facilitate reduction when adequate distraction is achieved. Weights should not exceed 6.75 kg in the adult. Stage II consists of a realignment of the traction vector to allow for extension once reduction is achieved. This keeps the posterior arch of C1 in close proximity of the anterior dens. Traction is then diminished gradually to 2.25 kg and the contemplation of stage III or spinal fusion begins.

Complications

Complications are uncommon during controlled treatment of these injuries. Neurologic compromise is rare in atlantoaxial fixation. Nevertheless, significant neurologic impairment and even death can occur (42). The risk of neurologic compromise is increased with Fielding types III and IV (42). Also, authors who advocate closed reduction under general or local anesthesia with direct lateral mass palpation through the oral cavity risk significant neurologic injury (52).

Approximately 50% of normal cervical rotation occurs at the atlantoaxial joint, and some loss of rotation is expected after C1-C2 arthrodesis. Interestingly, the rotation lost is less than predicted, and is usually functionally insignificant (42). Also, long-standing torticollis may cause facial asymmetry (plagiocephaly) in younger patients. Fortunately, the majority of these cases resolve following reduction and fusion (42). Of course, in cases of untreated or unreduced atlantoaxial rotatory subluxation, fixation results. It has been hypothesized that this fixation occurs initially with interposition of capsular and inflamed synovial tissue and articular damage with associated fractures, and later worsens with capsular contracture (42,58). In most cases, prompt reduction with traction avoids this unfortunate sequela. Appropriate treatment in cases of long-standing fixation unreducible by traction remains controversial. Successful outcomes have been reported with both in situ arthrodesis following traction and open reduction (42,64). Interestingly, recent reports of open reduction techniques have documented potential causes of fixation including abundant fibrous tissue, an entrapped segment of ruptured transverse ligament, and cross-union of the atlas and axis (64).

ATLAS FRACTURES

Atlas fractures account for approximately 4.7% to 6.6% of all acute cervical spine fractures (70,71). Approximately

50% of atlas fractures are associated with other cervical spine fractures (70,72). Most frequently associated are concomitant axis or odontoid fractures (71,73,74). Fracture of the posterior arch is the most common pattern and has the highest incidence of associated cervical injuries. Many atlas fractures are complicated by severe craniofacial trauma, which produces the typical hyperextension/axial load mechanism of injury.

The vast majority of atlas fractures occur by indirect violence. The atlas is compressed between the occipital condyles and the lateral masses of the axis. This axial compression may be combined with lateral bending, rotation, flexion, and extension to produce a variety of fracture patterns. Direct violence has been rarely documented as an etiology (71). Motor vehicle accidents and falls are the most common injuries, with diving accidents, hang gliding, waterskiing accidents, equestrian accidents, assault, and skateboarding accidents also being reported (70,74).

Fractures of the atlas, when complicated by other atlantoaxial injuries, are commonly paired as atlas-odontoid type II fractures (approximately 40%), followed by atlas-odontoid type III fractures (approximately 20%), and atlas-hangman's fractures (approximately 10%) (70,72,74). Other miscellaneous atlantoaxial fracture combinations and noncontiguous atlas-cervical spine fractures occur less commonly.

Fractures of the atlas are commonly associated with disruption of the transverse ligament with resultant instability in the AP plane. Disruption of the transverse ligament can occur by bony avulsion at its margins or by midsubstance tears (Fig. 14) (75). Osseous avulsions may complicate as many as 35% of atlas fractures (72). Obvious bony injury may distract the practitioner from an occult instability pattern if further diagnostic imaging techniques are not employed. A propensity for midsubstance tears has been reported by Fielding et al. (55), comprising 75% of cases in his cadaver study. However, most reviews indicate that injury occurs at

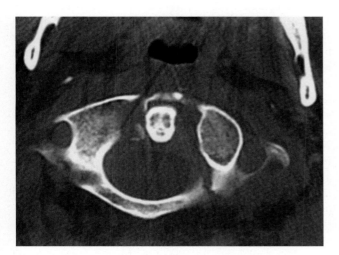

FIG. 14. CT image of an atlas fracture with associated transverse ligament avulsion fracture.

the ligamentous insertion into the medial tubercle of the atlas (72,76). Because the transverse ligament is actually a cruciform complex with extension cephalad to the occiput and caudad to the body of the dens, rupture of one arm of the transverse ligament potentially leaves several attachments secure. All of the above biomechanical studies with reproducing transverse ligament injury in the cadaver model showed maintenance of alar and capsular ligaments as well as the tectorial membrane (55,72,75,76). Each structure offers some degree of protection against frank atlantoaxial instability.

Neurologic deficits are unusual following atlantal fractures (71), and thought to be secondary to the capacious ring of the atlas and the propensity for centripetal displacement of its fragments. Neurologic deficits are most common in those atlas fractures with associated cervical injuries, especially odontoid fractures (70,71,74). Both complete and incomplete cord lesions have been reported (70,71). Neurologic injury is also related to the degree of energy imparted to the ring of C1 noted by the degree of lateral mass offset (52,55).

The diagnosis of atlas fractures can be difficult, and is frequently delayed. The primary symptoms are pain, muscle spasm, neck stiffness, suboccipital pain, limited range of motion, headaches, and a sense of instability (71,74,77). Neurologic manifestations are infrequent, and when present, may be obscured by concomitant head injuries. Neurologic symptoms may include cranial nerve palsies of cranial nerves VI, IX, X, XI, and XII due to their close proximity to the expanding displaced lateral masses. Scalp dysesthesias also may occur and are secondary to involvement of the greater occipital nerve as it passes through the atlantoaxial membrane. Late neurologic dysfunction has been noted to occur from cranial settling and basilar invagination (78). Patients with significant retropharyngeal swelling may also complain of difficulty swallowing.

Classification and Mechanism of Injury

Several classification schemes have been proposed for atlas fractures. Some have attempted to define groupings based on prognosis, and others on mechanism of injury. Ultimately, the similar treatment protocols and prognosis of all fracture types limit their overall utility (39). Figure 15 demonstrates the many possible fracture patterns.

Atlas fractures are associated with high-energy injuries and typically require an axial load vector. Concomitant or secondary bending forces in flexion, extension, or lateral deviation result in a variety of fracture patterns. Pure axial load is associated with the true burst fracture of C1 known as a Jefferson fracture (79). The lateral masses of C1 are wedge-shaped with the apex directed medially between the occiput above and the lateral mass of the axis below. Axial load causes an outward-directed force on the C1 lateral mass and centrifugal displacement. Fractures occur at the weakest area, typically in the thin anterior or posterior arches. It has been noted, however, that in Jefferson's original review none

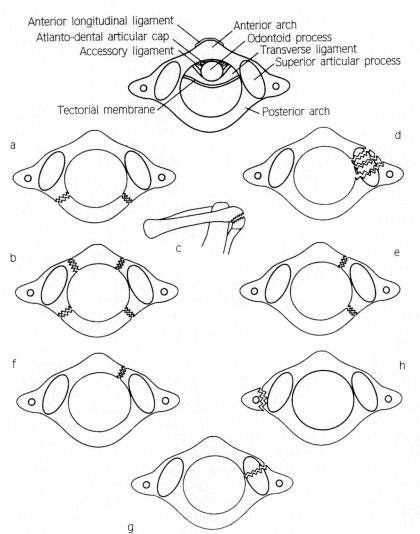

FIG. 15. Classification of several patterns of atlas fractures. **A:** Bilateral posterior arch injury. **B:** Four-part anterior and posterior arch fracture or burst fracture. **C:** Hyperextension avulsion fracture at the anterior arch. **D:** Comminuted lateral mass fracture. **E:** Ipsilateral anterior and posterior arch fractures with "floaty" lateral mass. **F:** Unilateral arch fracture. **G:** Lateral mass fracture. **H:** Transverse process fracture. (From ref. 192, with permission.)

of the four cases presented had the four-part fracture commonly associated with his name (80). They did, however, exhibit the characteristic lateral deviation of the C1 masses. When hyperextension forces are present, the posterior arch of C1 is compressed above by the occiput and below by the posterior elements of C2 producing posterior arch fractures (81). The addition of anterior or posterior shear forces or flexion/extension may result in associated fractures of the odontoid.

Landelis and Van Peteghem (71) have proposed a three-type classification. A type I fracture is confined to either the posterior or anterior arch and does not cross the equator of the atlas. Type II fractures involve both arches and cross the equator of the atlas. This type includes classic four-part Jefferson fractures. Type III fractures are primarily of the lateral mass with possible extension into one arch only. The authors found their classification useful in predicting neurologic deficit and long-term morbidity. The development of late symptoms was correlated best with the type II injury.

Levine and Edwards (82) have defined three types based on their mechanism of injury and position of the head at the time of injury. The first subgroup, type I, involves posterior arch fractures incurred by axial loading and hyperextension. Typically, these are bilateral breaks in the posterior ring. In type II injuries, lateral mass fracture occurs with fracture lines exhibited anterior and posterior to the involved lateral mass, which, in essence, isolates or disconnects one lateral mass. If further hyperextension occurs, then associated posterior arch fracture can be seen. Type III fractures consist of a burst fracture or Jefferson fracture resulting from axial compression.

Segal et al. (72) have recommended that the "comminuted fracture" be recognized as a distinct category with both diagnostic and prognostic importance. They define the comminuted fracture as a disruption of the ring both anterior and posterior to the lateral mass with an associated osteoperiosteal avulsion of the transverse ligament from the ipsilateral lateral mass. They propose that this pattern occurs when the head is deviated to the side of the fracture at the moment of impact.

As with any hyperextension injury, sudden traction on the anterior longitudinal ligament and supporting structures can result in avulsion of the anterior ring of the atlas. Stewart et al. (83) have described a horizontal fracture of the anterior atlantal arch, resulting from this proposed mechanism.

Radiologic Features

Quality lateral and AP open-mouth odontoid roentgenograms are necessary in the initial evaluation of suspected atlas fractures. The lateral projection allows evaluation of the posterior arch, ADI, and retropharyngeal swelling. A true lateral, however, superimposes left and right posterior arches, and a unilateral fracture may be obscured. Centering the tube over C3 results in a slightly oblique projection that demonstrates both left and right arches individually (77). The retropharyngeal soft tissue shadow seen in the lateral projection should be evaluated for swelling.

Elevation of soft tissue planes greater than 10 mm suggests an anterior arch, fracture, transverse ligament disruption, or odontoid fracture. Isolated posterior arch fractures have a normal, 5 mm or less, shadow (82).

Lateral mass displacement (LMD) as measured on the AP odontoid view is associated with atlas fractures. Normally, the lateral borders of the atlas and axis form a straight vertical line on the AP odontoid view. Total bilateral LMD greater than 6.9 mm suggests a tear of the transverse ligament, while LMD of less than 5.7 mm suggests that it is intact (84). Spence et al.'s (84) results were based on cadaveric studies and have been noted as a critical measurement in evaluating the odontoid view projection. Heller et al. (85), in 1993, noted that magnification of radiographs may exaggerate this stepoff. Lateral mass displacement of both sides greater than 8.1 mm is consistent with instability and loss of transverse ligament integrity. Bilateral lateral mass displacement is pathognomonic for Jefferson-type fractures (74). Unilateral displacement suggests a lateral mass fracture. The AP odontoid view should also be inspected for avulsion fragments of the transverse ligament. The ADI on flexion radiographs has proven to be the best indicator of a functional transverse ligament (86). ADIs greater than 3 mm in adults (4.5 mm in children) demonstrate functional incompetence of the transverse ligament (86) Two-plane tomography has proven to be a sensitive test for both anterior and posterior arch fractures (82). Lateral tomograms demonstrate posterior arch involvement, and AP tomograms are best for anterior arch evaluation.

Computed tomography is the radiographic study of choice for atlas fractures because of its ready availability, improved techniques, and imaging in the transverse plane (70). CT scanning provides excellent evaluation of both anterior and posterior arches, lateral masses, and bony avulsions of the transverse ligament. Nevertheless, a surprising number of atlas fractures missed by CT evaluation have been reported (82). Precise alignment of the gantry in the plane of the first cervical vertebra and a high-resolution scanner are require-

ments for obtaining an adequate study (81). Although inferior to CT imaging of bony structures, MRI provides incomparable resolution of the soft tissues about the atlas. It is ideal for evaluation of neural impingement and transverse ligament integrity (87).

Treatment

The treatment of atlas fractures is controversial. Most authors agree that the majority of atlas fractures are best treated nonoperatively (39,70,74,82). Atlas fractures complicated by other cervical spine injuries are usually best treated according to protocols for the associated fracture. Controversy exists surrounding the treatment of unstable injuries.

The majority of isolated C1 fractures without neurologic compromise are best managed nonoperatively (39,70,71,82). Those with LMD of less than 6.9 mm may be treated in less rigid cervical supports such as a Philadelphia collar or sternal occipital mandibular immobilization (SOMI) brace, or the more rigid halo brace, for a period of 8 to 12 weeks. Fractures with LMD greater than 6.9 mm ought to be managed with the more rigid halo brace for a period of 10 to 14 weeks. Interval clinical and radiographic evaluation is necessary to evaluate patient compliance and fracture union, and to tailor treatment duration. Physician-supervised flexion and extension studies should be performed at the completion of immobilization (70). Residual C1-2 instability requires late atlantoaxial fusion, or occipitocervical arthrodesis if the posterior arch of C1 is deficient.

Combined C1-2 fractures are generally best managed according to protocols for the associated fracture. Combination C1-odontoid type III, C1-hangman's, and other miscellaneous C1-2 fractures are successfully treated with halo immobilization for 8 to 14 weeks. The treatment of combination C1-odontoid type II fractures is determined by the amount of dens displacement. Those with dens displacement less than 5 to 6 mm can be managed in a halo brace. Those with dens displacement of greater than 5 to 6 mm have a high incidence of nonunion and should be considered for early surgical stabilization. Parameters established for age, degree, and direction of displacement and loss of reduction become critical in determining the indication for surgery based on the character of the odontoid fracture. The role of traction in atlas fractures is controversial. Successful reduction of fragments has been documented both clinically and in the laboratory (86). Reduction is likely due to the stabilizing effect of the major occipitocervical ligaments present, which when under traction limit the degree of fragment displacement. Maintenance of reduction, however, may require 6 to 8 weeks of immobilization, with traction weights of 20 to 25 lb often necessary (82). Patients who initially reduced and who are then placed in a halo vest may lose reduction (82). Furthermore, no long-term studies have demonstrated improved outcome following traction, and prolonged immobilization is fraught with its own complications. Halo vests alone are inadequate to produce the traction necessary for reduction and may exert compressive forces in some activities. Several authors have noted difficulty with adequate reduction of these fractures despite prolonged traction (71,82,88).

Operative indications for atlas fractures include neural impingement, combination C1-odontoid fractures with dens displacement greater than 5 to 6 mm, C1-2 instability despite adequate time of immobilization, and possibly Jefferson fractures with LMD greater than 6.9 mm when combined with a type II odontoid fracture (70,74).

The majority of operative atlas fractures involve instability of the atlantoaxial joint either secondary to a displaced odontoid fragment or late failure of transverse ligament healing. While C1-2 arthrodesis would seem the appropriate surgical intervention for atlantoaxial instability, this may be complicated in the presence of an atlas fracture with a floating posterior arch. Stability of the posterior arch must be considered prior to surgery. Lateral mass fractures and unilateral posterior arch fractures may retain sufficient arch integrity for successful arthrodesis (70). Bilateral posterior arch fractures preclude primary C1-2 arthrodesis, but may be approached with occiput-C2 arthrodesis, or delayed C1-2 arthrodesis following healing of the C1 arch fracture (89,90). The relative complications of each treatment should be weighed and tailored to the individual patient. Primary occipitocervical arthrodesis had been recommended by those who believed loss of this articulation would produce little clinical detriment (74). However, occiput-C2 fusion may result in as much as 80% to 90% loss of upper cervical rotation versus 20% to 50% in C1-2 fusions. McGuire and Harkey (80) noted two case reports in which unstable atlas fractures were treated successfully by direct transarticular screw fixation. Immediate rigid fixation of the lateral masses allows for stable atlantoaxial fusion, healing of the atlas fracture, and avoidance of halo immobilization. Given the past experience of significant success afforded by closed treatment of these injuries, potential residual instability can be addressed after failed immobilization.

Persistent widening of the lateral masses, however, may lead to incongruities of the occipitocervical and atlantoaxial articulation and contribute to later complication. For this reason, treatment of the unstable injury remains complex and controversial. Regardless of treatment, many patients with atlas fractures report long-term symptoms of scalp dysesthesia, neck pain, neck stiffness, and limited range of motion. Segal et al. (81) noted two-thirds of patients with good functional outcomes still complained of restricted range of motion, and in Levine and Edwards' (72) review 88% of patients had neck pain. The incidence of these complications is higher in combined C1-2 fractures (71). Fracture through the lateral masses may also predispose to long-term pain symptoms (91).

Nonunion of atlas fractures can occur and may or may not be symptomatic (77). Nonunion has been correlated with both fracture pattern and subjective functional outcome (72). The comminuted fracture pattern as described by Segal et al. has a propensity for nonunion. Rigid immobilization for an adequate period of time is recommended to avoid this com-

plication. Direct operative fixation of atlas nonunions has been reported, but its indications remain limited (92).

Basilar invagination has been reported as a late sequela of widely displaced Jefferson fractures. Day et al. (78) have reported on a 67-year-old man with a 2-year history of increasing myelopathy who had incurred a widely displaced Jefferson fracture at the age of 21. Radiographic evaluation revealed that the ring of C1 was so widely displaced as to allow the occipital condyles to articulate with C2 with subsequent tenting of the cervicomedullary junction over the dens. Kahanovitz et al. (93) have also reported entrapment of a posterior arch fragment within the foramen magnum following an initially undiagnosed and untreated fracture of the atlas.

FRACTURES OF THE ODONTOID

Fractures of the odontoid have long been both interesting and complex fractures with which to deal. The nature of the morphology of the dens with respect to the body of C2 is an anomaly that has become the characteristic feature of the upper cervical spine, and, along with its counterpart, the atlas, is distinct with respect to its shape, lack of intervening disc, anterior synovial articulation, and response to patterns of injury. The transition from the tip of the odontoid to a more normal-appearing base of the atlas mirrors it role as the liaison between the complex articulations in the upper cervical spine and the more consistent subaxial biomechanics. Because of its features, the overall assessment of odontoid injuries, their classification, their response to injury, and their treatment have been subject to initial frustration with high nonunion rates, fracture displacement, and high morbidity. However, with improved techniques in patient extrication/ evacuation from a trauma scene and transportation to the hospital for stabilization, a greater number of odontoid fractures have been identified and greater emphasis placed on their evaluation and treatment. Improvements in technology, radiographic assessment, and overall understanding of the biomechanics of these injuries have maximized their treatment and overall outcome.

The early literature favored closed techniques for treatment of many odontoid fractures, with poor distinction made between the different varieties of odontoid fractures that produced a great deal of frustration resulting from high nonunion rates—upward of 80% to 90%. This led in the 1970s to greater interest in studies of the mechanism of injury, and led further biomechanical investigations to develop a more clear consensus on the ideal treatment options (94–97). Schatzker et al.'s (96) dismal consideration of these fractures as the "unsolved problem" resulted from a poor correlation between their two-tier classification system and the success or failure of their outcomes. Fortunately, our ability to appreciate the nuances in their presentation has been refined, and review of the literature has facilitated better understanding of their treatment; however, they still remain controversial.

The incidence of odontoid fractures has been reported to be between 7% and 15%; however, these are often quoted from earlier studies in the literature. Due to the significant improvements in the prehospital extrication, handling of the patients, and their overall transport to and stabilization in the emergency room, the mortality of such injuries has diminished significantly over the years, so it would stand to reason that their incidence has trended upward (98,99). In clinical practice, it appears that odontoid fractures occur in the adult population in a bimodal pattern with violent trauma resulting in injuries to a younger population, typically from motor vehicle accidents. The second peak in its distribution occurs with relatively low-energy injuries occurring in the elderly population. Severe hyperextension forces from falls on the face or forehead typically produce a sheer vector that results in a posteriorly displaced fracture in this population. Relatively minor injuries are compounded and become significantly displaced fractures due to osteoporosis underlying medical illness (100). In cases of motor vehicle trauma, however, a high percentage of patients have associated injuries to the head and face, noncontiguous cervical spinal fractures, as well as intraabdominal visceral and other musculoskeletal injuries (101). Also, resulting from such an injury, many patients present with little neurologic loss given the space available for the cord at this level.

In 20% to 25% of cases, neurologic injury results in nerve root deficits, greater occipital neuralgia, and, in severe cases, respiratory paralysis and tetraplegia (101,102). Iatrogenic injury is at greatest risk in those patients who are neurologically intact and unconscious or intoxicated or with significant secondary injuries to complicate the resuscitative process. Morbidity and mortality rates are difficult to estimate throughout the literature due to the early emphasis on close treatments for all injuries with resultant nonunion and instability. The mortality rates for these injuries remain low, ranging from 3% to 8% of cases (103). Recent studies have emphasized the difficulties with these injuries in the elderly patient, noting mortality rates ranging from 20% to 40%, with the cause of death mostly related to respiratory compromise and concomitant medical illness (104,105). Prolonged nonoperative treatment with halo vest immobilization contributed to a diminished time to mobilization and a poor tolerance to such an orthosis, supporting the conclusion that early operative intervention minimizes the confines of an external orthosis.

Pediatric odontoid fractures, however, vary in their presentation as well as their healing potential. In children under 7 years of age, fractures of the dens account for up to 75% of cervical spinal injuries and typically occur at an average age of 4 years (99). The dramatic difference in incidence between adults and children correlates with both the anatomy of the occipitocervical junction in the pediatric patient and the individual anatomy of the dens. In children, the upper cervical spine is prone to greater force concentration due to the size differential between the occiput and the cervical spine. This makes the lever arm of the dens vulnerable to injury. Unfortunately, at the same location exists the synchondrosis or basilar physis between the odontoid ossification center and the body of the axis; although lower cervical spine fractures do occur in younger children, most involve this dens-axis interface. As in adults, motor vehicle injuries or high-energy injuries can cause these fractures; however, due to the nature of the synchondrosis, lower-energy accidents such as minor falls, and obstetrical trauma such as forceps deliveries are possible etiologies. Fortunately, however, neurologic integrity is often preserved, and reduction can be maintained easily with supine recumbency in mild hyperextension followed by halo immobilization or Minerva jacket or casting. With enlarged occipitocervical dimensions, a flexion vector is produced on the neck with lying in a supine position. To gain extension in the neck, an occipital recess must be made in the bed or backboard, or the child's torso needs to be elevated to allow for relative extension of the neck (106). Given the superb healing potential in children as well as the significant blood supply to the synchondrosis, healing occurs in most cases with excellent union by 12 to 16 weeks, and operative treatment is typically unnecessary. Spontaneous closure of the odontoid synchondrosis typically occurs between ages 7 and 10 years, and it is after this point that odontoid fractures take on more adult characteristics.

Irregularities of the odontoid process are known to exist. Os odontoideum is a developmental anomaly of the cervical spine that may predispose a patient to significant instability. Previously, it had been thought to be a congenital deformity, resulting from failure of the os terminale to fuse with the main portion of the odontoid or body of the axis (107–109). However, more recent descriptions initially supported by Fielding et al. (110), indicate that a traumatic etiology may be responsible for this anomaly, and that it is in fact an acquired lesion (Fig. 16) (111). Os odontoideum is by defini-

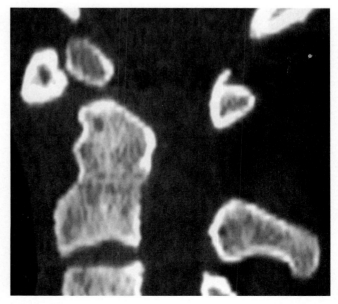

FIG. 16. CT sagittal reconstruction of an os odontoideum.

tion discovered well after its evolution, so its etiology is less important than the knowledge of its potential instability. When discovered even after trivial trauma such as on a screening lateral cervical spine x-ray, further investigation is needed with flexion and extension x-rays to determine the degree of instability associated with this abnormality. With flexion or extension of the head or neck, the os odontoideum will move typically with the ring of the atlas and result most often in anterior instability. However, posterior instability is possible with significant ramifications on spinal cord impingement and the space available for the cord (112). Indications for posterior spinal fusion include acute traumatic myelopathy, progressive myelopathy in the face of chronic findings, space available for the cord less than 13 mm, persistent local symptoms with demonstrable anterior or posterior translation, or patients without symptoms that have a significant degree of instability of greater than 5 to 10 mm of motion (110,113,114).

A discussion of the anatomy, embryology, and vasculature of the odontoid is critical in understanding the healing potential of these injuries and the relevance of their dysplasia. The tip of the odontoid process is distinct from the remainder of the atlas in that it originates from the fourth occipital sclerotome. The first cervical vertebral sclerotome produces the remainder of the odontoid process as well as the atlas. As this portion of the odontoid process enlarges, it cranially fuses with the tip of the dens and migrates caudally to fuse with the body of the axis, which arises from the second cervical sclerotome (115). During its development, five primary ossification centers appear in the axis: two for the odontoid process, one for the body, and two for the neural arches (107). At birth, the odontoid appears as an isolated structure separated from the axis body by the neurocentral synchondrosis or the physeal line that exists at the level of the superior articular facet of the axis. The physis is usually closed by 7 years of age (99). It is important to realize that the embryologic base of the odontoid actually forms a good portion of the body of the axis and is not located at the waist of the odontoid. Its presence as a persistent neurocentral synchondrosis appears below the level of the superior articular facets of the body of the axis. It is this level that will become important in differentiating and classifying fractures. In addition, the tip of the odontoid process has a separate ossification center known as the ossiculum terminale that typically does not appear until 3 years of age and eventually fuses with the remainder of the odontoid by age 12 (110).

The vasculature to the odontoid process has been well established and does not appear to be as tenuous as once thought (116–118). Schiff and Parke (118) demonstrated both anterior and posterior ascending arteries entering the axis at the base of the dens and traveled upward along the outside of the bone to form an apical arcade over the tip of the dens. There is also a contribution from a perforating artery of the carotid. This vasculature in an upward direction appeared to place the more cephalad odontoid in jeopardy of avascular necrosis if a transverse fracture occurred with sig-

nificant displacement. Additional vessels, however, were noted in later studies by Althoff and Goldie (116) and Schatzker et al. (119,120) to form a rich anastomosing network of both interosseous and extraosseous vessels about the axis that would likely prevent significant avascular necrosis if a fracture occurred. Such an end-vessel supply, therefore, does not exist; consequently, high nonunion rates with many odontoid fractures result from other factors, which may include degree of displacement, distraction, or soft tissue interposition from the local synovial tissues that encompass the atlantoaxial articulation (4,101). Schatzker et al. noted vascular supply via the apical and accessory ligaments to the cephalad portion of the odontoid, and in their canine model, if the odontoid was fractured above the insertion of the accessory ligaments, distraction typically occurred and poor healing resulted. When fractures were below the accessory ligaments, healing occurred in most cases.

The ligamentous attachments to the odontoid provide the only stabilization to this articulation. The transverse ligament also has superior and inferior or upper and lower bands that attach superiorly on the occiput and inferiorly on the inferior dens and add to their stabilizing power. It is this cruciform ligament that poses the greatest deterrent of hyperflexion at the atlantoaxial joint with posterior displacement limited mostly by bony articulation.

The odontoid is held in place up against the anterior arch of the atlas by the strong transverse ligament. The alar ligaments run from the tip of the odontoid to the two occipital condyles with a central apical ligament attaching to the foramen magnum from the tip of the odontoid. Accessory ligaments also exist anterior to the transverse ligament attachment to the atlas; they arise from both lateral masses and attach to the anterolateral surface of the dens. It is the contribution of these superior ligaments that stabilize the odontoid with respect to the atlas in all planes of motion, however, that may also be implicated due to their attachment and elasticity to maintain distraction or displacement of an odontoid fracture and contribute to potential nonunion.

Classification System

Odontoid fractures have been given a great deal of attention in the literature over the years, and there have been several classification systems of injury severity, potential for healing, and instability. Several of these systems are often noted in the literature; however, only the Anderson and D'Alonzo (121) system (Fig. 17) has been consistently used (96,117, 122–125). This classification was developed after a review of patients over 18 years at the Campbell Clinic. Previous authors referred to difficulties in treating these patients including delay in diagnoses, high degrees of nonunion, and delayed neurologic findings; however, they did so without a standardized means of evaluating fracture types. The location of the fracture was not specified in Schatzker's work beyond being either high or low and displaced anterior or posterior (96,126). Anderson and D'Alonzo's review, however,

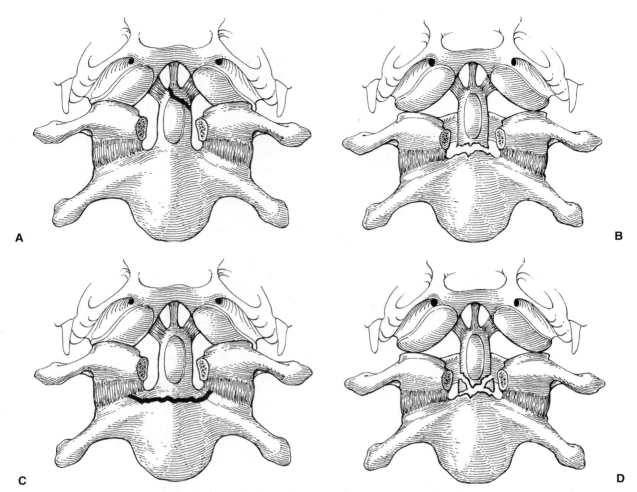

FIG. 17. A–C: Anderson and d'Alonzo (121) classification of odontoid fractures. **A:** Type I: avulsion fracture of the odontoid tip. **B:** Type II: mid-waist fracture at the junction of the odontoid process and the body of C2. **C:** Type III: fracture extending into the body of C2. **D:** Modification of type IIA proposed by Hadley (123), comminuted fracture of the odontoid waist.

formulated three distinct types of fractures and evaluated different modes of treatment and their results. Their primary objective was to establish a means of determining prognosis with respect to union of these fractures. Although limited by the constraints of a retrospective review, this classification appeared to have the most clinical relevance and has been the most consistent description in the literature.

The type I fracture, known as an avulsion fracture of the most cephalad tip of the odontoid, was described as an oblique fracture that appeared to result from disruption of the alar ligament attachment. This has been the least common variety of odontoid fractures in the literature and only two patients exhibited this in Anderson and D'Alonzo's study. There have been few reported cases in the literature of these injuries, with only four resulting in survival. In each of these cases, the fractures were considered stable injuries and isolated to the odontoid (33,73,121,127,128). Their low incidence as well as our greater understanding of upper cervical and atlantoaxial injuries have recently contributed to the assertion by several authors that the injury is ambiguous and

simple in its description and likely does not exist as an isolated entity. It also may potentially characterize the presence of a more worrisome and ominous occult atlantooccipital instability (33,129,130). Although these injuries are usually fatal, in survivors the avulsion fracture is typically minimally displaced and may be the only occult radiographic marker of such severe ligamentous disruption. It is unclear whether or not one alar ligament causes the avulsion or the apical ligaments–associated connection as well pulls off a larger fragment with both alar ligaments attached. Sharp, well-defined jagged borders usually help delineate this fracture fragment from an unfused secondary ossification center of the apex of the dens. Close inspection is required for soft tissue injury as well as of the atlantooccipital and occipitoatlantal relationships because serious complication and death may occur if such an injury is overlooked.

The type II fracture occurs with more regularity; however, it has an equally controversial and confusing history in the literature. It was originally described as occurring at the junction of the odontoid process with the body of the secondary cervical vertebra. These fractures are often significantly displaced either anteriorly or posteriorly and difficult to manage closed secondary to ligamentous attachments to the cephalad portion, maintaining slight distraction of the fracture fragment. As previously indicated, the blood supply was originally thought to contribute to nonunion; however, it is more likely to be associated with degree of displacement and fracture separation. Fractures in children are similar to type II; however, they occur through the neurocentral synchondrosis, which is lower in position than this "waist"-type fracture. The pediatric injuries have a high degree of union, making operative treatment unnecessary in most cases.

Much attention has been paid to the type II fractures of the odontoid, and attempts have been made to correlate fracture morphology with degree of nonunion. Hadley et al. (123) indicated that there may be a type IIA version of this fracture that presents with significant comminution at the fracture line. These multiple fracture fragments interfere with correct alignment and adequate reduction of the fracture via closed means, and it was postulated that they contribute to the degree of nonunion despite initial displacement. It is the authors' contention that with the demonstration of such fragmentation, closed reduction should be abandoned and operative intervention should be considered to maximize healing.

In the type III fracture the fracture line extends downward into the cancellous portion of the body and courses through one or both of the superior articular surfaces. This fracture has had the least amount of controversy with respect to its healing potential, which is likely due to the exuberant blood supply, fracture interdigitation, and excellent healing potential of cancellous bone in this location.

As with many injuries to the cervical spine, the primary method of diagnosis relies on accurate interpretation of plain radiographs, and it is important to have well-demonstrated open-mouth odontoid views to visualize the entire odontoid process and anterior body of the C2 vertebra to augment well-aligned lateral radiographs. Plain tomography has been replaced to a significant degree by CT with sagittal and coronal reconstructions. If axial cuts are processed in 1- to 3-mm increments, significant clarity can be obtained on these reconstructions. A review of minimally displaced type II odontoid fractures by Rubenstein et al. (131) indicated that computed axial tomography (CAT) scan section thickness, if reduced to 1 mm, improves the diagnosis of type II odontoid fractures and augments the efficacy of sagittal and coronal reformations and 3D reconstructions. Axial images have a finite degree of accuracy due to the parallel nature of the fracture plane and the image scans. It has also been noted in the literature that MRI may be useful in evaluation of injuries to the transverse ligament in such patients (98,132). Green et al. (132) postulated that the early diagnosis of transverse ligament is necessary so as not miss an atlantoaxial instability after healing of the odontoid fracture. Three cases of ruptured transverse ligaments were seen in patients with type II fractures in this study.

Mechanism of Injury

Several theories have been advocated based on clinical as well as autopsy studies. Moradian et al. (95) in 1978 had one of the larger studies, evaluating 34 cadaver models with varying forces applied in flexion, lateral deviation, extension, and rotation-extension. Flexion force tested in 16 specimens resulted in eight type III fractures of the odontoid. Lateral forces, however, resulted in a higher percentage of type II odontoid fractures. Moradian et al. could not produce an odontoid fracture with an extension force in their model; however, rotation and extension produced one type III fracture. The authors concluded that their model was not reliable for the production of odontoid fractures; however, it appeared that lateral loading caused the lateral mass of C1 to act as a hammer fracturing the odontoid. Review of the literature looking at the biomechanics of these fractures fails to find consistent theories. Schatzker et al. (96) came to the conclusion after such a review that the mechanism of injury responsible for odontoid process fractures was a combination of forces, with overall displacement resulting from the more dominant-sheering vector. Avulsion forces have been associated with distraction injuries of the occipitocervical junction and can be possibly related to type I injuries (4,33). Althoff's (117) study postulated, however, that axial compression or axial load with a component of vertical sheer was responsible for the majority of the injuries. A case report of a vertical fracture of the odontoid is consistent with such an axial load and needs to be considered when discussing various patterns of injury (125). A review of the literature reveals various mechanisms of injury, and overall displacement is likely related to the more dominant vector. Due to the anatomic position of the anterior aspect of the ring of C1, extension or posterior translatory forces certainly can contribute to fracture of the dens. With anterior or flexion forces, a taut transverse ligament would be the anatomic structure most likely to contribute to anterior odontoid displacement (39,133). Concomitant extension and axial load may also contribute to frequently associated atlas fracture (43). Although multiple vectors of energy transmission are responsible for these injuries, it is evident in the literature that anterior displaced fractures appear to be more common, up to seven times more frequently noted and posteriorly displaced fractures (39). The experience that the senior author (J.M.C.) has had at Thomas Jefferson University Hospital, however, indicates a greater degree of posterior displaced fractures in 61% of cases treated between 1988 and 1990 (39,134).

Treatment

As with any trauma patient careful evaluation of cardiorespiratory, hemodynamic, and intraabdominal injuries must be done along with the evaluation of skeletal integrity. Initial radiographic evaluation includes chest x-ray, pelvis, and the cross-table lateral cervical spine, which is often the only indicator of an upper cervical spine injury in a patient who is uncooperative, intoxicated, or unconscious. Identification of a fracture of the odontoid is typically made in this fashion, and when noted, prompt immobilization is necessary during the initial resuscitative efforts. Early immobilization can consist of a Philadelphia collar or similar rigid orthosis that is maintained until the patient's condition has stabilized to allow for reevaluation of the present injury and the possibility of concomitant, noncontiguous spinal injuries. Immediate immobilization prevents further displacement and neurologic compromise. In nondisplaced fractures, early halo immobilization can be completed successfully to maximize stability during transportation, nursing care, and the completion of secondary radiographic studies. If any displacement is seen or early halo placement is delayed, 5 lb of skeletal traction through cranial tongs can be used, with the patient in a rotating-type bed to maintain suitable traction, prevent displacement, minimize risk to the neural structures, and minimize the complications of recumbency.

Whenever cranial traction is applied, vigilant x-rays should be obtained after the addition of weights to ensure that overdistraction is not occurring. Overdistraction is especially ominous in type I fractures, which have been associated with atlantooccipital instability. The addition of cervical traction needs to be accomplished gradually up to 5 lb, and several radiographs should be taken in checking for overdistraction. Although more commonly associated with atlantoaxial disruption, longitudinal atlantoaxial dislocation has been seen with type III odontoid fractures in a recent case report, and the placement of 5 lb of skeletal traction resulted in marked neurologic deterioration (135).

Specific treatment options are available for each type of injury noted above. In type I injuries, although the previous literature has indicated that collar immobilization is necessary for healing, the recent trend associating avulsion fractures of the odontoid with occipitoatlantal instability warrants significant caution with this approach. When atlantooccipital instability is present, the degree of loss of ligamentous integrity is significant to interfere with proper healing. As with any cervical spine injury that is purely ligamentous in origin, late instability is common and is not well tolerated in this location. Careful evaluation should be done of occipitoatlantal bony parameters on plain radiography and CT, as well as of soft tissue indications for injury. If no evidence exists for such instability, a rigid cervical orthosis can be used for up to 3 months to allow for sufficient healing. At the completion of immobilization, flexion/extension radiographs are mandatory to ensure occult instability is not present.

Throughout the literature, type II fractures have proven to be the most troublesome. Nonunion rates range up to 88% when treated nonoperatively (116,117,121,123,126,136–138). Unfortunately, conservative treatment meant varying forms of braces and halos, with and without displacement noted, and varying degrees of traction instituted. Treatment of these fractures remains difficult because of the contradiction in the literature regarding advocating conservative versus nonoperative treatment. Bell and Meyer (136) in 1983 proposed the greatest success with nonoperative treatment of type II fractures by instituting skeletal traction for 6 weeks until alignment was secure, followed by bracing with a Somi orthosis for up to 3 months. This contradicted Ryan and Taylor's (128) study one year earlier, which reviewed the factors in the literature that were characteristically known to contribute to nonunion, including fracture type, ligamentous integrity, degree of displacement, traction, and adequacy of reduction. They subsequently based their management on these anatomic factors; they felt that skull traction to any degree typically increased the fracture gap, potentially increased displacement, and was detrimental in the overall care of these injuries. They recommended halo placement with alignment of at least 66% to 70% of fracture contact to maximize healing potential with near-anatomic alignment obtained on the AP view. If, however, the patient presented 2 weeks after the injury occurred, nonunion rates increased and surgery was indicated.

Other authors have advocated a more dogmatic approach to the treatment of these injuries, given the confusion in the literature. Degrees of displacement and angulation have been advocated for nonoperative versus operative treatment, based on the patient's age and general condition, and the instability and type of fracture. Anderson and D'Alonzo (121), who promoted the most common classification system discussed earlier, recommended that all type II fractures undergo posterior spinal fusion. Nonoperative treatment resulted in a 36% nonunion rate, and surgery was recommended; however, the physician must take into account age, associated injuries, and the general condition of the patient prior to undergoing operative intervention. It is also interesting to note that in their study only 80% of patients treated with posterior cervical fusion obtained a stable union.

In 1985, the largest multicenter study was published by Clark and White (137), who reviewed 144 odontoid fractures, 96 of which were type II injuries. They noted a 32% nonunion rate resulting from halo orthosis treatment. Significant displacement was considered to be 5 mm or more in either the anterior or posterior direction, and significant angulation was considered to be 10 degrees. Given these parameters, a chi-square analysis of these fractures reveal that nonunion or malunion was significantly related to these values. The authors also noted that rates of union were higher in patients who were younger than 40 years old; however, these numbers were not statistically significant. Fractures that were treated with posterior cervical fusion had the highest stability rate of 96%.

Various authors subsequent to these reports have noted increased nonunion rates with varying degrees of displacement from 4 to 6 mm on average (123,139,140). Age also continues to be a factor when considering operative versus nonoperative intervention. Although there have been reports where age does not appear to have a significant effect on nonunion rates (24,28), the majority of studies note poor results with conservative or nonoperative treatment in type II injuries in the elderly (140,141). Several authors have recommended operative intervention in patients older than 55 to 65 years (96,138,141–143). Confusion may occur when the literature notes a divergence of union rates occurring at approximately 40 years of age (100,139). This is most likely due to a different etiology of the injury; younger patients have a higher involvement in high-velocity motor vehicle accidents or falls, whereas the elderly suffer odontoid fractures with much less force imparted to their spine. It is not until the later decades, however, that true nonunion rates begin to be significantly altered. The management of the elderly continues to be debated in the literature because conservative treatment, even in nondisplaced fractures, has been shown to potentially increase skin decubiti, respiratory complications, and death (100). Bednar et al. (143a) in 1995 reported a prospective study of type II odontoid fractures treated with halo immobilization and noted a significant increase in mortality in the geriatric population, despite preservation of neurologic integrity. The elderly are difficult to mobilize, and certain debilitated patients with type II fractures may benefit from more aggressive surgical intervention to prevent the risks of recumbency and loss of vigor resulting from immobilization in a halo orthosis.

Assimilating all of this information from the literature is not an easy task in clinical practice. The senior author (J.M.C.) summarized the experience with treatment of type II odontoid fractures at Thomas Jefferson University Hospital, the Regional Spinal Cord Injury Center of the Delaware Valley. This information was also presented as a review by Craft et al. (134). Seventy consecutive patients between 1980 and 1990 were reviewed with a 43% nonunion rate. Those patients with type II fractures treated with halo immobilization went on to eventual nonunion in 75% of cases as compared to a 100% union rate in patients undergoing posterior spinal fusion primarily. Degree and direction of displacement were also significant factors associated with poor results. In patients who had posteriorly displaced fractures, 70% went on to nonunion despite reduction. This is significant when compared to a 33% nonunion rate for anteriorly displaced fractures. The degree of displacement was also significant, and, when over 5 mm, 81% of posteriorly displaced fractures and 100% of anteriorly displaced fracture failed to unite. In this review, anteriorly displaced fractures of less than 5 mm showed no signs of nonunion. The data gained from this retrospective review formed the basis of our treatment protocol. In displaced type II fractures of greater than 5 mm in any direction, risk factors for nonunion and primary indications for operative intervention include age over 60 years, instability, and loss of reduction. It was also noted that a delay of 10 days or longer increased the nonunion rate.

The method of close reduction and conservative treatment employed at Thomas Jefferson University warrants further discussion. Significantly displaced fractures of the odontoid that require reduction are not often sufficiently reduced by axial traction alone. Initial skeletal traction is used gradually, approaching 5 to 10 lb in the longitudinal direction for diminishing cervical spasm and neck pain as well as the potential for iatrogenic neurologic injury during transport. It is important to have a dedicated radiographic technician to provide portable, lateral cervical spine x-rays during the initiation and progression of traction to ensure that overdistraction and improper alignment are not occurring. A bivector apparatus is used to facilitate the reduction of posteriorly displaced fractures. Two simultaneous vector forces are used—one in the axial direction to produce disimpaction of the fracture fragments, and the other along a suitable tangent to this distraction force in the sagittal axis. The halo ring is first placed on the patient to allow for a halo traction device in the superior direction and attachment of the secondary device to the anterior aspect of the halo ring for the more anterior vector. A special slide or skid attached to the overhead frame of the patient's bed as seen in Fig. 18 facilitates the adjustment of this anterior vector to angulation necessary for appropriate reduction. When fractures are displaced anteriorly, axial traction in

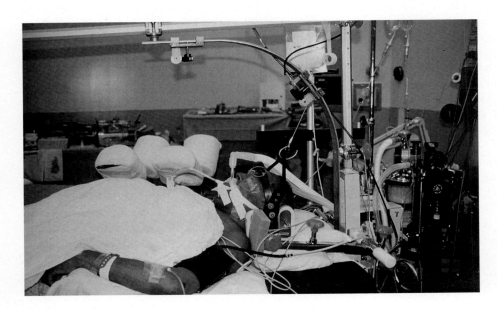

FIG. 18. Bivector traction is facilitated by utilizing an overhead track or skid, as seen in this photo, to position the anterior traction force.

the longitudinal direction with slight extension of the neck or slight posterior distraction is typically sufficient for obtaining reduction. Once reduction is obtained and found to be stable with diminishing traction weights, halo vest application is performed, and continued nonoperative or operative intervention is decided on based on the original characteristics of the fracture.

Type III fractures of the odontoid have traditionally been thought to be associated with high union rates due to the excellent blood supply, fracture interdigitation, and cancellous nature of the bone at the level of the body of C2. The literature is replete with reports of excellent union rates, from 80% to 100%, in these fractures (121,126,138). There has been evidence, however, in the literature that care must be taken when treating these fractures, and high union rates do not necessarily mean that malunion or loss of reduction with nonunion is impossible. Clark and White (137) were careful to note that type III fractures are not benign, and there is a potential for a significant rate of malunion when proper immobilization is not maintained. Nonunion certainly can occur with a cervical orthosis alone, and a halo device appears to be the most reliable form of immobilization to prevent inadequate healing. The authors reported that 13% of their patients with type III fractures went on to nonunion, with a 15% malunion rate. Other authors have also noted difficulties with immobilization, potentiating poor results with these fractures, and recommended longer periods of traction and immobilization to maximize healing (70,126,139). Apuzzo et al. (139) reported a 54% rate of nonunion in 13 patients with type III fractures, and they concluded that the elderly patient with greater than 4 mm of displacement is a candidate for primary posterior cervical fusion, despite the low level of fracture.

Cervical orthosis treatment can be initiated if impaction and nondisplacement of the fracture is obvious on radiographs. Burst fractures, however, show some degree of displacement, and the recommendation at Thomas Jefferson University Hospital is skeletal traction to obtain reduction for 2 to 6 weeks depending on stability, followed by halo immobilization for 3 months. As in any fracture of the cervical spine, completion flexion/extension x-rays at the end of this period of immobilization will determine whether or not stability has been achieved. This is especially true when odontoid fractures are associated with injuries to the ring of the atlas. Contiguous fractures of the atlantoaxial complex are not uncommon; however, their incidence remains significant but variable in the literature (70,74,81,121). The experience at Thomas Jefferson University Hospital has been shown to be as high as 23% of concomitant burst fractures at the atlas with odontoid fractures (16). The traditional mode of treatment when these injuries occurred together has been to obtain reduction of the odontoid fracture via closed means and maintenance of halo immobilization until the ring of the atlas has sufficiently healed. If flexion and extension x-rays then continue to show persistent instability at the atlantoaxial complex, operative intervention

is then undertaken, with sublaminar fixation now feasible with the healed posterior arch of C1. Although it could be argued to use primary occipital C2 fusion to avoid such prolonged immobilization; excellent results have been obtained despite the period of immobilization, limiting the operative intervention to the atlantoaxial complex, and thereby avoiding the loss of atlantooccipital range of motion (70,74,144).

Surgical Techniques

Preoperative planning for posterior cervical surgery requires a thorough understanding of the patient's pattern of fracture, displacement, and instability. Also, the surgeon must become familiar with the local neurovascular anatomy and bone morphology of the atlantoaxial interval, best assessed with CT techniques. Vertebral artery ectasia and malposition are potential threats to certain operative techniques, and the precise location of the vertebral artery needs to be appreciated prior to initiating dissection and internal fixation. A radiographic technologist needs to be present throughout the operation to provide fluoroscopic images in the lateral position. Prophylactic antibiotics are routinely given, and pneumatic compression stockings are used to diminish the risk of deep venous thrombosis. In traumatic cases with acute instability, reduction would most likely have been improved preoperatively with traction, and the patient is most efficiently treated with a preoperative halo vest that continues to be worn in the postoperative period. Surgery is facilitated with the use of a Stryker frame in the operating room if cervical traction is used during surgery to maintain alignment.

Although positioning remains the surgeon's preference, reduction and maintenance of odontoid fracture position can be facilitated with the use of the Mayfield frame and the halo ring adaptor (Fig. 19). Using this technique, the patient is logrolled in the prone position onto chest bolsters or "lami" rolls to adequately cushion bony prominences, and the head is positioned appropriately and affixed to the Mayfield frame in a sufficient manner to maintain reduction and preserve neurologic integrity. Neurologic integrity is also evaluated during positioning and during surgery with the use of somatosensory evoked potential monitoring by a neurophysiologist in the operating room. After careful positioning and securing the patient, a wake-up test can also be performed to ensure preservation of distal neurologic function. If the fracture has been reduced preoperatively and the patient is in a halo vest, after positioning the patient in the prone position the posterior shell is then removed to facilitate the approach to the posterior cervical spine. Prior to any surgical exposure, final positioning is confirmed with lateral fluoroscopic x-rays.

Soft tissue dissection then begins over the occipital cervical junction, and blood loss is minimized by maintaining the dissection within the avascular plane directly over the spinous processes. Limiting the dissection to the atlantoaxial complex, the occipital periosteum should be left intact to

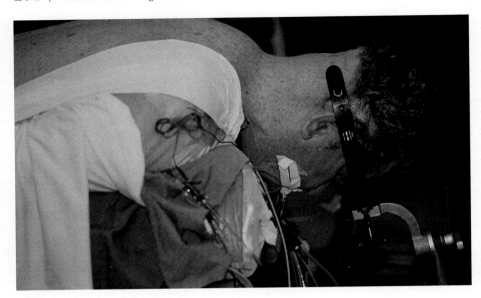

FIG. 19. Photograph of a patient positioned utilizing the halo ring adaptor to the Mayfield frame.

avoid superior extension of the fusion mass. Subperiosteal dissection of the spinous process of C2, its lamina, and the posterior elements of C1 needs to be performed for adequate visualization, and the dissection laterally at the atlantoaxial interval needs to proceed with caution because cavernous venous sinuses exist in this area and can result in significant blood loss. Hemostatic agents should be readily available, including Oxycel (Beckton and Dickson), and Gelfoam (Upjohn) moistened with thrombin is used in addition to bipolar electrocautery. Dissection of the posterior arch of C1 classically is limited to 1.0 to 1.5 cm lateral to the midline to avoid injury to the vertebral arteries as they course posteriorly prior to entrance through the occipitocervical fascia. Care is taken not to disrupt the fascia and facet capsule overlying the C2-3 interval as well as their interspinous ligaments to minimize the risk of postoperative junctional instability.

Posterior cervical fusion involving the atlantoaxial complex has been performed with various wiring techniques since the early 1900s. Gallie (145) in 1939 described a technique by which sublaminar C1 wires are used centrally to fix the posterior axis of C1 to C2, thereby preventing translation. Modifications have been made since this wiring technique, and the most common technique used is the modified Brooks fusion where a wedge-compression method of bone graft placement is used as well as sublaminar wires placed under C1 and C2, facilitating segmental fixation (Fig. 20) (146). Modification of this technique allows for distributing fixation both centrally and laterally on the lamina, resulting in a more stable construct. In cases with an incompetent posterior arch of C1 or when sublaminar passage at this location is contraindicated, Callahan et al. (147) use drill holes in the bony elements of C1 to afford purchase of the wires.

The technique of sublaminar wire placement in the upper cervical spine does not come without risks. Sufficient space available for the cord at this level allows for their use; however, the subaxial spine has not been amenable to this tech-

nique. Surgeon preference dictates the technique used for sublaminar wire placement; however, wire placement must be accompanied by continuous posteriorly directed forces on the undersurface of the lamina to prevent dural compromise or compression. Wire passage can be accompanied by kinks

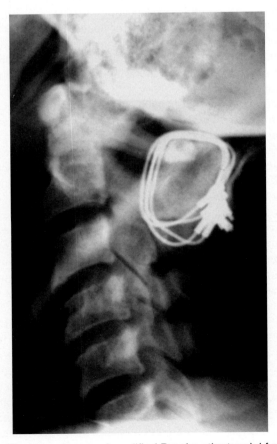

FIG. 20. Lateral x-ray of modified Brooks atlantoaxial fusion.

in the wire that may indent the spinal cord. Newer devices such as flexible cables diminish this risk.

Wire passage is performed from the caudad-to-cephalad direction to take advantage of the angulation of the lamina and insertion of the ligamentum flavum inferiorly. Sublaminar manipulation is performed after careful subperiosteal dissection of the ligamentum flavum off of both the superior and inferior surfaces of the lamina of C1 and C2. It is important to continue dissection laterally to the most lateral aspect of the lamina to facilitate placement of the wires at that location. The method of placement, two wires on either side of the midline under each lamina, is facilitated by looping a 16- to 24-gauge stainless steel wire and directing it under the lamina from inferior to superior with the assistance of a heavy, no. 1 silk suture previously placed with a curve-free needle. The needle is used in the reverse direction, with the sharp end of the needle removed with a wire cutter to avoid laceration of the dura. The looped end of the wire is then attached to the inferior aspect of the silk suture and pulled superiorly under the lamina of C2 and C1, taking care that the wire does not indent the dura, especially when transversing the C1 and C2 interval. A posteriorly directed force can be facilitated by the use of a Frazier right-angle dural elevator to maintain an upward force on the wire. The use of stainless steel or titanium cables, which are more flexible, will diminish the risk of dural compression.

Once the sublaminar wires are in position, cortical cancellous bone grafts are taken and fashioned to provide maximal cancellous surface on the posterior elements of C1 and C2. Two such grafts are fixed on either side of the spinous processes, and each graft is secured with two wires—one more centrally located, and the other displaced as far lateral as possible. Notches in the graft can be made to secure the position of the wires on the grafts. Both wires are seen in Fig. 21 on either side of the midline firmly securing the cortical cancellous bone graft to the posterior elements. In cases where the passage of sublaminar wires is contraindicated, several authors have advocated the interlaminar clamp; however, the size of this instrumentation limits the surface area available for bone grafting and may jeopardize the success of fusion (148,149). In addition, with any sublaminar wire technique, care must be taken not to overcompress the lamina of C1 and C2. This may inadvertently pull the arches of C1 and C2 together and posteriorly displace the odontoid fracture (150). A properly placed wedge compression graft in the Brooks-Jenkins technique allows for maximal surface area contact for graft incorporation and prevents excessive approximation of the posterior elements of C1 and C2 by the intervening cancellous bone in the atlantoaxial interval. The modified Brooks technique has been found to provide greater stability in flexion, extension, lateral bend, and rotation as compared to the Gallie technique (151–153).

Transarticular screw fixation to obtain rigid atlantoaxial stability was first introduced into the literature by Magerl and Seeman (154) in 1987. The advantages of this technique are clear in that it produces rigid immobilization of the atlantoaxial complex through three-column fixation and allows for direct facet arthrodesis. The biomechanical superiority of this technique has been noted in the literature; Grob et al. (155) in 1992 noted that Magerl transarticular screw fixation provided the most stable construct in lateral bending and axial rotation when comparing this technique to the Gallie, Brooks, and Halifax fixation systems (156). The original discussion by Magerl and Seeman included extensive exposure of the occipitocervical spine down to the cervicothoracic junction for placement of the screws; however, recent modifications of the procedure have allowed for percutaneous introduction of the screws through paramedian stab wounds and a much smaller midline incision (157,158).

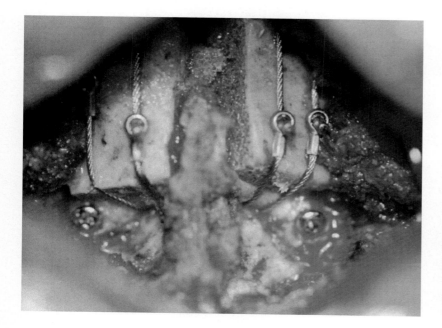

FIG. 21. Intraoperative photograph of posterior spinal fusion utilizing the modified Brooks technique. Note the large cortical cancellous bone grafts affixed on each side of the midline, each with two cables spread apart such as to distribute the purchase along the posterior elements of the atlantoaxial complex. In addition, note two inferior screws placed as transarticular fixation. This intraoperative photograph demonstrates the silk suture placed under the lamina of C1 and C2 to facilitate the introduction of sublaminar wires or cables.

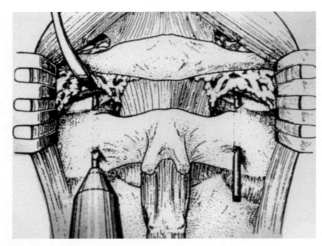

FIG. 22. Artist's rendition of Magerl screw insertion. (From ref. 161, with permission.)

The starting point of screw placement had been defined to be 2 mm cephalad to the C2-3 facet joint as well as 2 to 3 mm lateral to the junction of C2 lamina and C2 lateral mass (Fig. 22). A 2-mm burr is then used to make a starting hole, 1 to 2 mm deep in the cortex of the inferior aspect of the inferior articular process at this location. A long guidewire is used external to the body to determine the trajectory of the screw based on lateral fluoroscopic control. The preoperative position of the fluoroscope needs to be in position prior to draping to facilitate this technique (Fig. 23). In general, the trajectory needs to be guided superiorly and anteriorly toward the anterior ring of C1 to avoid inferior anterior vertebral artery injury. The starting point and the trajectory are general guidelines that need to be assessed based on intraoperative appreciation of the neural canal and subsequent fluoroscopic evaluation of screw direction. Once this trajectory is appreciated, small paramedian, 1- to 2-cm incisions are made in the cervicothoracic spine 3 to 4 cm lateral to the midline. Dissection is carried down bluntly to the muscular fascia, and a trocar with a large outer diameter sleeve is directed subfascially down into the cervical spine wound. The point of the trocar is then placed at the area of the starting hole that was previously made with the 2-mm burr (Figs. 24 and 25). The trajectory is then confirmed on lateral fluoroscopy, and intraoperative palpation of the medial isthmus of the C2 pedicle with the Penfield is maintained throughout drill and screw insertion. Calibrated drill bits and screwdrivers are used to obtain bicortical purchase in the lateral mass of C1, with screw lengths typically 40 to 50 mm in length. Successful parallel placement of two screws is achieved using this technique, and augmented with a modified Brooks fusion to maximize stability in flexion and extension (Fig. 26). The success of this procedure is contingent upon the atlantoaxial facet joint being reduced. If it does not appear to be reduced intraoperatively, manual reduction is necessary and can be performed prior to the placement of the screw. A

Due to the technical difficulty of this percutaneous screw placement and the demanding nature of the technique overall, Silveri and Vaccaro (158) readdressed the fine aspects of the McGuire technique and the preoperative and intraoperative preparation of the patient, and outlined the approach used for successful placement of these transfacet screws. After the dissection has been established as indicated previously, the C2-3 facet joint needs to be well established, with the inferior aspect of the inferior articular facet of C2 exposed to be palpated for proper anatomic landmarks. Dissection of the posterior elements of C2 also needs to include exposure of the isthmus of the C2 pedicle with subperiosteal dissection performed with a Penfield elevator as well as small cervical curettes. This also allows for palpation of the atlantoaxial facet joint posteriorly. It is this direct palpation of the facet joint that allows curettage of the articular surface to augment fusion.

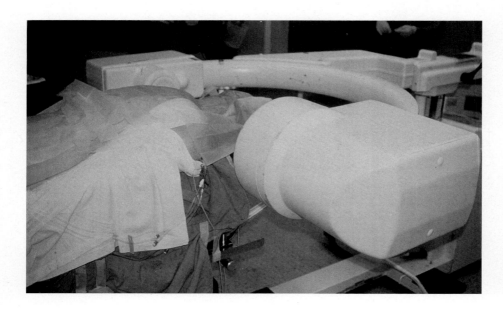

FIG. 23. Preoperative positioning of the patient and lateral fluoroscopy to facilitate transarticular atlantoaxial screw insertion.

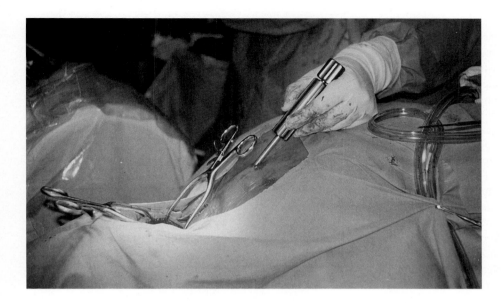

FIG. 24. Photograph of percutaneous placement of the cannulated sheaths for transarticular screw fixation.

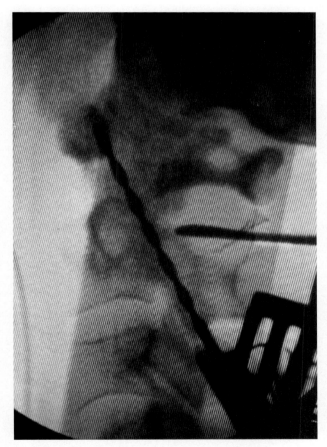

FIG. 25. Lateral fluoroscopic image of the drill in position along the transarticular trajectory.

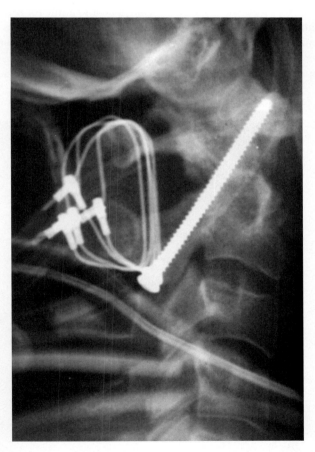

FIG. 26. Photograph of final placement of the transarticular screw fixation augmented by the modified Brooks sublaminar wire technique.

guidewire can be used to maintain reduction while the contralateral side is instrumented. Cannulated screw systems are not recommended as there is the potential for inadvertent advancement of the guidewire into the soft tissues of the neck anteriorly during drilling and screw placement.

Despite advances made in this technique to facilitate its completion and minimize exposure, it remains a very technically demanding procedure with significant risk to neurovascular structures. Despite a low incidence of these complications, injuries have been reported to the vertebral artery and anterior structures in the neck (154,155,159–161). Stereotactic image-guidance systems have been used both clinically and experimentally to diminish the risk of spinal canal navigation and placement of internal fixation (162). Silveri et al. (163) presented a study looking at risk assessment and bone morphology of the atlantoaxial complex when considering atlantoaxial transarticular screw fixation. Significant anatomic constraints were noted when constructing a "virtual" transarticular screw pathway. The greatest bony constraint was that of the pars interarticularis of C2. Image-guided spinal surgery would appear to allow for real-time anatomic localization of critical structures and minimize errors in trajectory that would place the spinal canal or vertebral artery at risk. It is also an excellent means of preoperatively evaluating the bone morphology and neurovascular anatomy of the area in a 3D fashion (Fig. 27). A final conclusion of the study was that significant variability existed between individuals for axial and sagittal angles of inclination as well as measurements for starting-point location for the ideal screw position. Consequently, a single set of guidelines for safe screw placement could not be established. It is vital, therefore, to use the tactile and visual landmarks intraoperatively, palpate the medial portion of the isthmus, and judiciously use fluoroscopic x-rays to direct the trajectory appropriately.

Anterior screw fixation of the dens is the only means of providing direct interfragmentary fixation of the fracture. The technique was described in 1982 by both Bohler (164) and Nakanishi et al. (165) in separate studies. The advantages of direct fixation of the odontoid fracture are that it provides rigid internal fixation with preservation of atlantoaxial rotational range of motion, diminishes risk of occipitocervical or subaxial instability from dissection, does not require formal bone grafting procedures, and does not entail the complications related to autogenous graft harvest. The procedure is performed through a typical anterior approach to the cervical spine used for most subaxial anterior cervical fusion surgery. The level of the incision is made at the level of the cricoid cartilage, and dissection is carried out superiorly once the prevertebral fascia is reached (164), which allows

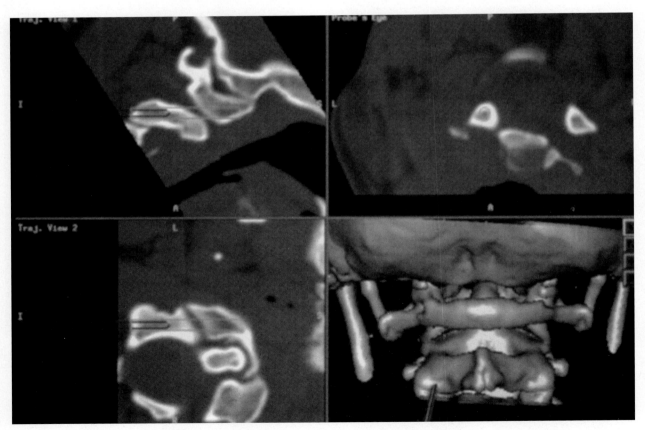

FIG. 27. Transaxial computer-generated images of the virtual ideal path of a atlantoaxial transarticular screw. (Courtesy of K. Foly, M.D. and the Danek Stealth Station Image Guidance System.)

successful cephalad trajectory of the instrumentation with appropriate inclination. Cannulated screw systems can also be used to simplify the drill, tap, and screw technique of stable internal fixation (166). Indications for this procedure include type II fractures and some cases of high type III fractures. Authors have also noted this technique to be ideal in cases of unreduced anterior fractures where the reduction can be performed manually intraoperatively (138,167). Other indications include posterior element deficiencies or fractures of the ring of C1, which would preclude sublaminar wire fixation. Contraindications, however, include oblique fracture configurations, especially with an anterior-inferior to superior-posterior plane of fracture, which parallel the direction of the intended screw placement and would not allow for stabilization. Pathologic fractures also have been cited as contraindicated secondary to poor bone stock as well as most nonunions (103,166). There are authors, however, who continue to advocate anterior and posterior techniques as well as isolated anterior fixation for specific nonunions (164,168).

To successfully utilize the technique, biplanar fluoroscopy is mandatory for proper visualization of screw trajectory in the open mouth (AP) and lateral planes (Fig. 28). Preoperative evaluation with CT needs to determine whether or not two screws can fit within the odontoid waist. Most early reports advocated that two screws be placed in parallel fashion; however, current trends are toward internal fixation with one screw with bicortical purchase (103,168). Biomechanics of single-screw fixation did not show any detriment as compared to two screws (169–171). Proper, reliable postoperative orthotic immobilization is necessary to maximize successive healing. Union rates as high as 88% to 100% have been reported in the literature (164,166). As with any internal fixation device, failure of fixation can oc-

cur, especially in the elderly patient, and requires revision surgery. Attention to detail during the surgical technique is mandatory to ensure adequate purchase in the caudad and cephalad fracture fragments. The appropriate insertion of the guidewire would be in the inferior border of the C2 endplate, and, if need be, a portion of the anterior C2-3 disc needs to be removed to gain the proper trajectory and purchase. Failure to do so could also result in fixation failure (Fig. 29), especially in the osteoporotic patient or in patients who do not maintain reliable external orthosis stabilization during the healing process (39,169). Other complications have been noted as well, such as nonunions, carotid injury, fracture redislocation, late myelopathy, and the formation of an esophagotracheal fistula (172). As with many techniques, significant complications can result if one is unfamiliar with the procedure. Although there are advantages to this technique, experience is needed for its application. If unfamiliar with the procedure, then the direct visualization of the posterior cervical techniques of sublaminar fixation, although difficult, will likely pose less risk. Difficult patient positioning, a barrel-chest deformity, or unreducible fracture will make anterior screw fixation of the dens less effective and should be abandoned. The overall success rate of anterior screw fixation relies first on an adequate reduction, and second on the technical aspects of screw position and purchase.

A little known anterior approach to atlantoaxial fusion was originally described by Barbour (173). A bilateral approach to the anterior aspect of the atlantoaxial joints is performed as described by Whitesides and Kelly (174). Dissection is carried out in the upper cervical spine at the level of the mastoid process coursing inferiorly along the border of the sternocleidomastoid. Dissection continues posterior to the sternocleidomastoid muscle and the carotid sheath, ele-

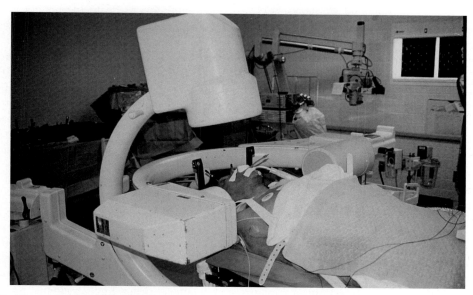

FIG. 28. Preoperative position of biplanar fluoroscopy used to obtain concurrent anteroposterior (AP) and lateral images during placement of anterior odontoid screw fixation.

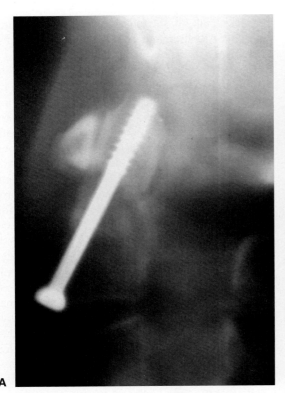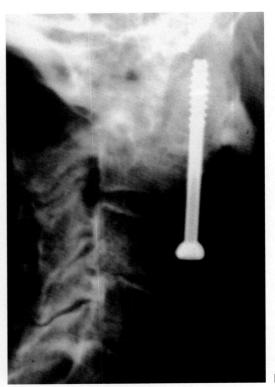

A   B

FIG. 29. A: Anterior odontoid screw fixation for a type II dens fracture in an elderly male. **B:** Insufficient bony purchase of the screw along the anterior cortex in an osteoporotic elderly male contributed to failure of fixation.

vating these structures anteriorly to expose the prevertebral fascia of the upper cervical spine and lateral masses. Once the lateral masses of C1 and C2 with their articulation are identified, the articular surface is curetted and bone is grafted as needed by making sure that one stays anterior to the intertransverse process membrane, which will protect the vertebral artery just posterior to it. Transarticular screws are then placed using a cannulated screw technique. Cortical screws, 3.5 mm in size, are placed tangentially from lateral to medial, directed 25 degrees inferiorly in the coronal plane and 10 degrees posteriorly in the sagittal plane, with the starting point located at the anterior base of the transverse process of the atlas. Guidewire placement is first done and radiographic evaluation follows to ensure proper positioning. Indications for such a bilateral exposure are few. The technique is reserved for complex nonunions of the odontoid or previous atlantoaxial fusions.

FRACTURES OF THE AXIS

Traumatic spondylolisthesis of the axis, or hangman's fracture, has long been a matter of both medical and judicial interest. Although now most commonly associated with motor vehicle accidents, this lesion was first described, studied, and indeed sought after in judicial hangings.

Judicial hanging has been a recognized form of capital punishment over the millennia. The historical pronounce-

ment "hanged by the neck until dead" gave little in terms of specific procedural instructions, with the result that death came by a variety of mechanisms and at widely varying rates. With a posterior, or suboccipital, noose, death came slowly by asphyxiation and at times required the hurried executioner to expedite matters by hanging weight from the victim's legs or perhaps standing on the condemned's shoulders. Furthermore, death was not always certain, and it was common for friends and loved ones to rapidly cut down the victim in an attempt at resuscitation.

Later efforts at increasing the efficiency of hanging included the introduction of the long drop. Experiments at various drop distances yielded a variety of deadly results, including decapitation, and subsequent efforts were made to devise appropriate drop height tables based on body weight (175,176). It was soon observed, however, that only with submental knot placement did one obtain an expeditious and efficient form of capital punishment.

In 1890, Paterson (177) examined the cervical spine of a man hanged with submental knot placement and reported bilateral interarticularis fractures of the axis. Wood-Jones (178) in 1913 reported two distinct fracture patterns incurred by hanging. He noted that both basilar skull fracture and fracture dislocation of the axis with cord transection resulted from submental knot placement. Subsequently, he and others recommended that English judicial hangings be performed with submental knots. Marshall (179,180) concurred and furthermore invented a collar that held the knot in this position during hanging.

Today, most traumatic spondylolistheses of the axis occur during motor vehicle accidents or falls (181). Schneider et al. (182) in 1965 noted the similarity of the lesions incurred in vehicular accidents to those of the hangman's noose and coined the term *hangman's fractures.* Garber (183) in 1964 chose the less colorful but more descriptive term *traumatic spondylolisthesis of the axis.*

Despite the ominous term *hangman's fracture,* most traumatic spondylolistheses of the axis are not complicated by neurologic compromise or death. The occurrence of cord transection is related to the mechanism of injury. Judicial hanging produces violent hyperextension-distraction forces that fracture the neural arch of the axis, disrupt the C2-C3 disc, and transect the spinal cord. While similar fractures of the neural arch and ligamentous injuries can be incurred in civilian injuries, they are rarely associated with the distraction required for cord transection. Furthermore, in the majority of cases they are canal expansive injuries, thus making neurologic compromise an infrequent complication.

The symptoms and signs of traumatic spondylolisthesis of the axis are nonspecific. The diagnosis should be suspected in any patient presenting with a history of the appropriate mechanism of injury. Most awake patients complain of suboccipital discomfort, neck pain and stiffness, and possibly apprehension or subjective neck instability (39). Occasionally, patients complain of occipital neuralgia (184). Many patients have facial or scalp contusions, abrasions, lacerations, and fracture. The presence of facial, head, or neck trauma should alert the physician to the possibility of a C2 fracture or other cervical spine injury. Neurologic signs are infrequent, but may include a spectrum from extremity paresthesias, to transient hemiparesis, to tetraplegia (185).

Associated injuries of the cervical spine are common. Most common are fractures of the atlas and odontoid fractures (184). Fractures of the lower cervical spine also commonly occur. Concomitant fractures of the thoracic and lumbar spine are also reported (184,186). Severe head, chest, and multiple injury patterns are also commonly seen (185). Mortality can occur secondary to the axis fracture or associated injuries (185,187).

Classification of traumatic spondylolisthesis of the axis has been well accepted in the literature. It is a three-part classification system originated by Effendi et al. (185) in 1981, and subsequently modified by Levine and Edwards (181) in 1985 (Fig. 30). Type I fractures are characterized by little or no fracture displacement (less than 3 mm) without significant angulation. It is a fracture bilaterally through the pars intraarticularis that is pathognomonic for these injuries. Levine and Edwards' review indicated that this type of fracture resulted most likely from hyperextension and axial loading and was associated with other fractures of the upper cervical spine including atlas fractures, Jefferson fractures, fractures of the lateral mass of the atlas, and odontoid fractures. The degree of trauma is typically not severe enough to

disrupt the intervening disc at C2-3 or compromise anterior or posterior longitudinal ligaments.

Type II fractures in the Effendi classification system are those with greater than 3 mm of displacement. Displacement is measured by the distance between the posteroinferior body of C2 with respect to the posterosuperior body of C3. Angulation also occurs at the C2-3 disc space, indicating disc injury and significant posterior longitudinal ligament injury (188). The mechanism of injury responsible for this subtype is initial hyperextension as in a sudden deceleration force in a motor vehicle accident with fracture of the bilateral pars intraarticularis followed by sudden secondary flexion forces that disrupt the C2-3 disc space and tear the posterior longitudinal ligament. The sudden flexion force can also produce an associated compression fracture of the anterosuperior end plate of C3. Significant flexion and anterior translation force also strips the anterior longitudinal ligament off the anterior portions of the C3 vertebral body, allowing for translation to occur.

Levine and Edwards' (181) modification of the Effendi classification system occurs with these type II fractures. They noted that a subset of these type II fractures termed type IIA result in significant angulation of the axis without noticeable displacement. The angulation is pivoted on an intact anterior longitudinal ligament with gross disruption of C2-3 disc space and posterior longitudinal ligament. The presumed mechanism of injury is flexion distraction to allow for failure intention of the posterior bony neural arch with subsequent secondary failure of disc and ligamentous structures. An intact anterior longitudinal ligament, therefore, upon providing longitudinal traction prevents gross displacement of the C2 body from the C3 body, but increases the angulation noted.

The final classification subtype is that known as type III, in which there is not only a bilateral interarticularis fracture of the body of C2 but also anterior facet joint dislocation, which could be unilateral or bilateral in nature and is associated with significant displacement. Several subtypes of this fracture have been noted by Levine and Rhyne (188) and can involve fractures within the pars interarticularis or through the posterior elements in the lamina and typically is associated with a combined mechanism of injuries, with flexion distraction producing the dislocation of the facet joints, and at some point a hyperextension injury causing the bony element fracture posteriorly. With this injury comes both posterior longitudinal ligament and anterior longitudinal ligament injuries, and attempts at closed reduction via ligamentotaxis are significant enough to reduce the dislocated facets. It is destined to failure. These fractures are extremely unstable and require careful monitoring during initial evaluation. Significant bony variations to these fracture patterns can occur, and CT evaluation of each injury is prudent to minimize underestimation of the degree of injury as seen in Fig. 31. In what appeared to be an innocuous, low-energy type I injury, CT scan revealed that the fracture line consisted of a unilateral pars defect with a fracture of the body of C2 anterior to

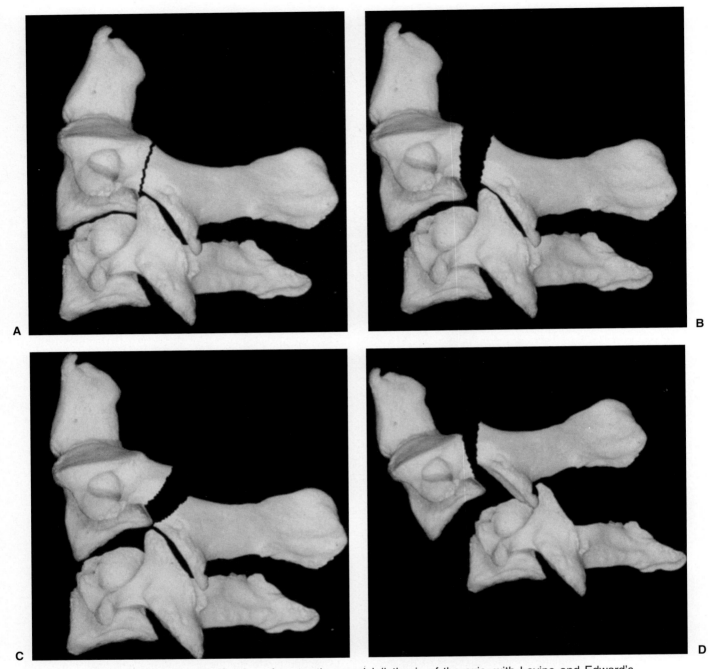

FIG. 30. Effendi's classification of traumatic spondylolisthesis of the axis, with Levine and Edward's modifications. **A:** Type I: pars interarticularis fracture with less than 3 mm of displacement and no angulation. **B:** Type II: pars interarticularis fracture with greater than 3 mm of translation and angulation. **C:** Type IIA (Levine and Edward's modification): fracture without translation exhibiting anterior angulation. **D:** Type III: fracture of the pars interarticularis with associated unilateral or bilateral facet dislocation of C2 or C3.

the isthmus. Such a fracture carries with it a greater degree of energy imparted to the upper cervical spine and should alert the physician to a higher incidence of noncontiguous spine injuries. In this example, evaluation of the cervicothoracic junction revealed a fracture dislocation of the lower subaxial spine. This fracture pattern is also one similar to those described by Burke and Harris (129) in 1989 and subsequently by Starr and Eismont (189) in 1993. When an atypical pattern exists, and the fracture line extends unilaterally or bilaterally into the body of C2, anterior displacement of the hangman's fracture results in the cervicocranium moving, anteriorly draping the spinal cord against the remaining

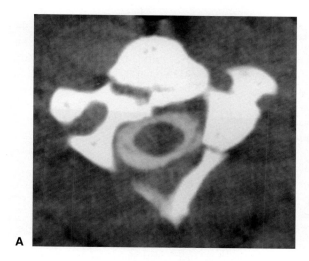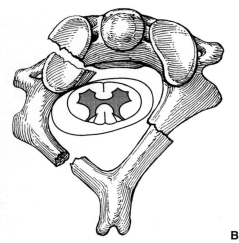

FIG. 31. A: CT axial image of a hangman's fracture variant as described by Starr (189). **B:** Line drawing of potential spinal cord compression, with displacement of such a variant of a hangman's fracture.

bony portion of the body of C2. This in turn causes significant canal and neural impingement, unlike a typical hangman's fracture where the total cross-sectional area of the canal is increased by the displacement (187).

Incomplete injuries to the axis can also result in posterior laminar fractures or lateral mass fractures, which are isolated and best evaluated on CT scans. Although typically stable fractures, flexion and extension x-rays in a cooperative patient are necessary to determine if instability is present and will likely dictate the duration of external immobilization. Burke and Harris (129) elucidated two distinct types of body fractures of the axis. The first fracture is a hyperextension avulsion injury to the inferoanterior aspect of the body of C2, commonly occurring in the elderly or osteoporotic patient. There is minimal soft tissue injury and it represents a relatively benign process. This hyperextension tear and drop avulsion fracture ruptured from the pull of the anterior longitudinal ligament and has a vertical height that Burke found to be equal to or greater than the horizontal length of the fracture fragment. This is in distinction to a higher energy of injury resulting from a hyperextension fracture dislocation through the body with significant soft tissue abnormality disruption of the C2-3 disc space with a transverse fracture whose width is greater than the fracture's vertical height. This high-energy injury is significantly unstable and warrants close attention.

Treatment

Treatment of traumatic spondylolisthesis of the axis is facilitated by understanding the pathomechanics behind the injury. Effendi et al. (185) were the first to indicate a correlation between fracture types and subsequent treatment. The Levine and Edwards modification, however, with a complete discussion of the differences in mechanisms of injury, helps to delineate the rationale behind individual fracture patterns

and their treatment. Prior to these classification systems, a variety of treatment protocols were used with variable results. These ranged from prolonged skeletal traction to primary surgical stabilization in all cases (182,190). The treatment has become more consistent with the knowledge of the mode of injury for each subtype, and given the high rate of neurologic preservation with these injuries, close treatment has resulted in significant success.

Type I injuries are considered by most clinicians to be stable with minimal displacement. Flexion and extension x-rays can be utilized to determine the exact nature of the injury and ensure that it is in fact a type I injury. With this knowledge, immobilization can be carried out in a cervical orthosis, and union is achieved by 3 months. Levine and Edwards note, however, that patients who are obese or who have short necks may experience skin decubiti and irritation from cervical orthoses, and in these cases a halo vest may be indicated.

Type II fractures are associated with significantly more soft tissue trauma and instability. Fractures with significant displacement and angulation need to be immediately immobilized in a cervical orthosis upon arrival at the emergency room to prevent iatrogenic injury and further displacement. Their classification based on x-rays then needs to be determined as to a type II or type IIA pattern. Fractures that are considered type II exemplify displacement secondary to the secondary flexion and compression forces on the head. Although hyperextension caused the bony element fracture, reduction maneuvers via cervical tongs and longitudinal traction need to be performed with a slight extension moment to reverse the deforming forces causing the displacement and angulation. This is best accomplished with the patient in the supine position with a roll placed under the midcervical spine to maintain an extension moment. Generally, 1 to 2 weeks of longitudinal traction is needed to maintain reduction, and weights of 4.5 to 9.0 kg have been advocated

(181,191). Care must be taken, however, in not progressing too quickly to halo-vest immobilization. Redisplacement can occur if early healing is not sufficient. To avoid this complication in patients who have significant fracture displacements of greater than 4 to 5 mm or 10 to 15 degrees of angulation as advocated by Levine and Edwards (181), prolonged longitudinal traction will likely be necessary. To determine whether or not the length of cervical traction is sufficient, the patient can be maintained in the supine position with the traction weights removed, and after a sufficient period of time a lateral x-ray is obtained to determine whether or not redisplacement or angulation has occurred. If the fracture appears stable, halo-vest application can ensue with x-rays obtained in the upright position. In their study, Levine and Edwards noted that despite cervical traction for 4 to 6 weeks to maintain reduction, final healing revealed, on average, 3 mm of residual fracture translation and 4.5 degrees of angulation in 16 of 22 patients treated. Healing occurs with either short- or long-term traction, provided attention to detail is maintained (181,184,186). Levine and Rhyne (188) recommended that immediate halo application be considered when translation is less than 4.5 mm or angulation is less than 15 degrees.

Type IIA injuries as previously stated result from a different mechanism of injury and consequently require a slightly varied treatment protocol. The fractures are primarily flexion-distraction injuries with an intact anterior longitudinal ligament. Therefore, closed reduction with longitudinal traction, as stated earlier, results in accentuation of the angular deformity. Stable in translation and unstable in angulation, these fractures are treated very efficiently in immediate halo-vest application with an extension and slight compression. Further reduction will be seen in time as gravity and the weight of the halo vest continue to compress the fracture.

Type III injuries are extremely unstable and are complex in that the posterior element fracture and displacement are associated with gross dislocation of one or both facet joints. Given this degree of injury and loss of ligamentotaxis, closed reduction is virtually impossible, and open reduction of the facet joints is recommended. Manual reduction of the facet joints at C2-3 is then followed by posterior spinous process or sublaminar wiring of C2-4 from C1 to C3 depending on the integrity of the posterior elements. This is followed by halo-vest immobilization to treat the pars interarticularis fracture as one would in a type I injury. Levine and Rhyne (188) note that, rarely, when a unilateral facet dislocation is associated with the pars fracture, closed reduction may be attempted with halo immobilization.

Traumatic spondylolisthesis is best treated by thorough understanding of the mechanism of injury. It is clearly not the result of pure hyperextension forces as was originally thought with submental nondisplacement and judicial hangings. A high success rate with nonoperative treatment and relatively low nonunion rates of 5% to 6% are easily obtained with a low rate of neurologic complication if the above principles are followed (181,184,185,188). At the completion of healing, long-term follow-up should include flexion and extension x-rays to monitor the viability of the C2-3 disc space. Significant degeneration is possible as well as instability and nonunion.

REFERENCES

1. Alker GJ Jr, Oh YS, Leslie EV. High cervical spine and craniocervical junction injuries in fatal traffic accidents. *Orthop Clin North Am* 1978;9:1003–1010.
2. Bell C. Surgical observations. *Middlesex Hosp J* 1817;4:469–470.
3. Nobel ER, Smoker WRK. The forgotten condyle: the appearance, morphology, and classification of occipital condyle fractures. *AJNR* 1996;17:507–513.
4. Bucholz RW, Burkhead WZ. The pathological anatomy of fatal atlantooccipital dislocations. *J Bone Joint Surg* 1979;61A:248–250.
5. Goldstein, SJ, Woodring JA, Young AB. Occipital condyle fracture associated with cervical spine injury. *Surg Neurol* 1982;17:350–352.
6. Bloom AI, Neeman Z, Slasky BS, et al. Fracture of the occipital condyles and associated craniocervical ligament injury, incidence, CT imaging, and implications. *Clin Radiol* 1997;52(3):198–202.
7. Cottalorda J, Allard D, Dutour N. Fracture of the occipital condyle. *J Pediatr Orthop* 1996;5B(1):61–63.
8. Stroobants J, Fidlers L, Storms J, Klaes R, Dua G, Van Hoye M. High cervical pain and impairment of skull mobility as only symptoms of occipital condyle fracture. *J Neurosurgery* 1994;81:137–138.
9. Bolender N, Cromwell LD, Wendling L. Fracture of the occipital condyle. *AJR* 1978;131:729–731.
10. Urculo E, Arrazola M, Arrazola M Jr, Riu I, Moyua A. Delayed glossopharyngeal and vagus nerve paralysis following occipital condyle fracture. *J Neurosurg* 1996;84:522–525.
11. Wessels LS. Fracture of the occipital condyle. *S Afr J Surg* 1990;28: 155–156.
12. Anderson P, Montesano P. Morphology and treatment of occipital condyle fractures. *Spine* 1988;13:731–736.
13. Bozboga M, Unal F, Hepgul K, Izgi N, Turantan I, Turker K. Fracture of the occipital condyle. *Spine* 1992;17:1119–1121.
14. S'harma BS, Mahagan RK, Bhaitia S, Khosla VK. Collet-Sicard syndrome after closed head injury. *Clin Neurol Neurosurg* 1994;96:197–198.
15. Bulas DI, Fetz CR, Johnson DC. Traumatic atlantooccipital dislocations in children. *Radiology* 1993;188:155–158.
16. Hosong N, Yonenobu K, Kawagoe K, et al. Traumatic anterior atlantooccipital dislocation. *Spine* 1992;18:786–790.
16a. Bell HS. Paralysis of both arms from injury of the upper portion of the pyramidal decussation. "Cruciate paralysis." *J Neurosurg* 1970;33: 376–380.
17. Bunders PA, Rechtine GR, Bohlman HH. Upper cervical spine injuries. *Orthop Rev* 1984;13:23–32.
18. Simeone FA, Lyness SS. Vascular complications of upper cervical spine injuries. *Orthop Clin North Am* 1978;9(4):1029–1038.
19. Boldrey CE. Role of atlantoid compression in etiology of internal carotid thrombosis. *J Neurosurg* 1956;13:127–139.
20. Dickman CA, Papadopoulos SM, Sonntag VKH. Traumatic occipitoatlantal dislocations. *J Spinal Disord* 1993;6:300–313.
21. Woodring J. Traumatic atlantooccipital dislocations with survival. *Am J Radiol* 1981;137:21–24.
22. Davis D, Bohlman H, Walker AE, Fisher R, Robinson R. The pathological findings in fatal craniospinal injuries. *J Neurosurg* 1971;34: 603–613.
23. Wholely MH, Bruwer AJ, Baker HL. The lateral roentgenogram of the neck. *Radiology* 1958;71:350–356.
24. Kathol MH, El-Khoury GY. Diagnostic imaging of cervical spine injuries. *Semin Spine Surg* 1996;8(1):2–18.
25. Wackenheim A. *Roentgen Diagnosis of the Craniovertebral Region*, 1st ed. New York: Springer-Verlag, 1974.
26. Harris JH Jr, Carson GC, Wagner LK, Kerr N. Radiologic diagnosis of traumatic occipital vertebral dissociation: normal occipitovertebral relationships on lateral radiographs of supine subjects. *Am J Radiol* 1994;162:881–886.
27. Powers B, Miller MD, Kramer RS, Martinez S, Gehweiter JA. Traumatic anterior occipital dislocations. *Neurosurgery* 1979;4:12–17.

28. Karol LA, Sheffield EG, Crawford K, Moody MK, Browne RH. Reproducibility in the measurement of atlantooccipital instability in children with Down syndrome. *Spine* 1996;21(21):2463–2467.

29. Bundschub CV, Allen JB, Ross M, Poncer IS, Gudera SK. Magnetic resonance imaging of suspected atlantooccipital dislocation. *Spine* 1992;17:245–248.

30. Naso WB, Cure J, Cuddy BG. Retropharyngeal pseudomeningocele after atlantooccipital dislocation: report of two cases. *Neurosurgery* 1997;40(6):1288–1290.

31. Przybylski, GJ, Clyde BL, Fitz CR. Craniocervical junction subarachnoid hemorrhage associated with atlantooccipital dislocations. *Spine* 1996;21(5):1761–1768.

32. Traynelis VC, Marano GD, Dunker RO, et al. Traumatic atlantooccipital dislocations. Case report. *J Neurosurg* 1986;65:863–870.

33. Scott EW, Haid RW, Pease D. Type I fractures of the odontoid process. Implications for atlantooccipital instability. *J Neurosurg* 1990;72:488–492.

34. Georgopoulos G, Pizzutillo PD, Lee MS. Occipitoatlanto instability in children. *J Bone Joint Surg* 1987;69A:429–436.

35. Wertheim SB, Bohlman HH. Occipitocervical fusion indications, techniques, and long term results in thirteen patients. *J Bone Joint Surg* 1987;69A:833–836.

36. Ransford AO, Crockard HA, Poro JL, et al. Craniocervical instability treated by contoured loop fixation. *J Bone Joint Surg* 1986;68A:193–197.

37. Roy-Camille R, Saillart G, Mazel C. Internal fixation of the unstable cervical spine by a post osteosynthesis with plates and screws. In: Sherk HH, Dunn EJ, Eisment FJ, et al. (eds). *The Cervical Spine,* 2nd ed. The Cervical Spine Research Society. Philadelphia: JB Lippincott, 1989:390–403.

38. Smith MD, Anderson P, Grady MS. Occipitocervical arthrodesis using contoured plate fixation. *Spine* 1993;18(14):1984–1990.

39. Vaccaro AR, Cotler JM. Traumatic injuries of the adult upper cervical spine. In: An HS, Simpson JM (eds). *Surgery of the Cervical Spine.* London: Martin Dunitz, 1994:227–266.

40. Sponseller PD, Cass JR. Atlantooccipital fusion for dislocation in children with neurologic preservation. *Spine* 1997;22(3):344–347.

41. Coutts MB. Atlanto-epistropheal subluxations. *Arch Surg* 1934;29:297–311.

42. Fielding JW, Hawkins RJ. Atlantoaxial rotatory fixation. *J Bone Joint Surg* 1977;59A:37–44.

43. Jacobson G, Adler DC. Examination of the atlantoaxial joint following injury: with particular emphasis on rotational subluxation. *AJR* 1956;76:1081–1094.

44. Corner ES. Rotatory dislocations of the atlas. *Ann Surg* 1907;45:9–26.

45. Leventhal MR, Maguire JK, Christian CA. Atlantoaxial rotary subluxation in ankylosing spondylitis. *Spine* 1990;15:1374–1376.

46. Phillips WA, Hensinger RN. The management of rotatory atlantoaxial subluxation in children. *J Bone Joint Surg* 1989;71A:664–668.

47. Robertson PA, Swan AP. Traumatic bilateral rotatory facet dislocation of the atlas on axis. *Spine* 1992;17:1252–1253.

48. Grisel P. Enucleation de l'atlas et torticolis naso-pharyngien. *Presse Med* 1930;38:50–53.

49. Parke WW, Rothman RH. The pharyngovertebral veins: an anatomical rationale for Grisel's syndrome. *J Bone Joint Surg* 1984;66A:568–574.

50. Fielding JW, Francis WR, Hawkins RJ, Hensinger RN. Atlantoaxial rotatory deformity. *Semin Spine Surg* 1991;3(1):33–38.

51. Jones ET, Loder RT, Hensinger RN. Fractures of the spine. In: Rockwood CA, Wilkins KE, Beatty JH (eds). *Fractures in Children,* 4th ed. Philadelphia: Lippincott-Raven, 1996:1047–1052.

52. Levine AM, Edward CC. Traumatic lesions of occipitoatlantoaxial complex. *Clin Orthop* 1989;239:53–68.

53. Wortzman G, Dewar FP. Rotatory fixation of the atlantoaxial joint: rotational atlantoaxial subluxation. *Radiology* 1968;90:479–487.

54. Sherk HH. Lesions of the atlas and axis. *Clin Orthop* 1975;109:33–41.

55. Fielding JW, Cochran GVB, Lawsing JF III, Hohl M. Tears of the transverse ligament of the atlas. A clinical and biomechanical study. *J Bone Joint Surg* 1974;56A:1683–1691.

56. Mazzara JT, Fielding JW. Effect of C1-C2 rotation on canal size. *Clin Orthop* 1988;237:115–119.

57. Fielding JW. Cineroentgenography of the normal cervical spine. *J Bone Joint Surg* 1957;39:1280–1288.

58. Price AE. Unique aspects of pediatric spine surgery. In: Errico TJ, Bauer RD, Waugh T (eds). *Spinal Trauma,* 2nd ed. Philadelphia: JB Lippincott, 1991:581–625.

59. Schneider RC, Schemm GW. Vertebral artery insufficiency in acute and chronic spinal trauma. *J Neurosurg* 1961;18:348–360.

60. Werne S. Studies in spontaneous atlas dislocations. *Acta Orthop Scand* 1957;23:1–150.

61. Wong DA, Mack RP, Craijnile TK. Traumatic atlantoaxial dislocation without fracture of the odontoid. *Spine* 1991;16:587–589.

62. Fielding JW, Stillwell WT, Chynn KY, Spyropoulos EC. Use of computed tomography for the diagnosis of atlantoaxial rotatory fixation. *J Bone Joint Surg* 1978;60A:1102–1104.

63. Fielding JW, Hawkins RJ, Ratzan SA. Spine fusion for atlantoaxial instability. *J Bone Joint Surg* 1976;58A:400–407.

64. Crockard HA, Rogers MA. Open reduction of traumatic atlantoaxial rotatory dislocation with use of the extreme lateral approach. *J Bone Joint Surg* 1996;78A:431–435.

65. MacEwen GD, King AGS, Bonnarens F, Heinrich SD. Fusion techniques for pediatric disorders. In: Cotler JM, Cotler HB (eds). *Spinal Fusion.* New York: Springer-Verlag, 1990:247–283.

66. Altongy JF, Fielding JW. Combined atlantoaxial and occipitoatlantal rotatory subluxation. *J Bone Joint Surg* 1990;72A:923–926.

67. Clark CR, Kathol MH, Walsh T, El-Khoury. Atlantoaxial rotatory fixation with compensatory counter occipitoatlantal sublimation. *Spine* 1986;11:1048–1050.

68. Sassard WR, Heinig CR, Pitts WR. Posterior atlantoaxial dislocation without fracture. Case report with successful conservative treatment. *J Bone Joint Surg* 1974;56A:625–628.

69. Moskovich R, Crocard HA. Post-traumatic atlantoaxial subluxation and myelopathy. Efficacy of anterior decompression. *Spine* 1990;15:442–447.

70. Hadley MN, Dickman CA, Browner CM, Sonntag VKH. Acute traumatic atlas fractures: management and long term outcome. *Neurosurgery* 1988;23:31–35.

71. Landelis CD, Van Peteghem PK. Fractures of the atlas: classification, treatment and morbidity. *Spine* 1987;13:450–452.

72. Segal LS, Grimm JO, Stauffer ES. Nonunion of fractures of the atlas. *J Bone Joint Surg* 1987;69A:1423–1434.

73. Eismont FJ, Bohlman HH. Posterior atlantooccipital dislocation with fractures of the atlas and odontoid process. Review of a case with survival. *J Bone Joint Surg* 1978;60A:397–399.

74. Kesterson L, Benzel E, Orrison W, Coleman J. Evaluation and treatment of atlas burst fractures (Jefferson fractures). *J Neurosurg* 1991;75:213–220.

75. Panjabi MM, Oda T, Crisco JJ, Oxland TR, Katz L, Nolte LP. Experimental study of atlas injuries I: Biomechanical analysis of their mechanisms and fracture patterns. *Spine* 16:S460–S465.

76. Dvorak J, Schneider E, Siadinger P, Rahn B. Biomechanics of the craniovertebral region. The alar and transverse ligaments. *J Orthop Res* 1988;6:452–461.

77. Sherk HH, Nicholson JT. Fractures of the atlas. *J Bone Joint Surg* 1970;52A:1017–1024.

78. Day GL, Jacoby CG, Dolan KD. Basilar invagination resulting from untreated Jefferson's fracture. *AJR* 1979;133:529–531.

79. Jefferson G. Fractures of the first cervical vertebra. *Br Med J* 1927;2:153–157.

80. McGuire RA, Harkey HL. Primary treatment of unstable Jefferson's fractures. *J Spinal Disord* 1995;8(3):233–236.

81. Levine AM, Edwards CC. Fracture of the atlas. *J Bone Joint Surg* 1991;73A:680–691.

82. Levine AM, Edwards CC. Treatment of injuries in the C1-C2 complex. *Orthop Clin North Am* 1986;17:31–44.

83. Stewart GC, Gehweller JA, Lalb RH, Martinez S. Horizontal fracture of the anterior arch of the atlas. *Radiology* 1977;122:349–352.

84. Spence KF, Decker S, Sell KW. Bursting atlantal fracture associated with rupture of the transverse ligament. *J Bone Joint Surg* 1970;52A:543–549.

85. Heller JG, Viroslav S, Hudson T. Jefferson fractures. The role of magnification artifact in assessing transverse ligament integrity. *J Spinal Disord* 1993;6:392–396.

86. Oda T, Panjabi MM, Crisco JJ, Osland TR, Katz L, Nolte LP. Experimental study of atlas injuries II: relevance to clinical diagnosis and treatment. *Spine* 1991;16:S466–S473.

87. Dickman CA, Mamourian A, Sonntag VK, Drayer BP. Magnetic resonance imaging of the transverse atlantal ligament for the evaluation of atlantoaxial instability. *J Neurosurg* 1991;75:221–227.

88. Levine AM, Edwards CC. Traumatic lesions of the occipitoatlantoaxial complex. *Clin Orthop* 1989;239:53–68.

89. Lipson SJ. Fractures of the atlas associated with fractures of the odontoid process and transverse ligament ruptures. *J Bone Joint Surg* 1977;59:940–942.

90. Wilber GW, Peters JG, Likavec MJ. Surgical techniques in cervical spine surgery. In: Errico TJ, Bauer RD, Waugh T (eds). *Spinal Trauma*. Philadelphia: JB Lippincott, 1991:145–158.

91. Bohlman HH. Acute fractures and dislocations of the cervical spine. *J Bone Joint Surg* 1979;61A:1119–1142.

92. Rogers MA, Ransford AO. Osteoplastic repair of the atlas. *J Bone Joint Surg* 1992;74B:880–882.

93. Kahanovitz N, Mehringer MC, Johansen PH. Intracranial entrapment of the atlas complicating an untreated fracture of the posterior arch of the atlas. *J Bone Joint Surg* 1981;63A:831–832.

94. Macman DJ, Larson SJ. Management of odontoid fractures. *Neurosurgery* 1982;11:471–476.

95. Moradian WA, Fietti VG Jr, Cochran GB, Fielding JW, Yaig J. Fractures of the odontoid. A laboratory and clinical study of mechanism. *Orthop Clin North Am* 1978;9:985–1001.

96. Schatzker J, Rorabeck CH, Waddell JA. Fractures of the odontoid process of the axis: an analysis of 37 cases. *J Bone Joint Surg* 1971;53B:392–405.

97. Schweigel JF. Halo-thoracic brace management of odontoid fractures. *Spine* 1979;4:192–194.

98. Chutkan NB, King AG, Harris MB. Odontoid fractures: evaluation and management. *J Am Acad Orthop Surg* 1997;5(4):199–204.

99. Sherk HH. Fractures of the atlas and odontoid process. *Orthop Clin North Am* 1978;9(4):973–984.

100. Pepin JW, Bourne RB, Hawkins RJ. Odontoid fractures with special reference to the elderly parent. *Clin Orthop* 1985;193:178–183.

101. Southwick WO. Management of fractures of the dens. *J Bone Joint Surg* 1980;62A:482–486.

102. Anderson LD, Clark CR. Fractures of the odontoid process of the axis. In: Sherk HH, Dunn EJ, Eismont FJ, et al. (eds). *The Cervical Spine*, 2nd ed. Cervical Spine Research Society. Philadelphia: JB Lippincott, 1989:325–343.

103. Duncan RW, Esses SI. Dens fracture: specifications and management. *Semin Spine Surg* 1996;8(1):19–27.

104. Bedman DA, Hummel J. Odontoid process fractures at the Hamilton General Hospital. Presented at McMaster University Orthopaedic Research Day, Hamilton, Ontario, Canada, April 1990.

105. Hanigan WC, Powell FC, Elwood PW, Henderson JP. Odontoid fractures in elderly patients. *J Neurosurg* 1993;78:32–35.

106. Sherk HH, Schut L, Lane JM. Fractures and dislocations of the cervical spine in children. *Orthop Clin North Am* 1976;7:593–604.

107. Bailey DK. The normal cervical spine in infants and children. *Radiology* 1952;59:712–719.

108. McRae DL. The significance of abnormalities of the cervical spine. *AJR* 1960;84:3–25.

109. Michaels L, Prevost MJ, Crang DF. Pathologic changes in a case of os odontoideum. *J Bone Joint Surg* 1969;51A:965–972.

110. Fielding JW, Hersinger RN, Hawkins RJ. Os odontoideum. *J Bone Joint Surg* 1980;624:376–383.

111. Ricciardi JE, Kaufer H, Louis DS. Acquired os odontoideum following acute ligament injury. *J Bone Joint Surg* 1976;58A:410–412.

112. Shirasaki N, Okada K, Hosono N, Ono K. Os odontoideum with posterior atlantoaxial instability. *Spine* 1991;16(7):706–715.

113. Forlin E, Herscovici D, Bowen JR. Understanding the os odontoideum. *Orthop Rev* 1992:1441–1447.

114. Spierings EH, Braakman R. The management of os odontoideum: analysis of thirty-seven cases. *J Bone Joint Surg* 1982;64B:422–428.

115. Parke WW. Development of the spine. In: Rothman RH, Simeone FA (eds). *The Spine*, vol 1, 3rd ed. Philadelphia: WB Saunders, 1992:3–33.

116. Althoff B, Goldie IF. The arterial supply of the odontoid process of the axis. *Acta Orthop Scand* 1977;48:622–629.

117. Althoff B. Fracture of the odontoid process: an experimental and clinical study. *Acta Orthop Scand Suppl* 1979;177:1–95.

118. Schiff DM, Parke WW. The arterial supply of the odontoid process. *J Bone Joint Surg* 1973;55A:1450–1456.

119. Schatzker J, Rombeck CH, Waddell JP. Nonunion of the odontoid process. *Clin Orthop* 1975;108:127–137.

120. Schatzker J, Rorabeck CH, Waddell JP. Fracture of the dens: analysis of thirty-seven cases. *J Bone Joint Surg* 1971;53B:392–405.

121. Anderson LD, D'Alonzo RT. Fractures of the odontoid process of the axis. *J Bone Joint Surg* 1974;56A:1663–1674.

122. Barros TP, Fielding JW. Traumatic spondylolisthesis of the axis with unusual distraction. *J Bone Joint Surg* 1990;72A:124–125.

123. Hadley MN, Browner CM, Liu SS, Sonntag VH. New subtype of acute odontoid fractures (type IIA). *Neurosurgery* 1988;22:67–71.

124. Johnson JE, Yang PJ, Seeger JF. Vertical fracture of the odontoid: case report. *Neurosurgery* 1996;38(1):200–202.

125. Kokkino AJ, Lazio BE, Perin NI. Vertical fracture of the odontoid process: case report. *Neurosurgery* 1996;38(1):200–202.

126. Husby J, Sorensen K. Fracture of the odontoid process of the axis. *Acta Orthop Scand* 1974;45:182–192.

127. Francavilla TL, Melisi J, Chappell ET. Type I odontoid fractures. *Neurosurgery* 1989;25:481.

128. Ryan MD, Taylor TF. Odontoid fractures: a rational approach to treatment. *J Bone Joint Surg* 1982;64B:416–421.

129. Burke JT, Harris JH. Acute injuries of the axis vertebrae. *Skeletal Radiol* 1989;18:335–346.

130. Harris JH, Edeiken-Monroe BH. *The Radiology of Acute Cervical Spine Trauma*, 2nd ed. Baltimore: Williams & Wilkins, 1987.

131. Rubinstein D, Escott EJ, Mestek MF. Computed tomographic scans of minimally displaced type II odontoid fractures. *J Trauma* 1996;40(2):204–210.

132. Green KA, Dickman CA, Marciano FF, Drabier J, Drayer BP, Sonntag VH. Transverse atlantal ligament disruption associated with odontoid fractures. *Spine* 1994;19:2307–2314.

133. McAfee PC. Cervical spine trauma. In: Froymoyer JW (ed). *The Adult Spine: Principles and Practice*. New York: Raven Press, 1991:1063–1106.

134. Craft DV, Cotler JM, Bauerle WB. A rational approach to the management of type II and type III odontoid fractures. Presented at the Annual Academy of Orthopaedic Surgeons Annual Meeting, Washington, DC, 1991.

135. Przybylski GJ, Welch WC. Longitudinal atlantoaxial dislocation with type III odontoid fracture. Case report. *J Neurosurg* 1996;84(4):666–670.

136. Bell W, Meyer P. Nonhalo/nonsurgical management of C1-C2 fractures. *Orthop Trans* 1983;7:481.

137. Clark CR, White AA. Fractures of the dens. *J Bone Joint Surg* 1985;67A:1340–1348.

138. Fujii E, Kobayashi K, Hirabayashi K. Treatment in fractures of the odontoid process. *Spine* 1988;13:604–609.

139. Apuzo MK, Heiden JS, Weis MH, Ackerson TT, Harvey JP, Kuze T. Acute fractures of the odontoid process. *J Neurosurg* 1978;48:85–91.

140. Hadley MN, Dickman CA, Browner CM, Sonntag VH. Acute axis fractures. A review of 229 cases. *J Neurosurg* 1989;71:642–647.

141. Dunn ME, Seljeskog EL. Experience in the management of odontoid process injuries. Analysis of 128 cases. *Neurosurgery* 1986;18:306–310.

142. Blockley NJ, Purser DW. Fractures of the odontoid process of the axis. *J Bone Joint Surg* 1956;38B:794–816.

143. Ekonj CU, Schwartz ML, Tator CH, Rowed DW. Odontoid fracture: management with early mobilization using a halo device. *Neurosurgery* 1981;9:631–637.

143a. Bednar DA, Parikh J, Hummel H. Management of type II odontoid process fractures in geriatric patients: a prospective study of sequential cohorts with attention to survivorship. *J Spinal Disord* 1995;8(2):166–169.

144. Meyer PR Jr, Cotler HB. Fusion techniques for traumatic injuries. In: Cotler JM, Cotler HB (eds). *Spine Fusion: Science and Techniques*. New York: Springer-Verlag, 1990:189–246.

145. Gallie WE. Fractures and dislocations of the cervical spine. *Am J Surg* 1939;46:495–499.

146. Brooks AL, Jenkins EB. Atlantoaxial arthrodesis by wedge compression method. *J Bone Joint Surg* 1978;60A:279–284.

147. Callahan RA, Rockwood R, Green B. Modified Brooks fusion for an os odontoideum associated with an incomplete posterior arch of the atlas. *Spine* 1983;8:107–108.

148. Cybulski GR, Stowe JL, Crowell RM. Use of Halifax interlaminar clamps for posterior C1-C2 arthrodesis. *Neurosurgery* 1988;22:429–431.

149. Holness RO, Huestis W, Howes WJ. Posterior stabilization with an interlaminar clamp in cervical injuries. Technical note and review of long term experience. *Neurosurgery* 1984;14:318–322.

150. Miz G. Cervical spine instability and biomechanics of treatment. In: Errico TJ, Bauer RD, Waugh T (eds). *Spinal Trauma,* 2nd ed. Philadelphia: JB Lippincott, 1991:123–140.
151. Hajek PD, Lipka J, Hartline P, et al. Biomechanical study of C1-2 posterior arthrodesis techniques. *Spine* 1993;18:173–177.
152. Hanley EH, Harvell JC. Immediate postoperative stability of the atlantoaxial articulation: a biomechanical study comparing simple midline wiring and the Gallie and Brooks procedures. *J Spinal Disord* 1992;5:306–310.
153. Sherk HH, Snyder BJ. An exceptional case analysis of upper posterior weak fusion. *Orthop Trans* 1979;3:125.
154. Magerl F, Seeman T. Stable posterior fusion of the axis and atlas by transarticular screw fixation. In: Kehr P, Widner P (eds). *Cervical Spine.* Strasbourg: Springer-Verlag, 1987:322–327.
155. Grob D, Crisco JJ, Panjabi MM, Wang P, Dvorak J. Biomechanical evaluation of four different atlantoaxial fixation techniques. *Spine* 1992;17:480–490.
156. Montesano PX, Juach EC, Anderson PA, Benson DR, Hanson PB. Biomechanics of cervical spine internal fixation. *Spine* 1991;16:510–516.
157. McGuire RA Jr, Harkey HL. Modification of technique and results of atlantoaxial transfacet stabilization orthopedics. *Orthopedics* 1995;18:1029–1032.
158. Silveri CP, Vaccaro AR. Posterior atlantoaxial fixation: the Magerl screw technique. *Orthopaedics* 1998;21(4):1–5.
159. Apfelbaum RI. Screw fixation of the upper cervical spine, indications, and technique. *Contemp Neurosurg* 1994;16(7):1–8.
160. Coric D, Branch CL, Wilson JA, Robinson JC. Arteriovenous fistula as a complication of C1-C2 transarticular screw fixation. Case report and review of the literature. *J Neurosurg* 1996;85:340–343.
161. Jeanneret B, Magerl F. Primary posterior fusion C1-C2 in odontoid fractures: indication, technique, and results of transarticular screw fixation. *J Spinal Disord* 1992;5:464–475.
162. Foley KT, Smith MM. Image guided spine surgery. *Neurosurg Clin North Am* 1996;7(2):171–186.
163. Silveri CP, Foley KT, Vaccaro AR, Shah S, Garfin SR. Atlantoaxial transarticular screw fixation: risk assessment and bone morphology using an image guidance system. Presented at Cervical Spine Research Society 25th annual meeting, December 1997, Rancho Mirage, CA.
164. Bohler J. Anterior stabilization for acute fractures and nonunions of the dens. *J Bone Joint Surg* 1982;64A:18–27.
165. Nakanishi T, Sasaki T, Tokita N. Internal fixation for the odontoid fracture. *Orthop Trans* 1982;6:176.
166. Etter C, Coscia M, Jaberg H, Aebi M. Direct anterior fixation of the dens fractures with a cannulated screw system. *Spine* 1991;16(3):525–532.
167. Geisler FH, Cheng C, Poka A, Brumback RJ. Anterior screw fixation of posteriorly displaced type II odontoid fractures. *Neurosurgery* 1989;28:30–38.
168. Esses SI, Bednar DA. Screw fixation of odontoid fractures and nonunions. *Spine* 1991;16:483–485.
169. Chang KW, Liu YW, Cheng PGB, et al. One Herbert double threaded compression screw fixation of displaced type II odontoid fractures. *J Spinal Disord* 1994;7:62–69.
170. Graziano G, Jaggers C, Lee M, et al. A comparative study of fixation techniques for type II fractures of the odontoid process. *Spine* 1993;18:2383–2387.
171. Sasso R, Doherty BJ, Crawford MJ, et al. Biomechanics of odontoid fracture fixation. Comparison of one and two screw technique. *Spine* 1993;18:1950–1953.
172. Worsdorfer O, Arnad M, Neugebauer R. Problems of anterior screw fixation of odontoid process fractures. Presented at the Second Common Meeting of the European and American Sections of the Cervical Spine Research Society, June 1988, Marseilles, France.
173. Barbour JR. Screw fixation in fracture of the odontoid process. *S Aust Clin* 1971;5:20–24.
174. Whitesides TE Jr, Kelly RP. Lateral approach to the upper cervical spine for anterior fusion. *South Med J* 1966;59:879–883.
175. Hammond DN. On the proper method of executing the sentence of death by hanging. *Med Rec NY* 1882;22:426.
176. Haughton S. On hanging, considered from a mechanical and physiological point of view. *Philos Magazine J Sci* 1866;32(4th series):23.
177. Paterson AM. Fracture of the cervical vertebrae. *J Anat* 1890;24:ix.
178. Wood-Jones F. The ideal lesion produced by hanging. *Lancet* 1913;1:53.
179. Marshall JD. Letter to the editor. *Lancet* 1913;1:194.
180. Marshall JD. Letter to the editor: the executioner surgeon. *Br Med J* 1913;2:1340.
181. Levine AM, Edwards CC. The management of traumatic spondylolisthesis of the axis. *J Bone Joint Surg* 1985;67A:217–226.
182. Schneider RC, Livingston KE, Cave AE, et al. Hangman's fracture of the cervical spine. *J Neurosurg* 1965;22:141–154.
183. Garber JN. Abnormalities of the atlas and axis vertebra—congenital and traumatic. *J Bone Joint Surg* 1964;46A:1782–1791.
184. Francis WR, Fielding JW, Hawkins RJ, Pepin J, Hensinger RN. Traumatic spondylolisthesis of the axis. *J Bone Joint Surg* 1981;63B:313–318.
185. Effendi B, Roy D, Cornish B, Dussault RG, Laurin CA. Fracture of the ring of the axis. A classification based on the analysis of 131 cases. *J Bone Joint Surg* 1981;63B:319–327.
186. Fielding JW, Francis WR, Hawkins RJ, Pepin J, Hensinger RN. Traumatic spondylolisthesis of the axis. *Clin Orthop* 1989;239:47–52.
187. Bucholz RW. Unstable hangman's fractures. *Clin Orthop* 1981;154:119–124.
188. Levine AM, Rhyne AL. Traumatic spondylolisthesis of the axis. *Semin Spine Surg* 1991;3:47–60.
189. Starr JK, Eismont FJ. Atypical hangman's fractures. *Spine* 1993;18:1954–1957.
190. Cornish BL. Traumatic spondylolisthesis of the axis. *J Bone Joint Surg* 1968;50B:31–43.
191. Meyer PR Jr, Heim S. Surgical stabilization of the cervical spine. In: Meyer PR Jr (ed). *Surgery of Spine Trauma.* New York: Churchill Livingstone, 1989:397–523.
192. An H, Simpson JM (eds). *Surgery of the Cervical Spine.* Baltimore: Williams & Wilkins, 1994:235.

Surgery of Spinal Trauma,
edited by J.M. Cotler, J.M. Simpson, H.S. An, and C.P. Silveri.
Lippincott Williams & Wilkins, Philadelphia © 2000.

CHAPTER 8

Fractures and Dislocations of the Adult Lower Cervical Spine

J. Michael Simpson

Acute injuries of the lower cervical spine and spinal cord remain among the most common causes of severe disability despite recent advances in research, patient assessment, early resuscitation, and rehabilitative processes. Although research continues in attempts to minimize or reverse spinal cord injury, treatment remains enigmatic. The incidence of spinal cord injury in the population has not changed despite preventive efforts and a decreased incidence of drunken driving. Such measures have decreased rates of injury from sports activities and vehicular trauma; however, spinal cord injury related to firearms has markedly increased.

The diagnosis of lower cervical spine injuries is often delayed and treatment is frequently inadequate, resulting in loss of further neurologic function and compromised rehabilitation (1–3). During the past two decades there has been renewed interest in treatment of, and research on, spine and spinal cord injuries. With the development of spinal cord injury centers, great strides have been made toward improving emergency care and surgical treatment. Newer surgical techniques improving decompression and stabilization of the spine, specifically anterior and anterolateral operative ap-

proaches to spinal injuries with improved internal fixation devices, have improved our ability to surgically intervene and help patients. This chapter discusses the principles of patient assessment, classification of injury, and treatment of cervical spine and spinal cord injuries.

EVALUATION OF THE SPINAL-INJURED PATIENT

Initial assessment of the traumatized patient must include maintenance of airway, breathing, and circulation. If necessary, intubation can be performed while holding the patient's head in a straight line with gentle manual traction. A few patients with a high neurologic level of injury may deteriorate in the first day or two posttrauma and require mechanical ventilation. Cervical cord–injured patients can develop neurogenic shock due to loss of sympathetic tone. Hemodynamically, they present with hypotension and bradycardia. Neurogenic shock is best treated with vasopressors and atropine. After the primary assessment, the secondary examination is completed to exclude other life-threatening injury. During this time an examination of the spinal column and neurologic status of the patient is assessed and documented carefully (4).

A high index of suspicion is required to prevent further neurologic injury during the evaluation and early treatment process. All patients with head or high-energy trauma, neu-

---

J. M. Simpson: Medical College of Virginia, Virginia Commonwealth University; Tuckahoe Orthopaedic Associates, Richmond, Virginia 23226.

rologic deficit, or complaints of neck pain must be assumed to have a cervical spine injury until proven otherwise (5).

Particular attention must be given to the unconscious patient, who may lack protective reflex muscular tone. The most effective method of patient transport is supine positioning of the patient on a spine board, combined with the use of a hard cervical collar and sand bags taped on either side of the head (6). The Philadelphia collar alone provides adequate control of flexion and extension, but fails to control cervical rotation.

A cursory neurologic examination is advisable prior to moving any patient suspected of having a cervical spine injury. Once the examination is completed, the cervical collar is placed and the patient log-rolled onto the spine board. During this process care is taken to maintain the head and neck in line with the body. Further movement of the patient should be prevented until the patient is evaluated by a physician and radiographs are obtained in the emergency room.

Prompt and accurate diagnosis of cervical spine injuries in the emergency room demands a continued high index of suspicion. In Bohlman's (2) review of 300 cervical spine fractures, he found that 100 were initially missed in the emergency room while resuscitative measures focused on more obvious or life-threatening injuries. The most common causes of missed cervical spine injuries in the emergency room include multiple trauma, multiple noncontiguous fractures, and altered consciousness due to coma or intoxication (2). As many as 3% to 16% of patients with evidence of cervical fracture will have a noncontiguous spine fracture, the most common pattern being a fracture of the C1-C2 complex and a second remote subaxial cervical spine fracture (7–10).

Throughout the emergency room process, patients with spinal cord injury are best managed through a team approach. Resuscitation is supervised by a member of the trauma service, while evaluation and treatment of the spine injury is completed by a three-member spinal cord team composed of orthopedic, neurosurgical, and physical medicine services. Each member of the team is responsible for evaluation of the patient. Detailed neurologic examination by all members is required and documented. The American Spinal Injury Association (ASIA) has developed standards for assessing and classifying spinal cord injuries (11). A standardized assessment form allows detailed reporting of the neurologic examination (Fig. 1). The level of neurologic function is defined by the ASIA Impairment Scale at the most caudal level with at least grade III motor function (Table 1). The overall motor function of the patient can by quantified using the motor score. The motor score ranges from 0 to 100 and is determined by the summation of bilateral manual muscle test score for 10 key muscle groups: elbow flexors (C5), wrist extensors (C6), elbow extensors (C7), finger flexors (C8), hand intrinsics (T1), hip flexors (L2), knee extensors (L3), ankle dorsiflexors (L4), long toe extensors (L5), and ankle plantarflexors (S1).

Radiographic Evaluation

All traumatized patients require anteroposterior chest, pelvic, and lateral cervical radiographs as part of the initial assessment. The initial lateral radiograph of the cervical spine must demonstrate the base of the skull, all seven cervical vertebrae, and the superior end plate of T1. The cross-table lateral radiograph is an excellent screening tool, which by itself will diagnose 70% to 79% of all cervical spine injuries (12). A complete cervical spine series consisting of lateral, anteroposterior, and open-mouth views will diagnose 90% to 95% of all cervical spine injuries (13–15). In large patients it can be difficult to visualize the C7-T1 junction on a lateral film. It may be necessary either to apply traction to the arms or to obtain a swimmer's view (16–18). Unconscious or uncooperative patients, and those with upper extremity injuries, may require computed tomography (CT) imagining to evaluate the cervicothoracic junction fully.

In evaluating the lateral radiograph, four lines are drawn or visualized to ensure normal anatomic relationships: the anterior spinal line, posterior spinal line, spinolaminar line, and the basilar line of Wackenstein (Fig. 2). The anterior and posterior spinal lines course along the anterior and posterior aspect of the vertebral bodies, respectively, forming continuous smooth lines. The overall contour should be a gently sloping lordosis. The spinolaminar line is drawn, connecting the posterior aspect of the foramen magnum to the anterior cortex of each spinous process and should also be a smooth lordotic curve. The interpreter must be aware of one normal variation in this line: the spinolaminar line of C2 may lie 2 to 3 mm posterior to that of C3. The basilar line of Wackenstein lies along the posterior surface of the clivus, and is a tangent to the posterior cortex of the odontoid tip. This relationship is important in evaluating craniovertebral relationships.

Lateral radiographic evaluation should also include scrutiny of vertebral body height, articular pillars, alignment of articular facets, interspinous widening, and spinous process fracture. The articular pillars are rhomboid in shape, and the two pillars of any one vertebra should be superimposed on a true lateral radiograph. With the absence of this normal relationship, one should be alerted to the possibility of fracture or facet dislocation. Interspinous distances below the level of C3 should be almost equal. An increased distance usually indicates posterior ligamentous injury. Vertebral body translations greater than 3.5 mm and angulation greater than 11 degrees, when compared to adjacent levels, are regarded as unstable (19,20) (Fig. 3).

The prevertebral soft tissues should also be evaluated on the lateral radiograph. Prevertebral soft tissue space measuring between 7 and 10 mm at C2 indicates a possible abnormality, and additional studies are warranted. When the soft tissue space is >10 mm, the patient must be considered to have a cervical injury and further workup required (21).

The role of flexion and extension radiographs in the emergency setting remains controversial. They may be useful in the alert, cooperative patient without neurologic deficit but

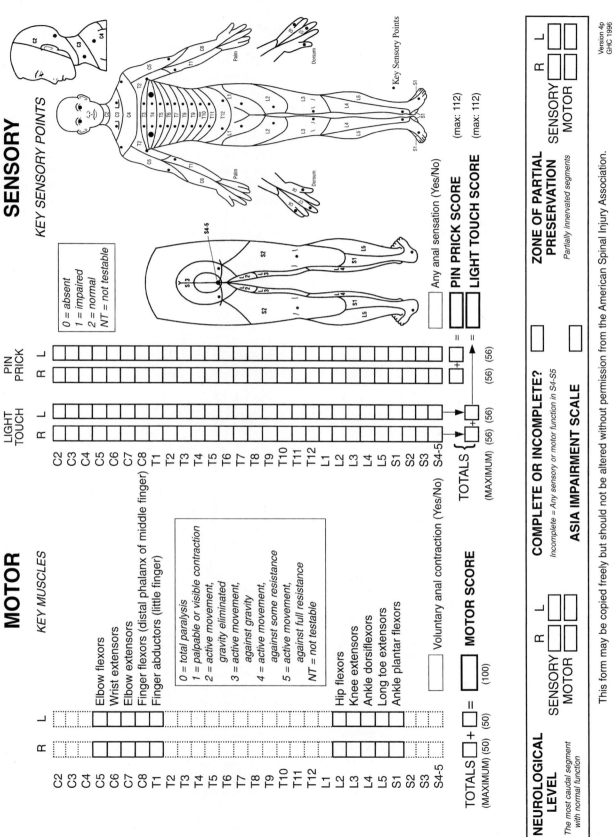

FIG. 1. American Spine Injury Association (ASIA) Spinal Cord Injury Assessment Form. (From ref. 11, with permission.)

TABLE 1. *American Spinal Injury Association (ASIA) Impairment Scale*

Grade on right	Muscle	Grade on left
5	C5	5
5	C6	5
5	C7	5
5	C8	5
5	T1	5
5	L2	5
5	L3	5
5	L4	5
5	L5	5
5		5
50		50

Total score 100

This motor index score, when used accurately, provides a numerical grading system to document improvement or deterioration of motor function.

Motor grading system
0 absent—total paralysis
1 trace—paipable or visible contraction
2 poor—active movement through range of motion with gravity eliminated
3 fair—active movement through range of motion against gravity
4 good—active movement through range of motion against resistance
5 normal

	Present	Absent
Bladder function		
Bowel function		

Motor index score adapted from scoring system by Lucas and Ducker.

with complaints of neck pain. Under these circumstances, a positive flexion-extension study has obvious clinical implications; however, a negative film does not rule out occult injury. Patients with acute cervical spine injury may have reflex muscular spasm masking instability for up to 2 to 3 weeks (22). As such, the treating physician must continue to have a high index of suspicion and protect the patient in a rigid cervical collar. Follow-up flexion-extension views are repeated at 2 to 3 weeks.

Computed tomography is an excellent method of evaluating patients with cervical spine injuries. Its advantages include speed, availability, supine position, axial imaging, and excellent cortical detail. It is traditionally used to identify the pathoanatomy of those fractures seen on plain radiographs. It can also be used to evaluate the lower cervical spine that cannot be adequately visualized on plain radiographs. Scanning should consist of 2- to 3-mm consecutive images and include one vertebra above and below the suspected level of injury.

Magnetic residence imaging (MRI) has become a popular modality in evaluating cervical trauma and has revolutionized our ability to determine the extent of cervical spine and spinal cord injury (23–25). It has generally replaced myelography as a diagnostic tool in cervical trauma. Advantages of MRI include its lack of ionizing radiation, direct multi-

axial imaging capabilities, ability to detect noncontiguous fractures, and, most importantly, its ability to determine the degree of soft tissue injury, including the intervertebral disc, spinal cord, and ligamentous structures. Recent studies have demonstrated that the incidence of disc injury complicating spinal trauma is significantly higher than previously thought. In some injury patterns the incidence of disc herniation is more than 50% (26–29). T2-weighted images are best for visualizing the spinal cord (30,31). Imaging signals consistent with intramedullary hematoma and/or spinal cord contusion associated with edema, encompassing more than one spinal segment, have been shown to be associated with more severe neurologic deficits, while less severe injuries have been correlated with either a normal spinal cord signal or edema encompassing one segment or less (30,31). MRI is indicated for (a) all patients with complete or incomplete

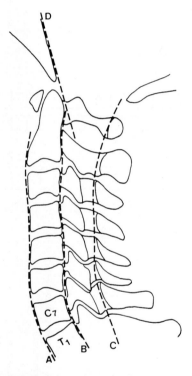

FIG. 2. Lateral view of the cervical spine with four lines drawn, demonstrating normal bony cervical relationships. Line A is the anterior spinal line that starts at the anterior aspect of C2, and continues inferiorly along the anterior surface of each vertebral body. This should be a smooth, uninterrupted line to C7. Line B is the posterior vertebral body surfaces, and this should also be smooth and uninterrupted. Line C represents the spinolaminar line, which connects the posterior aspect of the foramen magnum to the anterior cortex of each cervical spinous process. This should be a continuous, smooth, lordotic curve, with one possible exception: the spinolaminar line of C2 may lie 2 to 3 mm posterior to this curve, which is a normal variant. Line D is the basilar line of Wackenstein, which lies along the posterior surface of the clivus and is at a tangent to the posterior cortex of the odontoid tip. This is important in defining craniovertebral relationships. Normal soft tissue spaces are identified as <10 mm at C2, <4 mm at C3-4 and <15 mm at C5-7.

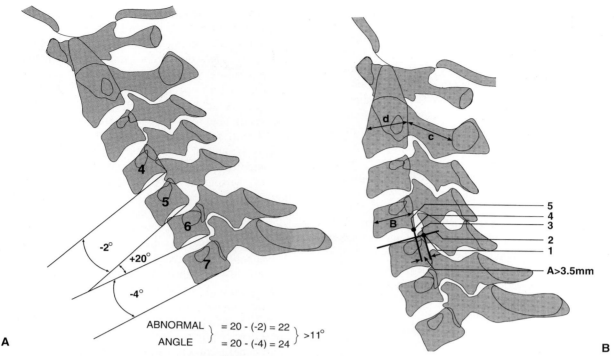

FIG. 3. A: The angulation between C5 and C6 is 20 degrees, which is >11 degrees than at either adjacent interspace. (Redrawn from ref. 107, with permission.) **B:** If the linear distance A is >3.5 mm, then it is considered unstable. If Pavlov's ratio (c/d) is <0.8, it is considered abnormal. (Redrawn from ref. 32, with permission.)

neurologic deficits, to search for and quantify the degree of spinal cord compression; (b) any patient in whom neurologic status deteriorates; and (c) patients who are suspected of having a posterior ligamentous injury, despite negative plain radiographs. The disadvantages of MRI include its relatively long acquisition time; limited availability; and contraindications in patients with pacemakers, aneurysm clips, metallic fragments in the eye or spinal cord, and severe claustrophobia.

EARLY MANAGEMENT OF CERVICAL SPINE INJURIES

Once the injured patient's medical status is secured, and diagnostic imaging studies completed, the stability of the injuries must be determined, deformity and subluxation reduced and immobilized, and complications associated with cervical spine injury avoided.

The concept of stability, in many respects, is vague. Radiographic measurements of translation and angulation are helpful but limited in their ability to recognize potential for neurologic injury. Spinal stability has been described by White and Panjabi (32) as "the ability of the spine under physiologic loads to maintain the relationship between vertebrae in such a way as there is neither initial or subsequent damage to the spinal cord or nerve roots." Based on multiple considerations, White et al. (20) have suggested that a checklist of dynamic and static radiographic criteria and neuro-

logic findings be utilized (Table 2). These criteria are particularly helpful in equivocal cases of stability but not required in the vast majority of presenting cervical spine injuries. In brief, any of the following situations must be considered an unstable injury of the cervical spine: anterior and posterior column injury, any structural injury associated with injury to the spinal cord, and gross deformity of the cervical spine with or without neurologic involvement.

The classification schemes described by Holdsworth (33), Allen et al. (34), and Denis (35) help determine the forces responsible for injury, the extent of structural damage, the extent of stability, and treatment options.

TABLE 2. *Checklist for the diagnosis of clinical instability*

Element	Point value
Anterior elements destroyed or unable to function	2
Posterior elements destroyed or unable to function	2
Relative sagittal plane translation >3.5 mm	2
Relative sagittal plane rotation >11 degrees	2
Posterior stretch test	2
Cord injury	2
Root injury	1
Abnormal disc narrowing	1
Congenital spinal stenosis	1
Dangerous loading anticipated	1
	>5 = clinical instability

Reduction and Immobilization of Cervical Injury

For any patient suspected of having a cervical injury, immobilization with a rigid orthosis is required while diagnostic images are completed. When an injury is identified, application of cervical skeletal traction is often preferred. For most injuries, the author prefers application of MRI-compatible Gardner-Wells tongs, with pins placed neutral to or 1 cm behind the external auditory canal and just above the pinna. Pins placed anterior to this point will exert an extension moment to the spine, whereas those placed posterior to this point will impart a flexion moment. The weight required for immobilization must be tailored to the individual injury, but in most cases 10 to 15 lb is sufficient. Once the patient is immobilized with the traction device, a lateral radiograph of the neck should be taken to check overall alignment. A complete neurologic exam should be repeated to ensure no change in neurologic status. In those cases where the timing and logistics of trauma resuscitation preclude thorough evaluation and application of traction, the patient should be maintained in a rigid cervical orthosis.

Spinal deformity resulting from trauma can cause injury to the spinal cord, but may also be responsible for ongoing neurologic compromise via a destructive cycle of vascular compromise and edema (36). As such, attempted closed reduction is attempted in any cervical spine injury that demonstrates shortening, angulation, or translation. The goal of closed reduction is restoration of normal spinal alignment, which may indirectly result in decompression of the spinal canal, and thus enhance neurologic recovery. There are many recent clinical and animal studies demonstrating that the extent of neurologic recovery is influenced by duration and degree of neurologic compression (37–43). Given these facts, closed reduction should be attempted as soon as possible.

Closed reduction must be completed in a closely supervised setting with vigilant radiographic and neurologic monitoring. The patient should be awake, alert, and cooperative to provide feedback to the physician during the procedure (29). Reduction is accomplished through a combination of skeletal traction, patient positioning, and postural bumps (39,44). While performing reduction maneuvers, it is preferable to have the patient on a Stryker frame using Gardner-Wells tongs as previously described. Attempt at reduction begins with 10 lb of applied traction, which is then increased by 10 lb in sequential fashion over 10- to 20-minute intervals. Evaluation of vertebral distraction/reduction is performed after each incremental change in the traction weight. A lateral radiograph is taken 5 to 10 minutes after weight change and the radiograph evaluated before determining the need for additional traction weight. The neurologic status must also be evaluated after each weight change. If the patient has intact bony structures but simply has a unilateral or bilateral facet dislocation, the weight is reduced to 10 to 20 lb after reduction is achieved. A final lateral radiograph is obtained to confirm maintenance of reduction. For burst fractures and osteoligamentous injuries, higher weights may be required to maintain acceptable reduction and correction of spinal deformity. MRI-compatible tongs are preferred, unless a high-weight reduction is anticipated. In such cases stronger stainless steel–tipped tongs should be used to prevent pin failure. The role of manipulation during closed reduction is controversial and should be reserved for those practitioners familiar with its indications and technique (45). The weight required for reduction of a cervical injury is variable. The maximum amount of weight that can be safely applied is not known (9). Attempted closed reduction must be discontinued when any of the following conditions has been met: (a) the spine is reduced, (b) more than 1 cm of distraction occurs at the zone of injury or any other location, (c) the patient's neurologic status deteriorates, or (d) the physician believes additional attempts have little or no chance of success. Closed reduction following this methodology has been successful in 90% to 95% of cases (46).

The halo-vest orthosis has been used to stabilize the cervical spine and is effective in restricting cervical motion when compared with more conventional cervical orthoses (47). The advantage of halo immobilization in patients with lower cervical injuries include both the physical and psychologic benefits of early immobilization when compared to prolonged bed rest and skeletal traction. Avoidance of complications associated with prolonged bed rest shortens hospitalization and rehabilitation stays. The halo device also has the advantage of more precise neck positioning to counteract the direction of instability. These advantages make the halo attractive for use in both nonsurgical and postsurgical management of lower cervical spine injuries. Nonsurgical management of the cervical injury in a halo, however, requires careful follow-up as failure rates may range from 10% to 40% depending on the specific injury pattern (48–53).

Halo-vest complications are frequent, most of them being related to pin loosening and pin tract infections (42–54). Such complications can be minimized if proper attention is directed to application and maintenance of the halo device. The halo ring should be positioned below the greatest circumference of the patient's skull, minimizing the potential for the ring to shift cephalad and out of position. The pins should be initially torqued to 6 to 8 lb and then retorqued to the same level 24 to 48 hours after application (54). The anterior pins should be placed in the safe zone just superior to the middle or lateral third of the orbit, thereby protecting the supraorbital nerve (54). If the pins loosen, they should be retorqued to the original level, assuming that bony resistance is appreciated within one to two turns. If no resistance is encountered, the pin site should be changed. Careful molding and fitting of the vest is also important to eliminate excessive motion.

Prevention of Complications

Spinal cord injury and patient immobilization, as with most trauma, predispose the patient to a host of associated medical complications: pulmonary dysfunction, venous thrombosis, peptic ulcer disease, and skin breakdown. Complications can most effectively be reduced through rapid intervention and patient mobilization. Prophylactic measures can minimize patient risk and include prevention of aspiration, aggressive pulmonary toilet, early enteral feeding, and use of H2 receptor blockers. Gastrointestinal bleeding has been reported to occur in 9% to 40% of patients and is most common in the first 14 days postinjury (2,3,55,56). The incidence of deep venous thrombosis in spinal cord injury has been reported in the range of 25% to 95% and is clinically relevant in 25% to 35% of patients (57,58). Current prophylaxis protocols call for adjusted low-dose heparin, antiembolic stockings and compression boots. Skin breakdown is best treated through prevention with vigilant nursing care and the use of rotating beds. Established skin ulcers must be aggressively treated through debridement, local wound care, and pressure relief.

Corticosteroids

Steroids have been shown to benefit patients with acute spinal cord injury by decreasing inflammation and minimizing neural tissue damage and dysfunction at the cellular level. The theoretical disadvantages include immunosuppression and gastrointestinal bleeding. Early studies, using relatively low doses of steroids administered over the course of several weeks, resulted in significant increases in both infection and gastrointestinal bleeding rates with little or no improvement in neurologic function (59–61). High-dose administration of methylprednisolone started within 8 hours of admission and administered over 24 hours has been shown to improve motor scores in patients with incomplete lesions (61). In this study, the effects of methylprednisolone were compared to those of a placebo or naloxone. Infection rates of 7.9% versus 3.6% and gastrointestinal bleeding rates of 4.5% versus 3% were noted in the steroid and placebo groups, respectively. However, the study included only those patients treated within 8 hours of blunt spinal cord injury, and did not include penetrating spinal cord injuries. Based on the relatively modest increase in complication rate in this more recent study, the recommended bolus of methylprednisolone is 30 mg/kg of body weight and is administered to all patients with acute (less than 8 hours) blunt spinal cord injury, followed by an infusion of 5.4 mg/kg/h over 23 hours.

SURGICAL TREATMENT OF UNSTABLE CERVICAL SPINE INJURIES

General Principles

Surgical decompression must be considered in all cases of radiographically demonstrable neurologic compression after realignment of the spine (61–65). Decompression is mandatory in cases of incomplete neurologic injury to promote recovery. With complete neurologic injuries, decompression may facilitate root recovery, which can significantly improve the patient's functional status (66,67). For patients with evidence of neurologic compression who remain intact neurologically, decompression may be completed as part of a surgical procedure designed to reconstruct spinal integrity.

The specific surgical approach for neural decompression is dictated by the anatomic location of neurologic compression. As the overwhelming majority of compression is caused by either vertebral body retropulsion or herniated disc material, most cervical decompressions are performed anteriorly. Laminectomy as a means of spinal cord decompression is contraindicated in cervical trauma; it has been shown to be of little therapeutic value, and predisposes the patient to late kyphosis, progression of neurologic deficit, and poor outcomes (33,68–71).

However, laminectomy can be used for the few patients with depressed laminar fractures causing posterior compression of the spinal cord, and for the rare patient with ankylosing spondylitis with a clinically significant epidural hematoma.

For most patients requiring stabilization and decompressive procedures, the author prefers the use of a Stryker type frame as the operative table. This frame incorporates a pulley to facilitate traction and allows for rapid and safe repositioning of the patient undergoing combined anterior-posterior surgical procedures.

The indications for spinal cord monitoring during surgery for acute cervical spine injuries are not well delineated. Somatosensory evoked potentials and motor evoked potentials may be useful for the neurologically intact patient and those with an incomplete spinal cord injury. This is particularly true when significant intraoperative manipulation of the spinal column is anticipated.

Despite the stability provided by cervical spine instrumentation, many patients remain candidates for halo-vest immobilization. This may be recognized as overtreatment for many injuries, but consideration must be given to patients with concomitant head injuries and those patients thought likely to disregard physician recommendations.

Timing of Surgery

Initial studies of early surgical intervention (less than 3 to 5 days) reported increased potential for mortality and neurologic deterioration, leading many authors to recommend a delay in operative intervention for 1 to 2 weeks (72,73). Experimental spinal cord injury in animals, however, has clearly shown that the degree of neurologic damage is affected by the duration of cord compression, leading most authors to recommend urgent decompression (37–43). There is no doubt that early decompression and stabilization of spine injuries offers the benefit of patient mobilization. In recent studies where spinal cord monitoring was utilized and improved anesthetic and surgical techniques have been employed, no increase in morbidity or mortality has been demonstrated following early surgical intervention (37,41, 74).

Classification

Plain radiographs, CT, and MRI provide accurate definition of structural injury. Many classification systems have been described to assess such injuries; however, none has been universally accepted (33–35,75). An accurate classification system is important in identifying common fracture patterns, determining prognosis, and assisting the physician in planning reduction maneuvers and determining proper treatment methods.

Holdsworth (33) was the first to attempt the classification of spinal injuries. In his system, the spinal column is divided into anterior and posterior columns. The anterior column is composed of the anterior longitudinal ligament, vertebral body, intervertebral disc, and posterior longitudinal ligament. The posterior column is composed of the pedicles, laminae, spinous processes, ligamentum flavum, capsular ligaments, and the supraspinatus and interspinous ligaments. He subsequently classified all spinal injuries into six categories: simple wedge compression fractures, dislocations, extension injuries, burst fractures, rotational fracture-dislocations, and shear injuries. For each injury type, a particular mode of failure is implied. Stable fractures had injuries associated to only one column, whereas unstable injuries had two-column involvement. This system, however, fails in its ability to determine stability accurately and its clinical adaptability is thereby limited.

White and Panjabi (32) have used cadaveric testing to determine parameters for clinical instability. They progressively sectioned ligaments from anterior to posterior and from posterior to anterior in cadaveric specimens. After each sectioning the spine was loaded and deformations measured. More than 3.5 mm of anteroposterior translation or more than 11 degrees of kyphotic angulation compared to adjacent cervical levels was considered to be clinically significant and represent unstable injuries (Fig. 3). To further aid the clinician, White has recommended the use of a checklist (Table 2). With this checklist each element is assessed and the total positive values calculated. If the value is >5, then the spine is probably unstable. Patients with values >5 do not necessarily require surgery but, at a minimum, are treated with a halo vest. This checklist is not uniformly accepted; however, it does provide an objective form for assessing clinical stability.

The classification system described by Allen et al. (34) represents a mechanistic analysis of spinal injury. This system is based on the position of the neck at the time of injury and/or the applied forces vectors. In this scheme, six categories or phylogenies of injury are described (Table 3). Each phylogeny is then subdivided in stages that represent severity of injury. The higher-numbered stages represent more severe forms of structural injury and imply a greater potential for neurologic injury. Injury designation is accomplished based on the mechanism of injury and review of plain radiographs. Critical to the differentiation of entry pattern is recognition that compressive loads result in a shortening of the vertebral column, whereas distraction results in length-

TABLE 3. *Allen et al. mechanistic classification of clinical injuries*

	Stages
Compressive flexion	1–5
Vertebral flexion	1–3
Distractive flexion	1–4
Compressive extension	1–5
Distractive extension	1–2
Lateral flexion	1–2

From ref. 34.

ening. Although this mechanistic classification is useful, it is not without limitations. The system is cumbersome and in many cases it is difficult to identify the proper fracture phylogeny. The six categories of described injury are compressive flexion, vertical compression, distractive flexion, compressive extension, distractive extension, and lateral flexion. In the following discussion of individual injury patterns, I will incorporate the mechanistic analysis of Allen et al. when clinically appropriate.

Distractive Flexion Injuries

Distractive flexion represents the most common injury pattern and is most often caused by motor vehicle accident and falls from a height. Injury between C5-C6 and C6-C7 is most commonly seen.

Distractive loads applied to the spine in a flexed position cause tensile failure through lengthening of the posterior ligamentous structures. Figure 4 depicts the four stages of distraction-flexion injury as described by Allen et al. (34), which include unilateral facet dislocation and bilateral facet dislocation represented by stages II and III in this scheme. With a unilateral facet dislocation there is approximately 25% subluxation of the vertebral body. In this injury posterior- and middle-column destruction is complete. Anterior-column ligamentous structures may remain intact. With bilateral facet dislocation approximately 50% of the vertebral body is translated anteriorly. The posterior articular surfaces of the superior vertebral articular processes lie against the anterior surface of the inferior articular processes. Stage IV is an uncommon injury pattern in which all ligamentous complexes are disrupted and full body translation has occurred.

Less severe posterior ligamentous injuries can result in facet subluxation, which is represented by stage I. These injuries are often missed with only subtle radiographic change. Many of these patients do not have severe onset of pain initially but note an increase in pain in the following days once the inflammatory response ensues. On examination, the physician will not recognize a palpable defect or widening between the spinous processes. On flexion-extension radiographs, more than 3.5 mm of translation or more than 11 degrees of angulation is considered unstable. MRI imaging is useful in identifying posterior ligamentous disruption. Find-

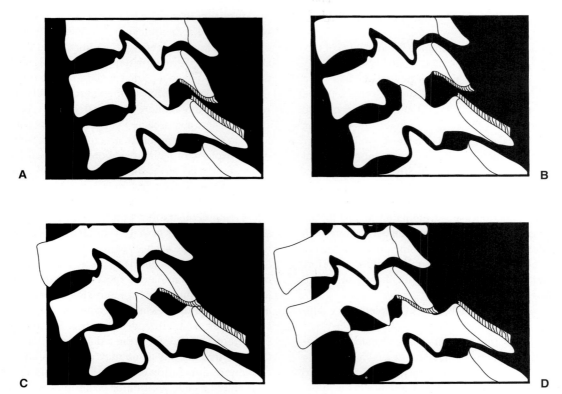

FIG. 4. A: Distractive flexion stage 1 (DFS1): with failure of the posterior ligamentous complex, subluxation of the facet joint occurs with interspinous widening and mild kyphosis. In the early stages, there may be a concomitant compressive failure of the anterior elements of the lowermost vertebrae in the injured motion segment. This may, in fact, resemble the initial stages of a compressive flexion phylogeny. **B:** Distractive flexion stage 2 (DFS2): this lesion represents a unilateral facet dislocation. Vertebral body translation with a unilateral facet dislocation is no more than 25%. Posterior and middle column disruption is complete. Anterior column ligamentous structures may remain intact. **C:** Distractive flexion stage 3 (DFS3): this lesion represents a bilateral facet dislocation with approximately 50% vertebral body width translation anteriorly. The posterior surfaces of the superior vertebral articular process lie against the anterior surfaces of the inferior articular processes. **D:** Distractive flexion stage 4 (DFS4): in this injury, full vertebral body width translation occurs with injury to all ligamentous complexes.

ings typically include high-intensity signals in the interspinous spaces or facet joints and discontinuity of the hypointense vertical lines that represent this ligamentous structure. CT imaging with sagittal reconstruction may additionally be helpful in isolating these injuries.

Unilateral facet dislocations may be associated with a fracture of the facet. Furthermore, there can be a fracture of the lateral mass with separation that results from fracture of the pedicle and lamina on the same side, creating a free-floating lateral mass. On the lateral view the involved lateral mass appears rotated compared to the opposite side and adjacent levels. On the anteroposterior view, the lateral mass is rotated and the pedicle fracture identified. MRI imaging demonstrates a 10% to 20% incidence of associated disc herniation in patients with a unilateral facet dislocation (76). Most patients with a unilateral facet dislocation are found to be neurologically intact. However, patients who have preexisting spinal canal narrowing may suffer significant spinal cord injury. More commonly, isolated nerve root impression at the involved level can be present in approximately 50% of cases.

Bilateral facet dislocation represents a highly unstable injury and is associated with ligamentous disruption of all posterior structures, the posterior longitudinal ligament, and the posterior annulus. The anterior longitudinal ligament often remains the only intact structure. The soft tissue injury is extensive and is associated with disc herniation in 30% to 50% of cases (77). Significant injury to the spinal cord occurs in the majority of cases secondary to direct compression between the inferior vertebral body and superior laminae and due to the tensile forces created in the cord from distractive forces.

Occasionally, patients present neurologically intact, particularly if the patient has a large spinal canal or if there is a concomitant fracture of the lamina with displacement. As noted earlier, a minimum 50% anterior vertebral body translation is appreciated on the lateral radiograph. Such injuries can often be missed if attention is not directed at the cervicothoracic junction. The first thoracic vertebra must always be visualized in trauma cases. Vertebral artery occlusion has been documented by Willis et al. (78) in 50% to 60% of patients with facet dislocation but has not been clinically correlated.

Closed reduction should be attempted for all stages of distraction flexion injuries as soon as the patient is medically stable. Greater recovery of neurologic deficit has been demonstrated in patients who were successfully reduced within 8 hours of injury (39). Several authors have offered formulas for determining the weight required for reduction of cervical spine dislocations, but none has proven effective. Some authors recommend using no more than 50 lb of weight for fear of overdistraction (79,80). High weight reduction, however, has been reported with significantly higher success rates (44–46). In a report of 81 consecutive attempted closed reduction using weights up to 110 lb, the reduction success rate was 91% (46). When performing such high weight reductions, however, it is imperative that the patient undergo serial neurologic and radiologic evaluation. With any evidence of overdistraction or change in neurologic status, the process is aborted.

Following reduction, an MRI scan is completed to evaluate for compressive pathology.

Patients with distraction flexion injuries treated by nonsurgical methods in a halo vest have up to a 64% incidence of late instability. Failure to achieve adequate reduction or to maintain reduction may be the result of fracture dislocation, with loss of normal bony restraints preventing anterior displacement. Primary posterior cervical fusion is preferred for patients in all unstable distraction flexion injuries when neurologically intact. Unsuccessful closed reduction requires open reduction and posterior cervical fusion. Patients with neurologic deficits may require anterior decompression and reconstruction before posterior stabilization. The decision for this type of operative intervention is dictated by radiographic evidence of anterior cord compression from an associated disc herniation.

As noted earlier a high percentage of the patients with distraction flexion injuries have an associated acute disc herniation at the level of injury. Several authors have reported catastrophic neurologic injury following closed reduction of this injury complex (77,81,82). Careful review of these studies, however, indicates that many patients underwent closed reduction under general anesthesia. In a series of 50 consecutive patients suffering either a unilateral or bilateral facet dislocation, a prereduction MRI scan demonstrated an associated disc herniation in 54% of patients (83). All patients in this study underwent emergent attempted closed reduction with a success rate of 80%. Despite the presence of an associated disc herniation, there was no case of neurologic deterioration in cases with unilateral or bilateral facet dislocation or fracture dislocation. In fact, four patients demonstrated clear and significant neurologic improvement. Based on the results of the study, the author continued to recommend conscious closed reduction of all cervical spine dislocations and severely comminuted fractures. Furthermore, MRI is not strongly recommended prior to routine reduction of such cervical injuries, as the delay associated with obtaining the scan may further compromise neurologic recovery. For patients in whom closed reduction fails, an MRI is a prerequisite to open reduction. Patients with an unreduced dislocation and associated disc herniation require combined anterior cervical decompression and a posterior stabilization procedure.

Surgical stabilization of the neurologically intact patient with unilateral or bilateral facet dislocation is best completed from a posterior approach. For those patients with a pure dislocation and intact articular structures, we recommend Bohlman's triple-wire technique. For a unilateral facet fracture dislocation, a posterior single-level fusion is recommended.

Because of the facet fracture there can be loss of rotational control, and thus interspinous wire fixation may be inadequate. Supplementation with an oblique facet wire as described by Edwards et al. (84) or lateral mass plating is recommended under such circumstances. Prior to surgery an MRI scan is recommended to assess the potential of a disc herniation. For a unilateral facet dislocation or fracture dislocation with spinal cord compression from a herniated disc, an anterior decompressive procedure is warranted followed by a posterior stabilizing procedure. For the patient with nerve root compression from a disc herniation or facet fracture, the treating physician may consider either an anterior decompression followed by an anterior interbody fusion with anterior plate fixation or posterior stabilization. Alternatively, a posterior foraminotomy and posterior fusion may be completed. In the unusual case of a failed closed reduction, an open reduction may be completed posteriorly by levering the facet joints, usually coupled with some manipulation of the involved spinous processes. Alternatively, removing a small amount of the superior articular facet facilitates joint reduction.

For bilateral facet dislocations with a complete or incomplete neurologic deficit, immediate closed reduction is the first line of treatment. If a postreduction MRI demonstrates continued spinal cord compression secondary to a disc herniation, an anterior discectomy and interbody fusion with autologous bone graft and plating can be performed.

Alternatively, a concomitant posterior arthrodesis may be done depending on surgeon preference. For patients without an associated disc herniation, an isolated posterior fusion can be completed using either an interspinous wiring technique or lateral mass plate fixation.

Vertical Compression Injury

Vertical compression injuries are most common following motor vehicle accidents, diving accidents, and direct blows to the top of the skull. The most common levels of injury are C6 and C7. These injuries result from a compressive force applied to the neutrally aligned spine, and lead to shortening of both anterior and middle columns. This injury pattern as described by Allen et al. (34) is seen in Fig. 5. In stages I and II there is simply a cupping of one or both of the end plates of the vertebral body, which represents only partial failure of the anterior column. The posterior ligamentous structures re-

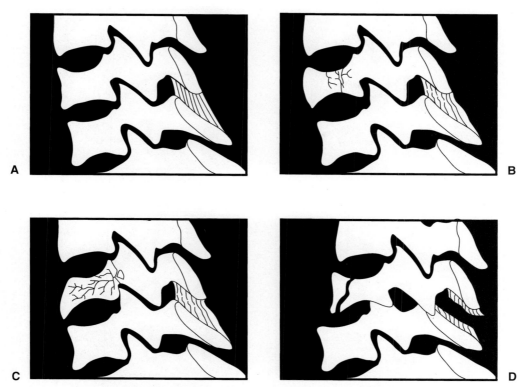

FIG. 5. A: Vertical compression stage 1 (VCS1): this lesion consists simply of a fracture of either the superior or inferior vertebral end plate, resulting in a cup-like deformity. The stage 1 lesion usually involves both the anterior and middle columns, but does not result in ligamentous failure. **B:** Vertical compression stage 2 (VCS2): both vertebral end plates are involved in a VCS2 lesion. Fracture lines may be demonstrated through the vertebral body, but displacement is minimal. Ligamentous structures remain intact. The spinal canal remains patent. **C:** Vertical compression stage 3 (VCS3): this lesion represents simply a progression of the vertebral body damage as seen in a VCS2 lesion. The vertebral body has become fragmented, and residual pieces displace peripherally in multiple directions. The posterior portion of the vertebral body bulges into the neural canal, potentially compressing the spinal cord. This lesion occurs without significant ligamentous disruption. **D:** VCS3 injury with ligamentous disruption through the anterior, middle, and posterior ligamentous columns, narrowing the neural canal by two mechanisms. Bone is retropulsed from the vertebral body, and approaches the lamina at the injured segment. Additionally, there is posterior translation through the motion segment, usually resulting in a complete neurologic injury.

main uninjured in these stages, and late kyphotic deformity is unusual. Therefore, patients can be managed in a rigid cervical orthosis or halo vest for a period of 6 to 8 weeks. For the unusual patient with any neurologic involvement, an MRI scan is done.

Stage III of vertical compression injuries usually involves fragmentation and displacement of the vertebral body, and is referred to commonly as a burst fracture. With such injury, the neural canal is narrowed by retropulsed bone. Skeletal traction may result in reduction of the fracture but not consistently. After reduction an MRI scan is done and the spinal canal assessed for residual anatomic compression. Most of these patients present with neurologic injury and require anterior decompression and reconstruction coupled with anterior plate fixation.

Alternatively, based on surgeon preference, posterior stabilization may be completed. The stage III injury may involve posterior ligamentous injury. These are highly unstable injuries and most often present with significant neurologic dysfunction. Anterior neurologic decompression coupled with either anterior or posterior stabilization is generally recommended.

Compressive Flexion Injury

Allen et al. (34) have described five stages of compression flexion forces. Many of the injury patterns seen in this category can be easily confused with those of vertical compression. Of the five stages represented and described in Fig. 6, most represent minor bony trauma and are of little clinical significance. However, these injury patterns may at times appear benign on initial evaluation but be associated with significant ligamentous injury, rendering them unstable. The most common levels of injury in this fracture pattern are at

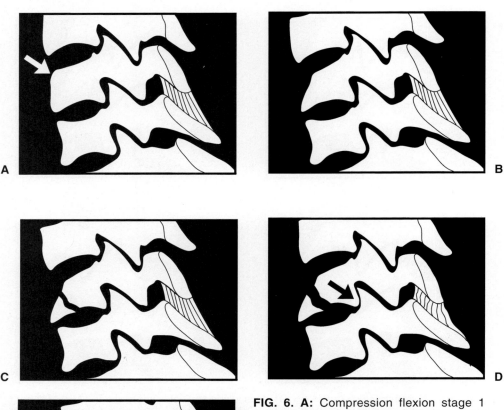

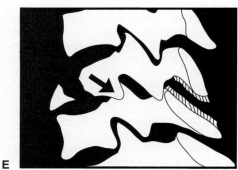

FIG. 6. A: Compression flexion stage 1 (CFS1): this represents the most minor injury as a result of a compressive load applied to the spine when held in a flexed position, and the lesion consists simply of rounding of the anterosuperior aspect of the vertebral body. There is no disruption of the posterior ligamentous structures. The middle and posterior columns are completely intact. B: Compressive flexion stage 2 (CFS2): there is now an obliquity to the anterior surface of the vertebral body, and concomitant loss of anterior column height. This results in a beaked appearance of the anteroinferior surface of the vertebral body. Again, ligamentous structures remain intact posteriorly. C: Compressive flexion stage 3 (CFS3): in this stage, a fracture line clearly passes obliquely from the anterior surface of the vertebral body, and extends through the inferior subchondral plate. In this diagram, the posterior ligamentous structures are shown to be intact, although they may be injured and require examination through magnetic resonance imaging (MRI). D: Compressive flexion stage 4 (CFS4): in addition to the fracture line seen in CFS3, this lesion includes translation of the inferoposterior vertebral margin into the neural canal at the involved motion segment. This is indicative of early ligamentous failure through the middle and posterior ligamentous complexes. The amount of posterior translation, however, is <3 mm. E: Compressive flexion stage 5 (CFS5): this lesion represents full ligamentous disruption of all columns with marked posterior translation in excess of 3 mm. It is a grossly unstable lesion.

C4-5 and C5-6. Compressive loads applied to the flexed spine result in compression of the anterior column with distraction of the posterior column. In stages III and IV (fracture of the vertebral body without displacement, and less than 3 mm of displacement, respectively), posterior ligamentous disruption is possible. These patients require evaluation by MRI to rule out posterior ligamentous disruption.

A disruptive posterior column renders the injured segment highly unstable.

Stages IV and V represent the commonly described "teardrop fracture," which involves posterior displacement of the vertebral body into the spinal canal and is frequently associated with injury to the spinal cord. The posterior longitudinal ligament is usually preserved and guides realignment during fracture reduction. These fractures need to be differentiated from a simply avulsion fracture at the anterior inferior corner of the vertebral body caused by hyperextension injury, which is usually benign. For the unstable injury without neurologic compromise, a posterior stabilization procedure followed by halo immobilization may be all that is required. Injuries associated with neurologic compression generally require anterior decompression followed by either anterior or posterior stabilization.

Compression Extension Injuries

Compression extension injuries may occur at all levels of the subaxial spine and may be associated with injuries to the C1-C2 region. Compression forces applied to the spine in extension will result in early failure of the posterior column followed by failure of the anterior column. The fracture pattern may not be obvious on the initial lateral radiograph. Oblique views or CT imaging may be necessary to establish the diagnosis. Stage I and II of a compressive extension type injury result in a single or multilevel posterior element fractures without vertebral body displacement (Fig. 7). These injuries are best managed with a rigid cervical orthosis or halo vest for the neurologically intact patient. Allen et al. (34) delineate five stages for this injury pattern, with the latter stages being relatively uncommon and representative of three-column ligamentous injury. These more stable injuries may potentially result in neurologic compromise. If neurologic in-

jury exist, preoperative MRI scan should be obtained followed by appropriate decompression and stabilization. Posterior stabilization procedures may be complicated by multiple fractures of the laminar surfaces. Plate screw constructs may be used for such situations.

Distractive Extension Injury

Distractive forces applied to the spine in extension will cause tensile failure and lengthening of both the anterior and posterior columns of the spine (Fig. 8). Failure can be through either the bony or ligamentous structures. MRI is often helpful in determining the extent of soft tissue injury. These are uncommon injuries. Injuries without evidence of vertebral body displacement on status flexion and extension views (distractive extension stage I) can be treated in a cervical orthosis or halo vest. Spontaneous ankylosis may occur. Alternatively, for anterior ligamentous injury, a primary anterior arthrodesis with plate fixation may be considered.

Vertebral body displacement represents failure of all three ligamentous complexes and potentially is associated with vertebral body displacement into the spinal canal. This may be a subtle abnormality on initial radiographs as the lesion reduces with the head held in a slightly flexed position. MRI scan usually can delineate the three-column ligamentous injury to the spine. This represents an unstable injury and requires anterior fusion with plate fixation. Posterior fusion can be added in extremely unstable cases.

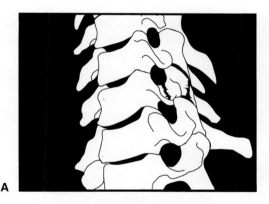

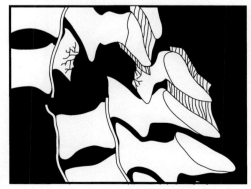

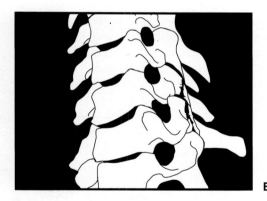

FIG. 7. A: Compressive extension stage 1 (CES1): this oblique view of the cervical spine demonstrates fracture through the pedicle and lamina of the injured vertebrae. The CES1 lesion consists of such fractures with or without rotatory vertebral body displacement. Laminar fractures are often difficult to see on plain radiographs. Oblique and pillar views will most reliably reveal CES1-type injuries. **B:** Compressive extension stage 2 (CES2): oblique projection demonstrating bilaminar fractures, which most commonly occur at contiguous multiple levels. There is no evidence of other soft tissue failure in the cervical motion segment. C: Compressive extension stage 5 (CES5): this lesion consists of bilateral vertebral arch fractures and ligamentous failure of all three columns. With such an injury, vertebral body translation is seen, and often results in a complete spinal cord injury.

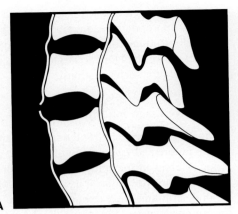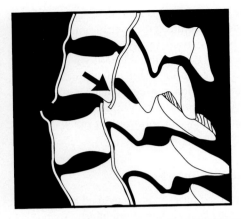

FIG. 8. A: Distractive extension stage 1 (DES1): this injury, alternatively, can occur through the anterior ligamentous complex or result from a transverse fracture through the vertebral body. Radiographically, there will be a widening of the disc space anteriorly at the injured segment without posterior vertebral body displacement. **B:** Distractive extension stage 2 (DES2): this lesion is characterized by failure of all three ligamentous complexes through the involved motion segment with posterior vertebral body displacement into the neural canal. As this lesion often reduces with the head held in flexion, plain radiographic features may be subtle. However, MRI will delineate a significant three-column injury to the spine.

Lateral Flexion Injury

Lateral flexion injuries occur most commonly following a motor vehicle accident and blows to the side of the head. The asymmetric nature of the force loads the spine in a coronal plane, resulting in tensile failure of one side of the spine and compressive failure of the opposite side (Fig. 9). Most of these injuries are of little clinical significance to the patient and can be treated with a cervical collar. More significant injuries may lead to unilateral ligamentous destruction and potential for displacement. These injuries are very uncommon and may require surgical stabilization. Preoperative MRI scan may be helpful in defining the extent of soft tissue injury.

SURGICAL TREATMENT

Anesthesia

Patients with unstable surgical spine injuries must be managed carefully to prevent iatrogenic injury during the processes of intubation and positioning. Awake, fiberoptically aided nasotracheal intubation is generally required, preferably with the patient secured with skeletal traction. We prefer to use a turning frame, such as a Stryker, as an operating table. This allows patient positioning while minimizing patient movement. An intraoperative lateral radiograph is taken to check cervical alignment. Visualization may be improved by pulling downward on the shoulders with tape. Any alignment correction is made before the neck and graft sites are

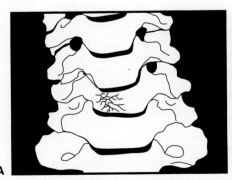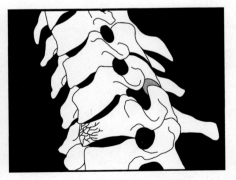

FIG. 9. A: Lateral flexion stage 1 (LFS1): this lesion simply consists of an asymmetric compression fracture of the vertebral body, and is often associated with an ipsilateral vertebral arch fracture. The asymmetric compression is most evident on the anteroposterior view. **B:** Lateral flexion stage 2 (LFS2): lateral asymmetric compression of the vertebral body occurs with contralateral ligamentous failure or vertebral arch fracture with displacement as seen on the anteroposterior radiograph.

surgically prepped. The surgeon must ensure that shoulder traction is not excessive through palpation of the shoulder girdle and brachial plexus. The face and orbits must also be checked for evidence of pressure.

Somatosensory and motor evoked potentials are not routinely used but advisable in cases where an operative reduction is planned or decompression is contemplated through a severely stenotic level. Succinylcholine should be avoided in the presence of an acute neurologic injury. This drug is associated with massage leakage of potassium from muscle cells and cardiac arrest.

Posterior Decompression

Cervical laminectomy is rarely indicated in acute cervical injury except in the rare case of depressed laminar fractures and for those patients with multilevel spondylosis suffering extension injuries with resultant central cord syndrome. In the past, laminectomy was used routinely for anterior compressive lesions but it fails to directly address the pathology. Furthermore, postoperative instability and kyphosis may further compromise neural function (85). In any trauma case where a laminectomy is required and completed, a concomitant arthrodesis should be performed and stabilized using lateral mass plates or facet wiring techniques. In the spondylitic spine, a multilevel laminectomy allows for posterior cord displacement. Cord displacement can lead to excessive cervical nerve root tension and resulting radiculopathy. The C5 nerve root is particularly susceptible and thus we advise completion of a foraminotomy to minimize the potential for iatrogenic injury. Foraminotomy may also be completed for those patients with facet fracture and resultant nerve root impingement. The occasional patient may have a symptomatic foraminal encroachment from degeneration or disc herniation.

Surgical Technique

Laminectomy

Once the patient is properly positioned on the frame and the neck region properly prepped, the involved spinous processes are exposed through a midline incision and hemostasis obtained. The appropriate levels can usually be identified by palpation of the prominent C2 spinous process. If there is any question, an intraoperative x-ray is taken. Dissection is then completed by exposing the appropriate laminae bilaterally. The involved spinous processes can be removed with a rongeur if preferred by the surgeon, and the laminectomy then performed in a piecemeal fashion similar to that carried out in the lumbar spine. This does tend to be time-consuming and requires passage of instruments central to the spinal canal, which may further compromise the spinal cord and potentiate neurologic injury.

We prefer an en bloc resection of the involved laminae. Two lateral troughs are created with the use of a round cutting burr just medial to the lateral border of the facet joint

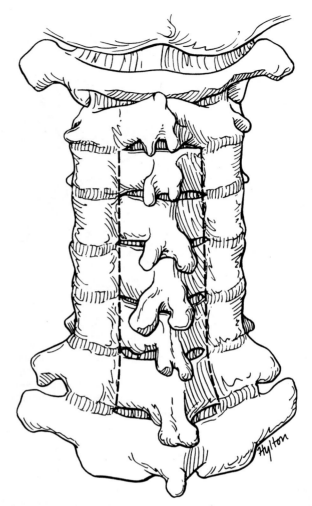

FIG. 10. Operative view of the posterior cervical spine for a patient undergoing a multilevel laminectomy. The vertical lines on each side of the laminae indicate the pathway for drilling and creation of the troughs. (From ref. 108, with permission.)

(Fig. 10). A diamond-cutting burr may be used, but tends to be slow and creates more heat. The drilling process is completed under loupe magnification, beginning at the lower lamina to be excised and extending in a cranial fashion. The surgeon encounters three layers of bone (Fig. 11). The outer cortical and middle cancellous layers of the lamina are removed with a burr. The inner cortical table is seen and thinned with the burr, although the cortical rim is not penetrated. Overaggressive drilling may cause injury to the dura or underlying nerve root. Continuous irrigation is advised to prevent thermal injury and maintain adequate operative visualization.

Once the troughs are thinned appropriately, a 1-mm Kerrison rongeur is used to complete the trough through resection of bone and accompanying ligamentum flavum. Once the troughs are completed, the ligamentum flavum must be resected at the proximal and distal poles of the laminectomy site. A towel clip is placed into the spinous processes of the

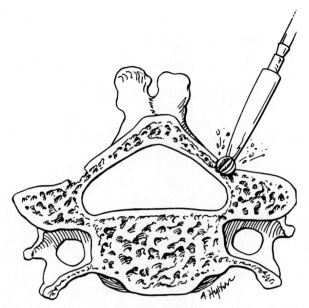

FIG. 11. The vertical line described in Fig. 10 shows the location of the trough. This trough is created using a round 4-mm cutting burr just medial to the lateral border of the facet joint. Drilling is completed in a caudal-to-cranial direction. Three layers of bone will be encountered during the drilling process. The inner cortical layer is thinned but not penetrated with the burr. Continuous irrigation is used to prevent thermal injury. (From ref. 108, with permission.)

most superior/inferior involved vertebral segments. The spinous processes are then lifted, and the ligamentum flavum dissected using a no. 12 scalpel blade or fine scissors (Fig. 12). Care must be taken not to allow any portion of the resected laminae to dip anteriorly compressing the spinal cord.

Once the ligamentum flavum is resected, the entire block of lamina is then excised. The lateral margins of the dura are visible, with the facet joints remaining intact. Lateral epidural veins are usually encountered and managed with bipolar cautery. Individual nerve roots should be palpated for adequate decompression.

Foraminotomy

While mechanical studies have shown that up to 50% of the facet joints may be removed without development of instability (86), in cases of trauma the possibility of instability is greatly increased and therefore an arthrodesis is always performed. The cervical foramen is located directly below and slightly cranial to the facet joint. If a laminectomy has not been completed, a 1- or 2-mm Kerrison rongeur is used to create a circular laminotomy defect measuring approximately 8 to 10 mm. Approximately half of this defect is placed on the superior lamina and the other half on the inferior lamina.

A high-speed air drill with a 3-mm diamond-tip burr is used to thin the facet joint bone directly over the nerve root. Usually the foramen can be palpated with a fine dental probe to help the surgeon identify the particular drilling pathway required for decompression (Fig. 13). The surgeon will encounter a hard outer rim of cortical bone followed by softer cancellous bone that is easily thinned. The inner cortical table is then encountered, and drilling must proceed slowly and cautiously as the nerve root is approximated. Drilling should be completed in a medial to lateral direction. Continuous irrigation is used to prevent thermal injury.

Once the anterior cortical rim is thinned appropriately, a fine angled curette is then used to chip off the thinned layer

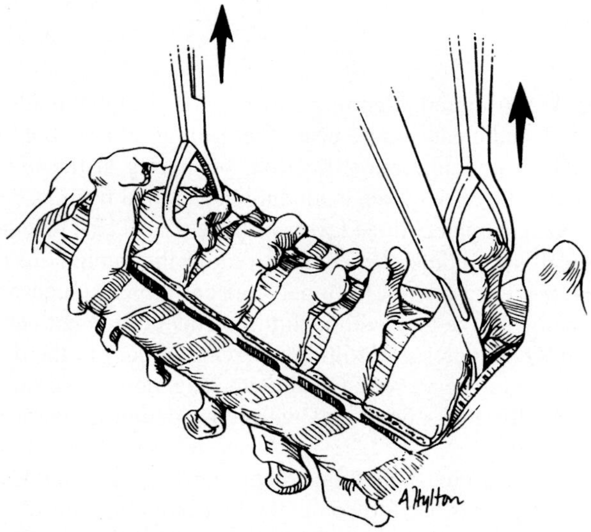

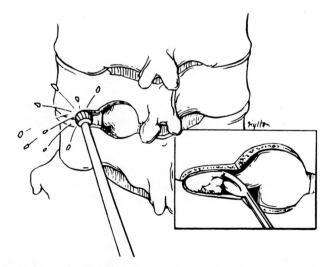

FIG. 12. Towel clips are placed in the spinous processes at the proximal and distal poles of the laminectomy. Gentle upward traction is applied as the ligamentum flavum is resected. (From ref. 108, with permission.)

FIG. 13. After the foramen is palpably identified, a 3-mm diamond tip burr is used to thin bone over the nerve root. Once the bone is adequately thinned, a fine angled curette is used to remove the remaining bone over the nerve root **(inset)**. (From ref. 108, with permission.)

of remaining bone in an anterior to posterior direction. The lateral extent of the foraminotomy is determined by passing a thin, blunt nerve hook or dental probe out the neural foramen. Proper lateral decompression of the nerve root generally requires approximately 5 mm of nerve root exposure. Cranial to caudal exposure should extend from pedicle to pedicle. After foraminotomy in the traumatic case, a posterior fusion is performed.

Posterior Cervical Fusion

Posterior cervical fusion is the most commonly performed operation for traumatic instability. The procedure is highly effective and safe with excellent long-term outcomes. Simpler, cost-effective wiring techniques can be used in the majority of cases. Newer techniques and devices may be costly but in some cases can provide biomechanical advantage.

Numerous studies have demonstrated biomechanical advantages of various posterior cervical fixation techniques (87–91). Interspinous wiring and Bohlman's triple-wire technique have sufficient stability for hyperflexion injuries but require an intact neural arch and facet articulations. Sublaminar wire techniques play little role in the posterior cervical spine. Passage of wires carries an unnecessary risk of neural impingement and biomechanically offers no added stability when compared to spinous process wiring. Halifax clamps perform poorly in cyclical loading secondary to screw loosening or dislodgment and should be avoided. Lateral mass plating has gained popularity and biomechanically has demonstrated increased resistance to rotational and axial loading forces and overall provides the stiffest cervical constructs.

For each case of cervical spine injury requiring posterior cervical stabilization, the particular surgical technique utilized depends on the specific pathoanatomy, biomechanical requirements of the injury, and the surgeon's expertise and experience. In most cases triple-wiring techniques should suffice.

Indications for the posterior approach include unstable injuries without need for anterior decompression. Posterior fusion may also be complete and an adjunct to an anterior decompression.

Interspinous Wire Technique—Bohlman's Triple Wire

Since Rogers (92) initially described a method of cervical wiring and fusion, many other techniques have been described in the literature (91,93–97). Wiring techniques are quite effective in preventing flexion but less effective in preventing extension or rotation. I favor Bohlman's interspinous process triple-wire technique, which compresses the bone grafts to the underlying lamina (Fig. 14). This triple-wire technique has been shown to be safe and effective and biomechanically superior to many other constructs (91,93).

Once the patient is positioned and alignment checked radiographically, the patient's cervical spine bone graft donor sites are prepped and draped. The skin and subcutaneous tissues are dissected to the midline fascia. A second radiograph is taken to identify surgical levels. Subperiosteal dissection is completed to expose the spinous processes, lamina, and necessary facet joints. Caution is necessary to avoid dissection beyond fusion sites and to prevent creeping fusion extension. A 3-mm burr is used to drill a hole at the base of the spinous process on both sides. The drill hole should be placed at the proximal aspect of the cephalad spinous process and at the distal aspect of the caudad spinous process. A towel clip is gently passed through the hole to create a tunnel for wire passage. A single 18- or 20-gauge wire is then passed through both spinous processes (for single-level fusion) and tightened appropriately. If more than one level is to be fused, figure of 8 wiring is used to incorporate the middle spinous process in the wiring construct. If the middle spinous process or lamina is fractured, wiring should be avoided at this level. The second and third wires are passed through the cephalad and caudal holes at the base of the processes, respectively. The lamina and facet joints are decorticated using the burr. Corticocancellous bone grafts of appropriate length are then harvested from the outer table of the iliac crest. Two drill holes are placed in each graft for passage of wires. The grafts

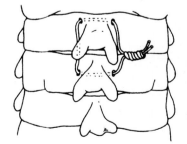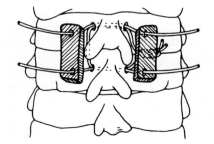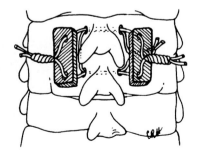

FIG. 14. A triple-wire technique with interspinous process wires. **Left:** A wire passed from the cephalad part of the superior spinous process to the inferior part of the caudad spinous process. **Middle:** The second and third wires are passed through the cephalad and caudad holes in the base of the processes, respectively. After decortication of the lamina and facets, corticocancellous bone grafts from the outer table of the iliac crest are placed. **Right:** Wires are tightened over the grafts and additional cancellous chips are laid down on the exposed lamina or facets. (From ref. 108, with permission.)

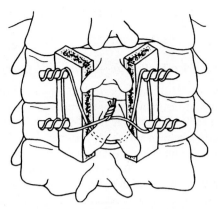

FIG. 15. Dewar technique. Kirschner wires are inserted at base of spinous processes using a lateral percutaneous technique. Bone grafts are then inserted over these wires and pecured with 18–20 gauge wire in a loop fashion. (From ref. 108, with permission.)

are then slid over the wires, and contact made between the graft and lamina. The posterior cortical edge of the graft should be placed under the bulbus spinous process to enhance stability of the construct and maximize graft-lamina contact. The wires on each side of the spine are then simultaneously tightened. Additional cancellous chips are placed on the exposed lamina or facets. The patient is usually kept in a cervicothoracic orthosis or halo vest for 6 weeks depending on the stability of the construct and compliance of the patient.

An alternative fixation is the Dewar procedure, in which Kirschner wires are inserted at the base of the spinous processes and secured with wire in a loop fashion (18,42,98) (Fig. 15). Another method involves Wisconsin button and wires with a Luque ring (Fig. 16). This technique provides good fixation without the use of sublaminar wires.

Facet fracture or subluxation can be managed with an oblique wiring technique or wire loop by passing the wire through the lateral mass (1,84,99). In the postlaminectomy condition requiring stabilization, interfacet wiring and fusion can be performed (100). The facet wire is passed by placing a small Penfield dissector into the facet joint. A 2-mm drill hole is then made in the facet in a superior-inferior direction; 20- or 22-gauge wires are then passed through the

hole. The facet wires are then placed at adjacent levels for multilevel facet stabilization. The facet wires are usually tied to the bone grafts for fusion but alternatively can be tied to metallic rods for additional stability. In the oblique wiring technique, the facet wire is passed in a similar fashion. The same wire is then passed around the inferior spinous process for one-level fusion. This is a very nice technique for unilateral facet dislocations (Fig. 17).

Complications associated with posterior interspinous wiring in the cervical spine are infrequent. Inadvertent penetration of the spinal canal and dural violation may occur during drilling or passage of wires. The most common complication associated with wiring is loss of fixation and recurring deformity. This complication is related to surgical technique and lack of proper postoperative immobilization. If a rigid construct is accomplished and patient bone quality sufficient, a Philadelphia collar or cervicothoracic orthosis may be adequate. However, if fixation is compromised or patient cooperation questioned, a halo vest should be utilized.

Lateral Mass Plate Fixation

Posterior stabilization of the cervical spine using screws and plates was first introduced by Roy-Camille et al. (95,101) in Paris. Louis (96) and Grob and Magerl (97) also designed similar posterior fixation devices using plate and plate-hook configurations with lateral mass screws. Anderson and associates (102) more recently reported on 30 patients with unstable cervical spine injuries who underwent a posterior arthrodesis with AO reconstruction plates. All patients developed solid unions without neurologic or vascular complications. Three patients had evidence of screw loosening without sequelae. Biomechanically, stability of these constructs has been shown to be superior to posterior wiring, particularly in extension and torsion modes.

Lateral mass screw placement is critical to the safety and efficacy of this fixation technique. Roy-Camille recommended starting the screw at the peak of the lateral articular mass directing the screw directly forward and 10 degrees laterally. Magerl recommended starting 1-2 mm medial and cranial to the center of the lateral mass directing the drilling

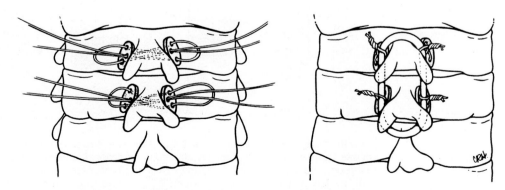

FIG. 16. Cervical spine fixation using Wisconsin buttons and spinous process wires. (From ref. 108, with permission.)

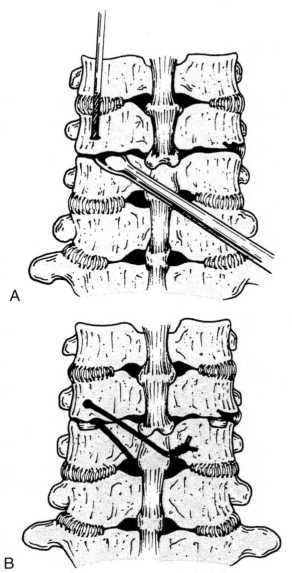

FIG. 17. A: Oblique wire technique. A drill or burr is used to make a hole passing from the lateral mass into the facet joint. To aid in drilling, the joint is gently distracted and a freer is placed into the joint to act as a backstop. **B:** A 20- to 22-gauge wire is passed around the caudal spine process and tightened. (From ref. 109, with permission.)

process 35 degrees cranially and 25 degrees outward (Fig. 18).

Biomechanical studies comparing the Roy-Camille technique to that of Magerl have demonstrated that the Magerl screws have significant better pullout strength (90). Gill et al. (87) further found that bicortical purchase greatly increases pullout strength.

The lateral mass of C7 represents a transitional zone for the cervicothoracic spine and as such the anatomy is widely variable. Identification of the starting point may be difficult or impossible and fixation compromised. Recently, placement of C7 pedicle screws has been advocated by many. Al-

ternatively, the Magerl hook-plate construct may be advantageous.

Surgical exposure for plate-screw construct requires visualization of the entire lateral mass to include the far lateral edge. The medial border is identified at the junction of the articular mass to the lamina. A "valley" is usually present at this anatomic junction to aid in the identification of this important landmark. The superior and inferior borders of the articular mass are defined by the cranial and caudal facet joints, respectively. Once this anatomy is well defined, a starting point for drilling is identified 1 to 2 mm medial to the center of the articular mass. Drilling is completed by one of the techniques described, based on the surgeon's preference. We prefer the technique described by Magerl; therefore, drilling proceeds in a direction parallel to the facet joints in the sagittal plane and directed laterally 25 degrees. Drilling continues to 20 mm or until bicortical perforation has occurred. The plate is the selected and screw holes tapped. Cancellous autogenous graft is inserted into the decorticated facet joint and along the lateral margins of the articular masses. Instrumentation ensues and radiographs are obtained to verify screw placement (Fig. 19).

Anterior Decompression and Fusion

Anterior decompression and fusion is indicated for patients with evidence of residual anterior spinal cord or nerve root compression and persistent neurologic deficit (103). Early surgical intervention is generally recommended to optimize conditions for neurologic improvement. In the majority of injuries, persistent compression is found ventral to the spinal cord. Thus, anterior decompression affords the most direct method to complete cord decompression while minimizing surgical trauma.

Late anterior decompression may also be completed in those spinal cord injuries where a neurologic plateau is obtained. Bohlman and Anderson (63,104) reviewed results of late anterior decompression in 109 patients with spinal cord injuries. The average time from the injury to surgery was 14 months. The follow-up period averaged 5.6 years, with a range of 2 to 14 years. Patients were divided into two groups based on neurologic function at the time of injury; 58 patients were found to have an incomplete motor quadriplegia (Frankel grades C and D) and 51 had complete motor quadriplegia (Frankel grades A and B). Twenty-nine of the 58 patients with incomplete motor quadriplegia became ambulators, and another six improved significantly on their preoperative ambulation capacity. Improvement in upper extremity function was demonstrated in 39 of 58 patients. In a group of patients with complete motor quadriplegia, only one regained capacity to ambulate. However, significant upper extremity root recovery and improvement in overall function was found to occur in 31 or 58 patients. Significant predictors of success included a patient age of less than 50 years, surgery within 12 months

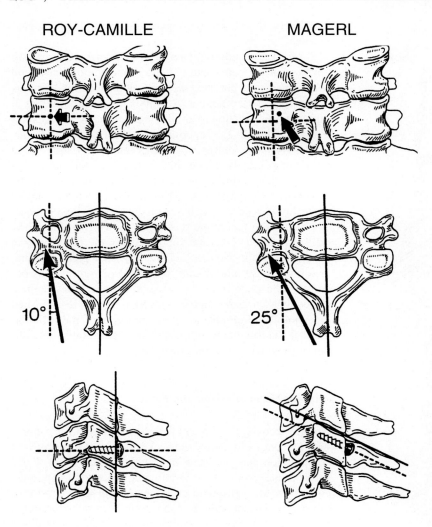

FIG. 18. Roy-Camille and Magerl techniques for lateral mass screw placement. (From ref. 110, with permission.)

of injury, and a greater degree of preoperative neurologic function.

Preoperative evaluation of patients with cervical spine injuries requiring anterior decompression have demonstrated anterior spinal cord compression on the basis of MRI or CT scanning. Prior to surgery the patient is maintained in cervical traction or alternatively placed in a halo vest with adequate reduction.

A Smith-Robinson approach is utilized and may be completed from either the right or left side according to the surgeon's preference (105). In most cases a transverse incision may be utilized extending from the midline to the border of the sternocleidomastoid muscle. Occasionally, an oblique incision may be preferred along the anterior border of the sternocleidomastoid, particularly in cases requiring more extensive visualization. The platysma muscle when encountered is split in line with its fibers, exposing the deep cervical fascia. This fascia is incised along the border of the sternocleidomastoid muscle and blunt dissection completed between the trachea and carotid sheath. The prevertebral fascia is then identified along the anterior surface of the cervical spine and intervertebral disc. This structure is divided completely, exposing the injured segment. An intraoperative radiograph is taken to verify the correct level. In surgical cases where corpectomy is planned, the disc above and below the injured segment is completely removed back to the posterior longitudinal ligament. The vertebral body is then removed in an anterior to posterior direction generally using an air-driven burr. Alternatively, a rongeur may be utilized; although this would not generally be advocated for acute injuries, it attempts to minimize the potential for further displacement of bone posteriorly into the spinal canal. Loupe magnification with a head lamp or operating microscope may facilitate this portion of the operation as the bony decompression continues back to the posterior cortical rim. This cortical shell can then be removed in a piecemeal fashion using a series of small curettes or Kerrison rongeur with a thin footplate. In patients with an associated disc herniation, the posterior longitudinal ligament may be resected to ensure adequate spinal cord decompression. Decompression is completed laterally until the dura or posterior longitudinal ligament obtains its convex appearance. This usually requires a 12- to 15-mm-wide decompression. Care must be taken to maintain orientation to the midline, thus avoiding injury to the vertebral artery (Fig. 20).

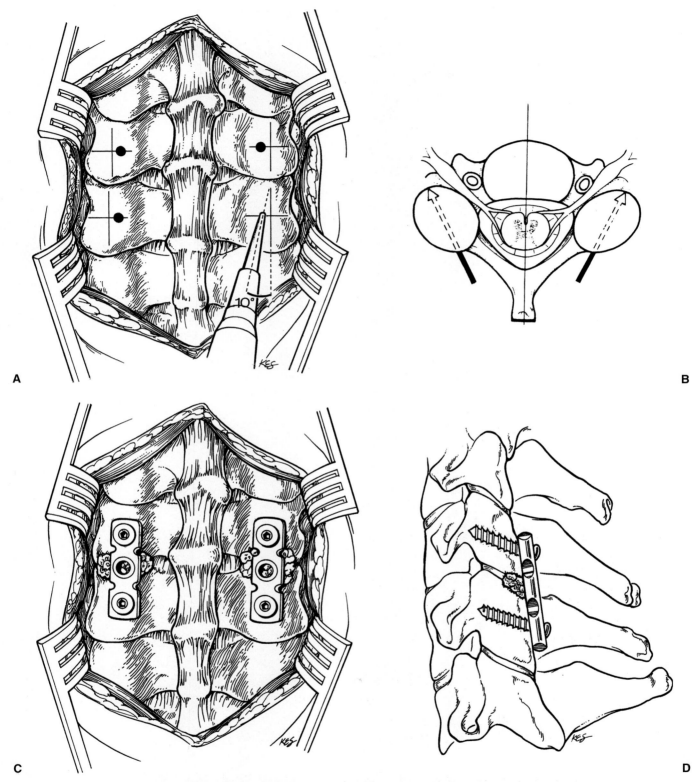

FIG. 19. A: Dorsal view of the cervical spine. The starting point for lateral mass screw placement is 1 to 2 mm medial to the center of the lateral mass. The screw is directed cranially 20 to 30 degrees and outward 10 to 20 degrees. **B:** Axial view of the cervical spine. Note the important landmark of the valley at the junction of the lamina and lateral mass. The vertebral artery and most dorsal extent of the nerve root are located directly anterior to this point. Screws must start lateral and angle outward to avoid neurovascular injury. (From ref. 111, with permission.) **C:** Lateral view after plate fixation with AO reconstruction plates. **D:** Dorsal view after lateral mass fixation. (From ref. 112, with permission.)

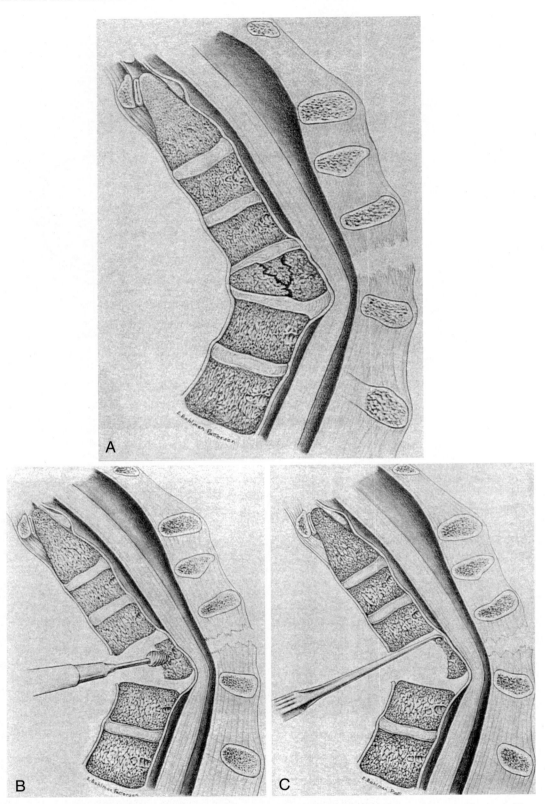

FIG. 20. A: Lateral view of burst type fracture with retropulsion of bone and disc into spinal canal. (From ref. 2, with permission.) **B:** In an anterior decompression, the disc and vertebral body are removed back to the posterior longitudinal ligament. The vertebral body is resected with rongeurs and an air driven burr. (From ref. 105, with permission.) **C:** Vertebral body resection continues until only a thin posterior wall remains. This wall can be removed easily with curettes. (From ref. 105, with permission.)

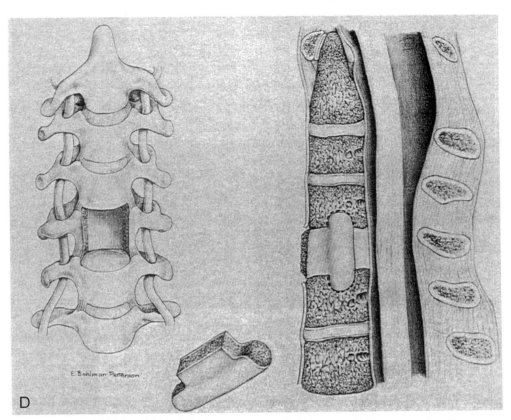

FIG. 20. *Continued.* **D:** Realignment is achieved with traction or use of distraction pins. Mortices are made in the end plate. An appropriate-length iliac crest graft is harvested and made into a T-shape, creating tenons. The tenons are seated into the mortices. (From refs. 2 and 112, with permission.)

The cartilaginous portion of the endplate is removed using a curette. A burr is used to contour subchondral bone into a mortise to accept the prepared bone graft. For a single-level corpectomy, a tricortical autogenous bone graft is harvested using an oscillating saw. The intervertebral body space is distracted maximally for the purposes of graft insertion. Careful measurement is made. The graft is contoured appropriately and tapped into the prepared surface. It is important to avoid posterior displacement of the graft into the spinal canal. In the majority of trauma cases, supplemental fixation in the form of an anterior cervical plate is added. Alternatively, based on the surgeon's preference, a concomitant posterior arthrodesis may be completed.

Anterior Cervical Plate Fixation

Multiple anterior cervical plating systems are now available commercially. The purpose of this instrumentation is to stabilize the spine, limit potential for pseudarthrosis or postoperative kyphosis, and obviate the need for posterior fusion techniques. Biomechanical studies have shown anterior fixation to be inferior when compared to the described posterior fixation techniques (40,84,90). Despite the apparent biomechanical limitations, clinical studies of patients treated with anterior cervical plates have shown good results with minimal potential for complication.

Anterior cervical plate fixation is started with selection of an appropriate plate, which must extend from the midportion of the superior and inferior uninvolved vertebrae. The plate is then contoured according to the anterolateral surfaces of the cervical spine, maximizing contact. When osteophytes are present on the vertebral bodies, they should be removed with a rongeur or high-speed burr to maximize bony contact and enhance stability of the overall construct.

Drilling ensues at the proximal and distal holes of the plate into the respective vertebral bodies. Drilling may be completed manually or with an air-driven drill with appropriate guide. Depending on the particular instrumentation system in Paris Orozco utilized, bicortical drilling may be necessary. The Caspar and Orozco plate systems generally require bicortical purchases to enhance stability and minimize potential for screw loosening (106). The surgeon is encouraged under these circumstances to partially drill and carefully palpate the hole to get a feel for posterior wall penetration. This repeated sequence of events is completed until the posterior wall is perforated. The hole is then tapped and a cortical screw placed; 3.5-mm-diameter screws are usually used in the cervical spine. The depth of this screw most frequently approximates 16 to 20 mm. Once all the screws are placed, an intraoperative x-ray is taken to verify the position and length of the screws. If, for any reason, there is less than adequate purchase into the vertebral body, the screw should be removed and redirected. If this procedure also fails, a small amount of methylmethacrylate may be used to enhance screw fixation. Complications associated with this technique include dural or spinal cord impingement from either the screw or drilling process. Subsequent loss of fixation may allow for loosening and displacement of screws with poten-

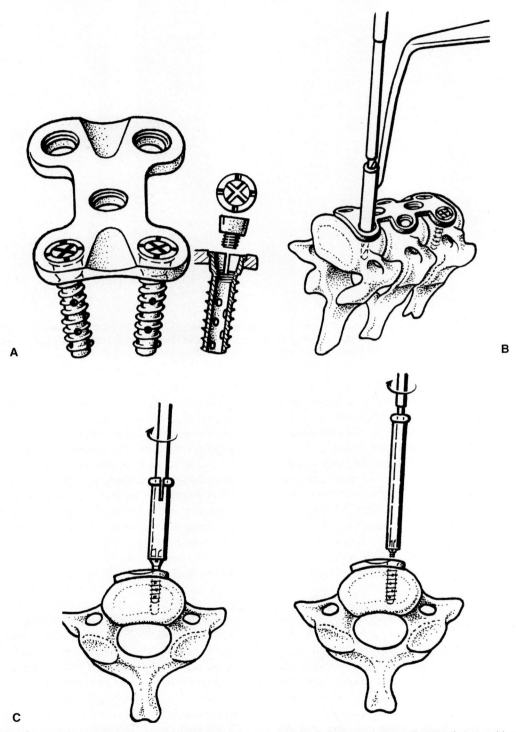

FIG. 21. A: AO-Morscher titanium cervical plating demonstrating screw design. (From ref. 111, with permission.) **B:** Drilling and tapping is completed with the plate appropriately centered over the vertebral body. (From ref. 111, with permission.) **C:** The screw is inserted followed by expansion screw. (From ref. 112, with permission.)

tial injury to surrounding soft tissues, most notably the esophagus.

The AO-Morscher pure titanium cervical plate has been designed to obviate the need for posterior cortical penetration. This system utilizes a 4-mm-diameter screw with an expansion head. The expansion screw itself fits into the hollowed-out cylindrical portion of the 4-mm screw, which, when tightened, widens the shoulder of the expansion head screw, locking it to the cervical plate. The benefit of this technique is avoiding the need for posterior cortical purchase. The stability of the construct, however, is dependent on screw purchase into the vertebral body. As most traumatic injuries tend to occur in the younger patient population, we find this particular technique to be advantageous.

Cervical Spine Locking Plate

The AO-Morscher locking plate has plate lengths available in sizes ranging from 16 to 55 mm. At one end of the plate, screw direction is set at a 12-degree angle to facilitate insertion of the screw where anatomy does not allow right-angle application. Screw sizes are 4.0 and 4.35 mm in 14-mm lengths. The screw heads are hollow as noted earlier to allow for an expansion screw to be inserted into the head, thus locking it to the plate.

The selected plate is placed on the spine and checked for position and length radiographically. The plate holes should be aligned in the midposition of the vertebral body and should not overlie an unfused disc. The plate is held firmly and a hole is then drilled with a 3.0-mm drill and drill guide. The drill is angled medially and 12 degrees cranially in the superior vertebra and medially and straightforward in the inferior vertebra. The drill guide allows for drilling to a depth of only 14 mm. The screws are then placed and tightened sequentially. The head of the screws should be flush into the cervical plate. The expansion screws are then inserted, locking the expansion head screw to the plate (Fig. 21). Postoperatively, patients are immobilized in a well-fitting Philadelphia collar or cervicothoracic orthosis.

CONCLUSION

A high index of suspicion must be exercised when evaluating any traumatized patient. To minimize iatrogenic injury, the patient must be properly transported and thoroughly evaluated in the emergency room. Attention to the described protocols will optimize patient treatment and outcomes. Once recognized, treatment is determined primarily on the basis of fracture morphology and neurologic status of the injured patient. The goals of treatment include to protect and maximize function of the neural tissue through immediate reduction, and to stabilize obvious fractures and dislocations associated with deformity. Based on recent studies, pharmacologic treatment with high-dose steroids appears to improve chances of neurologic recovery. The described surgical techniques of anterior decompression and fusion and interspinous wire fixation have excellent reported results and low complication rates when used appropriately. Proper postoperative immobilization as well should not be ignored. Despite the best surgical efforts, complications may arise from failed fixation possibly related to poor choice in external immobilization.

REFERENCES

1. Bohlman HH. Complications of treatment of fractures and dislocations of the cervical spine. In: Epps C (ed). *Complications of Orthopaedic Surgery.* Philadelphia: JB Lippincott, 1985:897—918.
2. Bohlman HH. Acute fractures and dislocations of the cervical spine: an analysis of 300 hospitalized patients and review of the literature. *J Bone Joint Surg* 1979;61A:1119–1142.
3. Bohlman HH, Zdeblick TA. Complications of treatment of fractures and dislocations of the cervical spine. In: Epps C (ed). *Complications of Orthopaedic Surgery.* Philadelphia: JB Lippincott, 1985:897–918.
4. Saul TG, Ducker TB. The spine and spinal cord. In: Wyatt J, et al. (eds). *American College of Surgeons: Early Care of the Injuries Patients,* 3rd ed. Philadelphia: WB Saunders, 1982:196–205.
5. Bohlman HH, Anderson PA. The neck. In: D'Ambrosia RD (ed). *Musculoskeletal Disorders, Regional Examination, Differential Diagnosis,* 2nd ed. Philadelphia: JB Lippincott, 1985:219–286.
6. Heckman JD (ed). *Emergency Care and Transportation of the Sick and Injured,* 5th ed. Chicago: American Academy of Orthopaedic Surgeons, 1992:334–349.
7. Bohlman HH. Surgical management of cervical spine fractures and dislocations. *Instr Course Lect* 1985;34:163–187.
8. Keenen TL, Antony J, Benson DR. Non-contiguous spinal fractures. *J Trauma* 1990;30:489–491.
9. Miller LS, Cotler HB, DeLucia FA, Cotler JM, Hume EL. Biomechanical analysis of cervical distraction. *Spine* 1987;12:731–837.
10. Vaccaro AR, An HS, Lin SS, Sun S, Balderston RA, Cotler JM. Non-contiguous injuries of the spine. *J Spinal Disord* 1991;5:320–329.
11. American Spinal Injury Association, ed. *Standards for neurologic and functional classification of spinal cord injury,* revised ed. American Spinal Injury Association.
12. Daffner RH, Deeb ZL, Rothfus WE. The posterior vertebral body line: importance in the detection of burst fractures. *AJR Radium Ther Nucl Med* 1987;148:93–96.
13. Galli RL, Spaite DW, Simmon RR. The cervical spine. In: *Emergency Orthopaedics.* East Norwalk, CT: Appleton and Lange, 1989:96–99.
14. More SE. Emergency evaluation of cervical spine injuries: CT versus radiographs. *Ann Emerg Med* 1985;14:973.
15. Stover SC. *Spinal Cord Injury. The Facts and Figures.* Birmingham, AL: University of Alabama, 1986.
16. Gisbert VL, Hollerman JJ, Ney Al, et al. Incidence and diagnosis of C7-T1 fractures and subluxations in multiple trauma patients: evaluation of the advanced trauma life support guidelines. *Surgery* 1989; 106:702–709.
17. Lodge T, Higgenbottom E. Fractures and dislocations of the cervical spine. *X-Ray Focus* 1966;7:2.
18. Scher A, Vambeck V. An approach to radiological examination of the cervicodorsal junction following injury. *Clin Radiol* 1977;28:24–43.
19. Bernhardt M, White AA, Panjabi MM, McGowan DP. Biomechanical considerations of spinal stability. In: Rothman RH, Simeon FA (eds). *The Spine,* 3rd ed. Philadelphia: WB Saunders 1992:1167–1195.
20. White AA, Soutwick WO, Panjabi MM. Clinical instability in the lower cervical spine. A review of past and current concepts. *Spine* 1970;1:15–27.
21. Templeton PA, Young JWR, Mirvis SE, Buddemeyer EV. The value of retropharyngeal soft tissue measurement in trauma of the adult cervical spine. *Skeletal Radiol* 1987;16:98–104.
22. Herkowitz HR, Rothman RH. Subacute instability of the cervical spine. *Spine* 1984;9:348–352.
23. Chakeres DW, Flickinger F, Bresnahan JC, et al. MR imaging of acute spinal cord trauma. *Am J Neurol Res* 1987;8:5.
24. Goldberg AL, Rothfus WE, Deeb ZL, et al. The impact of magnetic resonance on the diagnostic evaluation of acute cervicothoracic spinal trauma. *Skeletal Radiol* 1988;17:89.

25. Kulkami MV, McArdle CB, Kopanicky D, et al. Acute spinal cord injury. MR imaging at 1.5 T. *Radiology* 1987;164:837.

26. Harrington JF, Likavel MJ, Smith AS. Disc herniation in cervical fracture subluxation. *Neurosurgery* 1991;29:374–379.

27. Pratt ES, Green DA, Spengler DM. Herniated intervertebral disc associated with unstable spinal injuries. *Spine* 1990;15:662–665.

28. Raynor RB. Cervical cord compression secondary to acute disc protrusion in trauma. *Spine* 1977;2:39–43.

29. Rizzolo SJ, Piazza MR, Cotler JM, Balderston RA, Schaefer D, Flanders A. Intervertebral disc injury complicating cervical spine trauma. *Spine* 1991;16(suppl):S187–S189.

30. Cotler HB, Kulkarni MV, Bondurant FJ. Magnetic resonance imaging of acute spinal cord trauma: preliminary report. *J Orthop Trauma* 1988;2:1–4.

31. Schafer DM, Flanders A, Northup BE, Doan HT, Osterholm JL. Magnetic resonance imaging of acute cervical spine trauma: correlation with severity of neurologic injury. *Spine* 1989;14:1090–1095.

32. White AA, Panjabi MM. *Clinical Biomechanics of the Spine*, 2nd ed. Philadelphia: JB Lippincott, 1990.

33. Holdsworth FW. Fractures, dislocations and fracture-dislocations of the spine. *J Bone Joint Surg* 1970;52A:1534–1551.

34. Allen BL, Ferguson RL, Lehmann TR, O'Brien RP. A mechanistic classification of closed, indirect fractures and dislocations of the lower cervical spine. *Spine* 1982;7:1–27.

35. Denis F. The three column spine and its significance in the classification of acute thoracolumbar spinal injuries. *Spine* 1983;8:817–831.

36. Gooding MR, Wilson, CB, Hoff JT. Experimental cervical myelopathy. Effects of ischemia and compression of the canine cervical spine. *Neurosurgery* 1975;43:9–12.

37. Aebi M, Mohler J, Zach GA, Morscher E. Indication, surgical technique and results of 100 surgically treated fractures and fracture-dislocations of the cervical spine. *Clin Orthop* 1980;203:244–257.

38. Burke DC, Berryman D. The place of closed manipulation in the management of flexion-rotation dislocations of the cervical spine. *J Bone Joint Surg* 1971;53A:165–182.

39. Cotler JM, Nasuti J, Ditunno JF, An HS. Improvement of motor index score after rapid closed reduction of traumatic cervical spine dislocation using traction weights up to 130 pounds. Presented at the annual meeting of American Spinal Injury Association, Toronto, Ontario, Canada, 1992.

40. Dolan EJ, Tator CH, Endrenyi L. The value of decompression for acute experimental spinal cord injury. *J Neurosurg* 1980;53:749–755.

41. Levi L, Wolf A, Rigamonti D, Ragheb J, Mirvis S, Robinson WL. Anterior decompression of cervical spine trauma. Does timing of surgery affect outcome? *Neurosurgery* 1987;29:216–222.

42. Rorabeck CH, Rock MG, Hawkins RJ, Bourne RB. Unilateral facet dislocation of the cervical spine. An analysis of the results of treatment in 26 patients. *Spine* 1987;12:23–27.

43. Tarlov IM. Spinal cord compression studies. Time limits for recovery after gradual compression in dogs. *Arch Neural Neurosurg Psychol* 1954;71:588–597.

44. Cotler JM, Hervison FJ, Nasuti JF, Ditunno JF, An HS. Closed reduction of traumatic cervical spine dislocations using traction weights up to 140 pounds. Presented at the annual meeting of the Cervical Spine Research Society, Philadelphia, December 1991.

45. Cotler HB, Miller LS, DeLucia FA, Cotler JM, Davne SH. Closed reduction of cervical spine dislocations. *Clin Orthop* 1987;214:185–199.

46. Star AM, Jones AA, Cotler JM, Balderston RA, Sinha R. Immediate closed reduction of cervical spine dislocations using traction. *Spine* 1990;15:1068–1072.

47. Johnson RM, Hart DL, Simmons EF, Ramshy GR, Southwick WO. Cervical orthoses. *J Bone Joint Surg* 1977;59A:332–339.

48. Bucci MN, Dauser RC, Maynard FA, Hoff JT. Management of post-traumatic cervical spine instability: operative fusion versus halo-vest immobilization. Analysis of 49 cases. *J Trauma* 1988;28:1001–1006.

49. Bucholz RD, Cheung KC. Halo-vest versus spinal fusion for cervical injury: evidence from an outcome study. *J Neurosurg* 1989;70:884–892.

50. Cooper PR, Maravilla KR, Sklar FH, Moody SF, Clark WK. Halo immobilization of cervical spine fractures: indications and results. *J Neurosurg* 1979;50:603–610.

51. Holness RO, Huestis WS, Howes WJ, Langille RA. Posterior stabilization with an interlaminar clamp in cervical injuries: technical note and review of the long-term experienced with the method. *Neurosurgery* 1984;14:318–322.

52. Lind B, Sihbom H. Nordwall A. Halso-vest treatment of unstable traumatic cervical spine injuries. *Spine* 1988;13:425–432.

53. Whitehill R, Richman JA, Glaser JA. Failure of immobilization of the cervical spine by the halo-vest. *J Bone Joint Surg* 1986;68A:326–332.

54. Garfin SR, Botte MJ, Waters RL, Nickel VL. Complications in the use of the halo fixation device. *J Bone Joint Surg* 1986;68A:320–325.

55. Albert TJ, Levine M, Balderston RA, Cotler JM. GI complications in spinal cord injury. *Spine* 1991;16(suppl):S522–S515.

56. Leramo OB, Tator CH, Hudson AR. Massive gastroduodenal hemorrhage and perforation in acute spinal cord injury. *Surg Neurol* 1982;17:186–190.

57. Green D, Lee MY, Ito V, et al. Fixed versus adjusted dose heparin in prophylaxis of thromboembolism in spinal cord injury. *JAMA* 1988;260:1255–1258.

58. Merli GJ, Herbison GJ, Ditunno JF, et al. Deep venous thrombosis prophylaxis in acute spinal cord injury patients. *Arch Phys Med Rehabil* 1988;69:661–664.

59. Bailey RW, Badgley CE. Stabilization of the cervical spine by anterior fusion. *J Bone Joint Surg* 1992;42A:565–594.

60. Benzel EC, Larson SJ. Recovery of nerve root function after complete quadriplegia from cervical spine fractures. *Neurosurgery* 1986;19:772–778.

61. Bracken MB, Collins WF, Frieman DF, et al. Efficacy of methylprednisolone in acute spinal cord injury. *JAMA* 1984;251:45–52.

62. Benzel EC, Larson SJ. Functional recovery after decompressive spine operation for cervical spine fractures. *Neurosurgery* 1987;20:742–746.

63. Bohlman HH, Andersons PA. Anterior decompression and arthrodesis in patients with incomplete cervical spinal cord injury: long-term results of neurologic recovery in 58 patients. Part I. *J Bone Joint Surg* 1992;74A:671–682.

64. Bracken MB, Shepard MJ, Collins WF, et al. A randomized, controlled trial of methyprednisolone or naloxone in the treatment of acute spinal cord injury. Results of the second national acute spinal cord injury study. *N Engl J Med* 1990;322:1405–1411.

65. Bracken MB, Shepard MJ, Hefenbrane KG, et al. Methylprednisolone and neurologic function one year post spinal cord injury. *J Neurosurg* 1987;63:704–713.

66. Benzel EC, Larson SJ. Functional recovery after decompressive operation for thoracic and lumbar spine fractures. *Neurosurgery* 1986;19:772–778.

67. Bohlman HH. Late anterior decompression and fusion for spinal cord injuries: review of 100 cases with long term results. *Orthop Trans* 1980;4:42–43.

68. Holdsworth FW, Hardy A. Early treatment of paraplegia from fractures of the thoracolumbar spine. *J Bone Joint Surg* 1953;35B:540–550.

69. Morgan TH, Wharton GW, Austin GN. The results of laminectomy in patients with incomplete spinal cord injuries. *Paraplegia* 1971;9:14–23.

70. Schneider RC, Cherry G, Pantek H. The syndrome of acute central cervical spinal cord injury. Special reference to the mechanisms involved in hypertension injuries of the cervical spine. *J Neurosurg* 1954;11:546–577.

71. Stauffer ES, Wood W, Kelly EG. Gunshot wounds of the spine. The effects of laminectomy. *J Bone Joint Surg* 1979;61A:389–392.

72. Marshall FM, Reynolds GG, Fountains S, Wilmot C, Hamilton R. Neurologic prognosis after traumatic quadriplegia. *J Neurosurg* 1979;50:611–616.

73. Osterholm JL. *The Pathophysiology of Spinal Cord Trauma*. Springfield, IL: Charles C Thomas, 1978.

74. Krengel WF, Andersons PA, Hansen Y, Ayley JC. Early versus delayed stabilization after cervical spinal cord injury. Presented at the annual meeting of the North American Spine Society, Boston, 1992.

75. Roberts JB, Curis PH. Stability of the thoracic and lumbar spine in traumatic paraplegia following fracture of fracture-dislocations. *J Bone Joint Surg* 1970;52A:1115–1130.

76. Apple DF, McDonald AR, Smith RA. Identification of herniated nucleus pulposus in spinal cord injury. *Paraplegia* 1987;25:78–85.

77. Eismont FJ, Arena MJ, Green BA. Extrusion of an intervertebral disc associated with traumatic subluxation or dislocation of facets. *J Bone Joint Surg* 1991;73A:1555–1560.

78. Willis BK, Greiner F, Orrison WW, Benzel EC. The incidence of vertebral artery injury after midcervical spine fracture or subluxation. *Neurosurgery* 1994;34:435–442.

79. Bohlman HH, Ducker TB, Levine AM, McAfee PC. Spine trauma in adults. In: Rothman RH, Simeone FA (eds). *The Spine,* 3rd ed. Philadelphia: WB Saunders, 1992:973–1166.

80. Stauffer ES, Kaufer H, Kling TF. Fractures and dislocations of the spine. In: Rockwood CA, Green DP (eds). *Fractures in Adults.* Philadelphia: JB Lippincott, 1984:987–1093.

81. Raflin G, Jenneret B, Mageri F. Tetraplegia following cervical spine fusion. Presented at the annual meeting of the Cervical Spine Research Society, European Section, St. Gallen, Switzerland, 1989.

82. Walters RN, Adkins RH, Nelson R, Garland D. Cervical spinal cord trauma: evaluation and nonoperative treatment in halo immobilization. *Contemp Orthop* 1987;14:35–45.

83. Rizzolo SJ, Vaccaro AR, Cotler JM, Balderston RA, Ergener J, Dailey S. Incidence and clinical implications of disc injury in patients with acute cervical spine dislocations. Presented at the annual meeting of the American Academy of Orthopaedic Surgeons, San Francisco, February 1993.

84. Edward CC, Matz SO, Levine AM. The oblique wiring techniques for rotational injuries of the cervical spine. *Trans Orthop* 1985;9:142.

85. Bolesta MJ, Bohlman HH. Late complications of cervical fractures and dislocations and their surgical treatment. In: Frymoyer J (ed). *The Adult Spine—Principles and Practice.* New York: Raven Press, 1991:1107–1126.

86. Zdeblick TA, Zou D, Warden KE, et al. Cervical stability after foraminotomy: a biomechanical in vitro analysis. *J Bone Joint Surg* 1992;74:22–27.

87. Gill K, Paschal S, Corin J, et al. Posterior plating of the cervical spine. A biochemical comparison of different posterior fusion techniques. *Spine* 1988;13:813–816.

88. Cahill DW, Bellegarrigue R, Ducker IB. Bilateral facet to spinous process fusion: a new technique for posterior spinal fusion after trauma. *Neurosurgery* 1983;13:1–4.

89. Coe JD, Warden KE, Sutterlin CE, et al. Biomechanical evaluation of cervical spine stabilization methods in a human cadaveric model. *Spine* 1989;14:1122–1131.

90. Montesano PX, Juach EC, Anderson PA, et al. Biomechanics of the cervical spine internal fixation. *Spine Symp Intern Fixation* 1991;16:S10–S16.

91. Sutterlin CE, McAfee PC, Warden KE, et al. A biomechanical evaluation of cervical spinal stabilization methods in a bovine model. Static and cyclical loading. *Spine* 1988;13:795–802.

92. Rogers WA. Fracture and dislocations of the cervical spine. An end result study. *J Bone Joint Surg* 1957;39A:341–376.

93. McAfee PC, Bohlman HH, Wilson WL. The triple wire fixation technique for stabilization of acute cervical fracture-dislocations: a biomechanical analysis. *Trans Orthop* 1985;9:142.

94. Segal D, Whitelaw GP, Gumbs V, Pick RY. Tension band fixation of acute cervical spine fractures. *Clin Orthop* 1981;159:211–222.

95. Roy-Camille R, Mazel C, Saillant G. Treatment of cervical spine injuries by a posterior osteosynthesis with plates and screws. In: Kehr P, Weidner A (eds). *Cervical Spine.* Vienna, New York: Springer-Verlag, 1987:163.

96. Louis RP. *Surgery of the Spine.* Berlin: Springer-Verlag, 1983:49–83.

97. Grob D, Mageri F. Dorsal spondylosis of the cervical spine using a hooked plate. *Orthopaedics* 1987;16:55–61.

98. Davey JR, Rorabeck CH, Bailey SI, Bourne RB, Dewar FP. A technique of posterior fusion for instability of the cervical spine. *Spine* 1985;10:722–728.

99. Wilber RG, Peters JG, Likaver MJ. Surgical techniques in cervical spine surgery. In: Errico TJ, Bauer RD, Waugh T (eds). *Spinal Trauma,* 2nd ed. Philadelphia: JB Lippincott, 1991:145–158.

100. Callahan RA, Johnson RM, Margolis RN, Keggi KJ, Albright JA, Southwick WO. Cervical facet fusion for control of instability following laminectomy. *J Bone Joint Surg* 1977;59A:991–1002.

101. Roy-Camille R, Saillant G, Mazel C. Internal fixation of the unstable cervical spine by a posterior osteosynthesis with plates and screws. In: Sherk HH, Dunn EJ, Eismont FJ, et al., (eds). *The Cervical Spine,* 2nd ed. The Cervical Spine Research Society. Philadelphia: JB Lippincott, 1989:390–403.

102. Anderson PA, Henley MB, Grady MS, Montesano PX, Winn HR. Posterior cervical arthrodesis with AO reconstruction plates and bone graft. *Spine* 1991;15(suppl):S72–S79.

103. Bohlman HH. Indications for the anterior decompression and fusion for cervical spinal cord injuries. In: Tator CH (ed). *Early Management of Acute Cervical Spinal Cord Injury.* New York: Raven Press, 1982:315–333.

104. Anderson PA, Bohlman HH. Anterior decompression and arthrodesis in patients with motor complete cervical spinal cord injury. Long-term neurologic recovery in 52 patients. Part II. *J Bone Joint Surg* 1992;74A:683–692.

105. Bohlman HH, Eismont FJ. Surgical techniques of anterior decompression and fusion for spinal cord injuries. *Clin Orthop* 1981;154:57–56.

106. Caspar W, Barbier DD, Klara PM. Anterior cervical fusion and Caspar plate stabilization for cervical trauma. *Neurosurgery* 1989;25:491–502.

107. White AA, Johnson RM, Panjabi MM, Southwick WO. Biomechanical analysis of clinical stability in the cervical spine. *Clin Orthop* 1975;109:85.

108. An HS, Simpson JM. *Surgery of the Cervical Spine.* Baltimore: Williams & Wilkins, 1994.

109. Bucholz RW. Lower cervical spine injuries in skeletal trauma. In: Browner BD, Levine AM, Jupiter JB, Trafton PG, eds. *Fracture Dislocation and Ligamentous Injuries.* Philadelphia: WB Saunders, 1992:699–728.

110. Heller JG, Carlson GD, Abitbol JJ, et al. Anatomic comparison of the Roy-Camille and Magerl techniques for screw placement in the lower cervical spine. *Spine* 1991;16:S552–S557.

111. Aebi M, Webb JK. The spine. In: Allgower M, ed. *Manual of Internal Fixation,* 3rd ed. Berlin: Springer-Verlag, 1991:627–682.

112. An HS. *Principles and Techniques of Spine Surgery.* Baltimore: Williams & Wilkins, 1998.

Surgery of Spinal Trauma,
edited by J.M. Cotler, J.M. Simpson, H.S. An, and C.P. Silveri.
Lippincott Williams & Wilkins, Philadelphia © 2000.

CHAPTER 9

Injuries of the Cervicothoracic Junction

Paul A. Anderson

Assessment	Posterior Surgical Approach
Early Treatment	**Methods**
Definitive Treatment	**Surgical Technique**
Surgical Treatment	Cervical Lateral Mass Screws
Surgical Anatomy	C7 Pedicle Screws
Vascular Structures	Thoracic Pedicle Screws
Lymphatic Structures	**Results**
Neurologic Structures	**Discussion**
Anterior Surgical Approaches	

Injuries of the cervicothoracic spine (C7-T1) are enigmatic due to the difficulty in diagnosis and to a lack of proven efficacious treatment methods (Table 1). These injuries are thought to be rare but occur in 5% to 10% of all cervical spinal injuries (1,2). In published reports 50% to 60% of patients have had delayed diagnoses (3). This is due to overlying shoulder artifact on lateral radiographs, which leads to failure to visualize the cervicothoracic junction. Although special radiologic techniques are now available, they are more difficult to interpret. Injuries in the upper thoracic spine between T1 and T3 are much rarer than those at the cervicothoracic junction and are nearly impossible to visualize on standard lateral roentgenograms.

The cervicothoracic spine is a transition, and therefore may be subjected to excessive forces similar to other transition zones such as the craniocervical and thoracolumbar junctions. Numerous fixation systems have been developed for the cervical or thoracic spine, but none for this region. Spinal hooks that can be safely used in the thoracic spine have much less appeal in the cervical spine. Anterior plate and screws have proven efficacious in the cervical spine, but are difficult to insert across the cervicothoracic junction and may be clinically associated with poor results. Simple wire fixation in the upper thoracic spine is rarely sufficient. Newer techniques of instrumentation such as plates and screws can be used but may be associated with increased neurovascular risk.

P. A. Anderson: Department of Orthopaedic Surgery, University of Washington, Seattle, Washington 98122.

This chapter reviews the anatomy of the cervicothoracic junction, describes common injury patterns and their diagnoses, reviews the early and late treatments of injuries, and describes the technique and results of fixation across the cervicothoracic junction.

ASSESSMENT

Patients with cervicothoracic injuries usually complain of pain, unless they are experiencing altered states of consciousness from intoxication or closed head injury. Common mechanisms are deceleration injuries during vehicular trauma, and direct blows such as occur in logging accidents. In these cases there may be significant associated thoracic trauma, including flail chest and pulmonary contusion. Additionally, there may be abrasions seen over the dorsum.

Physical examination includes palpation of all spinous processes from the occiput to the sacrum. Tenderness at the cervicothoracic junction may be elicited, as well as a significant step-off in patients with C7-T1 dislocations. A palpable gap or crepitation is indicative of a highly unstable injury. The neurologic examination should include manual muscle testing in all muscles groups in the arms and legs. Of particular importance in the cervicothoracic junction are the intrinsic muscles, which are best assessed by finger abduction and grip strength.

Patients who present with trauma should have a complete cervical spine radiographic evaluation, including lateral, open mouth, and anterior/posterior. The lateral view should

TABLE 1. *Differences in injuries at the cervicothoracic junction compared to lower cervical spine*

Delayed or difficult diagnoses
Incidence of 5% to 10%
Difficult closed reduction using tong traction
Increased difficulty assessing alignment
Comminution of fractures, especially in those patients with direct blow mechanisms
Limited fixation techniques, e.g., pedicle screw
Larger spinous processes for interspinous wire fixation
Anterior approach difficult with limited ability to place internal fixation
Concentration of larger forces at cervicothoracic junction

TABLE 2. *Techniques to evaluate the cervicothoracic junction*

Standard three-view plain radiographs (lateral occiput–T1, anteroposterior, open mouth)
Pull-down lateral radiographs
Swimmer's lateral radiograph
Trauma oblique radiograph
Polytomography
Limited computed tomography (CT)
Magnetic resonance imaging (MRI)

visualize the superior aspect of T1 so that alignment at C7-T1 can be determined. This is often difficult due to overlapping of the shoulders (Fig. 1). This inability to obtain clear images has led to a high incidence of missed injuries at the C7-T1 level (4). Other factors that are associated with missed or delayed diagnoses include altered states of consciousness secondary to drugs or alcohol; closed head injury; advanced age and unknown mechanism of injury; ankylosing spondylitis; and higher levels of spinal fractures (3). To aid in visualizing the cervicothoracic junction, several additional radiographic views have been described (Table 2).

The bilateral arm traction lateral radiograph is a standard technique to depress the shoulder, allowing visualization of the C7-T1 junction. Ohiorenoya et al. (5) found that it was effective in only 7.7% of cases if the midbody of C7 was not visualized on the initial lateral radiographs. Bilateral arm traction views are contraindicated in those patients with upper extremity trauma. Evans (1) and Chapman et al. (6) have recommended swimmer's radiograph, which is obtained by placing one of the patient's arms in an abducted position and aiming the x-ray beam over the contralateral shoulder, angling upward 10 to 15 degrees toward the ipsilateral axilla where the x-ray film is located. These views can be obtained in most patients but are at times difficult to interpret due to the overlying scapula.

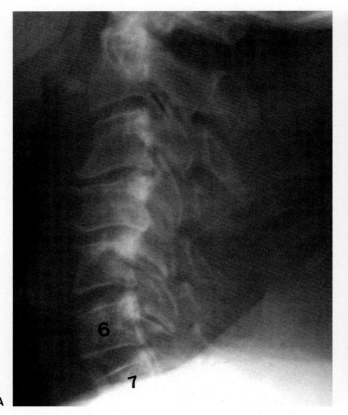

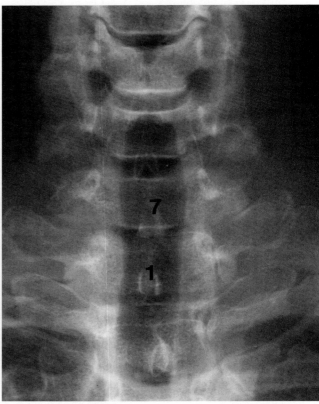

FIG. 1. A: A 32-year-old man presented with multiple injuries and complained of neck pain. He was neurologically intact. Initial lateral radiograph is negative but the cervicothoracic junction is not visualized. **B:** Anteroposterior radiograph is unremarkable.

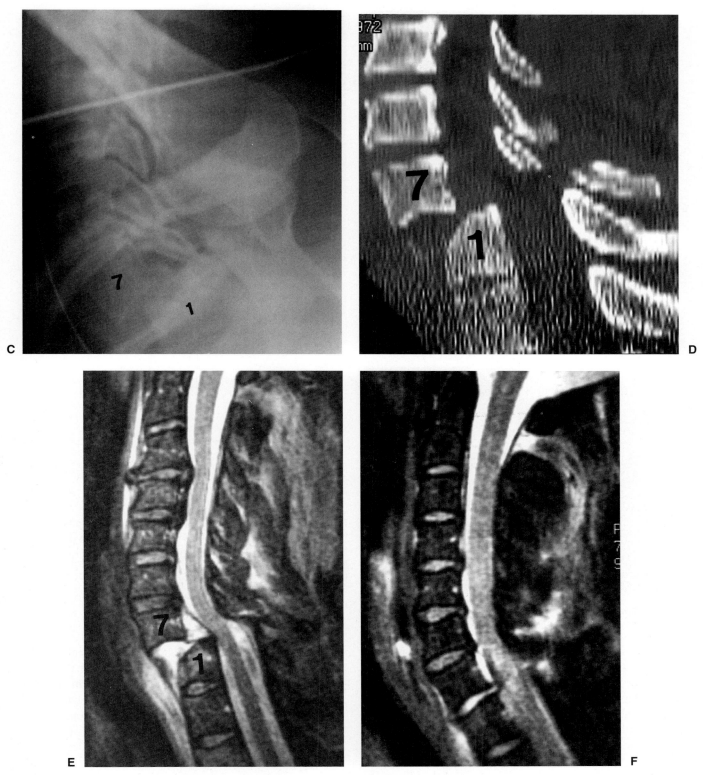

FIG. 1. *Continued.* **C:** A bilateral facet dislocation is seen on the lateral swimmer's radiograph. **D:** Computed tomography (CT) sagittal reconstruction clearly demonstrates the bilateral facet dislocation. Displaced laminar and spinous process fractures of C7 probably prevented spinal cord injury. **E:** Magnetic resonance imaging (MRI) prior to reduction was obtained. No disc herniation was noted; therefore, closed reduction was carried out. **F:** Postreduction MRI. No disc herniation is present and alignment is excellent. Increased signal is visualized in the posterior elements indicating extensive soft tissue injury.

(continued)

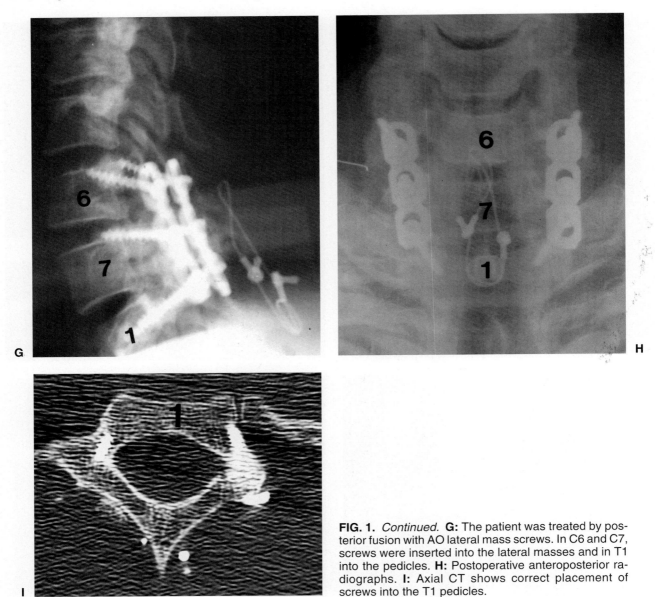

FIG. 1. *Continued.* **G:** The patient was treated by posterior fusion with AO lateral mass screws. In C6 and C7, screws were inserted into the lateral masses and in T1 into the pedicles. **H:** Postoperative anteroposterior radiographs. **I:** Axial CT shows correct placement of screws into the T1 pedicles.

Trauma supine oblique radiographs are obtained by positioning the patient supine with a plate behind the head and neck and obliquely angling the x-ray beam 45 degrees. This radiograph outlines the facet articulations, including those at the cervicothoracic junction. Theoretically, facet fractures and dislocations can be identified. Mann et al. (7) performed *in vitro* analysis of cadaveric specimens studying radiographs in varying degrees of rotation. They found that the trauma supine oblique radiograph had a high incidence of false-positive and false-negative results.

Polytomography is an excellent means of identifying the cervicothoracic junction; however, it is rarely available today and requires lateral positioning of the patient, which decreases its safety. Limited computed tomography (CT) scan

has been shown to be effective (8) (Fig. 1). Helical scanners allow short acquisition times and reformations that can readily identify sagittal plane alignment, as well as the position of the facet articulation. This is the author's preferred technique for evaluating the cervicothoracic junction. Tehranzadeh et al. (9) found three patients with occult C7-T1 injuries in whom limited CT failed to visualize C7-T1. Although thought to increase costs, limited CT may actually be less expensive than plain radiographic techniques because of its speed and the avoidance of multiple repeat radiographs that tie up a radiologic suite in the emergency department. Newer modalities such as digital imaging, fluoroscopy, and magnetic resonance imaging (MRI) may become state of the art, but require further investigation.

EARLY TREATMENT

The goals of treatment in patients with unstable cervicothoracic spine are to protect the spinal cord from further injury, reduce fractures or dislocations, stabilize the spine, and provide a long-term functional spinal unit. Once an injury has been identified, the patient should continue on spine precautions, including immobilization in a collar and placement on a bed. Log rolling every 2 hours is indicated to prevent decubitus for those patients with spinal cord injuries.

Patients with spinal cord injuries should have adequate oxygenation, via nasal cannula, and maintain a systemic pressure of at least 90 mm Hg to adequately perfuse the spinal cord. Because of spinal shock, the patient may present with hypotension and bradycardia, requiring the use of atropine and anticholinergic medications.

The initial goal of treatment of the spinal condition is to achieve rapid reduction using tong traction. Even fractures in the upper thoracic spine can be reduced if traction is applied using the rigid protocol. Injuries at the cervicothoracic junction require larger weights than higher level injuries; therefore, they require close monitoring to avoid iatrogenic injury (1,10). The timing of reduction is critical and should proceed immediately in patients with neurologic deficits to increase the likelihood of neurologic recovery. We have observed six patients who had reversal of quadriplegia due to facet dislocation by immediate traction instituted within 2 hours of injury.

Closed reduction is performed after application of Gardner-Wells tongs. We prefer titanium pins to allow MRI after reductions. Initially, 10 to 20 lb of traction weight are applied, and then increments of 10 to 15 lb are added every 15 minutes. After each weight application, the pins are checked to make sure they are still engaged in the skull, a repeat neurologic examination is performed, and a lateral radiograph is obtained. The lateral radiograph is scrutinized for signs of overdistraction, such as diastasis of disc spaces or facet joints. If there are concomitant injuries at C2, such as a hangman or odontoid fractures, traction is contraindicated and the patient requires an open reduction.

We have utilized weights up to 70% of total body weight before obtaining reductions in patients with cervicothoracic injuries. Cotler et al. (11) have reported a similar use of large weights without neurologic complications, if the technique is used according to a rigid protocol. Indications for emergent surgery are failure to achieve reduction in patients with significant neurologic deficits and neurologic progression. Methylprednisolone is given according to the National Acute Spinal Cord Injury (NACIS-2) protocol (12). A loading dose of 30 mg per kg is given and a maintenance dose of 5.4 mg per kg per hour is continued for 23 hours.

DEFINITIVE TREATMENT

No classification or biomechanical studies are available to guide treatment; therefore, principles that apply to the cervical spine are extrapolated in their use to the cervicothoracic junction. Fracture stability can be assessed using the method of White et al. (13). White recommends a clinical checklist that is summed to obtain a value. When values are greater than 5, then the patient has an unstable injury. Stable injury patterns at the cervicothoracic junction are primarily localized to one column of the spine and are not associated with vertebral body subluxation. Fracture types include isolated spinous process, facet or laminar fractures, vertebral body compression fractures, and avulsion of the anterior longitudinal ligament; however, beware of the patient with a compression fracture and a posterior osseoligamentous injury, as this combination proves to be highly unstable and frequently results in progressive deformity (14).

Stable fractures are treated with a cervicothoracic brace for 6 to 8 weeks. Prior to discharge, a lateral radiograph is obtained to ensure adequate alignment. The patient is then followed serially with repeat radiographs every 2 to 3 weeks. Flexion/extension films are obtained at the end of healing.

Unstable injuries, such as bursting type fractures, comminuted fractures at multiple levels, and facet fracture dislocations, are best treated surgically. Nonoperative treatment methods such as halo vest are associated with poor outcome (15,16). Additionally, other means such as recumbent traction are associated with a high mortality in patients with spinal cord injuries at the cervicothoracic junction (1).

SURGICAL TREATMENT

The anterior aspect of the cervicothoracic spine is limited by the clavicles and sternum. Although discectomy can be performed at C7-T1 in a majority of patients with a low anterior Smith-Robinson incision, fixation with plates and screws is difficult. Additionally, a high rate of failure of anterior plate constructs has been reported in constructs that end at the cervicothoracic junction. If an anterior approach is indicated due to persistent anterior cord compression and residual neurologic deficits, decompression can be performed by one of three techniques: a low anterior cervical Smith-Robinson approach (17), a high transthoracic approach through the bed of the third rib (18), or a combined anterior cervical and thoracic approach. This combined approach can be either via a transthoracic incision (19), or through exposure of the superior mediastinum through partial manubrial excision or midline sternal splitting (20–22). Because these approaches are infrequently performed, and the spine is deep and in a narrow opening, they are best avoided in acute traumatic situations unless absolutely indicated. In most cases anterior surgery can be avoided by the institution of early traction that will achieve adequate canal indirect decompression. If anterior decompression is performed, reconstruction is performed with a strut graft. Either during the same procedure or at a second procedure, the patient should then undergo posterior stabilization.

Posterior fusion with or without instrumentation is indicated in a majority of the patients with unstable cervicothoracic injuries. Interspinous wires are the simple and most efficacious treatment and are indicated for patients with pure dislocations or ligamentous injuries. This technique is facilitated at the cervicothoracic junction because of the enlarged spinous processes. If there is comminution of the posterior elements, or bursting type fractures, other forms of fixation should be utilized.

Callahan et al. (23) described the use of facet wires for cases when lamina are fractured or missing. This technique, in which long rib struts are tightened over multiple facet wires, has proven effective, but it requires a postoperative halo vest for 10 to 12 weeks. Luque rods or rectangles affixed to the spine with sublaminar wires have been described for use at the cervicothoracic junction. They have the disadvantage of requiring canal intrusion with risk of neurologic damage. Biomechnically, Luque rods lack rigidity, especially in the axial direction.

Pediatric hook-rod constructs have been placed across the cervicothoracic junction, but also involve canal intrusion with risk of neurologic injury (24). Posterior-cervical plate and screw fixation has been used due to its increased biomechanical strength (25–27). Unfortunately, neurologic complication occur in up to 7% of screws, especially with screws placed into the C7 lateral mass (28). Extension of lateral mass fixation into the thoracic spine is feasible based on morphologic studies of thoracic pedicles (29,30). Fortunately, screws can also be placed laterally into the rib head with little risk of iatrogenic injury. We have found that the unstable injuries of the cervicothoracic spine can be treated successfully with AO reconstruction plates utilizing cervical lateral mass screws and thoracic pedicle screws (6).

SURGICAL ANATOMY

The approach to the anterior aspect of the cervicothoracic spine is through the thoracic inlets. It is bounded anteriorly by the sternum and sternoclavicular joints, laterally by the first rib, and posteriorly by the first thoracic vertebra. From a surgical perspective, the anterior approach is blocked by the sternum and sternoclavicular joints. Many important vascular, neurologic, and visceral structures are at risk of injury in anterior approaches to the cervicothoracic junction.

Vascular Structures

The brachiocephalic or innominate veins form from the subclavian vein and internal jugular veins and are located immediately below the manubrium and sternoclavicular joints. At the level of the angle of the sternum these combine to form the superior vena cava. Lying deep and somewhat inferior to the left brachiocephalic vein is the aortic arch. Three major arteries divide from the arch: the brachiocephalic trunk, left common carotid artery, and left subclavian artery. The brachiocephalic trunk passes superiorly and laterally and divides beneath the right sternoclavicular joint into the right common carotid artery and right subclavian artery. The

common carotid artery, internal jugular vein, and the vagus nerve pass cranially together in the carotid sheath lying lateral on each side to the trachea.

Lymphatic Structures

The thoracic duct is a lymphatic organ that leaves the thorax behind the left subclavian artery. At or above the C7 level it is located behind the carotid sheath anterior to the scalenus anterior muscle. At this location it turns and empties into the left internal jugular vein, left subclavian, or left brachiocephalic vein.

Neurologic Structures

The vagus nerves are well protected in the thoracic inlet being enclosed in the carotid sheath. The left recurrent laryngeal nerve branches from the vagus at the aortic arch, passes behind the arch to the left of the ligamentum arteriosum, and ascends between the esophagus and trachea. The right recurrent laryngeal nerve arises from the right vagus as it passes in front of the right subclavian artery. The right recurrent laryngeal nerve loops under the subclavian artery, passing behind it, and ascends between the esophagus and trachea. The right recurrent laryngeal nerve often takes a more anomalous course and frequently passes obliquely from lateral to medial. In this location the nerve is at risk during a right-sided approach to the anterior cervicothoracic spine.

Anterior Surgical Approaches

Three anterior approaches have been described for cervicothoracic junction: the low anterior cervical Smith-Robinson approach, the transsternal or modification of transsternal, and the high thoracic thoracotomy. The vertebral bodies of the upper thoracic spine may also be approached by the costotransversectomy procedure. A standard Smith-Robinson approach can gain access to C7, T1, and T2 in some patients. Beveling off the anteroinferior corner of the cranial body can increase access.

Transsternal or partial-sternal splitting approaches have been described and allow access to T3 or T4 but are limited in caudal extent by the left brachiocephalic vein, which crosses the field. Sternal splitting has been associated with increased mortality and wound healing problems, and thus are less preferred (18). For better exposure, resection of the medial third of the clavicle and left side of the sternum opens the thoracic inlet (31,32). If the costoclavicular ligaments and some of the sternoclavicular ligaments can be spared, then shoulder stability does not seem to be a long-term problem.

The transthoracic approach through the third rib bed provides exposure between T1 and T5. The azygos vein on the right side and the hemiazygos vein on the left side must be protected or controlled. Division of the rhomboids, trapezius, and latissimus dorsi muscles are required for this approach and can cause short-term shoulder disability. Extension to the cervical spine is minimal with this technique.

Posterior Surgical Approach

The cervicothoracic spine is easily approached from a posterior midline incision. Fixation can be applied with sublaminar hooks, sublaminar wires, or with screws. In the upper thoracic spine, screws can be safely placed in the pedicles using bony landmarks and by direct visualization via a laminotomy and exposure of the pedicle. Screws placed laterally to the pedicle enter the rib head and in general are safe but not as biomechanically efficacious. At C7, screws can be placed laterally into the lateral masses, as described for lateral mass fixation, or transpedicularly. Because the C7 lamina and lateral mass are thin, and the lateral mass is poorly formed, pedicle fixation of C7 is often required and may be safer (33). The C7 pedicles angle downward 10 to 15 degrees and medially 30 to 40 degrees. Laminotomy at C6-7 can aid screw insertion. From C3 to C6, screw fixation, if desired, is performed in the lateral masses as described by Anderson et al. (25).

METHODS

Stabilization of the lower cervical spine with AO reconstruction plates has proven efficacious. Without a suitable alternative, we began to extend the lateral mass fixation across the cervicothoracic junction, utilizing thoracic pedicle screws (6). Twenty-three consecutive patients with unstable injuries from C7 to T4 were treated by stainless steel AO reconstruction plates. All patients were treated at Harborview Medical Center (Seattle, WA) and had autogenous iliac crest bone grafting.

The diagnosis of injury was made by plain radiographs or CT. Fine-section CT with reconstructions was extremely important in the radiographic evaluation of these injuries. Once a diagnosis was made, patients were placed in traction and had reduction by application of serial increasing weight. Injuries at the cervicothoracic junction may require large amounts of weight, at times up to 70% of body weight. Radiographs with special views confirm reduction, although CT or MRI was required in some patients. Methylprednisolone was given according to the NACIS-2 protocol in patients with spinal cord injuries. Operations were performed 3 to 7 days following admission.

SURGICAL TECHNIQUE

The patients were intubated by an awake nasotracheal technique using a fiberoptic scope. They were then placed prone on a Stryker frame and had a repeat neurologic examination. A midline incision was made with dissection carried out to the edge of the cervical lateral masses and to the tips of the transverse processes of the thoracic levels to be arthrodesed.

The nuchal ligaments at adjacent nonfused levels were carefully spared, as were nonfused facet joint capsules.

Cervical Lateral Mass Screws

Lateral mass screws are placed in the lower cervical spine, according to the technique of Anderson et al. (25). The starting point for screw insertion is 1 mm medial to the center of the lateral mass, and the screw is oriented 10 to 15 degrees laterally and 20 to 30 degrees upward, attempting to parallel the facet joint. At C7 the lateral mass is often poorly defined or thin, which may require placement of a C7 pedicle screw (see below) (24).

At the correct starting point, a 2-mm Kirschner wire (K-wire) is started 1 mm medial to the center of a mass and directed outward and upward. An adjustable drill guide is set for 14-mm depth and the drill is advanced. The hole is then checked for perforation with a smaller K-wire and the drill guide is readjusted to allow another 1 to 2 mm of advancement. The process is repeated until the far edge of lateral mass is perforated or until a depth of 18 to 20 mm. This process prevents iatrogenic plunging of the drill bit and possible neurovascular injury. The hole is then tapped with a 3.5-mm tap.

C7 Pedicle Screws

Abumi et al. (33) first reported the use of cervical pedicle screws. In general, these are not warranted between C3 and C6 because of the risk of neurovascular injury; however, due to differences in vertebral artery anatomy, they may be safely placed at C2 and C7. Accurate placement of C7 pedicle screws is improved by direct pedicle palpation via a C6-7 laminotomy. The starting point is just below the C6-7 facet and approximately at the midjoint level. From this point, a 2-mm drill with an adjustable drill guide is angled 30 to 40 degrees medially and slightly downward. The drill is advanced and the hole is thoroughly checked for perforations. Palpation of the medial side of the pedicle helps ensure proper screw placement. Once a depth of 20 to 22 mm is achieved, the hole is tapped with a 3.5-mm tap.

Thoracic Pedicle Screws

The thoracic pedicles in the upper thoracic spine are small, elliptical in shape, and angulated medially and downward (34). Lateral placement of screws into the rib is acceptable and decreases the risk of iatrogenic injury, although this placement is associated with decreased biomechanical strength. Unlike the C7, upper thoracic screws can be placed without laminotomies and direct visualization of the pedicle, although this technique can facilitate insertion. The starting point for thoracic pedicle screw placement is on the midfacet line and just below the superior facet (Fig. 2). Drilling is performed with a 2-mm drill and adjustable drill guide with the drill initially set to depth of 14 mm. The drill is advanced medially 5 to 10 degrees and downward 10 to 20 degrees. The

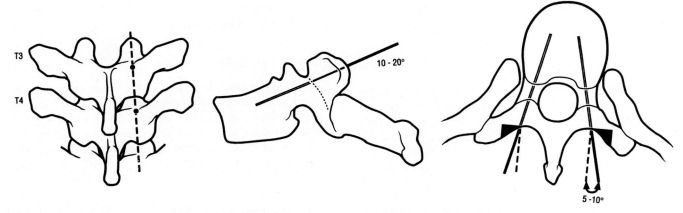

FIG. 2. The orientation of upper thoracic pedicles. **Left:** Dorsal view. **Middle:** Lateral view. The pedicles are oriented 10 to 20 degrees downward. **Right:** Axial view. The screws are directed 15 to 20 degrees medially.

hole is checked for perforations with a small K-wire and the drill guide is readjusted to allow an additional 2 mm of drilling depth. This process is repeated until a drilling depth of 22 to 24 mm has been achieved. The hole is then tapped with a 3.5-mm tap.

Malleable templates are then used to assess which plate best fits the patient's anatomy and to determine the degree of lordosis/kyphosis required. The proper plate is chosen, either an 8- or 12-mm hole spacing using the AO system, sectioned to length and contoured to proper lordosis. The intervening

facet joints are decorticated and packed with autogenous iliac crest bone graft. K-wires are placed into the drill holes and the plate is slid down over the wires ensuring proper placement (Fig. 3). The plate is then fixed with 3.5- or 4-mm screws of appropriate length. Unfortunately, intraoperative radiographs through this region are seldom useful. Spinous process wiring using the Rogers (35) technique may be performed in cases where the posterior elements are not damaged. Postoperatively, the patient is immobilized in a cervicothoracic brace for 2 months.

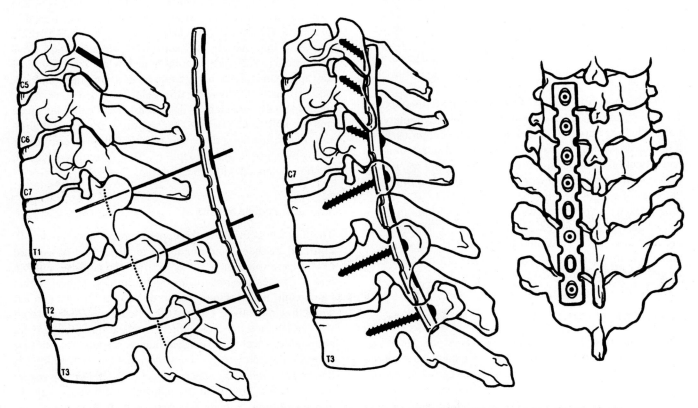

FIG. 3. Drawings demonstrate application of cervicothoracic plate. **Left:** Kirschner wires (K-wires) are placed in holes placed in thoracic pedicles to help align plate. **Middle:** Lateral view. **Right:** Anteroposterior view.

RESULTS

The mean age of patients was 47 with a range of 27 to 73 years. There were 15 males and 8 females. Nineteen had acute fractures, including six burst-type fractures, five fracture dislocations, and three pure bilateral facet dislocations. Five had multilevel fractures at three or more levels. Two patients had failed previous surgeries, and two patients had pathologic fractures secondary to metastatic disease. Neurologically, four patients were intact, five had isolated upper extremity radiculopathies, seven had complete paraplegia, and seven had incomplete paraplegia. The surgical procedures attempted to arthrodese as few levels as possible, although extra levels in the upper thoracic spine were often sacrificed. An average of four levels, with a range of two to nine, were permanently arthrodesed.

Follow-up averaged 15 months with a range of 6 to 41 months in surviving patients. Two patients died at 2 months and 4 months, respectively, from their multiple injuries. One patient died of unrelated causes 18 months after surgery.

Neurologically all patients initially intact and with radiculopathy were normal. Three patients with Frankel grade D deficits became grade E. Two of four patients with grade C became grade D, and the two others with grade C became grade E. One patient who was a complete grade A improved to grade C, and one to grade B, while five others had no improvement.

Flexion/extension radiographs were obtained in all patients; however, they were difficult to interpret due to overlying shadow. We could detect no motion in non–flexion/extension films in any patient. Two patients had persistent pain and had their hardware removed and fusion mass was explored, which showed solid arthrodesis in both cases.

DISCUSSION

The management of injuries at the cervicothoracic junction is difficult for many reasons. The diagnosis based on plain radiographs is often delayed or missed altogether. Newer imaging techniques such as limited CT or MRI allows excellent view on the sagittal projection. Once diagnosed, no accepted classification system is available to direct treatment. We recommend using the principles defined by White et al. (13) to determine stability. The treatment is complicated because closed reduction requires significantly larger traction weights. Alignment during closed or open reduction is often not visualized unless CT is obtained. Nonoperative methods utilizing either cervicothoracic braces or the halo vest are less useful than in other regions of the cervical spine.

Surgical treatment goals are to maintain alignment, provide stability to mobilize patients, and produce long-term arthrodesis. In patients with spinal cord injury, complete decompression of the spinal cord should be achieved. Anterior approaches are limited by the thoracic inlet, depth of the wound, and vascular structures. Reconstruction with internal fixation following anterior decompression is technically demanding and associated with a high failure rate.

Lower cervical spine stabilization with plate and screws was initially described by Roy-Camille et al. (26). We have utilized a modification of this technique and reported a 100% fusion rate and low complication rate. Extending this approach to across the cervicothoracic spine is possible by combining cervical lateral mass screws with upper thoracic pedicle screws. We have found this approach to be the most efficacious for treatment of unstable injuries to the cervicothoracic junction.

REFERENCES

1. Evans DK. Dislocations at the cervicothoracic junction. *J Bone Joint Surg* 1983;65B:124–127.
2. Nichols CG, Young DH, Schiller WR. Evaluation of cervicothoracic junction injuries. *Ann Emerg Med* 1987;16:640–642.
3. Bohlman HH. Acute fractures and dislocations of the cervical spine: an analysis of 300 hospitalized patients and review of the literature. *J Bone Joint Surg* 1979;61A:1119–1142.
4. Woodring JH, Lee C. Limitations of cervical radiography in the evaluation of acute cervical trauma. *J Trauma* 1993;34:32–39.
5. Ohiorenoya D, Hilton M, Oakland CDH, McLauchlan CAJ, Cobby M, Hughes AO. Cervical spine imaging in trauma patients: a simple scheme of rationalising arm traction using zonal divisions of the vertebral bodies. *J Accid Emerg Med* 1996;13:175–176.
6. Chapman JR, Anderson PA, Pepin C, Toomey S, Newell DW, Grady MS. Posterior instrumentation of the unstable cervico-thoracic spine. *J Neurosurg* 1996;84:552–558.
7. Mann FA, Wilson AJ, McEnery KW, Nuelle D. Supine oblique views of the cervical spine: a poor proxy for the lateral view. *Emerg Radiol* 1995;2:214–220.
8. Woodring JH, Lee C. The role and limitations of computed tomographic scanning in the evaluation of cervical trauma. *J Trauma* 1992;33:698–708.
9. Tehranzadeh J, Bonk RT, Ansari A, Mesgarzadeh M. Efficacy of limited CT for nonvisualized lower cervical spine in patients with blunt trauma. *Skeletal Radiol* 1994;23:349–352.
10. Chapman JR, Anderson PA. Posterior plate fixation of the cervicothoracic junction. *Tech Orthop* 1994;9:80–85.
11. Cotler JM, Herbison GJ, Nasuti JF, et al. Closed reduction of traumatic cervical spine dislocation using traction weights up to 140 pounds. *Spine* 1993;18:386–390.
12. Bracken MB, Shepard MJ, Collins WF, et al. A randomized, controlled trial of methylprednisolone or naloxone in the treatment of acute spinal cord injury: results of the second National Acute Spinal Cord Injury study. *N Engl J Med* 1990;322:1405–1411.
13. White AA, Southwick WO, Panjabi MM. Clinical instability in the lower cervical spine. A review of past and current concepts. *Spine* 1976;1:15–27.
14. Webb JK, Broughton RBK, McSweeney T. Hidden flexion injury of the cervical spine. *J Bone Joint Surg* 1976;58B:322–327.
15. Whitehill R, Richman JA, Glaser JA. Failure of immobilization of the cervical spine by the halo vest. A report of 5 cases. *J Bone Joint Surg* 1986;68-A:326–332.
16. Glaser JA, Whitehill R, Stamp WG, et al. Complications associated with the halo-vest. A review of 245 cases. *J Neurosurg* 1986;65:762–769.
17. Fielding JW, Stillwell WT. Anterior cervical approach to the upper thoracic spine. *Spine* 1976;1:158–161.
18. Hodgson A, Stock FE, Fang HSY, et al. Anterior spinal fusion: the operative approach and pathological findings in 412 patients with Pott's disease of the spine. *Br J Surg* 1960;48:172–178.
19. Micheli LJ, Hood RW. Anterior exposure of the cervicothoracic spine using a combined cervical and thoracic approach. *J Bone Joint Surg* 1983;65A:992–997.
20. Kurz LT, Purset SE, Herkowitz HN. Modified anterior approach to the cervicothoracic junction. *Spine* 1991;16(suppl 10):542–547.
21. Cauchoix J, Binet JP. Anterior surgical approaches to the spine. *Ann R Coll Surg* 1957;21:237–243.
22. Sundaresan N, Shah J, Feghali JG. A transsternal approach to the upper thoracic vertebrae. *Am J Surg* 1984;148:473–477.

23. Callahan RA, Margolis RM, Keggi RN, Albright KJ, Southwick WO. Cervical facet fusion for control of instability following laminectomy. *J Bone Joint Surg* 1977;59A:991–1002.

24. An HS, Vaccaro A, Cotler, JM, et al. Spinal disorders at the cervicothoracic junction. *Spine* 1994;19:2557–2564.

25. Anderson PA, Henley MB, Grady MS, et al. Posterior cervical arthrodesis with AO reconstruction plates and bone graft. *Spine* 1991;16(suppl 3):72–79.

26. Roy-Camille R, Saillant G, Berteaux D, Serge MA. Early management of spinal injuries. In: McKibbin B (ed). *Recent Advances in Orthopaedics*. Edinburgh: Churchill Livingstone, 1979: 57–87.

27. Cooper PR, Cohen A, Rosiello A, et al. Posterior stabilization of cervical spine fractures and subluxations using plates and screws. *Neurosurgery* 1988;23:300–306.

28. Heller JG, Silcox DH, Sutterlin CE. Complications of posterior cervical plating. *Spine* 1995;20:2442–2448.

29. Misenhimer GR, Peck RD, Wilse LL, et al. Anatomic analysis of pedicle cortical and cancellous diameter as related to screw size. *Spine* 1989;14:367–372.

30. Ebraheim N, An HS, Jackson WT, et al. Internal fixation of the unstable cervical spine using posterior Roy-Camille plates: preliminary report. *J Orthop Trauma* 1989;3:23–28.

31. Kurz LT, Pursel SE, Herkowitz HN. Modified anterior approach to the cervicothoracic junction. *Spine* 1991;16:S542–S547.

32. Sundaresan N, Shah J, Foley KM, et al. An anterior surgical approach to the upper thoracic vertebrae. *J Neurosurg* 1984;61:686–690.

33. Abumi K, Itoh H, Taneichi H, Kaneda K. Transpedicular screw fixation for traumatic lesions of the middle and lower cervical spine: description of the techniques and preliminary report. *J Spinal Disord* 1994;7:19–28.

34. Zindrick MR, Wiltsie LL, Doomik A, et al. Analysis of the morphometric characteristics of the thoracic and lumbar pedicles. *Spine* 1987; 12:160–166.

35. Rogers WA. Fracture and dislocations of the cervical spine. An end result study. *J Bone Joint Surg* 1957;39A:341–376.

Surgery of Spinal Trauma,
edited by J.M. Cotler, J.M. Simpson, H.S. An, and C.P. Silveri.
Lippincott Williams & Wilkins, Philadelphia © 2000.

CHAPTER **10**

Thoracic Spine Fractures

Stephen J. Pineda, Wayne Bauerle, and Paul C. McAfee

Fractures of the central segment of the thoracic spine (T2–T10) are distinct injuries. Commonly, these injuries are incorrectly grouped with fractures of the cervicothoracic or thoracolumbar junctions. These fractures can be broadly classified into those due to traumatic injury and those occurring in pathologic bone. Epidemiologic data reveal that spine fracture occurs in an estimated 65 in 100,000 people with approximately 15% of these fractures occurring within the confines of the rib cage (1,2). These fractures occur in a bimodal age distribution with peak incidences occurring between the ages of 25 and 30 and over 70. Males have a slightly higher incidence of fracture until the geriatric age population, at which time women outnumber men (2).

Motor vehicle accidents account for about 55% of traumatic thoracic spine fractures, with falls from heights, direct blows, and other miscellaneous trauma accounting for 21%, 12%, and 10%, respectively (3). Falls from heights generally result in axial loading injuries such as compression fractures, while motor vehicle accidents result in a variety of fracture patterns. In patients over 50, osteoporosis, metastatic disease, and multiple myeloma are responsible for 50%, 25%, and 4%, respectively, of thoracic level fractures (4).

Associated injuries frequently occur in patients with thoracic spine fractures requiring careful and complete physical examinations. Hanley and Eskay (1) reported that as many as

50% of patients with thoracic spine fractures had concomitant head trauma with alterations in mental status. Other authors have likewise shown that 20% of trauma patients may have a spine fracture that is initially unrecognized (5). A widened mediastinum may be indicative of a thoracic fracture rather than an aortic injury (6). Other frequently associated injuries include those to the chest and abdomen. Additional osseous trauma may be seen with secondary spine fractures, with foot and ankle complex injury being the most common.

Finally, the intimate association of the musculoskeletal and neurologic systems must be considered in the thoracic spine. Neurologic injury occurs in approximately 50% of these fractures (7–12). The frequency and type of neurologic injury is shown in Fig. 1 (1). Clearly, the more severe and higher energy injuries have a higher frequency of neurologic deficit. Prehospital immobilization and transport as well as emergency department evaluation must be performed with great diligence and care to ensure that maximal neurologic function is preserved.

ANATOMY

The anatomy of the thoracic spine and related structures is unique and merits discussion. The region is inherently stable because the rib cage and facet joint orientation confer significant stability on the spine. Narrow disc spaces, overlapping lamina, and rib abutment limit movement of the thoracic spine. Holdsworth (13) originally described a two-column theory of the spine. Denis (14) later expanded this to include

    S. J. Pineda and W. Bauerle: Springfield Clinic, Springfield, Illinois 62703.
    P. C. McAfee: Departments of Orthopaedic Surgery and Neurosurgery, Johns Hopkins University School of Medicine, Baltimore, Maryland 21204.

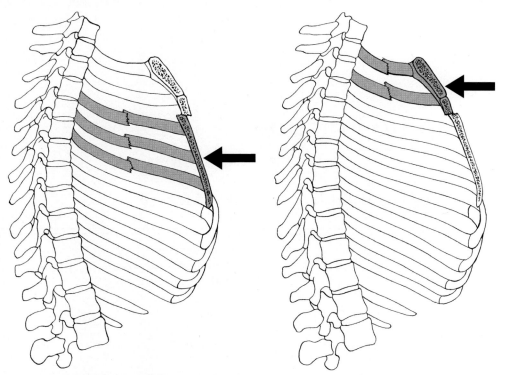

FIG. 1. The consequences of injury to the fourth column of the spine. Progressive kyphosis may develop in the presence of fracture involving both the ribs and sternum. (Adapted from ref. 16.)

a third column. The anterior column includes the anterior longitudinal ligament, the anterior annulus, and the anterior one-half of the vertebral body. The middle column includes the posterior annulus, vertebral body, and the posterior longitudinal ligament. The posterior column includes the remaining posterior structures including the pedicle, lamina, facet joints, and spinous processes.

The sternal-rib complex has been proposed as a fourth column in the thoracic spine. The current literature rarely discusses these structures' contribution to spinal stability. The association between thoracic spine and sternal and rib fractures has been described by multiple authors dating back to the 1950s (15,16). Other authors have likewise described the association of severe kyphotic deformity with compression-type sternal fractures in patients with either osteoporosis or metastatic disease of the sternum (17). The ribs articulate with both the sternum and the spine forming a circumferential cage around the chest. Berg (18) described two patients who had compromise of the spine and the sternal-rib complex who developed progressive hyphotic deformity with nonoperative treatment (Fig. 1). Therefore, concomitant evaluation of both the spine and chest must be performed in these patients.

Neurologic injury frequently occurs with significant spine trauma (8,19,20). In the midthoracic spine, there is limited free space for the neural elements. Even small amounts of retropulsed bone into the spinal canal may be compromising and result in significant neural injury (21). The intercostal

nerves are not as functionally important as the cervical or lumbar nerve roots, making spinal cord injury the sole concern in the thoracic spine. In Bohlman et al.'s (8) series, the majority of incomplete spinal cord–injured patients have an anterior cord syndrome, with a significantly smaller number of patients suffering from a central cord syndrome or other incomplete injury.

CLASSIFICATION

When classifying these fractures, one must address both the osseous and neurologic injury. A comprehensive yet straightforward system was initially proposed by Magerl (22) in 1991 and was later modified by the Scoliosis Research Society, the International Society for the Study of the Lumbar Spine, the Cervical Spine Research Society, the North American Spine Society, and the Orthopaedic Trauma Association. A schematic diagram of the classification is shown in Table 1 and Fig. 2 (23). In the classification, there are three primary injury patterns, which are then further divided into three subcategories. Type A injuries are compression injuries of the vertebral body. The mechanism of injury is usually axial loading with or without a flexion component. The resultant deformity is either a wedge-shaped vertebra or a vertebra that has a global loss of height. When the flexion component is significant, posterior-column injury may occur, which in turn creates a significant destabilized construct. The subtypes of this injury are (1) pure compression, (2)

TABLE 1. *Comprehensive classification of thoracic lumbar fractures*

Type	Group
Compression	Impaction (wedge)
	Split (coronal)
	Burst (complete burst)
Distraction	Through the soft tissues posteriorly (subluxation)
	Through the arch posteriorly (Chance fracture)
	Through the disc anteriorly (extension spondylosis)
Multidirectional with translation	Anteroposterior (dislocation)
	Lateral (lateral shear)
	Rotational (rotational burst)

Adapted from ref. 23, with permission.

compression with an associated sagittal or coronal fracture, and (3) burst injuries.

Type B fractures occur when the spine rotates around an axis that is either anterior or posterior to the rotational axis of the spine. Group 1 represents a seat belt or flexion/distraction type of injury with the posterior ligamentous complex. In group 2, the disruption occurs through the osseous structures and is often referred to as a Chance fracture. Group 3 injuries represent an extension-type injury with disruption primarily traversing the disc space.

Type C injuries also have failure of all three spinal columns with associated vertebral translation. The direction of the translation determines the subtype, with group 1 being translated in the anteroposterior (AP) direction and group 2 in the lateral direction, and group 3 represents rotational translation.

The neurologic injury is well classified by either the American Spinal Injury Association (ASIA) or the Frankel grading system (12). The former focuses on the anatomic location of the injury in the spinal cord, while the latter provides a more functional assessment.

RADIOLOGIC FEATURES

Multiple radiologic modalities are available to physicians when evaluating spine fractures. High-quality plain radiographs should be first completed and evaluated. The radiographs should be surveyed for signs of metabolic or neoplastic disease. Specific features of a compression fracture include a loss in height of the vertebral body and increased separation of the posterior spinous processes. The presence of widened pedicles, compromise of the posterior cortex of the vertebral body, or laminar fracture suggest that a burst fracture has occurred. Computed tomography (CT) scans provide a more accurate assessment of the middle column.

Magnetic resonance imaging (MRI) provides the most accurate evaluation of the neural elements and soft tissue. T1-weighted images provide the sharpest anatomic detail. The T2 sequence, by contrast, is best in demonstrating pathologic edema. Because the T2 sequence has a prolonged acquisition time, anatomic detail may be obscured. To avoid this, hybrid sequences such as turbo- or fast-spin echo can be employed; however, one must perform these with fat suppression to avoid bright signal from both adipose and edematous tissue. The images should be scrutinized for intramedullary edema, disc herniation, canal compromise, and integrity of ligamentous structures, especially the posterior interspinous ligament. Disruption of this structure in a flexion-distraction type injury implies a three-column injury (11).

TREATMENT

Treatment options for these injuries range from simple observation to brace treatment to surgical reconstruction. The primary objectives of treating these fractures are to obtain a stable vertebral column, preserve and/or improve neurologic function, and return the patients to their maximal functional capacity as soon as possible. To achieve these goals, the treating physician must consider not only the spine fracture but also the mechanism of injury, the presence of associated injuries, and the general medical health status of the patient.

The majority of thoracic spine fractures can be treated nonoperatively. If the fracture is truly stable, such as a compression of a single vertebral level with less than 50% loss of height, and there are no associated rib or sternal injuries, the fracture can be treated with observation. These patients should be followed with periodic radiographs to ensure that the patient does not develop progressive kyphosis. This is especially important in the elderly, who may develop spontaneous sternal collapse, which could exacerbate a kyphotic deformity (17,24,25).

If the spine has sustained a two- or three-column injury or if there are three or more compression fractures, especially with marked kyphosis, the fractures may be treated with a molded brace such as a thoracolumbar spinal orthosis (TLSO), providing that the sternal-rib complex is intact. If the injury is above the T6 level, a cervical extension is used. Capen et al. (9) retrospectively reviewed 49 patients with an average age of 29 years treated nonsurgically at their institution in 2 to 6 weeks followed by immobilization in a TLSO. Patients with either penetrating injuries or neoplastic disease were excluded; however, all fracture patterns were otherwise included. In this series, 29 patients had a complete neurologic deficit, 16 had an incomplete deficit, and four had normal neurologic function. In the series, all fractures healed. However, there were significant complications, which included a 24% incidence of deep venous thrombosis, a 16% incidence of pressure sores and skin injury, a 20% incidence of pulmonary complications, and a 6% incidence of gastrointestinal (GI) bleeding. None of the incomplete patients improved neurologically and one of the incomplete patients lost neurologic function (9).

In patients with complete paraplegia, operative therapy is not generally indicated. Place et al. (26) compared operative

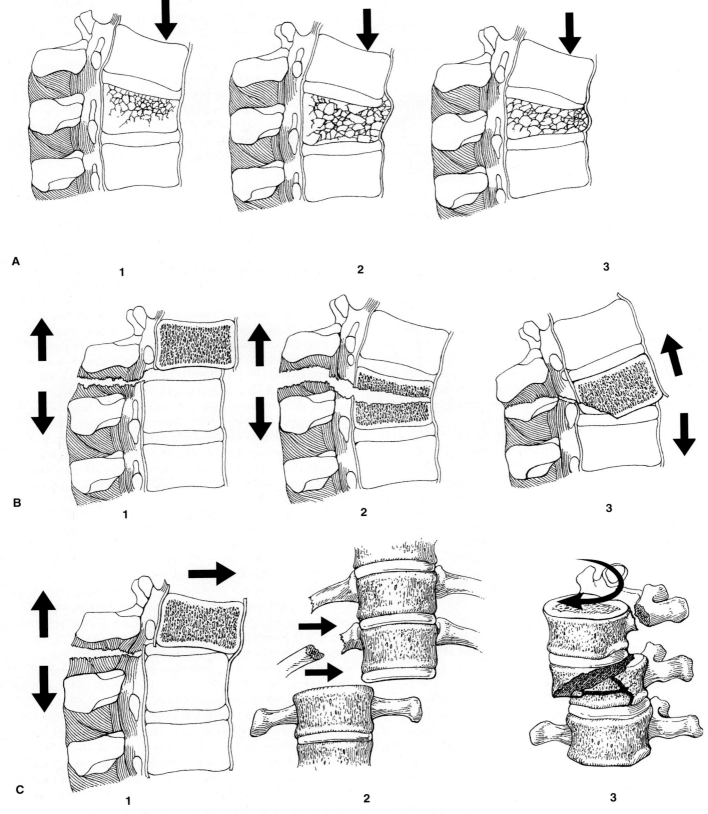

FIG. 2. A–C: Schematic drawings of each of the patterns in Table 1. (Adapted from ref. 23.)

and nonoperative treatment in patients with complete (Frankel grade A) paraplegia. The surgically stabilized group (posterior spinal fusion) had significantly shorter inpatient hospital stays than patients treated with laminectomy. The posterior spinal fusion group also had shorter stays than the nonoperative group; however, the difference was not significant. The surgically treated group, however, had significantly more complications than the nonoperative group (Table 2), allowing the authors to conclude that nonoperative treatment is usually more advantageous in patients with complete paraplegia.

Operative treatment should be considered for patients who have either a grossly unstable spine or for those who have an incomplete neurologic deficit with spinal canal compromise. When stability is the only issue, posterior spinal fusion with instrumentation is the appropriate treatment. The most common instrumentation systems employ rods that are fixed to the spine using either hooks, screws, or wires. Most of these rigid instrumentation systems allow the surgeon to apply reduction forces to the spine, reducing dislocations while restoring vertebral column height and sagittal plane balance. In 1978, Harrington's group (11) reported on 95 patients stabilized with their system. While 40% of their neurologically injured patients had some functional improvement, the authors did not distinguish between thoracic and lumbar injuries, making it difficult to draw precise conclusions from the results. Gertzbein et al. (3) reported significant loss of reduction with progressive kyphotic deformity occurring in individuals treated with Harrington instrumentation. Their opinion was that anterior column support was needed when significant anterior column injury was present for Harrington instrumentation to be successful. Current instrumentation systems are much more rigid and allow for segmental spinal fixation. Such use of instrumentation with multiple hook constructs is much more resistive to kyphotic forces. Nevertheless, external brace support or anterior column reconstruction should be considered to augment posterior constructs.

TABLE 2. Complications

	Operative (n = 65)	Nonoperative (n = 48)
Wound healing	3	0
Scoliosis	3	2
Lumbar Charcot	1	0
Reoperation	6	0
Pulmonary embolism	2	0
Death	0	1
Cerebrospinal fluid leak	1	0
Spasticity	1	0
Severe back pain	1	3
Head injury	0	1
Total	18 (27.7%)*	7 (14.6%)*

* $p < .10$.
Adapted from ref. 26, with permission.

In the presence of incomplete neural injury combined with spinal canal narrowing, anterior surgery provides the best opportunity for recovery of neurologic function. (Decompression of the spinal canal from the posterior approach would require an extensive laminectomy and manipulation or retraction of the spinal cord. These procedures are associated with significant morbidity and should not be performed when treating these injuries.) Bohlman et al. (8) reported on their experience with transthoracic decompression of the spine. In their series, each patient treated with anterior decompression and fusion had at least one Frankel grade of neurologic improvement.

SURGICAL TECHNIQUES
Posterior Spinal Fusion

Preoperative planning for this surgery should include spinal cord monitoring and cell saver blood retrieval. The patient should be positioned on either chest rolls or a Hall-type frame. A midline incision is made and carried down to the posterior spinous process. The distance between the posterior spinous process is noted and the interspinous ligaments are inspected for hematoma to determine the integrity of the posterior column. The paraspinal muscles are stripped from the spine using subperiosteal technique; however, the interspinous ligaments are left undisturbed. The hook placement sites are identified and prepared. Hook location options with most instrumentation systems include the lamina, pedicle, and transverse process. A claw configuration is preferred at the proximal and distal hardware anchor sites, which are usually situated two levels above and two levels below the fractured vertebrae. In most thoracic spine constructs the upper claw configuration includes thoracic pedicle hooks that go up, countered with either a transverse process that goes down or a laminar hook. Some surgeons prefer to stagger the placement of these hooks from right to left to minimize spinal canal encroachment and limit the potential for iatrogenic neurologic injury. This is particularly true in those patients who are neurologically intact or who have incomplete neurologic injuries. The surgeon must be particularly careful inserting in the thoracic spine laminar hooks that go down. The shoe of the hook must fit snugly against the undersurface of the lamina to prevent significant canal encroachment.

Furthermore, when compressing the claw construct, there can be a tendency to push the shoe of this hook further into the spinal canal. In the majority of surgical patients with good bone quality, transverse process hooks are utilized, while laminar hooks are reserved for those with notable osteopenia. In the lower thoracic spine (T10-T12), thoracic laminar hooks that go down can generally be placed safely and contoured and installed utilizing three-point bending principles in the majority of injuries. Appropriate compression or distraction forces are then applied to the spine. While the Harrington group (11) reported that overdistraction was unusual because of the tethering effect of the anterior longitudinal ligament, the authors' experience suggests that this method is not reliable and that reduction forces must be carefully applied and the vertebral height and spinal alignment be identified with intraoperative x-rays. Decortication and bone grafting are then performed and the wound is then closed.

Costotransversectomy

The costotransversectomy allows the surgeon to approach and instrument the posterior elements of the spine while also providing some limited access to the anterior elements. The preoperative requirements are the same as the posterior approach. The patient is positioned in the lateral position. While either a midline or paravertebral hockey stick incision can be used, the midline is preferable because it allows access to the posterior elements for stabilization. After the appropriate level to be decompressed has been verified, the paraspinal muscles are divided horizontally and the transverse process, rib, and costotransverse joints are exposed as shown in Fig. 3. The periosteum is stripped from the rib and the rib then divided approximately 3 cm lateral to the transverse process. The transverse process is then removed as needed and the pleura and its underlying contents are swept anteriorly (Fig. 4). The vertebral body is now exposed (27).

Transthoracic Decompression

Transthoracic decompression can be performed by either open or thoracoscopic methods. The open procedure has been described by Bohlman et al. (8) and will be summarized

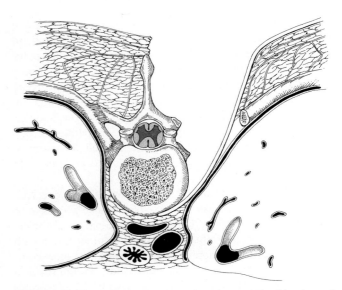

FIG. 4. The final dissection exposing the vertebral body and allowing access to the spinal canal. (Adapted from ref. 27.)

here. The patient is placed in the lateral position and the bed is broken so that the patient's convex side is facing up. The right-side approach is preferred so as to avoid the aorta. The appropriate rib is identified, stripped of its periosteal attachments and then removed. The pleural cavity is entered, the ribs are spread and the lung is retracted out of the field. The segmental vessel is identified in the fascia overlying the midportion of the vertebral body and then ligated. The intercostal nerve is traced into the vertebral foramen. The base of the rib is then removed and then the fractured vertebral body fragments are removed. At this point, the dura should be easily visualized. The proximal and distal end plates are prepared (after removal of the discs) and a tricortical bone graft is placed within the defect. Anterior instrumentation can then be applied to the spine. The chest is closed with a chest tube in place (Fig. 5).

Several authors have described anterior thoracic decompression using thoracoscopy (13,28). This is a demanding procedure that requires specialized training and instrumentation and should be performed with the assistance of an experienced thoracoscopic surgeon. McAfee et al. (29) reported on their series of thoracoscopic decompression, which included three patients who had burst fracture of the thoracic spine. Each of these patients improved from a Frankel grade D to grade E. Because current technology for bone grafting and instrumentation using this procedure is limited, posterior spinal instrumentation is frequently required prior to the anterior decompression.

COMPLICATIONS

Numerous complications may result from thoracic spine injury and it is not possible to review each one in this chapter. Complications can be broadly divided into con-

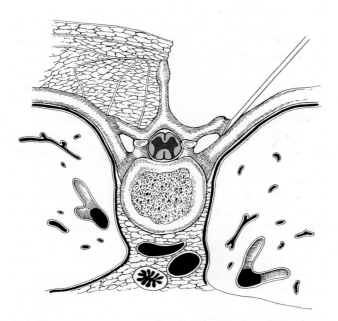

FIG. 3. The plane of dissection during costotransversectomy. The interval between the transverse process and the rib is developed. (Adapted from ref. 27.)

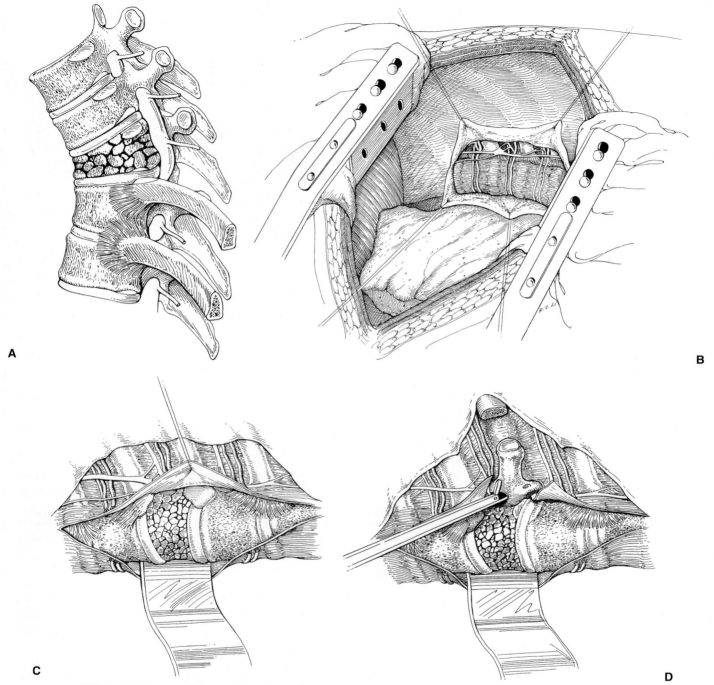

FIG. 5. A: Schematic drawing of a burst fracture with bone and soft tissue compressing the spinal cord. **B:** Exposure of the vertebral column. The segmental vessels have been tied off. **C:** The intercostal nerve has been followed into the intervertebral foramen. **D:** The rib head and near pedicle are removed.

Continued

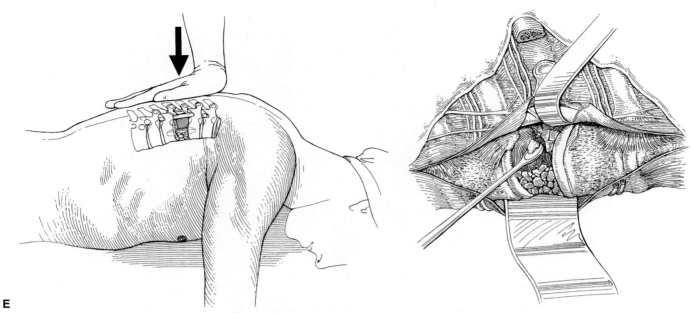

E

FIG. 5. *(Continued)* **E:** The fracture fragments are then removed exposing the dura.

sequences of injury and consequences of treatment. The initial evaluation of the suspected spine-injured patient must be extremely thorough. When the injury occurs in the setting of trauma, standard trauma life support protocols should first be implemented. The treating team of physicians must ensure that all injuries are identified and handled appropriately. For the patient with a thoracic spine injury, a complete neurologic examination is required. Follow-up serial examinations are needed to evaluate for change in neurologic functions. Patients with thoracic spine trauma have been reported to have fractures at multiple spinal levels as well as axial skeletal fractures. Additionally, injury to the great vessels, lungs, as well as the esophagus and lymphatic structures are possible and must not be overlooked during an initial evaluation (30).

Complications resulting from surgical treatment can be separated into medical and surgical problems. The medical problems have been well described and are similar to those traditionally encountered in orthopedic surgery such as cardiac and pulmonary failure, deep venous thrombosis, pulmonary embolism, ileus, ulcer, and related gastrointestinal disorders and urinary dysfunction. The most common surgical complications include loss of neurologic function, failure to obtain a solid fusion, and the development of late kyphosis. To minimize these, the surgeon must endeavor to minimize blood loss and maintain adequate blood pressure to prevent spinal cord ischemia, avoid spinal cord manipulation, and minimize canal encroachment by surgical hardware. Careful attention to the preparation of a fusion bed with iliac crest bone graft should help achieve a solid fusion and prevent late kyphosis.

PATHOLOGIC FRACTURES

Pathologic fractures are the most common thoracic spine fractures in individuals older than 50 years. Osteoporosis is the most common etiology, accounting for approximately 50% of the fractures with 30% and 5% being due to metastatic disease and multiple myeloma, respectively (4). When a painful thoracic spine fracture is identified after minimal or no trauma, an appropriate history and physical searching for signs of metabolic and neoplastic disease is performed.

The plain radiographics are inspected for lytic or blastic changes. In the absence of these changes, the patient is treated expectantly for a period of 6 weeks. A brace may be added to provide additional support. If symptoms persist, a metastatic disease evaluation is performed. The most common tumors to metastasize to the spine are breast, prostate, lung, kidney, and thyroid. If the findings remain equivocal, the vertebra may be biopsied and appropriate medical treatment undertaken (31).

If a tumor is identified and it compresses the spinal cord, the patient is treated with chemotherapy, steroids, and radiation based on the tumor's responsiveness to these modalities. (An MRI scan is always obtained prior to treatment to determine the extent of the tumor.) Surgical treatment is reserved for refractory cases and then undertaken; it involves spinal cord decompression and spinal column stabilization. The surgical approach is chosen based on the location of the tumor mass, which is usually anterior.

If osteoporosis is identified, the patient's bone density is measured and a therapeutic protocol is initiated based on the recommendations of the patients primary care physician (32,33).

CONCLUSION

Fractures occurring between T2 and T10 need to be treated separately from those occurring at either the cervicothoracic or thoracolumbar junctions. These injuries may result from major trauma or occur in the presence of pathologic bone. These fractures are classified based on the traditional three-column theory; however, the sternum and rib cage form a fourth column that confers additional stability to this portion of the spine. Treatment must address both osseous and neurologic injury. In the absence of neurologic deficit, stable fractures can be managed either expectantly or with a brace. In complete injuries, the authors favor nonoperative treatment unless the spine is grossly unstable and prevents rehabilitation. The incomplete neurologic injury requires reduction of vertebral dislocation followed by surgical stabilization. If spinal cord compression is present, we favor anterior transthoracic spinal cord decompression. Anterior column stabilization can be performed with bone graft and plating, or posterior instrumentation can be used if severe instability exists.

RADIOGRAPHIC CASES

Case 1

These x-rays demonstrate a compression fracture sustained in a fall. There is minimal wedging of the vertebral body and no evidence of middle column compromise. The fracture was treated expectantly and healed without incident.

Case 2

This patient has multiple myeloma metastatic to multiple levels of the thoracic spine. The preoperative x-rays demonstrate a pathologic fracture of the T7 vertebral body. The MRI scan demonstrates spinal cord compression at the same level. The patient underwent video-assisted thoracoscopic decompression with bone grafting and instrumentation. The entire procedure except for the bone graft harvest was performed endoscopically. The postoperative x-rays are shown.

Case 3

These x-rays demonstrate a pathologic fracture from metastatic tumor. Multiple vertebral levels are involved. Cord compression from tumor and fracture fragments is evident. This patient underwent anterior thoracic decompression with iliac crest bone graft followed by posterior spinal fusion. Segmental instrumentation with a rod and hook construct was used. The construct spanned many vertebra in anticipation of future metastatic disease.

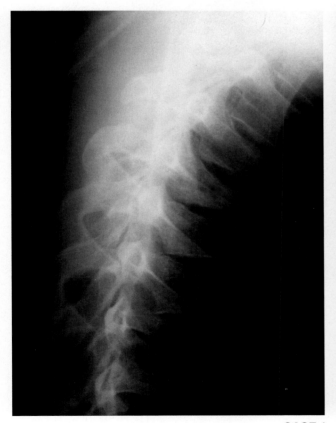
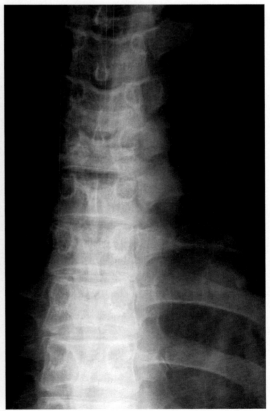

CASE 1.

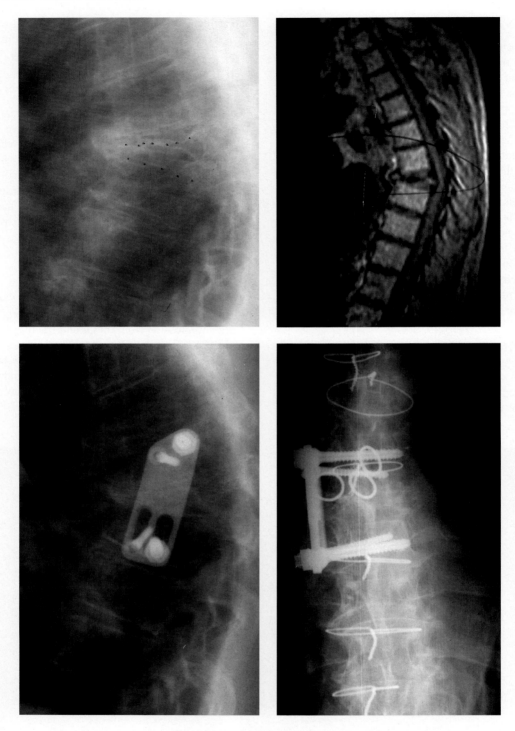

CASE 2.

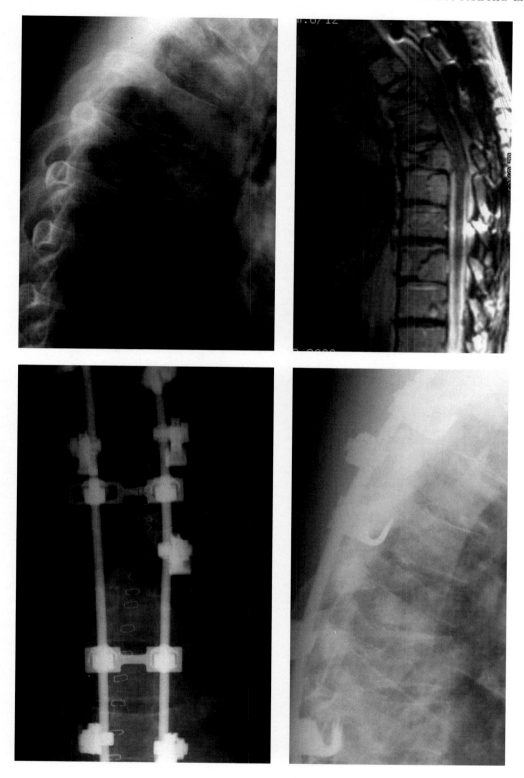

CASE 3.

REFERENCES

1. Hanley EN, Eskay ML. Thoracic spine fractures. *Orthopedics* 1989; 12(5):689–696.
2. Hu R, Cameron AM, Burns C. Epidemiology of incident spinal fracture in a complete population. *Spine* 1996;21(4):492–499.
3. Gertzbein SD, Macmichael D, Tile M. Harrington instrumentation as a method of fixation in fractures of the spine. *J Bone Joint Surg* 1982;64B;526–529.
4. Biyani A, Ebraheim NA, Lu J. Thoracic spine fractures in patients older than 50 years. *Clin Orthop* 1993;328:190–193.
5. Meldon SW, Moettus LN. Thoracolumbar spine fracture: clinical presentation and the effect of altered sensorium and major injury. *J Trauma* 1995;39(6):1110–1114.
6. Bolesta MJ, Bohlman HH. Mediastinal widening associated with fractures of the upper thoracic spine. *J Bone Joint Surg* 1991;73A:447–450.
7. Bohlman HH. Treatment of fractures and dislocations of the thoracic and lumbar spine. *J Bone Joint Surg* 1985;67A:165–169.
8. Bohlman HH, Freehafer A, Dejak J. The results of acute injuries of the upper thoracic spine with paralysis. *J Bone Joint Surg* 1985;67A:360–369.
9. Capen DA, Gordon ML, Zigler JE, Garland DF, Nelson RW, Nagelberg S. Nonoperative management of upper thoracic spine fractures. *Orthop Rev* 1994;10:818–821.
10. Dickman CA, Yahiro MA, Lu HTC, Melkerson MN. Surgical treatment alternatives for fixation of unstable fractures of the thoracic and lumbar spine. *Spine* 1994;19;2266S–2273S.
11. Dickson JH, Harrington PR, Erwin WD. Results of reduction and stabilization of the severely fractured thoracic and lumbar spine. *J Bone Joint Surg* 1978;60A;799–805.
12. Frankel HL, Hancock DO, Hyslop G, et al. The value of postural reduction in the initial management of closed injuries of the spine with paraplegia and tetraplegia. *Paraplegia* 1969;7:179–192.
13. Hertlein H, Hartl WH, Dienemann H, Schurmann M, Lob G. Thoracoscopic repair of thoracic spine trauma. *Eur Spine J* 1995;4;302–307.
14. Denis F. The three column spine and its significance in the classification of acute thoracolumbar spinal injuries. *Spine* 1983;8;817–831.
15. Fowler AW. Flexion/compression injury of the sternum. *J Bone Joint Surg* 1957;39B:487–497.
16. Jones KH, McBride GG, Mumby RC. Sternal fractures associated with spinal injury. *J Trauma* 1989;29(3);360–364.
17. Itani M, Evans GA, Park WM. Spontaneous sternal collapse. *J Bone Joint Surg* 1982;64B:432–434.
18. Berg EE. The sternal-rib complex. *Spine* 1993;18(13):1916–1919.
19. Korovessis P, Sidiropoulos P, Dimas A. Complete fracture dislocation of the thoracic spine without neurologic deficit: a case report. *J Trauma* 1994;36(1):122–124.
20. Lilkenqvist U, Halm H, Castro WHM, Mommsen U. Thoracic fracture-dislocations without spinal cord injury: a case report and literature review. *Eur Spine J* 1995;4:252–256.
21. Gertzbein SD. Neurologic deterioration in patients with thoracic and lumbar fractures after admission to the hospital. *Spine* 1994;19:1723–1725.
22. Magerl F. A new classification of spinal fractures. *Orthop Trans* 1991;15:728–729.
23. Gertzbein SD. Spine update classification of thoracic and lumbar fractures. *Spine* 1994;19;626–628.
24. Nash CL, Schatzinger LH, Brown RH, Brodkey J. The unstable thoracic compression fracture. *Spine* 1977;2(4):281–283.
25. Stahlman GC, Wyrsch RB, McNamara MJ. Late-onset sternomanubrial dislocation with progressive kyphotic deformity after a thoracic burst fracture. *J Orthop Trauma* 1995;9(4):350–353.
26. Place HM, Donaldson DH, Brown CW, Stringer EA. Stabilization of thoracic spine fractures resulting in complete paraplegia. *Spine* 1994; 19(15):1726–1730.
27. Kostuik JP. Surgical approaches to the thoracic and thoracolumbar spine. In: Frymoyer JW, ed. *The Adult Spine.* New York: Raven Press, 1991:1243–1266.
28. Goldstein JA, McAfee PC. Video-assisted thoracic surgery of the spine. *Curr Opin Orthop* 1996;7(11):54–60.
29. McAfee PC, Regan JR, Fedder IL, Mack MJ, Geis WP. Anterior thoracic corpectomy for spinal cord decompression performed endoscopically. *Surg Laparosc Endosc* 1995;5(5):339–348.
30. Baker FC, Patka P, Haarman HJTM. Combined repair of a traumatic rupture of the aorta and anterior stabilization of a thoracic spine fracture. A case report. *J Trauma* 1996;40(1):128–129.
31. An HS, Andreshak TG, Nguyen C, Williams A, Daniels D. Can we distinguish between benign versus malignant compression fracture of the spine by magnetic resonance imaging? *Spine* 1995;20(16):1776–1782.
32. Liberman UA, Weiss SR, Broli J, et al. Effect of oral alendronate on bone mineral density and the incidence of fractures in postmenopausal osteoporosis. *N Engl J Med* 1995;333(30):1437–1443.
33. Moro M, Hecker AT, Bouxsein ML, Myers ER. Failure load of thoracic vertebra correlates with lumbar mineral density measured by DXA. *Calcif Tissue Int* 1995;56:206–209.

Surgery of Spinal Trauma,
edited by J.M. Cotler, J.M. Simpson, H.S. An, and C.P. Silveri.
Lippincott Williams & Wilkins, Philadelphia © 2000.

CHAPTER 11

Fractures and Dislocations of the Thoracolumbar Junction

Jeffrey S. Fischgrund and Harry N. Herkowitz

The thoracolumbar junction represents the most common area of injury to the axial skeleton because of the forces generated between the long lever arm of the stiff thoracic spine and the mobile lumbar spine following a traumatic incident. The thoracolumbar junction is also neurologically unique, because it represents a transitional zone between the spinal cord and cauda equina. Neurologic injuries can present with either spinal cord injuries or cauda equina lesions.

The fracture patterns seen in this region range from minor compression fractures, burst fractures with retropulsed bone and soft tissue into the spinal canal, to fracture-dislocations. Considerable controversy has existed over the operative indications for burst fractures when bone or soft tissue retropulsion occurs into the spinal canal in the neurologically intact patient. This chapter outlines the radiographic evaluation, classification, mechanisms, fracture patterns, and nonoperative and operative treatment of injuries occurring at the thoracolumbar junction.

RADIOGRAPHIC EVALUATION

The initial radiographic assessment of the patient with a possible thoracolumbar fracture includes anteroposterior and cross-table lateral radiographs. Anteroposterior radiographs

---

J. S. Fischgrund and H. N. Herkowitz: William Beaumont Hospital, Royal Oak, Michigan 48073.

should be examined for transverse process or rib fractures, as well as loss of vertebral body height. Malalignment in the anterior-posterior plane suggests the possibility of fracture-dislocation. Generally the spinous processes should be aligned in the midline in the patient who has no history of scoliosis. Visualization of the pedicles should reveal their normal oval appearance, with no signs of cortical disruption.

Lateral radiographs easily reveal the loss of body height in burst and compression fractures. The posterior cortical wall should be carefully examined for signs of retropulsion, indicative of a burst fracture. Malalignment again suggests fracture-dislocation. The spinous processes should be carefully examined, as any evidence of interspinous process widening indicates disruption of the posterior ligamentous complex (1).

The use of plain tomograms has largely been replaced by computed tomography (CT). Tomograms are still useful when evaluating flexion-distraction injuries, since these horizontal fractures can be missed on transaxial images. In these specific injuries, tomograms can often help distinguish between ligamentous and osseus injuries. CT is very helpful when determining the stability of the various fracture patterns. In compression and burst fractures, an important determinant of stability is the integrity of the posterior structures. The osseus ring surrounding the spinal canal is in the same plane as the CT axial image, thus optimally evaluating the neural arch (2). Facet subluxation and laminar fractures

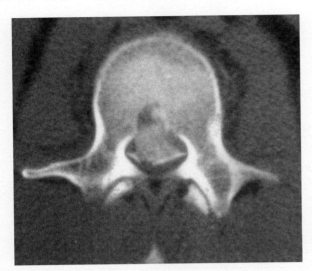

FIG. 1. Axial computed tomography (CT) image demonstrating approximately 80% compression of the spinal canal due to a large retropulsed fragment.

are easily seen on axial images. The degree of bone retropulsion from burst fractures can also be calculated from these images (Figs. 1 and 2). Sagittal reconstruction is helpful for visualization of flexion-distraction injuries, since transaxial images can miss injuries in the horizontal plane.

With severe fracture-dislocation, CT imaging in the axial plane may demonstrate two vertebral bodies on the same axial image (Fig. 3), or discontinuity of the canal from one level to the next. The degree of vertebral body comminution can also be assessed by axial images and sagittal reconstructions.

In an effort to further evaluate thoracolumbar fractures, some authors have recommended the use of magnetic resonance imaging (MRI) (3,4). Advantages of MRI include the following: (a) multiplanar views are possible without patient repositioning (axial, coronal, and sagittal); (b) trauma to the spinal cord can be visualized, as well as the presence of epidural hematomas or disc disruptions; and (c) information regarding the integrity of the spinal ligaments (anterior longitudinal ligament, posterior longitudinal ligament, and posterior interspinous ligaments) can be obtained. Although MRI is obviously superior for visualization of the posterior ligamentous complex, it has not yet been shown that the determination of the integrity of these ligaments significantly affects the clinical decision-making process.

Magnetic resonance imaging may be used in detecting the integrity of the soft tissue attachments to the retropulsed bone fragment. Disruption of the fibers of the posterior annulus (5,6) may indicate potential failure of reduction of this retropulsed bone by distraction methods (indirect reduction). MRI is most useful for evaluating the patient with a significant neurologic deficit that does not correspond to the osseous injury demonstrated by plain radiographs and/or CT.

CLASSIFICATION

Management of thoracolumbar fractures can be greatly assisted by the use of an accurate classification scheme. Ideally, the classification of fractures should assist the clinician in the decision-making process regarding treatment and provide useful information for future research studies (7). A comprehensive classification scheme should include most

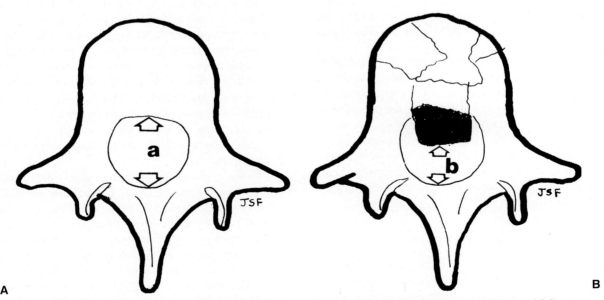

FIG. 2. A: The normal sagital diameter of the spinal canal. **B:** The diameter of the spinal canal following a burst fracture. The percent canal compromise can be determined by dividing the area remaining in the spinal canal at the level of maximal compression by the normal sagittal diameter of the spinal canal (*b* divided by *a*).

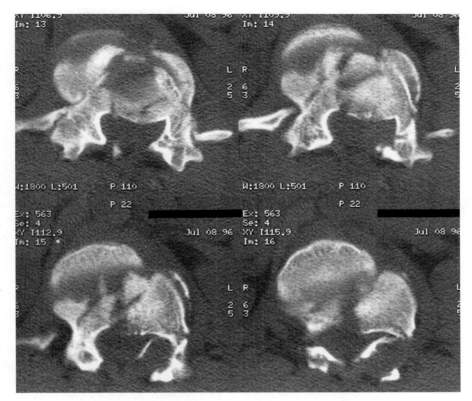

FIG. 3. CT scan of a fracture-dislocation. Note the axial cuts, which demonstrate two vertebral bodies on the same axial slice.

common injuries, be easy to apply, and be used consistently by a majority of spinal surgeons.

One of the earliest classification systems of spinal fractures was described by Watson Jones (8) in 1931. This early system focused primarily on the diagnosis and treatment of flexion injuries. Holdsworth (9), motivated by poor outcomes following the treatment of traumatic paraplegia, recognized the importance of the posterior ligamentous complex and its contribution to spinal stability. He proposed the following classification system based on the mechanism of injury: 1, flexion; 2, flexion and rotation; 3, extension (rare in the lumbar spine); 4, compression.

Holdsworth noted that a flexion moment on the thoracolumbar spine usually leaves the posterior ligamentous structures intact and results in a wedge compression fracture. Flexion rotation often ruptures the posterior ligaments and results in spinal dislocation if the flexion moment is sufficiently high. A compressive force along the line of the vertebra transmits force along the vertebral end plates and body, resulting in the classic burst fracture. Based on this classification scheme, injuries were considered unstable only if the posterior ligamentous complex was rendered incompetent by the initial trauma.

This two-column theory of spinal stability was modified by Denis (10) in 1983, with the addition of a third or middle column. Evolution of the three-column spine concept was based on the biochemical work performed by Nagel et al.

(11), who, by testing fresh human cadaver at the first and second lumbar vertebrae, determined that "the interspace does not displace significantly under physiological loads with progressive disruption of the posterior elements until the anulus fibrosis is disrupted."

The three-column spine (Fig. 4), as defined by Denis (10), is as follows: The posterior column is formed by the posterior arch, as well as the posterior ligaments (including the supraspinatus and interspinous ligaments), joint capsule, and ligamentous flavum. The middle column is formed by the posterior longitudinal ligament, posterior anulus fibrosus, and the posterior wall of the vertebral body. The anterior column is formed by the anterior longitudinal ligament, the anterior anulus fibrosus, and the anterior part of the vertebral body. Using this three-column definition, Denis retrospectively reviewed over 400 thoracolumbar spine fractures and proposed the following comprehensive spinal fracture classification system:

Compression Fracture

A compression fracture is defined by failure of the anterior column by compressive forces. The middle column acts as a hinge and remains intact, thereby reducing the risk of neurologic compromise. The failure of the posterior column under tension may occur with severe trauma. Radiographic findings include normal height of the posterior vertebral body,

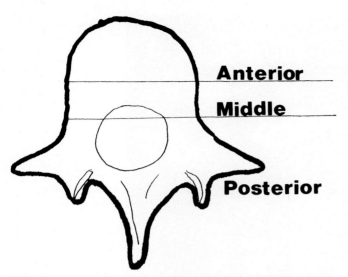

FIG. 4. The three-column spine as described by Denis (10) (see text for explanation).

wedging anteriorly, and proportionate posterior interspinous widening. CT scan demonstrates the anterior fracture without evidence of retropulsion (Fig. 5).

Burst Fracture

Axial loading of the spine may lead to failure of both the anterior and middle columns, resulting in a burst fracture. Lateral radiographs typically demonstrate loss of height of the posterior cortex with varying degrees of retropulsion. Lateral radiographs should also be carefully examined to determine the degree of interspinous widening, which is indicative of posterior column disruption. Anterior/posterior radiographs classically demonstrate an increase in the interpedicular distance, while CT scans not only demonstrate the body fracture, but also define the degree of retropulsion, the splaying of the posterior joints, and the presence or absence of a vertical lamina fracture.

Subclassification of burst fractures into types A, B, and C may be described based on endplate deformation (determined by lateral radiographs). Type A is due to a pure axial load and results in fracture of both endplates. The most common subtype (type B) is defined as a fracture of the superior endplate only. Type C fractures are rare and defined as inferior endplate fractures. Types D and E are due to rotation and lateral flexion forces, respectively, in combination with axial loading.

Seat-Belt–Type Injuries

Flexion distraction (seat-belt injuries) of the thoracolumbar spine were first described by Chance (12) in 1948, who reported on three cases in which the fracture line extended transversely through the posterior neural arch and exited through the posterior/superior endplate. Howland et al. (13) in 1965 noted the association of this type of injury with improperly positioned seat-belts. Several classification systems for this injury have been proposed. Denis (14) proposed four types based on osseous versus ligamentous disruption and one- versus two-level injury. Triantafyllou and Gertzbein (15) reported seven subtypes, and Gertzbein and Court-Brown (16) were the first to describe the association of burst fractures with flexion distraction injuries.

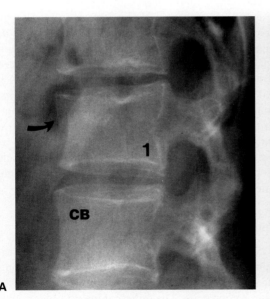
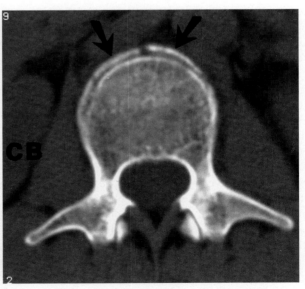

FIG. 5. A: Lateral radiograph demonstrating an L1 compression fracture. Note the loss of height of the anterior cortex, as well as no evidence of disruption of the posterior cortex scan. **B:** Axial CAT scan demonstrates the anterior fracture (arrows) with no disruption of the posterior cortex.

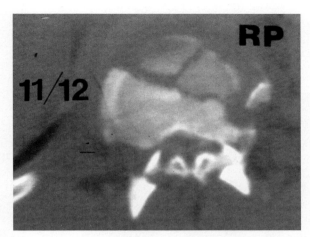

FIG. 6. Axial CT scan demonstrating a T11-12 fracture-dislocation. Note fracture of the anterior and middle columns, as well as dislocation of the facet joints.

Fracture-Dislocations

Failure of all three columns under either compression, tension, rotation, or shear leads to the most unstable spine injury, a fracture-dislocation (Fig. 6). Radiographs usually reveal either subluxation or dislocation in association with rib or transverse process fractures. Fracture-dislocations have been subdivided into three groups by Denis (10): (a) Flexion-rotation: this injury may result in retropulsion of the posterior body into the canal. However, unlike the burst fracture, the posterior longitudinal ligament is usually torn, resulting in increased instability and difficulty in obtaining an indirect reduction. (b) Shear: this extension injury begins with an anterior injury that progresses from an anterior longitudinal ligament tear to complete disc disruption. Continued shear forces then result in translation of the upper vertebrae in relation to the lower vertebrae. (c) Flexion-distraction: this injury is similar to a seat-belt injury, but additional trauma leads to disruption of the anterior annulus, resulting in vertebral subluxation or dislocation.

A new classification scheme with emphasis on the severity of the injury in relationship to fracture categories was proposed by Magerl et al. (17) in 1990. This scheme was modified by members of the leading spine societies: the Scoliosis Research Society, the International Society for Study of the Lumbar Spine, the Cervical Spine Research Society, the North American Spine Society, and the Orthopaedic Trauma Association. Final recommendations of this committee were published by Gertzbein (7) in 1994.

Fractures are classified into three main categories: type A, compression; type B, distraction; and type C, multidirectional with translation. Each main category is then subdivided into three groups, according to comminution and/or displacement. Fractures are increasingly unstable and the chance of neurologic deficit is higher as one progresses through the classification scheme.

Type A fractures are due to axial loading with or without a flexion force. Group 1 is a wedge compression fracture (Fig. 7). Group 2 is defined by a sagittal or coronal split (Fig. 8) of the vertebral body. Group 3 is a burst fracture (Figs. 9 and 10). All Type A fractures are associated with loss of vertical height without disruption of the posterior soft tissues.

Type B injuries result from distractive forces across the anterior and posterior elements. Groups 1 (Fig. 11) and 2 (Fig. 12) are similar to a Denis (10) flexion-distraction

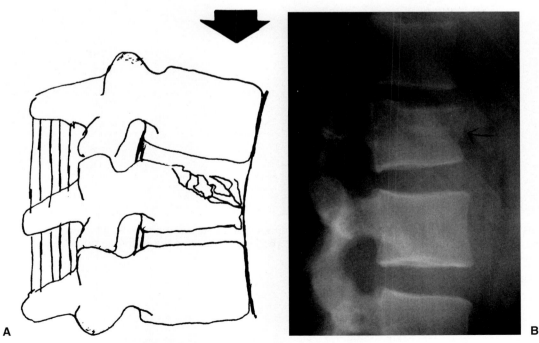

FIG. 7. A: Drawing of a wedge compression fracture (A-1). **B:** Lateral radiograph of a type A-1 fracture.

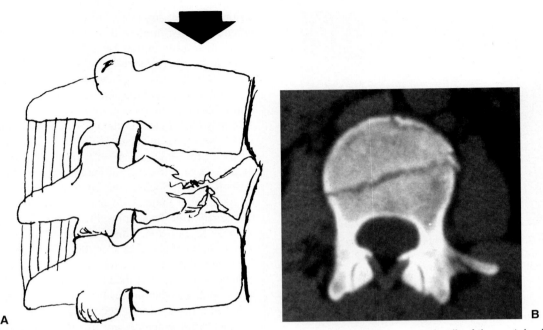

FIG. 8. A: Line drawing of a type A-1 fracture. **B:** CT scan demonstrates a coronal split of the vertebral body.

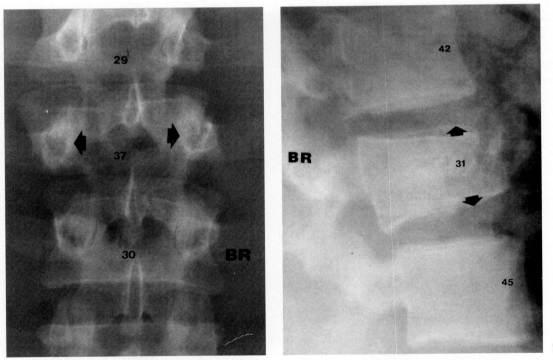

FIG. 9. A: Anteroposterior (AP) radiograph of an L2 burst fracture demonstrates interpedicular widening compared to the normal adjacent segments. **B:** Lateral radiographs of the same patient demonstrates loss of anterior height.

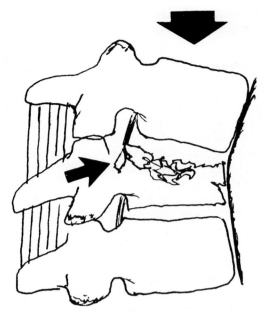

FIG. 10. A type A-3 injury. The smaller arrow demonstrates retropulsion of the posterior vertebral body.

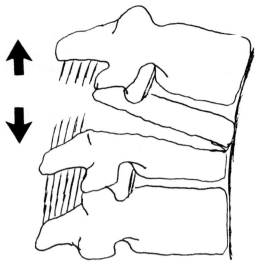

FIG. 12. A type B-2 injury.

injury, with disruption occurring through either the soft tissues posteriorly (group 1) or the bony arch (group 2). Extension-distraction forces may result in a group 3 injury (Fig. 13), with the fracture beginning anteriorly through the disc and extending posteriorly through either the posterior bony arch (extension spondylolysis) or soft tissues (posterior subluxation).

Type C injuries are defined by significant translation and are generally considered unstable. In Group 1 (Fig. 14), translation is in the anterior posterior plane; group 2 (Fig. 15) demonstrates lateral translation; and group 3 (Fig. 16) is due to rotational deforming forces. Axial loading may be associated with either a group 1 or group 3 injury, resulting in compression or burst fracture of the vertebral body.

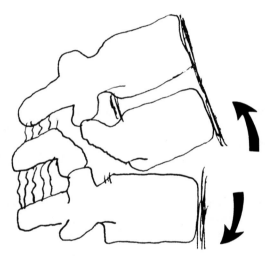

FIG. 13. A type B-3 injury.

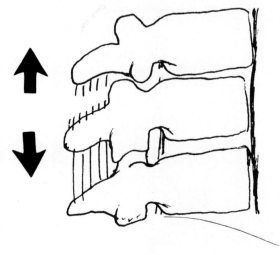

FIG. 11. A type B-1 injury.

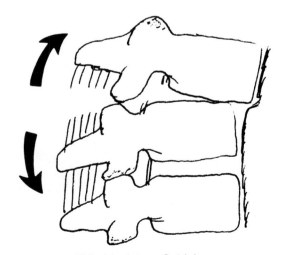

FIG. 14. A type C-1 injury.

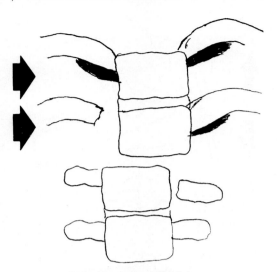

FIG. 15. A type C-2 injury.

BIOMECHANICS

Careful review of the previously described classification scheme frequently leads to confusion among treating physicians as to whether or not a fracture is stable or is in need of operative stabilization. Clinical stability has been defined by White and Panjabi (18) as "the inability of the spine under physiologic loads to maintain relationships between vertebrae, so that there is neither initial nor subsequent neurologic deficit, no major deformity, and no severe pain." Clinical instability as defined by either the two-column theory of Holdsworth or the three-column theory of Denis has been the object of numerous biomechanical investigations.

Willen et al. (19) in 1984 first reported on the experimental reproduction of lumbar burst fractures. This was accomplished by dropping a 10-kg weight a distance of 2 m onto a block of foam placed on a vertebral specimen. The resulting fracture consisted of a comminuted body with fractured end plates, prolapsed disc nucleus, bone fragments encroaching upon the spinal canal, and facet joint laxity. Both the superior and inferior end plates were noted to be disrupted in all cases, while neither the anterior longitudinal ligament nor the posterior longitudinal ligament showed evidence of transverse rupture. Biomechanical testing of the fractured vertebra revealed the flexion-extension range to be considerably increased. Based on these biomechanical results, it was concluded that these crushed fractures should be regarded as unstable, with a risk of progressive flexion deformity, neurologic deficit, and pain.

Reproduction of burst fractures was also performed by James et al. (20), who performed a standardized series of osteotomies on the first lumbar vertebral body with an oscillating saw. The anterior body was then crushed to keep the anterior longitudinal ligament intact. Biomechanical testing and flexion was performed following a series of sequential disruptions of the anterior middle and posterior columns, as defined by Denis (10). The deforming force tested was flexion since this is a primary force associated with kyphotic progression. Disruption of the anterior column led to a statistically significant increase in the angulation and translation, compared to the intact specimen, and was the largest contributor to the final amount of instability created in each specimen. More importantly, it was found that compromise of the middle column contributed least to the final instability; the posterior column contributed almost twice as much as the middle column to the end degree of instability. The authors concluded that these biomechanical data cast doubt on the importance placed on the middle-column integrity compared with the posterior column in determining burst fracture stability.

James et al.'s (20) results were similar to those of a previous study performed by Haher et al. (20a). By progressively performing spinal column destruction at L2 and then testing

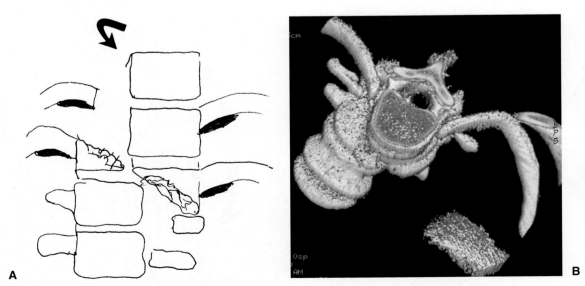

FIG. 16. A: Drawing of a type C-3 injury. **B:** 3-D reconstruction of a CAT scan, demonstrating a rotational fracture-dislocation (type C-3).

an entire specimen (T11 to the sacrum) in torsion, Haher et al. concluded that the annulus was the most effective structure in resisting torsion. However, this model destabilized the spine to produce an injury similar to a flexion-distraction injury. Also in this model the axis of rotation was defined by the testing apparatus and not by the specimens (21), and the specimens were tested only in torsion. Therefore, these results cannot be extrapolated to determine stability in the patient with a burst fracture.

A more recent biomechanical study by Panjabi et al. (21) reproduced burst fractures using a high-speed trauma model. Fracture patterns were confirmed by computed axial tomography (CAT) scan and were classified as Denis type B (superior end-plate fracture). Biomechanical testing was performed using a multidirectional flexibility testing protocol that does not impose any axis of rotation. In both the axial compression and flexion compression specimens, the integrity of the middle column was found to be the primary determinate of mechanical stability/instability. Additionally, the flexion compression specimen showed more severe damage to all three columns. Panjabi et al. felt that this was the first comprehensive objective evidence to validate the three-column theory.

NONOPERATIVE TREATMENT

Unfortunately, as evidenced by contradictions in the literature, evaluation of the above-mentioned biomechanical studies often leads to confusion. It is often difficult, if not impossible, to use relevant biomechanical studies to determine the need for surgical intervention in the patient with the thoracolumbar fracture. Perhaps the most controversial topic regarding operative treatment of thoracolumbar fractures are the indications for surgical intervention in the neurologically intact patient with a thoracolumbar burst fracture (Table 1).

To determine the efficacy of operative management of these fractures, the outcome of nonoperative management must be examined. Based on the White and Panjabi (18) definition of instability, the potential complications of nonoperative treatment include (a) development or progression of a neurologic deficit, (b) chronic pain, and (c) deformity. Nonoperative treatment outcomes must also be analyzed with respect to functional outcome, i.e., work and restrictions in activities of daily living.

Perhaps the most severe potential complication is the development of a neurologic deficit in the patient who is initially neurologically intact. The risk of this complication is difficult to determine from the literature since most severe burst fractures are often treated initially with surgery. Denis et al. (22) noted that of 29 nonoperatively treated burst fractures, six patients (20.7%) developed a neurologic deficit related to the fracture during follow-up. Contrarily, Reid et al. (23) reported on 21 patients with a burst fracture, none of whom developed neurologic deficit requiring operative intervention. Similarly, Canter et al. (24) reported on 18 patients with a burst fracture and no posterior column disruption, and noted no neurologic deficit at follow-up.

A progressive or new neurologic deficit can develop if kyphosis progresses in the weeks following the initial injury. Progressive kyphosis will cause the neural elements to be stretched over the posterior retropulsed bone following a burst fracture (Fig. 17). The gross distortion of the spinal canal produced by large bone fragments may also produce symptoms of spinal stenosis at a later date. However, follow-up CT imaging of patients treated nonoperatively have demonstrated that the vertebrae and bone fragments undergo substantial remodeling. Fidler (25) reported on two patients who had CT scans performed 18 months following injury. Both patients demonstrated restoration of the spinal canal to approximately 75% of normal. Similarly, Cantor et al. (24) noted that all patients who had follow-up CT scans at 1 year had at least 50% resorption of the bone in the canal. Four of these eight patients with initial canal compromise of 25% to 60% had complete resorption of the bone in the canal.

A prospective study by Mumford et al. (26) followed 41 patients who were neurologically intact with a burst fracture confirmed by CT imaging. In this carefully controlled study, the initial kyphosis, (range 0–47 degrees, mean 16 degrees) anterior body height loss (range 6–76%, mean 38%), and canal compromise (range 16–66%, mean 37%) did not influence the patients' initial treatment; all neurologically intact patients were treated with bed rest followed by ambulatory bracing. Only one patient (2%) required subsequent surgery for neurologic deficit. The above-reviewed literature does demonstrate that neurologic deterioration can occur following nonoperative treatment for burst fractures, although the range of occurrence is anywhere from 0% to 20%.

The known possibility of residual deformity following thoracolumbar fracture often leads to the initial recommendation of surgical intervention to restore normal alignment. The incidence of chronic low back pain has been suggested to correlate with the severity of residual kyphosis. Analysis of this correlation was performed by Weinstein et al. (27), who reported the longest follow-up of conservatively treated

TABLE 1. *Authors' indications for surgical treatment of neurologically intact patients with a thoracolumbar burst fracture*

Bohlman (83)	40% loss of body height
Denis (22)	Severe type B burst fracture
	Severe neural canal obstruction
Anderson (84)	25-degree kyphosis
	40–50% loss of height
	50% canal stenosis
	Posterior column disruption
Reid (85)	35-degree kyphosis
	60% loss of height
Canter (24)	35-degree kyphosis
	50% loss of height
	Posterior column disruption
Frederickson (22)	25-degree kyphosis
	50% stenosis

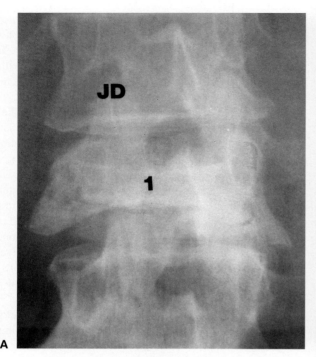 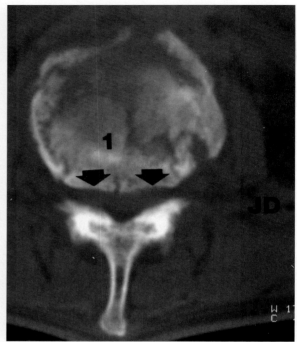

FIG. 17. A: AP radiograph of an L1 burst fracture. Progressive kyphosis at 6 weeks following the injury led to development of significant leg pain and weakness. **B:** CT scan demonstrates significant compression of the neural elements.

thoracolumbar burst fractures from a single institution. Forty-two patients were examined, with an average follow-up of 20 years. At final follow-up, neither the amount of kyphosis nor the extent of translation correlated with patient pain reported. The overall kyphosis angle (average 26 degrees in flexion and 17 degrees in extension) resulted in a nonanatomic result, which did not correlate with a poor functional result. Additionally, Weinstein et al. reported on the long-term functional outcome of these patients. The typical patient had mild to moderate complaints of back pain, while 10% reported no pain at all at 20 years following injury. With regard to employment status, 70% were employed full time at follow-up, while 88% eventually returned to their preinjury occupation.

Weinstein et al.'s (27) results have been confirmed by additional studies (23,28,29). Reid et al.'s (23) report of 21 patients, who were neurologically intact following a burst fracture, noted that although average kyphosis increased from 8 to 13 degrees during the follow-up period, there was no correlation between kyphosis and subsequent pain scores. All patients at final follow-up had a satisfactory pain score, with 75% of patients having a satisfactory work score (working full time).

Nonoperative treatment options include postural reduction, bed rest (with or without bracing), and ambulatory bracing. The duration of immobilization and bed rest varies, and usually needs to be adjusted to the patient's pain tolerance as well as concomitant injury. Holdsworth (9) initially recommended 8 to 12 weeks of recumbency in a plaster

jacket for unstable fractures. More recent recommendations (26) include 4 weeks of bed rest, followed by 12 weeks of bracing. As the emphasis continues to shift to cost containment in the hospital environment, inpatient days for bed rest will likely continue to decrease.

NEUROLOGIC DEFICIT

Neurologic injury at the thoracolumbar junction can produce various deficits. Although the spinal cord usually ends at L1, there may be variations in the position of its termination (conus medullaris). Injuries in this area can produce an upper motor neuron injury, lower motor neuron injury, or a combination of both (30). Holdsworth and Hardy (31) have described these neurologic deficits as follows: (a) complete division of the sacral spinal cord and lumbar nerve roots, (b) complete division of the sacral spinal cord with escape of the lumbar nerve roots on one or both sides, and (c) incomplete division of the sacral spinal cord with escape of the lumbar nerve roots to varying degrees.

Trauma to the neural elements usually occurs at the instant of initial injury. Transient translation of the vertebrae may occur at the time of impact and may be substantially greater than what is demonstrated on initial radiographs, due to recoil of soft tissues (32). Retropulsed bone fragments may add to neural element compression; this correlation between degree of canal compromise and subsequent neurologic deficit has been studied. Hashimoto et al. (33) investigated 122 consecutive patients with lower thoracic or lumbar burst fractures documented by CAT scans. They found that patients with burst fractures at T11 or T12 and greater than 35% canal compromise were at significant risk for neurologic injury. Canal compromise at L1 greater than 45% and at L2 or below greater than 55% was also associated with an increased risk of neurologic deficit. A small bony fragment retropulsed into the spinal canal brought about a greater incidence of neural damage at the cord level than at the cauda equina level, most likely due to the increased sensitivity of the spinal cord to damage. Additionally, a significant association between disruption of the posterior elements and neurologic involvement was noted. These results were confirmed by Gertzbein (32), who reviewed a large study sponsored by the Scoliosis Research Society. He noted that at the conus medullaris level there was a significant correlation of both the midsagittal diameter and cross-sectional area of the compromised spinal canal with neurologic status. This relationship was also found to be true at the cauda equina level.

Nerve root deficits may also occur from spinal trauma. Cammisa et al. (34) theorized that with axial loading, the pedicles and posterior elements splay laterally, as the posterior cortex of the body is retropulsed into the spinal canal. If a vertical laminar fracture occurs during the initial injury, the dura can be forced to protrude between the laminar fracture fragments. As the axial load is then dissipated, the dura and nerve rootlets can be entrapped between the laminar fragments (34). They reported on 60 patients with burst fractures, 30 of whom had concomitant laminar fracture; 11 of 30 were noted to have a dural laceration, and in four of the patients the neural elements were entrapped in the laminar fracture. Recognition of this fracture pattern (Fig. 18) with associated nerve root deficit may influence decisions regarding anterior versus posterior operative intervention.

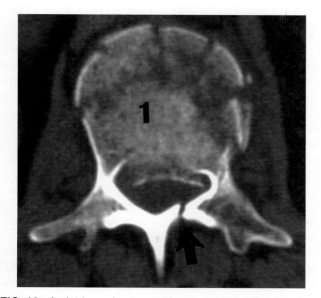

FIG. 18. An L1 burst fracture with an associated laminar fracture.

TABLE 2. *Frankel grading scale for neurologic deficits*

A: Complete motor and sensory loss
B: Sensory sparing, complete motor loss
C: Nonuseful motor function
D: Useful motor function
E: Normal motor, sensory and anatomic function

Operative intervention is often recommended for the patient who presents with a thoracolumbar fracture and a neurologic deficit. The goal of the operative procedure should be decompression of the affected nerve roots, theoretically improving potential for neurologic recovery. Review of the literature, however, does not strongly support this hypothesis. Dickson et al. (35) reported on 95 patients following reduction and stabilization of thoracolumbar fractures and noted that 75% of incomplete paraplegic patients improved at least one Frankel grade (Table 2). However, these results were no better than nonoperative results reported by earlier studies (30–33,35–37), as well as later studies (38).

These earlier reports of operative decompression often relied upon Harrington distraction rods or spinous process plates (Meuring-Williams) to achieve neural decompression and spinal stabilization. Rarely was there adequate documentation of the efficacy of this decompression. Later reports by McAfee et al. (39) and Bradford and McBride (40) on the utilization of direct anterior decompression noted that the degree of neurologic recovery following decompression appears more favorable than previous reports on the utilization of posterior stabilization or nonoperative treatment.

When reviewing reports of neurologic deficits, one must differentiate between spinal cord and nerve root injuries. Unlike injuries to the spinal cord and conus medullaris, a cauda equina lesion is similar to a peripheral nerve injury with regard to potential for recovery. Andreychik et al. (28) reported on a subgroup of patients who had isolated traumatic lesion of the cauda equina. All 10 patients who had single nerve root paralysis had substantial improvement regardless of the method of treatment (operative or nonoperative). However, those patients that presented with multiple nerve root paralysis appeared to benefit, in regard to restoration of motor, bowel, and bladder functions, from some type of operative decompression.

OPERATIVE TREATMENT

Surgical options for thoracolumbar fractures include anterior decompression and fusion (with or without instrumentation), posterior decompression (direct and indirect), and fusion with instrumentation, or a combined procedure. Anterior instrumentation options include both rod and plate constructs, while posterior instrumentation options include traditional rod-hook systems, transpedicular instrumentation, or hybrid constructs.

Posterior Decompressive Procedures

Laminectomy alone is rarely indicated as a method of treatment for neurologic deficit following a thoracolumbar fracture. Neurologic compression is usually anterior to the neurologic structures secondary to an anterior bone fragment from the retropulsed vertebral body fragment. Due to the resultant fracture kyphosis, the thecal sac is usually stretched over the anterior bone fragments. This anterior deformity must be reduced to provide neurologic decompression. A laminectomy alone provides only posterior decompression. Additionally, excision of posterior ligamentous structures will only further destabilize the spine (41).

Indirect Reduction

The technique of indirect reduction of the retropulsed fragment implies no direct manipulation of the bone fragment that encroaches upon the spinal canal. Although this method has been used clinically for almost 30 years, early proponents of surgical intervention for thoracolumbar fractures believed that the restoration of normal spinal anatomy (with reduction of kyphosis) promoted return of neural function. With the relatively recent widespread use of CT scans for pre- and postoperative imaging of the traumatically injured spine, the role of the displaced middle column has been recognized as the primary cause of neural element compression.

According to Edwards (42,43), indirect decompression requires (a) restoration of anatomic alignment, (b) distraction to reduce retropulsed fragments via ligamentotaxis, and (c) maximum lordosis to concentrate the distractive forces across the vertebral body and to shift the residual fragments anteriorly away from the cauda equina. The reduction of the fragment by ligamentotaxis was initially thought to be due to tensioning the posterior longitudinal ligament (PLL). The PLL, if intact, can act like a taut bowstring and generate an anterior directed force that then acts on the retropulsed fragments (44).

Later experimental studies by Frederickson et al. (5,6) have shown that the posterior longitudinal ligament complex provides only a minor contribution to the reduction of the fracture. The main contributor to the reduction of the fracture are fibers of the posterior annulus. These fibers, which originate from the midportion of the vertebral body above, run posteriorly/inferiorly to attach to the lateral margins of the fracture fragment. It is tension through these fibers that provides reduction of the fragment. Additionally, biomechanical studies have shown that application of distraction forces was the most effective in reduction of the intracanal fragment.

This distraction can be achieved by either hook-rod or pedicle screw construct. Numerous studies have shown that canal clearance is most effective with an indirect reduction if the surgical procedure is performed within 4 days of the initial injury (43,45–47).

Indirect reduction remains the method of choice for posterior decompression of the neural elements. Advantages of this procedure over direct reduction of the retropulsed fragments include (a) no manipulation of the neural elements, thereby decreasing the possibility of iatrogenic neurologic compromise; and (b) no removal of posterior bone or ligaments, thereby eliminating compromise of spinal stability.

Direct Reduction

Certain circumstances may make the likelihood of successful indirect reduction low, and if the decision has been made to proceed only with posterior procedure, then a direct reduction may be necessary. Criteria for direct reduction include (a) delayed operative treatment for thoracolumbar fractures (greater than 4 to 5 days), (b) severe injuries with major displacement and rotation of the retropulsed fragments (48), (c) lack of integrity of the posterior annular attachments to the intracanal fragments (5) (as assessed by MRI), or (d) continued neurologic compression noted at the time of surgery by either intraoperative myelogram or sonography (49).

Surgical Technique

Posterior direct decompression is usually accomplished by laminectomy in conjunction with body decompression via the transpedicular approach. Following identification of the pedicles, a power burr or curette is used to remove the central portion of the pedicle, leaving the cortical shells intact (48). The medial wall of the pedicle is then removed, with care being taken not to injure the exiting nerve root (50). A trough is then made in the posterior body, leaving a thin shell of retropulsed bone. The retropulsed bone may then be directly reduced by using either reversed-angle curettes or specialized impactors (51) (Fig. 19).

Posterior Instrumentation: Harrington Distraction Rods

One of the earliest instrumentation systems used for stabilization of the thoracolumbar junction was the Harrington hook-rod system. The use of dual rods, with one upper and one lower hook, spanning several levels above and below the fracture can apply either axial compressive or distractive forces. Compressive forces can be used to reduce fracture-dislocations in the presence of an intact anterior column. Distractive forces can restore the height loss associated with burst fractures while avoiding overdistraction, which is prevented by the intact anterior longitudinal ligament.

Successful outcomes with this system has been noted by several authors (35,52), with a high fusion rate. Initial reports described a technique utilizing hooks two levels above and two levels below the injured segment. After the initial introduction of this technique, biomechanical studies (53) have found that moving the upper hook site to three levels above the fractured segment significantly reduced the likelihood of instrumentation failure.

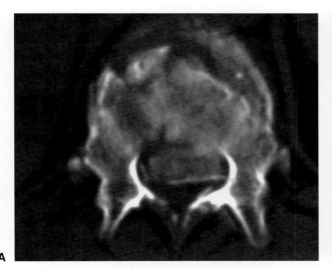 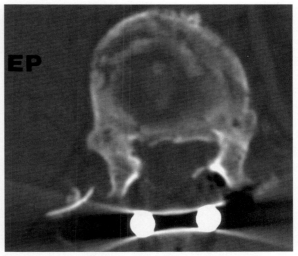

FIG. 19. A: Preoperative CAT scan for burst fracture showing severe canal compromise. **B:** Postoperative CAT scan following direct reduction of the retropulsed fragment. In this case, a transpedicular decompression was not performed, and the fragment was impacted back into the vertebral body with the aid of a hockeystick type retractor.

As Harrington rod-hook distraction instrumentation has become more widely used by spinal surgeons, several deficiencies have been noted. Loss of the initial reduction of the burst fracture has been noted on follow-up radiographs (54). When the anterior column is deficient (as in the case of burst fractures), the Harrington distraction rods are unable to successfully counteract the forces of bending and tension, leading to hook-lamina dislodgment, hook-rod dislodgment, and kyphosis.

Deficiencies of the Harrington rod-hook system can be addressed with the addition of Edwards rod sleeves or use of alternative systems that allow multiple hook use, such as the Cotrel-Dubousset (CD) and Texas Scottish Rite Hospital (TSRH) systems.

Spinal rod sleeves (42) are spacers that fill the potential space between the rod and posterior elements. The sleeves are composed of high-density polyethylene and are designed to fit between the base of the spinous process medially and between the facets laterally. The addition of rod sleeves confers anterior, mediolateral, and rotational stability. This anteriorly directed force (a) corrects posttraumatic kyphosis, (b) pushes the fractured vertebral body anteriorly away from the cord, and (c) bends the spinal rod within its elastic range to provide for a dynamic anterior force (Fig. 20). Use of the Edwards instrumentation system requires that the hooks be located between 3 and 5 cm from the end of the rod sleeve, which usually translates into two levels above and one level below the fracture, in the middle and upper lumbar spine. Reports on the use of this short rod-sleeve construct have shown satisfactory correction and maintenance of reduction at 2-year follow-up (55).

Segmental hook-rod systems (CD, TSRH, Isola) allow placement of multiple hooks along a single rod. The hooks, in various combinations, can provide both distractive and compressive forces. The use of cross-links in these systems provide for rotational stability. Additionally, the rods can be either prebent or bent *in situ* to reduce fracture kyphosis. Such segmental points of fixation may obviate the need for postoperative bracing under some circumstances, without increasing the risk of instrumentation failure (56–58).

Hook Insertion

Hook placement options in the thoracic and lumbar spine include the lamina (supralaminar and infralaminar), pedicle, and transverse process. Infralaminar hooks can be placed throughout the thoracolumbar spine and must be inserted between the ligamentum flavum and the undersurface of the lamina. This interval can be developed with either curettes or a Penfield retractor. Frequently, the inferior border of the lamina is curved and Kerrison rongeurs must be used to square off the lamina to provide for proper hook seating (Fig. 21). The infralaminar hook used must have a throat diameter that is sufficient to cradle the lamina, while not impinging on the spinal canal. Hook placement with an enlarged throat size will lead to spinal canal compromise, as shown in Fig. 22. Additionally, placement of two hooks at either the infralaminar or supralaminar position may abut in the midline, leading to either improper hook placement or spinal cord compression. Care should be taken to select proper hooks that are thin enough to allow placement of two hooks at the same level (Fig. 23).

Supralaminar hooks can also be placed at most levels in the thoracic and lumbar spine. The proper placement of supralaminar hooks often requires partial removal of both the inferior lamina above and superior lamina below. Frequently, the ligamentum flavum needs to be removed in its entirety. This interlaminar window should be made large

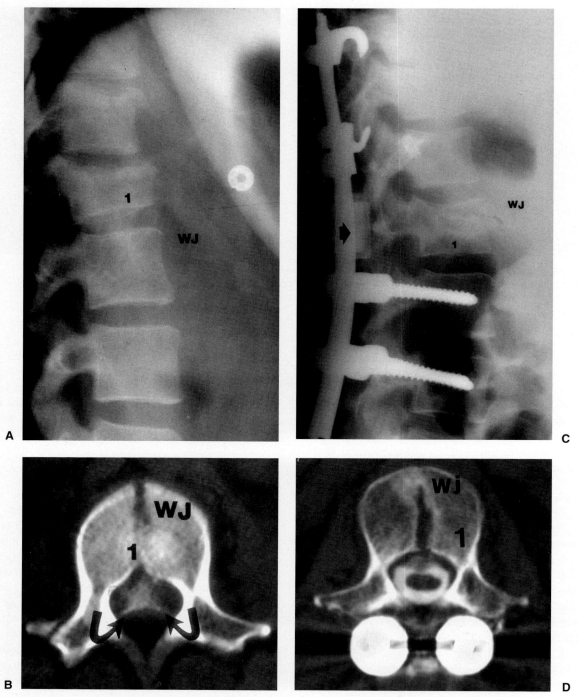

FIG. 20. A: Preoperative lateral radiograph demonstrates an L1 burst fracture. **B:** Axial CT scan demonstrates significant canal compromise. **C:** Postoperative lateral radiograph demonstrates a combination pedicle screw and hook construct, with a rod sleeve at the level of the fracture. Note good restoration of body height, as well as normal sagittal alignment. **D:** Postoperative CT myelogram with rod sleeves at the level of the fracture demonstrates significant reduction of the retropulsed fragment.

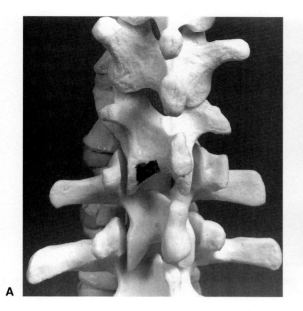

A

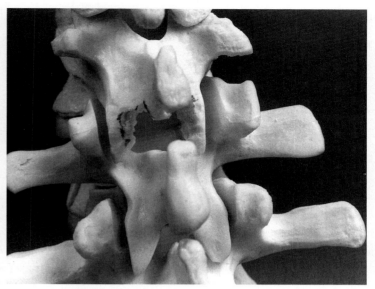

B

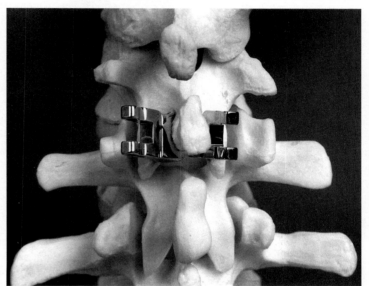

C

FIG. 21. A: Spine model with a shaded area demonstrating the proper place for infralaminar hook placement. B: A small portion of the inferior lamina has been removed with the Kerrison rongeur. C: Proper seating of two infralaminar hooks.

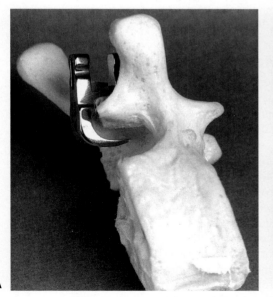

A

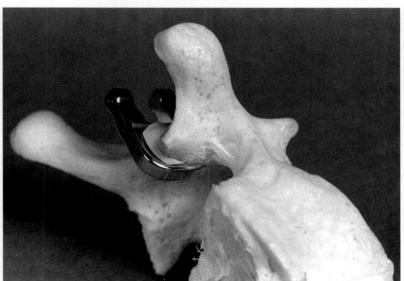

B

FIG. 22. A: An infralaminar hook placed with an enlarged throat size that penetrates the spinal canal. B: Proper infralaminar hook placement.

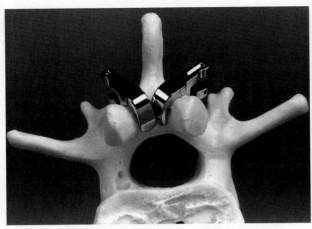
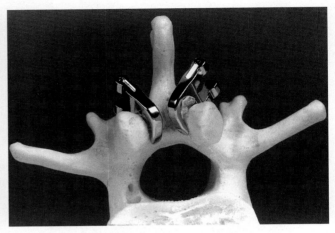

FIG. 23. Placement of two hooks at the same level should be done to ensure that they are not overlapping in the midline, which can result in spinal cord compression, as well as unequal distribution of hook-bone forces. **A:** Improper hook placement. **B:** The placement of thinner hooks that do not overlap in the midline.

enough so that the hook can be placed directly underneath the lamina without the shoe of the hook being angled down into the spinal cord during placement. Additionally, care should be taken not to disrupt the interspinous ligament or the facet capsules above the instrumented level, since this could lead to late development of supradjacent kyphosis (Fig. 24).

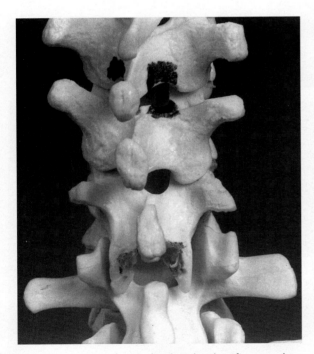

FIG. 24. Placement of supralaminar hooks often requires removal of portions of the inferior lamina above, and portions of the superior lamina below. The *shaded area* on the spine model indicates the amount of lamina that frequently needs to be removed.

Pedicle hooks can be placed in the thoracic spine between T1 and T10. Prior to hook insertion, a small portion of the inferior articular facet must be removed to allow for proper seating. After its removal, the cartilage of the facet frequently needs to be removed with a small curette. The exact location of the pedicle can be determined by the use of a probe. Pedicle hook placement below T10 is usually difficult due to the orientation of the facet joints (Fig. 25).

The combination of pedicle hooks and transverse process hooks leads to more rigid fixation than a single infralaminar hook alone. The combination of a hook that goes up and one that goes down is termed a claw construct. When this construct spans more than one level, an indirect claw construct is produced. Options for indirect claw constructs include infralaminar and supralaminar hooks at adjacent levels, as well as pedicle hooks and transverse process hooks at adjacent levels (Fig. 26).

Pedicle Screw Systems

The evolution of spinal instrumentation during the 1980s led to the use of pedicle screw instrumentation for stabilization of thoracolumbar fractures. Early proponents of these systems correctly identified the major deficiency of traditional rod-hook systems: the need for multiple-level fixation and fusion, often as many as four motion segments. Pedicle screw constructs, if successful, would require stabilization only one level above and one level below the injured vertebra, thus decreasing the length of the fusion necessary in the uninjured lumbar spine.

Early encouraging results (59–63) using the AO spinal internal fixator led to widespread use of numerous transpedicular instrumentation systems for the treatment of thoracolumbar fractures. This early enthusiasm, however, has given way to the reality of hardware failure, loss of initial reduction, and development of kyphosis (64–68).

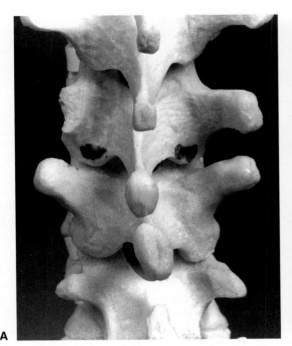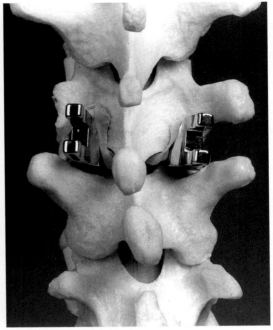

FIG. 25. Pedicle hook placement. **A:** The amount of bone that needs to be removed for pedicle hook placement. **B:** Proper pedicle screw placement. Note the more lateral position of the hooks, compared to the infralaminar position.

Reports by Kramer et al. (69), McLain et al. (65), and Gertzbein et al. (70) have shown that although pedicle screw systems can obtain initial early correction of kyphosis, follow-up radiographs often reveal loss of this reduction, often back to the original fracture kyphosis. This loss of reduction is most likely due to the inherent deficiency of the anterior column of the spine following a burst fracture. Pedicle screw systems utilize two-point fixation to provide lordotic and distractive forces, via manipulation of the uninjured vertebral body above and below the fractured vertebra. The lack of a posterior third point in fixation concentrates stresses and bending moments on the screw-bone interface, which is where bending and screw failure usually occurs.

To reduce the incidence of implant failure and progressive

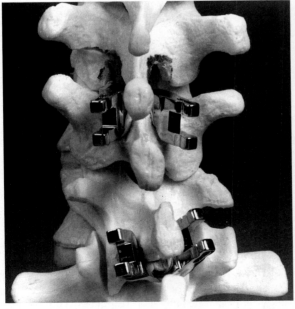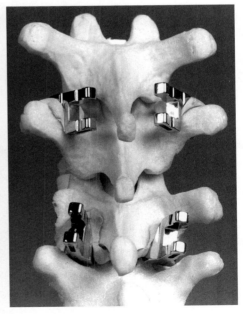

FIG. 26. A: A supralaminar/infralaminar indirect claw construct. **B:** An indirect pedicle-transverse process hook construct.

kyphosis, either the instrumentation must be modified (50) or the anterior column must be restored. Both Krag (71) and Carl et al. (64) have suggested segmental pedicle fixation two levels above the fractures to avoid implant failure. Alternatively, anterior column restoration can be accomplished by either transpedicular discectomy and disc space bone grafting, or transpedicular vertebral body bone grafting, as described by Daniaux et al. (50). Also, the anterior column may be reconstructed by an additional procedure utilizing anterior strut grafting.

McCormack et al. (72) have suggested that the anatomy of the fracture itself is more important than the pedicle screw construct used, when identifying features that lead to hardware failure. A point system based on load sharing classification was developed that grades (a) the amount of damaged vertebral body (Fig. 27), (b) the spread of the fragments in the fracture site (Fig. 28), and (c) the amount of traumatic kyphosis (Fig. 29). Using this point system, all fractures could be graded from a minimum total of three points to a maximum total of nine points. All spine injuries that showed screw failure at follow-up had preoperative point scores totaling seven or more. In contrast, no screw failure developed in patients whose fractures had total points of six or less. Similar findings had been reported by Kramer et al. (69).

Based on this scoring system, the best candidates for short segment posterior instrumentation are patients with flexion-distraction injuries with an intact anterior column or patients with mild burst fractures or fracture-dislocations with a point score totaling six or less.

Hybrid Constructs

To decrease the incidence of screw and implant failure following short segment pedicel screw fixation for thoracolumbar fractures, augmentation with laminar hooks has been recommended. Infralaminar hooks can be placed at the lower level of the construct without fusing additional lumbar spinal segments. Supralaminar hooks can be placed at the level above the cephalad instrumented vertebra. Although this requires an additional spinal segment to be fused, clinical relevance is generally insignificant, since this usually involves the thoracic spine. Chiba et al. (73) have shown that supplemental laminar hooks significantly increased construct stiffness and absorbed some portion of the construct strain, thereby reducing pedicle screw bending moments. Theoretically, this should decrease the likelihood of pedicle screw or construct deformation and clinical failure.

The failure rate of pedicle screw systems following short

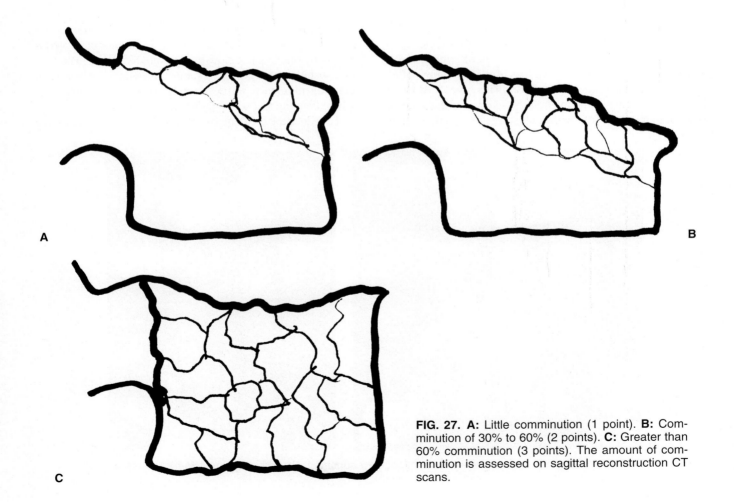

FIG. 27. A: Little comminution (1 point). B: Comminution of 30% to 60% (2 points). C: Greater than 60% comminution (3 points). The amount of comminution is assessed on sagittal reconstruction CT scans.

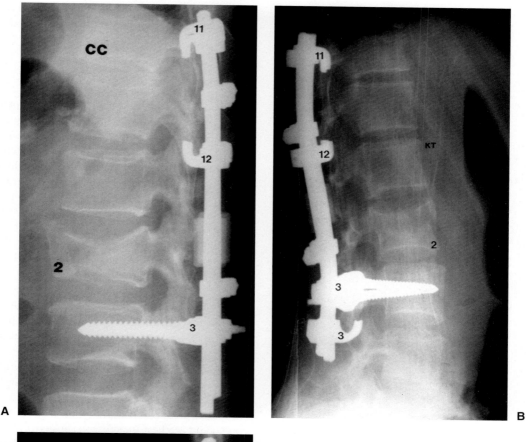

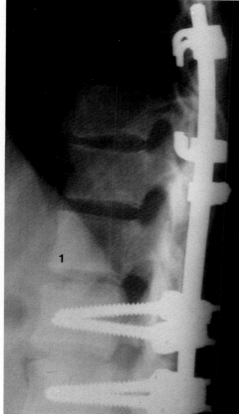

FIG. 30. A: A hybrid construct demonstrating pedicle screws below the fracture and an indirect claw above the fracture. **B:** A hybrid construct with a pedicle screw and an infralaminar hook below the fracture and an indirect claw above the fracture. **C:** Fixation with pedicle screws two levels below the injury and an indirect claw above the fracture.

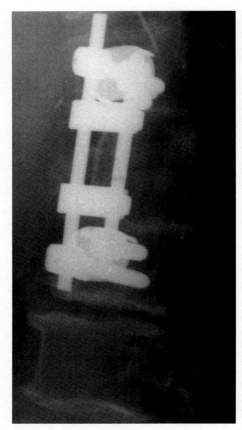

FIG. 31. Kaneda instrumentation following an L1 corpectomy and iliac crest bone grafting.

the load to failure. Additionally, screws should be inserted parallel to the disc space with bicortical purchase, with care being taken not to enter the disc space.

Treatment of Seat-Belt–Type Injuries

Rapid automobile deceleration can cause hyperflexion of the spine over a lap belt, which acts as a fulcrum. Lumbar fracture and deformity can then result from tension failure of the spine (78). The injury proceeds from a posterior to anterior direction and may include osseus and/or ligamentous injuries. This injury is most common between L1 and L3; radiographic features include posterior element disruption and separation, absent or minimal vertebral body height loss, and forward or lateral translation of the vertebral bodies (15). Intraabdominal injuries frequently accompany these fractures, with the incidence ranging from 15% to 65% of cases.

Evaluation of the injury pattern is critical as purely osseous injuries can often be adequately treated with extension casting or bracing. Lateral tomograms are often helpful to define the fracture pattern. Retropulsion of bone to the spinal canal, noted by CAT scan, indicates an associated burst fracture pattern, and also significantly influences surgical options. Finally, associated intraabdominal injury may preclude the use of casting or bracing, secondary to abdominal compression.

Flexion-distraction injuries with a significant ligamentous component are best treated with posterior fixation systems. If there is no burst component to the fracture, posterior com-

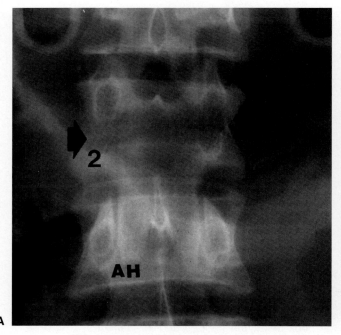

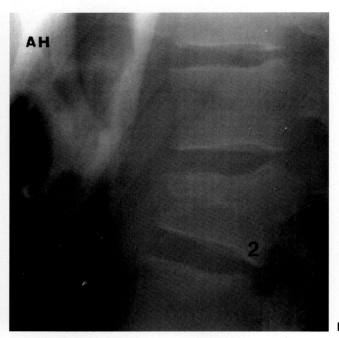

FIG. 32. A: AP radiograph demonstrates an L2 chance fracture. Note the separation of the posterior elements. **B:** Lateral radiograph demonstrates kyphosis at the fractured level. This kyphosis could not be reduced despite attempts at reduction and bracing.

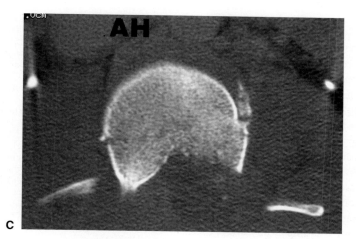

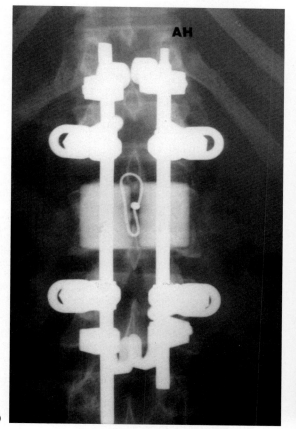

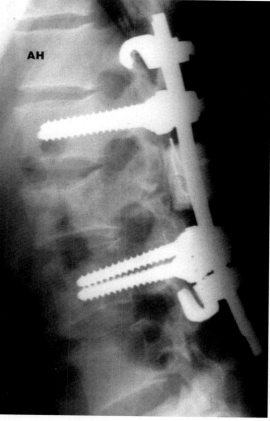

FIG. 32. *Continued.* **C:** CT scan of the L2 chance fracture demonstrates fractures at the base of the pedicles bilaterally. **D** and **E:** Postoperative AP and lateral radiographs demonstrate reduction of the fracture. Fixation was obtained by using a pedicle screw-laminar hook construct above and below the fracture. Provisional fixation was obtained by interspinous process wiring. Rod sleeves at the level of the fracture provides additional lordosis.

pression systems will often adequately reduce the fracture. Compression constructs should be avoided if there is a burst component, as additional compression may cause further retropulsion of bone into the spinal canal. Reduction of the deformity can be aided through the use of intraspinous wires, which are grad-

ually tightened to reapproximate the fractured spinous processes. Posterior instrumentation systems may be either a hook-rod or a pedicle screw construct, often requiring only one level of fixation below the injury and one to two levels of fixation above the injury (Fig. 32).

Gunshot Wounds

Gunshot wounds are a leading cause of traumatic paraplegia, second only to motor vehicle accidents. Low-velocity, low-energy wounds seen in the urban setting are generally less destructive than high-velocity missiles seen in a military setting. Most vertebrae fractured following gunshot wounds are considered stable, and generally there are few indications for operative intervention. Stauffer et al. (79) reviewed 185 patients who were victims of gunshot wounds to the spine with a resultant neurologic deficit. Fifty-six patients with a complete injury underwent a laminectomy, with only one patient having a partial return of function (sensory). Patients with incomplete injuries usually demonstrate improvement in their neurologic status whether or not a laminectomy was performed. Those patients who underwent a laminectomy had a complication rate of 10%, with spinal instability developing in six of these patients. Stauffer et al. concluded that surgical visualization of the cord did not contribute to the progression of neurologic recovery. These results have been confirmed by additional studies; Simpson et al. (80) were unable to demonstrate any benefits of surgery following penetrating injuries of the spine.

Vertebral or paravertebral infections following low-velocity gunshot wounds have been noted following intraabdominal injury (81,82). Ramanick et al. (81) reviewed 20 patients who had fractures at the thoracolumbar junction, following intraabdominal gunshot wounds. All patients underwent exploratory laparotomies at the time of admission and received broad-spectrum antibiotics for a minimum of 2 days. No infection was noted in the patients whose gastrointestinal tract was not perforated. Of the four patients who had either stomach or small bowel perforation by the bullet prior to vertebral column penetration, none developed any infection. However, infection did develop in seven of eight patients in whom the bullet perforated the colon before it hit the vertebra. The authors concluded that injuries that perforate the colon prior to vertebral fracture impaction may be candidates for early debridement of bullet fragments and nonviable bone. A similar study was performed by Roffi et al. (82). They found that early bullet removal did not appear to be a significant factor in the prevention of infection, and an extended course of broad-spectrum antibiotics combined with bed rest appeared to significantly reduce the risk of spinal or paraspinal infection, following lower GI tract penetration and vertebral fracture.

REFERENCES

1. Arigtuaco EJ, Binet EF. Radiology of thoracic and lumbar fractures. *Clin Orthop Rel Res* 1984;189:43–57.
2. McAfee PC, Yuan HA, Frederickson BE, Lubicky JF. The value of computed tomography in thoracolumbar fractures. *J Bone Joint Surg* 1983;65A:462–473.
3. Brightman RP, Miller CA, Rea GL, Chakeres DW, Hunt WE. Magnetic resonance imaging of trauma to the thoracic and lumbar spine. *Spine* 1991;17:541–550.
4. Petersilge CA, Patharia MN, Emery SE, Masaryk TJ. Thoracolumbar burst fractures: evaluation with MR imaging. *Radiology* 1995;199:49–54.
5. Frederickson E, Edwards W, Rauschning W, Bayley J, Yuan H. Vertebral burst fractures: an experimental, morphologic, and radiographic study. *Spine* 1988;17:1012–1021.
6. Frederickson E, Mann K, Yuan H, Lubicky J. Reduction of the intracanal fragment in experimental burst fractures. *Spine* 1988;13:267–271.
7. Gertzbein SD. Classification of thoracic and lumbar fractures. *Spine* 1994;19:626–727.
8. Watson Jones R. Manipulative reduction of crush fractures of the spine. *Br Med J* 1931;300–310.
9. Holdsworth FW. Fractures, dislocations and fracture-dislocations of the spine. *J Bone Joint Surg* 1963;45B:6–20.
10. Denis F. Spinal instability as defined by the three-column spine concept in acute spinal trauma. *Clin Orthop Rel Res* 1983;189:65–76.
11. Nagel DA, Koogle TA, Piziali RL, Perkash I. Stability of the upper lumbar spine following progressive disruptions and the application of individual internal and external fixation devices. *J Bone Joint Surg* 1981;63A:62–70.
12. Chance CQ. Note on a type of flexion fracture of the spine. *Br J Radiol* 1948;21:452–453.
13. Howland WJ, Curry JL, Buffington CB. Fulcrum fractures of the lumbar spine. *JAMA* 1965;193:240–241.
14. Denis F. The three column spine and its significance in the classification of acute thoracolumbar spinal injuries. *Spine* 1983;8:817–831.
15. Triantafyllou SJ, Gertzbein SD. Flexion distraction injuries of the thoracolumbar spine: a review. *Orthopedics* 1992;15:357–363.
16. Gertzbein SD, Court-Brown CM. Flexion distraction injuries of the lumbar spine. *Clin Orthop Rel Res* 1988;227:52–60.
17. Magerl F, Harms J, Gertzbein SD. A new classification of spinal fractures. Presented at the Societe Internationale Orthipedie et Traumatologie meetings, Montreal, Canada, 1990.
18. White AA, Panjabi MM. *Clinical Biomechanics of the Spine,* 2nd ed. Philadelphia: JB Lippincott, 1990.
19. Willen J, Lindahl S, Irstam L, Aldman B, Nordwal A. The thoracolumbar crush fractures. *Spine* 1984;9:624–631.
20. James KS, Wuger KH, Schlegal JD, Dunn HK. Biomechanical evaluation of the stability of thoracolumbar burst fractures. *Spine* 1994;15:1731–1740.
20a. Haher TR, Felmy W, Baruch H, et al. The Contributions of the three columns of the spine to rotational stability. A biomechanical model. *Spine* 1989;14:663–669.
21. Panjabi MN, Oxland TR, Kifune M, Arard M, Wen L, Chen A. Validity of the three column theory of thoracolumbar fractures. *Spine* 1995;20:1122–1127.
22. Denis F, Armstrong GW, Searls K, Matta L. Acute thoracolumbar burst fractures in the absence of neurologic deficit. *Clin Orthop Rel Res* 1984;189:142–149.
23. Reid DC, Ho R, Dans LA, et al. The nonsurgical treatment burst fractures of the thoracolumbar junction. *J Trauma* 1988;28:1188–1194.
24. Canter JB, Lebwohl NH, Garvey T, Eismont FJ. Nonoperative management of stable thoracolumbar burst fractures with early ambulation and bracing. *Spine* 1993;181:971–976.
25. Fidler MW. Remodelling of the spinal canal after burst fracture. *J Bone Joint Surg* 1988;70B:730–732.
26. Mumford J, Weinstein JN, Spratt KF, Goel CK. Thoracolumbar burst fractures: the clinical efficacy and outcome of nonoperative management. *Spine* 1993;181:955–970.
27. Weinstein JN, Collalto P, Lehmann TR. Thoracolumbar burst fractures treated conservatively: a long-term follow-up. *Spine* 1988;13:33–38.
28. Andreychik DA, Alander DH, Senica KM, Stauffer ES. Burst fractures of the second through fifth lumbar vertebrae. *J Bone Joint Surg* 1996;78A:1156–1166.
29. Chow GH, Nelson BJ, Gebbard JJ, Brugman JL, Brown CW, Donaldson DH. Functional outcome of thoracolumbar burst fractures managed with hyperextension casting or bracing and early mobilization. *Spine* 1996;21:2170–2175.
30. Wood EG, Harley EW. Thoracolumbar fractures: an overview with emphasis on the burst injury. *Orthopedics* 1992;15:319–323.
31. Holdsworth FW, Hardy A. Early treatment of paraplegia from fractures of the thoracolumbar spine. *J Bone Joint Surg* 1953;35B:540–550.
32. Gertzbein SD. Sclerosis Research Society: multicenter spine fracture study. *Spine* 1991;17:528–540.
33. Hashimoto T, Kaneda K, Abomi K. Relationship between traumatic spinal canal stenosis and neurologic deficits in thoracolumbar burst fractures. *Spine* 1988;13:1268–1272.

34. Cammisa FP, Eismont FJ, Green BA. Dural laceration occurring with burst fractures and associated laminar fractures. *J Bone Joint Surg* 1989;71A:1043–1952.

35. Dickson JH, Harrington PR, Erwin WD. Results of reduction and stabilization of severely fractured thoracic and lumbar spine. *J Bone Joint Surg* 1978;60A:799–805.

36. Frankel HL, Hancock GH, Melzak J. The value of postural reduction in the initial management of closed injuries of the spine with paraplegia and tetraplegia. *Paraplegia* 1969;7:179–192.

37. Burke DC, Murray DD. The management of thoracic and thoracolumbar injuries of the spine with neurological involvement. *J Bone Joint Surg* 1976;58B:72–78.

38. Davies WE, Morris JH, Hill V. An analysis of conservative (non-surgical) management of thoracolumbar fractures and fracture-dislocations with neural damage. *J Bone Joint Surg* 1980;62A:1324–1328.

39. McAfee PC, Bohlman HH, Yuan HA. Anterior decompression of traumatic thoracolumbar fractures with incomplete neurological deficit using a retroperitoneal approach. *J Bone Joint Surg* 1985;67A: 89–104.

40. Bradford DS, McBride GG. Surgical management of thoracolumbar spine fractures with incomplete neurologic deficits. *Clin Orthop* 1987; 218:201–216.

41. Jacobs RR, Asher MA, Snider RK. Thoracolumbar spinal injuries. *Spine* 1980;5:463–477.

42. Edwards C, Levine A. Early rod-sleeve stabilization of the injured thoracic and lumbar spine. *Orthop Clin North Am* 1986;17:121–145.

43. Edwards CC. Reconstruction of acute lumbar injury. *Oper Tech Orthop* 1991;1:106–122.

44. Harrington RM, Bodorick T, Hoyt J, Anderson PA, Tercer AF. Biomechanics of indirect reduction of bone retropulsed into the spinal canal vertebral fracture. *Spine* 1993;18:692–699.

45. Gertzbein SD, Crowe PJ, Schwartz M, Ronald D. Canal clearance in burst fractures using the AO internal fixator. *Spine* 1992;17:558–560.

46. Willen J, Lindhal S, Irstam L, Nordwall A. Unstable thoracolumbar fractures. *Spine* 1984;9:214–219.

47. Yazici M, Gulman B, Sen S, Koksal T. Sagittal contour restoration and canal clearance in burst fractures of the thoracolumbar junction (T12-L1): the efficacy of timing of the surgery. *J Spinal Dis* 1995;9:491–498.

48. Hardaker WT, Cook WA, Friedman AH, Fitch RD. Bilateral transpedicular decompression and Harrington rod stabilization in the management of severe thoracolumbar burst fractures. *Spine* 1992; 17:162–171.

49. Eismont FJ, Green BA, Berkowitz BM. The role of intraoperative ultrasonography in the treatment of thoracic and lumbar spine fractures. *J Bone Joint Surg* 1982;63A:1123–1136.

50. Daniaux H, Seykora P, Genelin A, Lang T, Kathrein A. Application of posterior plating and modifications in thoracolumbar spine injuries. *Spine* 1991;16:125–133.

51. Mimatsu K, Katho F, Kawakami N. New vertebral body impactors for posterolateral decompression of burst fracture. *Spine* 1993;18:1366–1368.

52. Flesch JR, Leider LL, Erickson DL, Chou SN, Bradford DS. Harrington instrumentation and spine fusion for unstable fractures and fracture-dislocations of the thoracic and lumbar spine. *J Bone Joint Surg* 1977;59A:143–153.

53. Purcell GA, Markolf KL, Dawson EG. Twelfth thoracic–first lumbar vertebral mechanical stability of fractures after Harrington rod instrumentation. *J Bone Joint Surg* 1981;63A:71–78.

54. Gertzbein SD, MacMichael D, Tule M. Harrington instrumentation as a method of fixation in fractures of the spine. *J Bone Joint Surg* 1982;64B:526–529.

55. Levine AM, Friedman C, Edwards CC. The use of a short rod sleeve construct for fixation of thoracolumbar spine trauma. Presented at the Orthopaedic Trauma Association annual meeting, 1990.

56. Benzel EC. Short segment compression instrumentation for selected thoracic and lumbar spine fractures: the short-rod/two-claw technique. *J Neurosurg* 1993;79:335–340.

57. Stambough JL. Cotrel-Dubousset instrumentation and thoracolumbar spine trauma: a review of 55 cases. *J Spinal Dis* 1994;7:461–469.

58. McBride GG. Cotrel-Dubousset rods in surgical stabilization of spinal fractures. *Spine* 1993;18:466–473.

59. Aebi M, Etter C, Kehl T, Thalgott J. Stabilization of the lower thoracic and lumbar spine with the internal spinal skeletal fixation system. *Spine* 1987;12:544–551.

60. Dick W. The fixateur interne as a versatile implant for spine surgery. *Spine* 1987;12:882–890.

61. Esse SI. The AO spinal internal fixator. *Spine* 1989;14:373–378.

62. Esse SI, Botsford DJ, Kostoilz JP. Evaluation of surgical treatment for burst fractures. *Spine* 1990;15:667–673.

63. Aebi M, Etter C, Kehl T, Thalgott J. The internal skeletal fixation system. *Clin Orthop Rel Res* 1987;227:30–43.

64. Carl Al, Tromanhauser SG, Roger DJ. Pedicle screw instrumentation for thoracolumbar burst fractures and fracture-dislocations. *Spine* 1992;17:S317–S324.

65. McLain RF, Sparling E, Benson DR. Early failure of short-segment pedicel instrumentation for thoracolumbar fractures. *J Bone Joint Surg* 1993;75A:162–167.

66. Speth MJ, Oner FC, Judic MA, Deklerk LW, Verbout AJ. Recurrent kyphosis after posterior stabilization of thoracolumbar fractures. *Acta Orthop Scand* 1995;66:406–410.

67. Chang KW. A reduction-fixation system for unstable thoracolumbar burst fractures. *Spine* 1992;17:879–886.

68. Benson DR, Burkus JK, Montesano PX, Sutherland TB, McLain RF. Unstable thoracolumbar and lumbar burst fractures treated with AO fixateur interne. *J Spinal Dis* 1992;5:335–343.

69. Kramer DL, Rodgers WB, Mansfield FL. Transpedicular instrumentation and short segment fusion of thoracolumbar fractures. *J Orthop Trauma* 1995;9:499–506.

70. Gertzbein S, Robbins S, Chow D, Rowed D, Schwartz M, Fazl M. Preliminary results of the AO internal fixator for spinal fractures. *J Orthop Trauma* 1989;3:162–163.

71. Krag MH. Biomechanics of thoracolumbar spinal fixation: a review. *Spine* 1991;16:584–599.

72. McCormack T, Karaikovic E, Gaines RW. The load sharing classification of spine fractures. *Spine* 1994;19:1741–1744.

73. Chiba M, McClain RF, Yerby SA, Moseley TA, Benson DR. Short-segment pedicle instrumentation. *Spine* 1996;21:288–294.

74. Harris MB. The role of anterior stabilization with instrumentation in the treatment of thoracolumbar burst fractures. *Orthopedics* 1992;15:347–350.

75. Becker G, Jacobs R. Improved correction and stabilization in anterior fusion with internal fixation. Presented at the 22nd Scoliosis Research Society meeting, 1987.

76. Dunn H. Anterior stabilization of thoracolumbar injuries. *Clin Orthop* 1984;189:116–124.

77. Kaneda K, Abumi K, Fujiya M. Burst fractures with neurologic deficits of the thoracolumbar-lumbar spine. *Spine* 1984;9:788–795.

78. Anderson PA, Henley MB, Rivara FP, Maier RV. Flexion-distraction and chance injuries to the lumbosacral spine. *J Orthop Trauma* 1991; 5:153–160.

79. Stauffer ES, Wood RW, Kelly EG. Gunshot wounds of the spine: the effects of laminectomy. *J Bone Joint Surg* 1979;61A:389–391.

80. Simpson RK, Verger BH, Narayan RK. Treatment of acute penetrating injuries of the spine: a retrospective analysis. *J Trauma* 1989;29:42–46.

81. Ramanick PC, Smith TK, Kopaniky DR, Oldfield D. Infection about the spine associated with low velocity missile injury to the abdomen. *J Bone Joint Surg* 1985;67A:1195–1201.

82. Roffi RP, Waters RL, Adkins RH. Gunshot wounds to the spine associated with perforated viscus. *Spine* 1989;14:808–811.

83. Bohlman HH. Current concepts review: treatment of fractures and dislocations of the thoracic and lumbar spine. *J Bone Joint Surg* 1985; 67-A:165–169.

84. Anderson PA. Non-surgical treatment of patients with thoracolumbar fractures. *The American Academy of Orthopaedic Surgeons Instructional Course Lectures* 1996;45:57–65.

Surgery of Spinal Trauma,
edited by J.M. Cotler, J.M. Simpson, H.S. An, and C.P. Silveri.
Lippincott Williams & Wilkins, Philadelphia © 2000.

CHAPTER 12

Traumatic Injuries of the Lower Lumbar Spine

Antoine G. Tohmeh and Charles C. Edwards

Surgical treatment of fractures involving the third, fourth, and fifth lumbar vertebrae (i.e., the lower lumbar spine) is substantially different from more proximal spinal injuries. The high degree of mobility (1) in this spinal segment not only subjects it to a multitude of injury force vectors but also makes the selection of fusion levels even more critical. Lumbar lordosis (2), which is 30 to 60 degrees between L1 and S1, increases significantly in the more caudal lumbar spine (3). It averages 13 degrees at L3-4, 20 degrees at L4-5, and 28 degrees at L5-S1. This prohibits the use of sublaminar hooks due to an unacceptably high dislodgment rate, especially at the lumbosacral junction (4). For these reasons, injuries of the lower lumbar spine warrant special attention.

PREVALENCE

Fractures involving the third, fourth, and fifth lumbar vertebrae are relatively uncommon. In Denis' (5) retrospective

study of 412 thoracolumbar injuries, only 12.8% of all compression type fractures were found to occur to the L3 to L5 levels. In this same series, 25% of all burst fractures occurred in this region, with only 6.7% and 3.3% involving the L4 and L5 vertebrae, respectively. In various series, one-level seatbelt injuries involved the L3 vertebra in 15% to 30% (6,7), 0% to 15% occurring at L4 and none at L5. Two-level seatbelt injuries occurred at L2, L3, and L4 in 37% of the cases and none occurred at a more caudal level (7). In Denis' series, 4% of fracture dislocations occurred at L3-4 with none occurring at more caudal levels. In our institution, pure facet dislocation was seen in only one of 30 injuries involving L4-5 or L5-S1 (8). In fact, L5-S1 dislocation is so uncommon that it has been the subject of few case reports (9,10).

NONOPERATIVE TREATMENT

As with other fractures of the thoracolumbar and lumbar spine, operative treatment, for the most part, depends upon loss of neurologic integrity, impending loss of neurologic integrity, instability, or potential instability of the injured segment. Specifically in the lumbar spine, kyphosis, to a large extent, is the most significant predictor of the need for surgi-

    A. G. Tohmeh: Orthopaedic Specialty Clinic, Spokane, Washington 99218.
    C. C. Edwards: Division of Orthopaedic Surgery, University of Maryland Hospital, Baltimore, Maryland 21201.

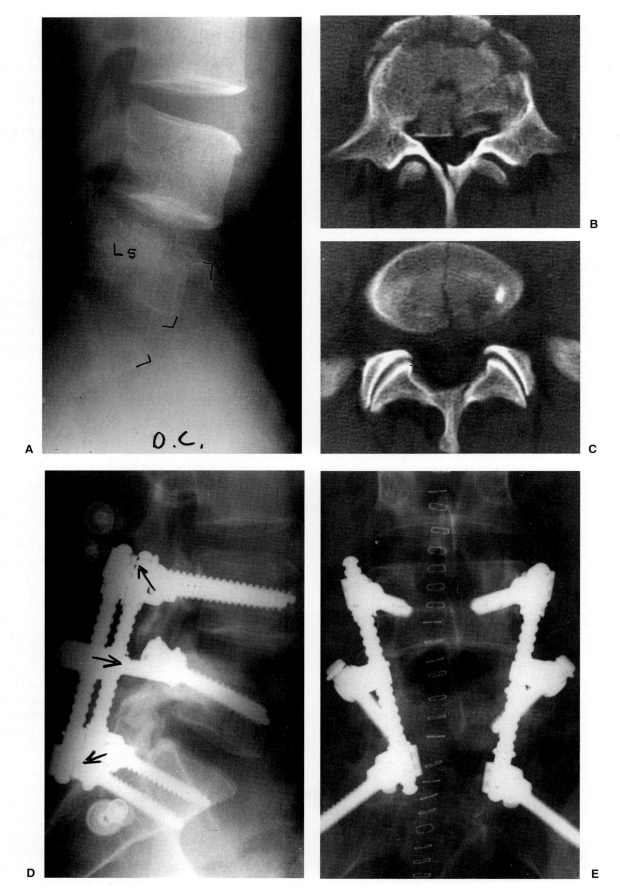

cal intervention, as in many cases neurologic injury is minimal due to the durability of the lumbar nerve roots. Certainly if there is neurologic compromise and significant deformity, surgical intervention should be considered. However, in those cases where neurologic integrity is preserved, nonoperative treatment may be a viable option if the degree of deformity is minimal and the body habitus of the patient, as well as the medical condition of the patient, are amenable to nonoperative treatment. Attempts have been made in the literature to establish guidelines for nonoperative versus operative treatment; however, they vary, both in the threshold for loss of vertebral body height, degree of angulation in kyphosis allowed, and extent to which retropulsion of the fracture fragments is tolerated. Most of the literature concerns thoracolumbar fractures, which clearly can tolerate a degree of postfracture kyphosis with good results long-term. In the lower lumbar spine, however, posttraumatic kyphosis is much less tolerated and all attempts should be made to restore or improve the sagittal lordotic curve. Although most of the guidelines for operative treatment involve 40–50% loss of vertebral body height, greater than 50% canal compromise and 30° of total kyphosis as preoperative indicators, these values certainly are too liberal for the lower lumbar spine. (10a,10b,10c,10d) More stringent criteria allowing only 15° of kyphosis with 50% loss of vertebral height at 25° of kyphosis with canal compromise of more than 50% have been recommended to minimize the post-deformity symptoms of the flattened lumbar spine. (10e).

The remainder of this chapter will discuss the operative intervention for those patients who are neurologically compromised or whose fracture characteristics result in an unstable lumbar spine. For the purposes of this discussion, injuries of the lower lumbar spine will be categorized as burst fractures, flexion-distraction (seat-belt injuries), fracture dislocation, and sheer injuries. Specific surgical treatment options for each are discussed.

BURST FRACTURES

Fracture Characteristics

Burst fractures affecting the L4 and L5 vertebrae have a characteristic fracture pattern (Fig. 1B,C). In a series of 22 patients treated and reviewed at our institution (11), the superior half of the vertebral body was comminuted with a sagittal plane split in the lower half. In most cases the pedicles remained intact. This is in contrast to burst fractures of the upper lumbar and thoracolumbar spine where varying degrees of pedicle comminution and disruption of the pedicle/body junction routinely occur. This should be kept in mind when surgery is contemplated and various fixation constructs considered. Burst fractures occur secondary to axial loading and involve at least the anterior and middle columns. It is generally agreed that the mechanism of injury in L5 burst fractures is vertical compression without significant rotational forces due to the position of this vertebra below the pelvic brim (12).

Historical Perspective

Frederickson et al. (12) first reported on the treatment of four patients with L5 burst fractures. Three of the four patients in this limited series were treated surgically. The authors concluded that there was no advantage to instrumentation.

Court-Brown and Gertzbein (13) treated three patients and concluded that L5 burst fractures should be treated conservatively, with 6 weeks of bed rest followed by bracing for an average of 3 months. These early reports are of minimal value due to the limited number of cases and the use of only distractive instrumentation, now known to result in lumbar kyphosis (flat back deformities).

An et al. (14) reviewed 31 burst fractures of the lower lumbar spine (L3 to L5) and compared casting to various instrumentation systems including Harrington rods, the Luque system, and Steffee plates. The common factors among patients with persistent back pain were long fusions and loss of lordosis. In an attempt to reduce the number of fusion levels, Mick et al. (15) compared conservatively treated patients with L5 burst fractures to those treated with Cotrel-Dubousset or Steffee pedicle screw systems. They concluded that nonoperative treatment yielded better results in young patients with minimal canal compromise. Should decompression be indicated, they recommended simultaneous fixation with a screw system to restore stability.

Although pedicle screw systems developed by Roy-Camille et al. (16), Cotrel-Dubousset, Steffee, and TSRH reduce the number of fused levels, they depend on postural reduction and implant contouring to restore sagittal plane contours. The drawback of rod contouring is the difficulty in achieving the correct bend in both rods at the optimal location and with appropriate rotation to achieve anatomic lordosis. Rod contouring also depends on a single point of contact between the rod and the posterior arch, which is greatly

FIG. 1. L5 burst in a 23-year-old man who was involved in a motor vehicle accident and sustained multiple injuries including fractures of the femur and radius as well as brachial plexus injury. **A:** The preoperative lateral x-rays showing reduced vertebral height and posterior retropulsion of bone. **B** and **C:** Computed tomography (CT) scan showing the typical findings in a lower lumbar burst. The upper body cut **(B)** shows well-preserved pedicles, while the lower cut **(C)** shows the sagittal split in the vertebral body. **D** and **E:** Postoperative lateral **(D)** and anteroposterior **(E)** films showing a distraction-lordosis construct with restoration of height and lordosis.

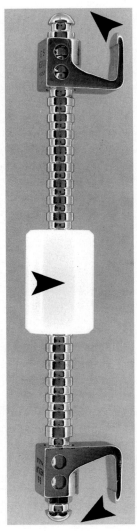

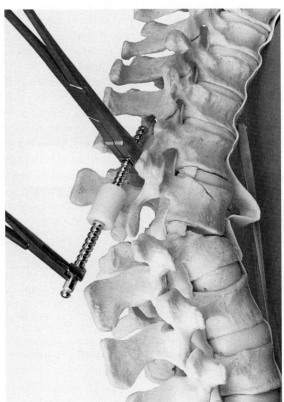

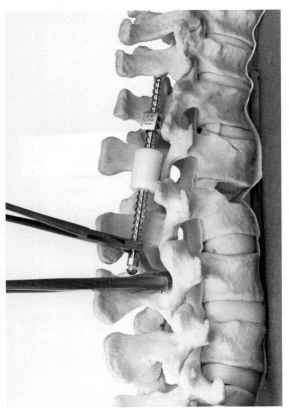

FIG. 2. A: Standard rod-sleeve construct. The hooks exert a distraction moment and pull posteriorly while sleeves push anteriorly to impart lordosis. **B–E:** Rod-sleeve assembly and reduction. **B:** A universal rod with sleeve is passed proximally through the upper hook. Note the distraction washer *(w).* **C:** The initial reduction is accomplished by pushing down on the distal end of the rod while pulling up on the distal end of the hook.

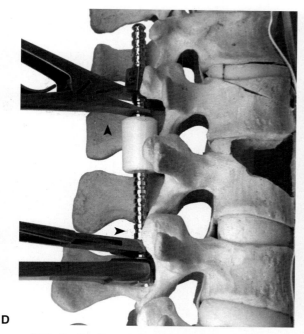

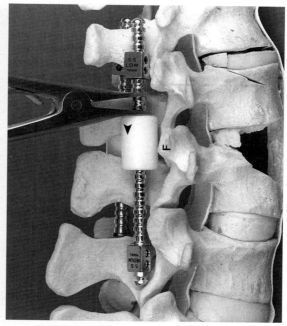

FIG. 2. *Continued.* **D:** The distal hook is engaged by advancing the rod with a spreader while holding the reduction. **E:** The spreader is reversed to move the sleeves down the rod until they are centered on the superior facet *(F)* and disrupted interspace.

compromised if the latter is injured or removed. To counteract the vector forces in burst injuries, simultaneous distraction and extension moments are required. This can be achieved by using the Synthes Internal Fixator or the Olerud pedicle screw system by instrumenting one level above and one level below the fractured vertebra. The disadvantage of these systems, however, lies in the fact that anterior translation and maximal lordosis at the injured level cannot be achieved. These factors are extremely important in achieving maximal indirect canal decompression and in preventing future kyphosis (17). The distraction-lordosis (DL) construct of the Edwards modular system (EMS) was designed to address all of these variables simultaneously. It minimizes fusion levels to one level above and below the fractured vertebra; restores height, lordosis, and translation; and achieves rigid fixation. Rosenthal et al. (11) treated eight patients with L4 and L5 bursts using the EMS and found significant improvement over other fixation modalities.

Indications for Surgery and Construct Selection

Burst fractures resulting in neurologic deficit or significant deformity and collapse should be treated surgically (14). A basic principle in the fixation of most spinal injuries is the selection of a surgical construct that will apply corrective forces in a direction opposite to the primary injury vector. This will restore alignment and stability and achieve indirect decompression.

The rod-sleeve (RS) construct of the EMS was designed for injuries of the thoracolumbar spine distally to the L3 vertebra (Fig. 2). The rationale of the rod-sleeve method is to achieve simultaneous distraction and extension by loading straight universal rods within their elastic range to maintain long-term lordosis. This construct can be used for L3 burst fractures without pedicle comminution and an intact posterior arch (Fig. 3). The latter is absolutely necessary since the extension fulcrum rests on the posterior elements through

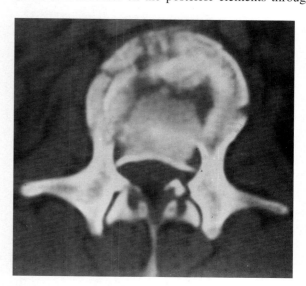

FIG. 3. Burst fracture of L3 with stable posterior arch. The anterolateral force applied by sleeves will widen the pedicles and allow reduction of the trapped central fragment.

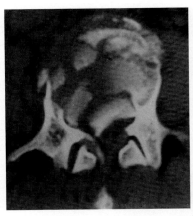

A, B

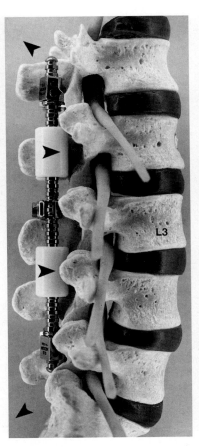

FIG. 4. A: L3 burst fracture with a completely displaced left pedicle. Whereas the sleeve could be placed over the right arch, the unstable left side requires bridging. This fracture can be alternatively treated with an anterior corpectomy and an L2 to L4 fusion. **B:** Lateral view of a bridging-sleeve construct showing that the sleeves are centered over the superior facets of L2 and L4. An indirect extension moment is applied at L3, resulting in correction of kyphosis. **C:** Anteroposterior view.

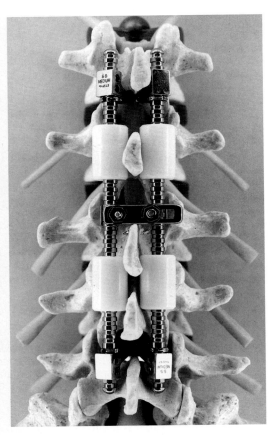

C

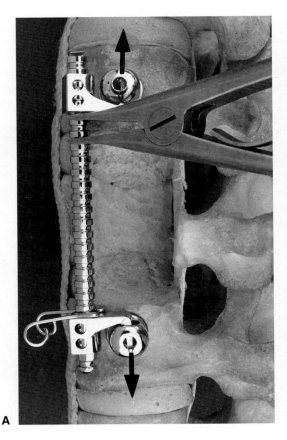

A

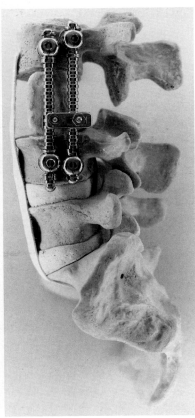

B

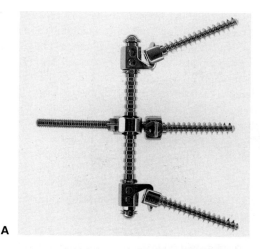

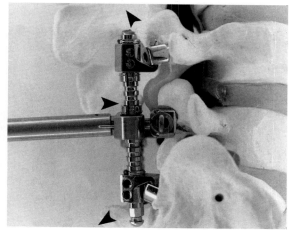

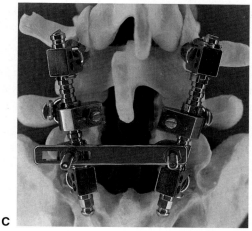

FIG. 6. Components of the distraction-lordosis construct. **A:** Angled slot screws maintain lordosis during distraction. The pedicle connector on the middle screw can be lengthened to translate the vertebral body anteriorly and increase lordosis. **B:** Lateral view of a distraction-lordosis construct model. This construct provides short-segment distraction and lordosis via spinal screws. **C:** Anteroposterior view. Note the cross-lock to enhance rigidity.

polyethylene sleeves. In this instance, an L1-L4 instrumentation/fusion is carried out with sublaminar hooks at L1 and L4. Should the L3 posterior arch be fractured but the pedicles preserved, a DL construct from L2 to L4 can be used. This requires pedicle screw instrumentation at L2, L3, and L4, thus the necessity of an intact L3 pedicle.

An L3 burst fracture with comminuted pedicles and posterior neural arch poses a dilemma (Fig. 4A). Due to posterior element comminution, neither of the two above-mentioned constructs can be used. A bridging sleeve construct, a modification of the standard RS method, using fulcrums at L2 and L4 can be used (Fig. 4B,C). In this instance an L1 to L5 instrumentation and a posterolateral L2-4 fusion are carried out. The disadvantages of this instrument-long, fuse-short method include the need for additional surgery to remove hardware and the potential for arthritic degeneration of instrumented but unfused facet joints (18–20). Additionally,

kyphotic collapse at the fracture site can occur after instrumentation removal. Another surgical approach for this specific injury pattern includes an anterior decompression and strut grafting coupled with anterior internal fixation from L2 to L4 (Fig. 5). Although this has the advantage of saving fusion levels, this procedure is associated with an increased morbidity, which could be critical in the multiply injured patient.

Burst fractures involving L4 and L5 typically leave the pedicles intact and thus allow for transpedicular fixation (Fig. 1). The DL construct (Fig. 6), utilizing fixation points at the injured level and immediate adjacent vertebral levels, maximizes restoration of lordosis and vertebral body height, while allowing for direct anterior translation and subsequent canal decompression. In this instance the posterior body of the fractured vertebra is translated anteriorly, away from the cauda equina, and the achieved lordosis allows the dura and

FIG. 5. Anterior neutralization construct. **A:** Kyphosis is corrected by gradually distracting between the spinal screws with an outrigger composed of two medium anatomic hooks and a universal rod. **B:** After placement of a large iliac or cadaver graft filled with cancellous bone, a universal rod is placed through the straight-hole screws and compression is applied with a spreader to lock the graft in place. Final position is maintained by crimping washers on the outside of each screw.

its contents to fall posteriorly, away from the retropulsed posterior body fragments.

SURGICAL TECHNIQUES

The EMS system is composed of six primary components or modules (Fig. 7). These components can be assembled into various surgical constructs, depending on the anatomic level and biomechanical needs of each case.

1. Universal rods. The fully ratcheted rods permit ratcheting in both directions for segmental compression or distraction. The fine 1/16-inch ratchets allow precise positioning, which is maintained with wide or narrow C-washers. Universal rods have the same 1/4-inch outside diameter as earlier rods, but the larger minor diameter and the lack of a discrete stress-riser make the Edwards universal rod less susceptible to late fatigue (Fig. 7A).
2. Anatomic hooks. These hooks are L-shaped to distribute load across both the edge and the under surface of the proximal lamina to minimize resorption, loosening, and dislodgment. Seating for distal hooks is improved by a round, rather than square, body and a tapered, rather than rectangular, shoe. These design changes have reduced hook dislodgment from 8% with standard C-shaped hook to less than 2% (4).

   The L-shape design also directs the shoe of the hook against the under surface of the lamina to limit canal pro-

trusion once the hook is loaded. Hooks are available in three heights (low, medium, and high) to secure a snug laminar fit and limit rod prominence (Fig. 7B).
3. Sacral/spinal screws. Screws are self-tapping with a ball-tip to minimize insertion risk (Fig. 7C). To keep breakage under 1%, a seating reamer is used to provide lateral head support, the proximal minor diameter is tapered, and a hook or connector linkage between the screw and rod absorbs peak impact loads. The linkage also makes it possible to insert the screw in any direction. Slotted screws are designed to accept hooks or connectors while holed screws accept the rods directly. In addition, standard or angled configurations accommodate different geometric/anatomic situations (Fig. 7C).
4. Rod sleeves. Polyethylene spacers provide translational and rotational control once wedged properly between the facets and spinous processes. These are available in four sizes to accommodate thoracic, thoracolumbar, lumbar, and lower lumbar spinal anatomy (Fig. 7D).
5. Adjustable connectors. These linkages between rods and screws can be gradually lengthened to restore lower lumbar lordosis or shortened to correct posttraumatic kyphosis. These are available in 90- and 105-degree foot angles to accommodate anatomic geometry. They are also available either as a closed or open ring. The latter can be snapped onto the rod *in situ* (Fig. 7E).
6. Rod cross-locks. Rod cross-locks fix the position of one spinal rod to another and enhance rigidity of the construct. The Edwards cross-locks are designed for simple

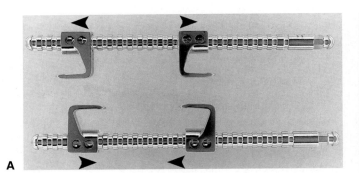

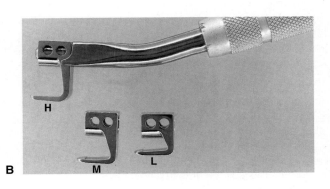

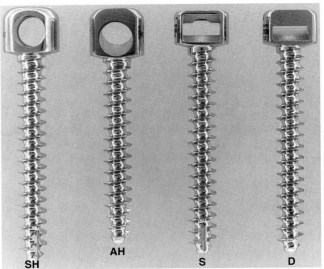

FIG. 7. Components of the Edwards modular system. **A:** Bidirectional ratcheted rods allow compression or distraction by simply reversing the hook orientation. **B:** Anatomic hooks with three sizes—low, medium, and high—to accommodate various laminar heights. **C:** Four different spinal screw configurations *(left to right)*: straight holed, angled holed, standard, and distraction.

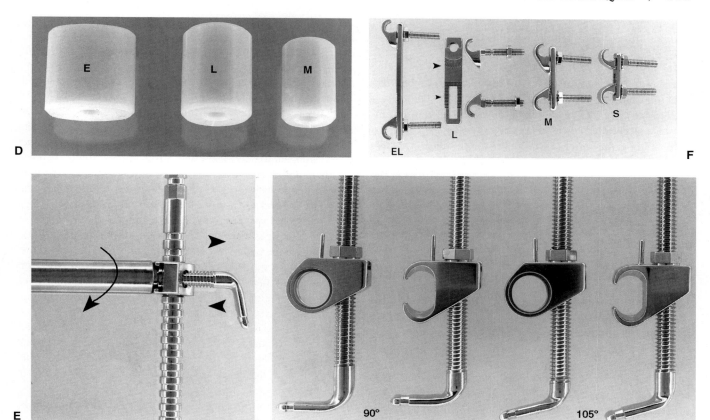

FIG. 7. *Continued.* **D:** Polyethylene sleeves: small (not shown) for thoracic, medium for thoracolumbar, large for high lumbar, and elliptical for midlumbar applications. **E:** Adjustable connectors *(left to right)*: 90-degree closed and open, and 105-degree closed and open. **F:** Rod cross-locks: these are available in four different lengths to accommodate various anatomic situations. The radial jaw *(large arrow)* accommodates angulation while the straight jaw *(small arrow)* adjusts for length. The angled jaw (not shown) was designed to be used when more than 10 degrees of rod divergence exists.

insertion following instrumentation. The cross-lock consists of a small slotted plate with jaws for rod attachment. One jaw accommodates rod angulation while the other adjusts for varying distances between rods. Each jaw has grooves that articulate directly with the universal rod (Fig. 7F). To assemble a cross-lock, the jaws are fitted about the rods and tightened into place with a standard modular system socket wrench; the wrench is then tilted to break off the threaded stems.

Standard Rod-Sleeve (RS) Construct (Fig. 2): L3 Burst with Intact Pedicles and Posterior Arch

Polyethylene sleeves are centered directly over the superior facets of the fractured vertebrae, spanning the spinous processes above and below the injured segment. In the sagittal plane, the sleeves wedge between the rods and facets. They work in conjunction with the anterior longitudinal ligament to restore maximum lordosis and correct any anterior-posterior translational deformity. In the coronal plane, sleeves

wedge between the facets and spinous processes to correct medial-lateral translation. The sagittal-coronal wedge effects provide rotational alignment and stability as well (21–23). The result is anatomic alignment for most thoracic and lumbar injuries.

If surgery is performed within several days of injury, sleeves facilitate indirect decompression of retropulsed fragments. Sleeves wedge the superior facets and pedicles apart to untrap central retropulsed fragments, which are then reduced by distraction ligamentotaxis. Sleeves also generate localized hyperlordosis to translate the fractured vertebral body and any residual retropulsed fragments anteriorly away from the cord and nerve roots (21).

Other features of the RS construct are responsible for superior late maintenance of alignment (17,24). First, anatomic hooks have a broad laminar contact area for less laminar resorption and hook loosening. Second, laminar resorption from the rod is eliminated by the large contact area and similar stiffness between the polyethylene sleeve and laminar bone (4,21). Third, sleeves of the appropriate size bow the rods within their elastic range. This dynamic lordotic force compensates for anterior ligament relaxation, maintaining full lordosis and stable fixation until fusion (21,22).

Because the RS method generates considerable corrective force, length of instrumentation can be much shorter than with previous rod techniques. The standard sleeve construct spans only three interspaces for lumbar injuries and four interspaces for thoracic injuries.

In surgery, the patient is placed over two transverse rolls to facilitate postural reduction. The surgeon identifies the facets opposite the fractured endplate; these will be at the level of ligamentous disruption and midway between the widened spinous processes. The superior endplate is disrupted in most of burst fractures, and the inferior endplate alone will be disrupted in only 7% (5). The surgeon selects the largest sleeve that fits comfortably between the superior facet and adjacent spinous process, generally small (2 mm) for midthoracic, medium (4 mm) for thoracolumbar, large (6 mm) for upper lumbar, and elliptical (8 mm) for midlumbar placement (Fig. 7D). A burr is used to remove any bony prominences and/or to narrow the sleeves as needed for a snug fit between the facets and spinous processes.

Anatomic hooks are inserted into the first interspace, 3 to 4 cm on either side of the sleeves. For a L3 burst fracture this typically translates to an infralaminar hook at L1. The infralaminar hook is inserted at the junction of the lamina and medial edge of the facet. To insert this hook the ligamentum flavum and medial aspect of the facet capsule is detached with a small curette. The laminar edge is squared off at the facet-laminar junction with an osteotome or burr to provide a flat seat for the hook. The surgeon then clears any remaining medial facet capsule or ligamentum flavum from the underside of the lamina with a no. 3 Penfield. The lowest hook that will clear the lamina is selected; low hooks provide 4 mm of clearance, medium 7 mm, and high 10 mm. The hook is mounted on the two-prong hook pusher, angled 15 degrees toward the midline, and inserted under the lamina.

Distal hooks are placed 3 to 4 cm below the sleeve, typically on the first lamina below the fracture. For an L3 burst this would be the L4 vertebra, resulting in an L1-L4 construct. To insert a distal hook, a large angled Kerrison rongeur is used to remove the overhanging edge of the adjacent proximal lamina and fully expose the ligamentum flavum. The ligamentum flavum is detached from the superior edge of the distal lamina. A Kerrison rongeur is used to form an 8-mm-wide seat for the hook at the laminar ridge where the ligamentum flavum inserts distally. Again, the lowest hook that will fit around the lamina is used and placed on the hook holder. The hook is then placed into the laminotomy site and directed cranially until the hook is fully seated. Both right and left distal hooks should be placed concurrently to ensure that the laminotomies are sufficient to laterally accommodate both hooks under one lamina. Remember,

however, to leave sufficient lateral bone to preserve a strong pars interarticularis.

To assemble the standard RS construct instrumentation, first slide a sleeve over the universal rod. Crimp a narrow washer into the rectangular groove ½ inch from the octagonal end of the rod. Slide the rod through the upper hook, while gently rocking the hook back and forth with a hook holder (Fig. 2B). Position the sleeve just proximal to the apical facet.

To reduce a kyphotic deformity, grasp the distal end of the rod adjacent to the washer with a rod holder. Gradually push down (anteriorly) with about 50 lb of force on the rod while pulling up posteriorly on the distal hook until the octagonal end of the rod is opposite the hole in the distal hook (Fig. 2C). Using a spreader, advance the rod into the lower hook while rocking the hook until it engages the washer (Fig. 2D). Assemble the second rod in the same manner, then move the sleeves with a spreader until they are centered directly over the superior facet of the fractured vertebrae (Fig. 2E). This completes the reduction and should produce a slight bow in the rod. Finally, apply incremental distraction for 20 minutes. This should be limited to one finger breadth on either side. Apply narrow or wide washers to precisely fix the final hook positions. If the end of the rod is within 1 cm of the upper hook, apply a narrow washer to prevent hook-rod disengagement.

After instrumentation is completed a lateral radiograph is obtained to confirm reduction. For incomplete paraplegics, indirect decompression should be documented with intraoperative myelography or ultrasonography. A posterolateral fusion is completed with autogenous iliac crest bone graft. Ambulation begins once drains are removed and a total contact polypropylene orthosis fitted. When bracing is not possible or when treating patients with osteoporotic bone, consider supplemental fixation with a proximal bilaminar claw construct.

Results

Results of 44 unstable burst fractures (17) with a 7-year average follow-up were previously presented. Anterior grafting was not performed in any case, yet there was an average reconstitution of 91% of vertebral body height. Average kyphosis across the fractured vertebrae and disc space was limited to only 3 degrees.

Bridging Rod-Sleeve Construct (Fig. 4B,C): L3 Burst with Disrupted Arch and/or Pedicles

This technique is similar in principle to the standard rod-sleeve method. Since direct pressure on a fractured neural arch is contraindicated, two pairs of sleeves are centered over the facets of the first intact posterior arch above and below the fractured vertebra. For an L3 burst fracture, sleeves are centered over L2 and L4, and hooks are placed under the L1 and L5 laminae, respectively. The rest of the procedure is completed in similar fashion as described for the standard rod-sleeve technique (Fig. 2).

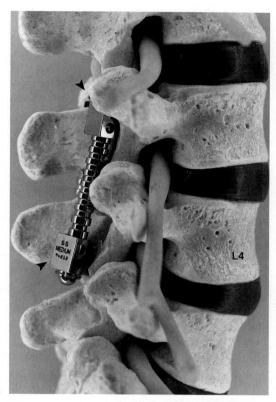 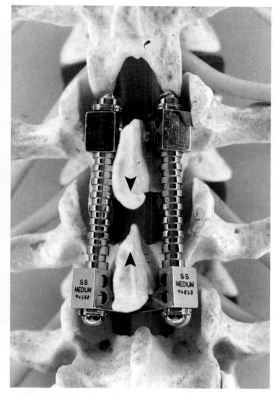

FIG. 8. Model of hook-hook compression construct. While this is feasible in the proximal lumbar spine, it is not recommended below L4. **A:** Lateral view. **B:** Anteroposterior view.

Anterior Neutralization (Fig. 5): Chronic L3 and L4 Burst with Canal Occlusion and Incomplete Paraplegia, and L3 Burst with Comminuted Arch and Pedicles

The anterior neutralization construct consists of a universal rod attached directly to the vertebral body above and below a fractured vertebra or corpectomy site fixed with spinal screws. It is used in conjunction with a compressible bone graft (Fig. 5B). The ratcheted universal rod is first distracted to reduce deformity and facilitate corpectomy decompression. Compression is then applied across a bone graft spacer to stabilize the segment until the fusion heals (25).

Straight-hole screws are placed anterolateral to posterolateral across the vertebral bodies above and below the fracture. Washer spacers are placed under the screw heads as needed to align the screw holes. Distraction is then applied with a temporary outrigger to provide surgical access for corpectomy and spinal cord decompression. To assemble the outrigger, insert the shoes of high anatomic hooks in the spinal screw holes and then slide a universal rod through the hooks oriented into distraction. Apply distraction with the universal rod to eliminate any kyphosis and facilitate placement of a large anterior graft (Fig. 5A). Fresh frozen femoral allograft packed with autologous cancellous bone has worked well as an anterior graft spacer. After placing the graft, the

outrigger is removed and the universal rod is inserted directly through the straight-hole screws. Gentle compression is then applied across the graft using a spreader on the outside of the distal screw. Compression is maintained by crimping washers on the outside of the spinal screws (Fig. 5B). When additional stability is required, two rods are used and joined with short rod cross-locks. Postoperative bracing is recommended. Experience with the anterior neutralization construct is limited, but results to date are encouraging.

Distraction-Lordosis (DL) Construct (Fig. 6): L3 Burst with Disrupted Arch but Intact Pedicles and L4 and L5 Burst

Fractures in the lower lumbar spine require distraction for fragment reduction and maintenance of height during ambulation. Lordosis is needed to restore lumbosacral alignment, maintain fixation, and counteract the flexion moment generated by the weight of the upper body. Short segment distraction and lordosis are achieved by the DL construct. Midposition connectors are extended to restore lordosis, and the proximal hooks are ratcheted to restore height. Connectors are then further extended to translate the fractured vertebral body, together with any residual retropulsed fragments, anteriorly away from the cauda equina (Fig. 6B).

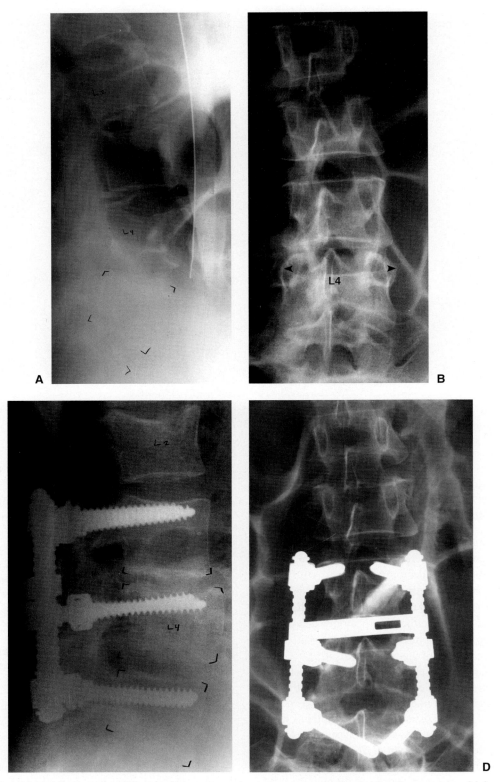

FIG. 9. L4 burst fracture in a 35-year-old woman who was an unrestrained driver in a motor vehicle accident. She also sustained facial injuries, sacral fractures, and a stable L2 burst. She had slight weakness of her left gastrocnemius and great toe extensors, paresthesias in the L5 and S1 dermatomes and depressed deep tendon reflexes, and was unable to void. The latter deficit was felt to be secondary to her sacral injury. **A** and **B:** Preoperative lateral and anteroposterior films. **C** and **D:** Postoperative films.

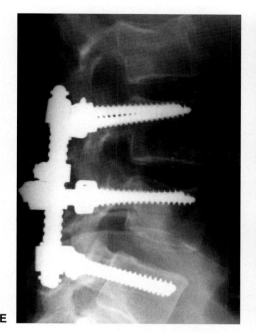
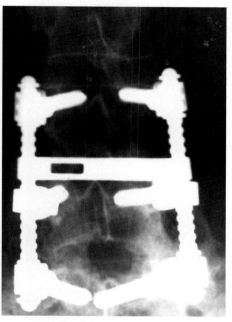

E

F

FIG. 9. *Continued.* **E** and **F:** X-rays 4 years after the injury. At 2 months after injury she had no back pain and her strength had improved. In addition, she had recovered completely from her bladder deficit. At 7 months postinjury she had normal strength and had a remodeled fusion mass. (Courtesy of Aleksander Curcin, M.D.)

To reduce an L5 burst fracture, for example, screws are placed into the pedicle of L4 and L5 and across the sacral ala at S1. The L4 screws are directed proximally and medially to avoid the L3-L4 facet capsules. The L5 screws are directed caudally, because in the typical case vertebral body comminution is limited to the proximal portion of the body (11). The sacral screws enter at the base of the L5-S1 facets and are directed 35 degrees laterally across the anterior cortex of the ala for secure bicortical fixation. Fixed-angled distraction screws are used both proximally and distally to maintain lordosis during distraction (Fig. 1).

Straight universal rods are attached to the screws via low anatomic hook linkages at L4 and S1. Adjustable connectors are snapped onto the rods and attached to the L5 screws. The proximal hooks are distracted and the L5 connectors lengthened under image control to restore height and lordosis (Fig. 6).

Patients with neurologic deficits resulting from lower lumbar burst fractures may benefit from laminectomy before or after spinal instrumentation is completed (Fig. 6C). This may free nerve roots entrapped by a greenstick-type laminar fracture. More commonly, however, partial or complete laminectomy allows the surgeon to confirm bony reduction, and permits removal or impaction of bone fragments that do not reduce. After reduction, decompression, and fixation, a transverse process iliac graft fusion is performed.

Results

The DL construct has been used by members of the Spinal Fixation Study Group in over 100 cases. Results from 40 cases with over 1-year of follow-up document good maintenance of height and lordosis, with a 90% union rate and no permanent root deficits associated with the procedure (Fig. 9).

Indications for Anterior Reconstruction Augmenting Posterior Instrumentation

While the above constructs are considered a standard for a given injury pattern it is important that the surgeon carefully analyze each individual injury and the biomechanical properties of the selected construct. While a specific construct may result in an adequate reduction of a fracture, it may be at a mechanical disadvantage, predisposing the spinal segment to late loss of reduction and nonunion (Fig. 10A,B). This is usually seen in three-column injuries in the lower lumbar spine with a particularly severe burst component. The axial forces acting on the deficient anterior column force the spinal segment in kyphosis and subject the posterior construct to cantilever bending moments. We therefore recommend anterior grafting with a strut when there is extreme comminution with wide displacement in both sagittal and transverse planes (Fig. 10B,C) for injuries at or below L3. The use of additional anterior instrumentation is dictated by the structural integrity of the involved spinal segment (Fig. 10B–G). This can be done as a second stage unless adequate posterolateral decompression is not possible and immediate anterior decompression is required.

Treatment of Late Deformity

The kyphoreduction construct is highly effective in reducing resistant or late posttraumatic kyphosis, generally without the need for anterior release. Even deformities present for months or years are consistently corrected with the kyphoreduction construct as long as anterior autofusion has not occurred. The construct is indicated to arrest progressive

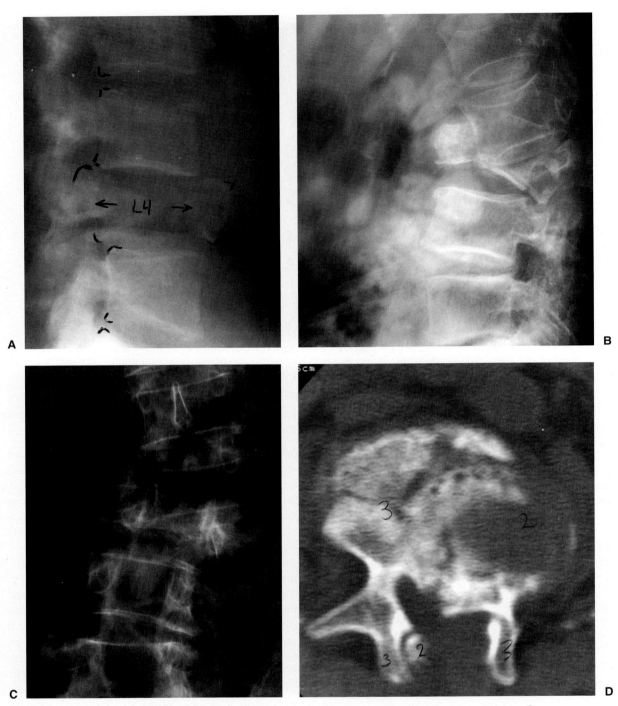

FIG. 10. A: Lateral view of an L4 burst fracture showing severe collapse and retropulsion. Severe anterior comminution predisposes the vertebra to late collapse and kyphosis. In this situation we recommend an anterior procedure for added structural support to negate anterior compressive forces. **B–H:** L3 burst with multiplanar instability. An 84-year-old woman who had a laminectomy for spinal stenosis 7 months prior to her injury. She was referred to us with progressive collapse and a severe neurologic deficit manifested by 2/5 (knee extension with gravity eliminated) left quadriceps strength and inability to walk. **B and C:** Preoperative x-rays showing a severe L2/3 kyphotic deformity with L3 body comminution and lateral listhesis. **D:** Preoperative CT scan showing the burst component and compression of the left neural elements explaining her deficit. The patient underwent posterolateral decompression, instrumentation, and fusion through a posterior approach.

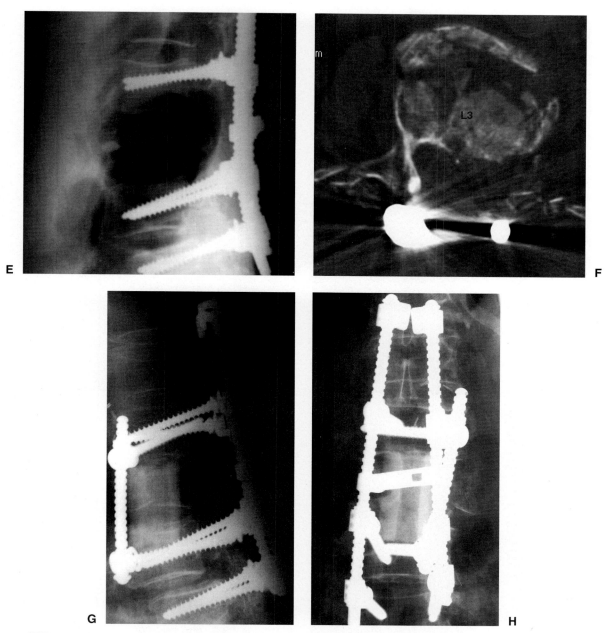

FIG. 10. *Continued.* **E:** Postoperative lateral film showing restoration of alignment and L3 vertebral body height. Since this is an injury with multiplanar instability in an osteoporotic patient, a more rigid construct was selected. A T12-L2 proximal claw was created using supralaminar hooks at T12 and pedicle screws at L2. The distal claw at L4-L5 was created by using pedicle screws. Distraction was achieved between the claws over contoured rods. **F:** Postoperative CT scan shows adequate decompression. **G** and **H:** Anterior buttress using a femoral shaft allograft and a neutralization construct. This was done through a second-stage retroperitoneal approach to negate the anterior compressive forces and to protect the posterior instrumentation from failure. The patient improved her deficit dramatically and was ambulating independently with a cane at 3 months.

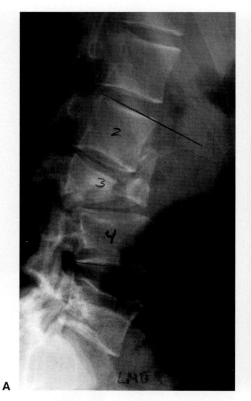

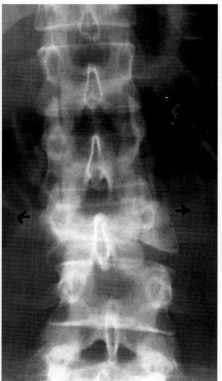

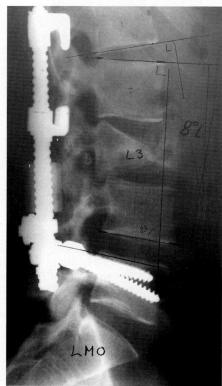

FIG. 11. L3 burst in a 19-year-old woman who sustained multiple injuries in a motor vehicle accident. The patient sustained closed head injury, posterior hip dislocation, a closed humeral, and rib fractures. Her hip was reduced and treated in traction and her humerus internally fixed with rush pins at another institution. She was referred to us 10 weeks later because of progressive deformity and back pain. She had common peroneal nerve palsy attributable to her hip dislocation; otherwise she had no neurologic deficit. **A** and **B:** Preoperative lateral **(A)** and anteroposterior **(B)** films showing widening of the L3 vertebral body, 16 degrees of absolute kyphosis at L2 to L4, and L3/4 retrolisthesis. **C:** Postoperative film following kyphoreduction showing 8 degrees of lordosis, indicating 23 degrees of correction. Note the proximal bilaminar claw and the sleeve at the L3-L4 joint.

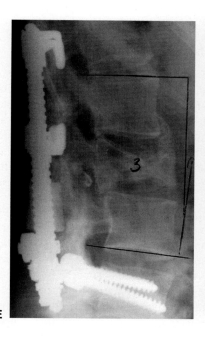
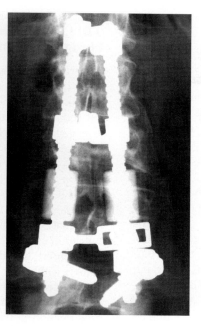

D, E

FIG. 11. *Continued.* **D** and **E:** Lateral **(D)** and anteroposterior **(E)** films 1 year after surgery showing maintenance of reduction. The patient had no symptoms referable to her spine at her 6 months postoperative visit.

kyphosis, correct excessive deformity, and relieve anterior neurologic impingement. Kyphoreduction alone can completely decompress the cord if the cross-sectional area of the canal at the point of maximum impingement is greater than the cross-sectional area of the cord on computed tomography (CT) or magnetic resonance imaging (MRI) evaluation. If fixed retropulsed fragments leave the canal area excessively compromised, then anterior corpectomy should be performed. In cases of mild kyphosis, the anterior neutralization construct will suffice for reduction of deformity and stabilization. In cases of extreme kyphosis, combined posterior kyphoreduction with anterior corpectomy and neutralization construct fixation are sometimes necessary.

The kyphoreduction construct makes use of viscoelastic stress relaxation to increase the amount of correction possible without an anterior release or vertebrectomy. Stress relaxation is facilitated by the very gradual application of an extension moment over several hours. This is followed by compression to shorten the posterior column and promote axial loading.

Lumbar Kyphoreduction (Fig. 11): Late Posttraumatic Kyphosis

Prior to surgery, flexion-extension films or tomograms are performed to rule out either an anterior bridge or substantial retropulsion. If either is found, a preliminary anterior surgical resection is performed. Otherwise, only posterior instrumented reduction is necessary.

At surgery, the patient is placed over transverse rolls for maximum postural reduction. If the posterior column has fused, a chevron osteotomy is performed in addition to partial facetectomies at each level to be instrumented. Proximal fixation is achieved with bilaminar hook claws centered 5 to

7 cm proximal to the apex of the spinal deformity (Fig. 11C). Distal fixation is achieved with pedicle screws in the lumbar spine. Sleeves of the appropriate size are passed over the rods and centered over the apical facets. Adjustable connectors are assembled between the rods and distal pedicle screws. Connectors are sequentially shortened over a 1- to 3-hour period, depending on the rigidity of the deformity. After three-point loading is complete, compression is applied with the ratcheted universal rods to shorten the posterior column. A central rod cross-link is added to enhance construct stability.

FLEXION-DISTRACTION INJURIES

Flexion-distraction injuries truly describe a spectrum of injury whose pathoanatomy depends on the location of the instantaneous axis of rotation at the time of injury and whether flexion or distraction force predominate. When the latter predominates, as occurs with a seatbelt against the abdomen, the spine hinges about the anterior longitudinal ligament resulting in tensile failure of all three spinal columns. Two major injury patterns are seen including the classic Chance fracture.

With these injuries the fracture line extends through the spinous process, laminae, pedicles, and the vertebral body. Patients with such predominant bony injuries and minimal ligamentous damage can be adequately treated with a hyperextension cast and immediate mobilization.

Alternatively, a pure ligamentous rupture may occur, with disruption of the interspinous ligaments, facet capsules, and posterior annulus. Although most of these patients remain neurologically intact, the annulus and posterior ligaments are replaced by scar that has no structural integrity; thus, late pain and instability are common. These injuries are best addressed surgically with a posterior compression construct.

When flexion predominates over distraction, the upper spine is driven anteriorly, resulting in facet dislocations. The posterior ligaments, annulus, and facet capsules are ruptured. The anterior longitudinal ligament is stripped from the lower vertebral body and the anterior cortex remains intact (8). While most of these patients sustain severe neurologic deficits with injury in the thoracolumbar spine, those with lower lumbar facet dislocation usually develop only root deficits. A posterior compression construct counteracts the deforming forces and maintains facet reduction. A significant concern with compression constructs when the annulus is ruptured is posterior disc herniation. In neurologically intact patients and those with incomplete deficits suffering thoracolumbar facet dislocations, a rod-sleeve construct is employed to exert a continuous extension moment, preserving lordosis and facet reduction without the risk of disc herniation. In the lower lumbar spine where the canal is relatively wider, we recommend a compression construct combined with discectomy for patients with partial or no neurologic deficit. In patients with complete neurologic deficits we recommend a compression construct irrespective of the injury level since neurologic recovery is unlikely. Significant disc bulging is unlikely following compression instrumentation for either posterior ligamentous rupture or Chance fractures and is, therefore, the preferred technique for these injuries regardless of neurologic status (22).

Surgical Technique: Screw Compression Construct (Fig. 12) of Chance Fractures, Posterior Ligamentous Disruption, and Bilateral Facet Dislocations

Posterior compression alone will achieve reduction of posterior ligamentous disruptions and Chance fractures. Bilateral facet dislocations, however, require preliminary manual reduction of the locked facets. First, the facets are disengaged by slightly distracting with a laminar spreader. After removing just the tip of the superior facet, a small elevator is used as a lever to reduce the facet dislocation. Reduction is completed with a short compression construct (Fig. 12C–E).

While anatomic hooks can be used for L3-L4 injuries (Fig. 8), spinal screws are recommended for attachment distal to L4 and in cases of spinal stenosis (Fig. 12A,B). For pedicle screw insertion, first remove the posterior cortex over each pedicle with a burr. A T-handled pedicle probe is used to locate the center of the pedicle and 2-mm drill bits are inserted into the pedicle. Intraoperative radiographs or fluoroscopy is used to confirm the insertion point and orientation. Palpate all four quadrants of the hole with a depth gauge to ensure that there is no pedicle cortex penetration. For vertebral bodies, select a screw length that will approach, but not penetrate, the anterior cortex. For sacral fixation, drill a screw hole from the base of the L5-S1 facet 35 degrees laterally and approximately 25 degrees caudal and parallel to the S1 endplate. Place drill-bit markers and confirm orientation radiographically. Carefully penetrate the anterior cortex with a

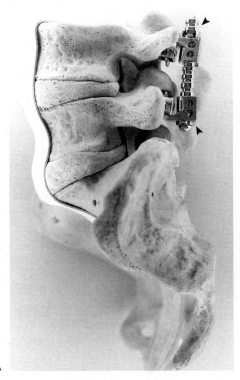
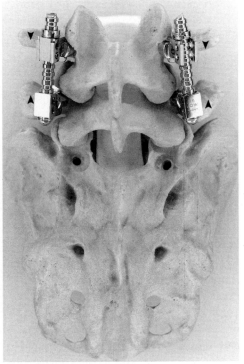

FIG. 12. A and **B:** Screw compression construct demonstrated on a model.

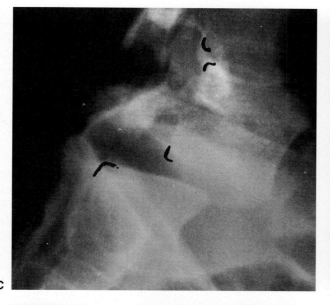

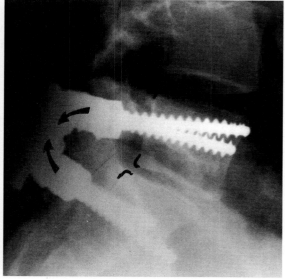

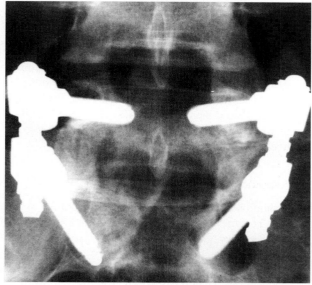

FIG. 12. *Continued.* **C–E:** Spinal screws are attached to a universal rod with low anatomic hooks oriented into compression. Lumbosacral facet dislocation. **C:** Bilateral facet dislocation at L5-S1. **D** and **E:** After manual facet disengagement, reduction is completed and stabilized with a screw-to-screw compression construct, which consists of spinal screws attached to a universal rod with low anatomic hooks oriented into compression.

hand drill, and select a screw length to provide bicortical alar fixation. A special reamer is used to prepare a seat for the screw head prior to inserting either pedicle or sacral screws with a standard hex screwdriver.

After placing screws, we recommend lateral decortication and insertion of a bone plug across each facet joint. To assemble the compression construct, pass the octagonal end of a universal rod cephalad through the body of the proximal hook, which is linked to the proximal screw. Crimp a narrow washer into the groove at the end of the rod to fix it in the hook. Place a second hook over the distal end of the rod, and insert it into the distal screw slot. After assembly of both rods, use a spreader on the distal end of the lower rod to apply compression. After balancing the compressive loads between both rods, apply a wide or narrow stop washer and cut off any excess rod.

Results

Flexion-distraction injuries treated with a short-segment compression construct have been reviewed by several authors. Levine and Edwards (26) noted that the compression construct maintained excellent reduction of bilateral facet dislocations and promoted early union in all cases. Fifty-two spinal injuries have been treated by members of the Spinal Fixation Study Group with a compression construct. Results demonstrate good maintenance of correction and a union rate exceeding 90%.

FRACTURE-DISLOCATIONS

These injuries occur when the spine is subjected to flexion and compressive forces. When the former predominates, the upper segments rotate into hyperflexion, creating an anterior column fracture of the lower vertebral body. As the upper spine rotates further, the vector of injury becomes more axial, creating a burst fracture. The severe flexion force also disrupts the posterior ligaments, thus resulting in anterior subluxation or dislocation of the upper spine. These are exceedingly unstable injuries involving all three columns, resulting in not only anteroposterior instability but also rotational instability. The surgical construct in these cases should counteract the injury forces by exerting extension and distraction moments. In the lower lumbar spine, this can be achieved by the DL construct as described earlier.

SHEAR INJURIES

These rare but exceedingly unstable injuries result from a sustained translational force that ruptures the anterior ligament and annulus and fractures the facets. These are unstable in all planes and present with significant translation in both the anteroposterior and lateral projections coupled with major neurologic deficits. These injuries are best addressed with segmental screw compression constructs as they represent three-column failure where maximal stability is needed.

Screws are typically placed at one vertebra above and two vertebrae below the disrupted level. Most lumbar shear injuries present with a retrolisthesis deformity. They can be easily reduced using a unilateral DL construct with proximal and distal low hook linkages oriented in distraction with a midposition connector (27). The surgeon first applies minimal distraction to restore disc-space height and then shortens the connector to reduce the anteriorly displaced middle vertebrae. A distal claw is then assembled on the opposite side using low hook linkages facing each other in the screw slots. Only one vertebra is instrumented above the disruption. The proximal hooks are oriented distally in the final construct. When two proximal vertebrae are instrumented, a claw is utilized. Finally, the initial unilateral DL construct used for reduction is replaced with a segmental neutralization configuration to match the opposite side. The rods are interlocked to enhance rigidity.

COMPLICATIONS

Pedicle Screw Insertion

Pedicle screws cause root injury in 3.2% of spinal injury cases. Exiting nerve roots wrap around the medioinferior aspect of the pedicle. If a pedicle screw is too large for the pedicle, the fracture fragments from the pedicle may impinge upon the adjacent root. If the screw is misdirected, the screw threads may cut into the root. Pedicle screw misplacement can be recognized with a postoperative CT scan. Removal of the screw often relieves radicular pain since roots are rarely severed.

Misplacement of lumbar pedicle screws can be prevented by the following technique: The middle of the pedicle is roughly indicated by the intersection of lines bisecting the transverse processes and the lateral margin of the facet joints. After opening the posterior cortex at this point with a burr, a pedicle finder is used to probe the pedicle. A 2-mm drill bit is placed in the hole and the position is confirmed with x-rays. A depth gauge is used to feel all four quadrants of the hole to make sure it has not broken out of the pedicle. This technique has evolved after the senior author's several years of experience and significantly reduces the risk of breakout.

Dural Leakage

Dural tears may result from the spinal injury or intragenic trauma. Surgical causes include misplacement of pedicle screws or attempts at fracture fragment removal. With iatrogenic tears, cerebrospinal fluid (CSF) pressure can keep the tear open and lead to either fistula or meningocele formation. Therefore, surgical closure of the dura is recommended when a tear is recognized. If leakage occurs postoperatively, a percutaneous subarachnoid catheter over 4 days will relieve CSF pressure and permit healing in 80% of cases.

Hook Dislodgment

As mentioned earlier in this chapter, hook dislodgment rates increase dramatically as distal hook placement approaches the sacrum. From a series of 206 unstable spine fractures treated with hooks and distraction rods, the senior author found dislodgment in only 4% of cases with distal hook placement proximal to L4, 7% with hooks at L4, 11% with hooks in L5, and 29% in the sacrum (28).

Nonunions

Nonunions may be asymptomatic for months or years and then become symptomatic and angulate following increased activity or pregnancy. These problems can be prevented by the proper selection and execution of instrumentation, careful grafting, and postoperative brace protection. Treatment requires reinstrumentation to correct the deformity with additional direct decompression in some cases to relieve neural impingement.

Postreduction Narrowing of the Canal

This is most often seen following compression instrumentation for bilateral facet dislocation. It was discussed extensively under flexion-distraction injuries.

REFERENCES

1. White AA, Panjabi MM. *Clinical Biomechanics of the Spine.* Philadelphia: JB Lippincott, 1978.
2. Bernhardt M, Bridwell KH. Segmental analysis of the sagittal plane alignment of the normal thoracic and lumbar spines and thoracolumbar junction. *Spine* 1989;14:717.
3. Stagnara P, DeMauroy JC, Dran G, et al. Reciprocal angulation of vertebral bodies in a sagittal plane: approach to references for the evaluation of kyphosis and lordosis. *Spine* 1982;7:335.

4. Edwards CC, York JJ, Levine AM, Weigel MC. Determinants of spinal hook dislodgment. *Orthop Trans* 1986;10:8.
5. Denis F. The three-column spine and its significance in the classification of acute thoracolumbar spine injuries. *Spine* 1983;8:817–831.
6. Gertzbein SD, Court-Brown CM. Flexion-distraction injuries of the lumbar spine. *Clin Orthop* 1988;227:52–60.
7. Gumley G, Taylor TKF, Ryan MD. Distraction fractures of the lumbar spine. *J Bone Joint Surg* 1982;64B(5):520–525.
8. Levine AM, Bosse M, Edwards CC. Bilateral facet dislocations in the thoracolumbar spine. *Spine* 1988;13:630–640.
9. Connolly PJ, Esses SI, Heggeness MH, Cook SS. Unilateral facet dislocation of the lumbosacral junction. *Spine* 1992;17(10):1244–1248.
10. Davis AA, Carragee EJ. Bilateral facet dislocation at the lumbosacral joint. A report of a case and review of the literature. *Spine* 1993;18(16):2540–2544.
10a. Bohlman HH. Current concepts in review: treatment of fractures and dislocations of the thoracic and lumbar spine. *Journal Bone Joint Surgery* 1985;67A:165–169.
10b. Willen J, Lindahl S, Nordwall A: Unstable thoracolumbar fractures: A comparative clinical study of conservative treatment and harrington instrumentation. *Spine* 1985;10:111–122.
10c. Dennis F. Acute thoracolumbar burst fractures in the absence of neurologic deficit: A comparison between operative and non-operative treatment. *Clinical Orthopaedic-Related Research* 1984;189:142–149.
10d. Kropinger WJ: Conservative treatment of fractures of the thoracic and lumbar spine. *Orthopaedic Clinics North America* 1986;17:161–170.
10e. Thoracolumbar spine fractures without neurologic deficit. In Stauffer ES: *American Academy of Orthopaedic Surgeons Monograph Series.* Rosemont, Illinois, 1993, AAOS.
11. Rosenthal MR, Levine AM, Edwards CC. Burst fractures in the low lumbar spine. *Orthop Trans* 1988;12:231.
12. Frederickson B, Yuan H, Miller H. Burst fractures of the fifth lumbar vertebra. *J Bone Joint Surg* 1982;64A(7):1088–1094.
13. Court-Brown CM, Gertzbein SD. The management of burst fractures of the fifth lumbar vertebra. *Spine* 1987;12(3):308–311.
14. An H, Vaccaro A, Cotler J, Lin S. Low lumbar burst fractures. Comparison among body cast, Harrington rod, Luque rod and Steffee plate. *Spine* 1991;16(8):S440–S444.
15. Mick C, Carl A, Sachs B, Hresko T, Pfeifer B. Burst fractures of the fifth lumbar vertebra. *Spine* 1993;18(13):1878–1884.
16. Roy-Camille R, Saillant G, Mazel C. Plating of thoracic, thoracolumbar, and lumbar injuries with pedicle screw plates. *Orthop Clin North Am* 1986;17:147–159.
17. Edwards CC, Rhyne AL, Weigel MC, Levine AM. 5–10 year results treating burst fractures with rod-sleeve instrumentation and fusion. *Orthop Trans* 1991;15:728.
18. Kahanovitz N, Arnoczky SP, Levine DB, et al. The effect of internal fixation on the articular cartilage of unfused canine facet joint cartilage. *Spine* 1984;9:268.
19. Kahanovitz N, Bullough P, Jacobs RR. The effect of internal fixation without arthrodesis on human facet joint cartilage. *Clin Orthop* 1984;189:204.
20. Casey M, Jacobs RR, Asher M. The rod long-fuse short technique in the treatment of thoracolumbar and lumbar spine fractures. *Orthop Trans* 1985;9:121.
21. Edwards CC, Levine AM. Early rod-sleeve stabilization of the injured thoracic and lumbar spine. *Orthop Clin North Am* 1986;17:121–146.
22. Edwards CC. Reconstruction of acute lumbar injury. *Oper Tech Orthop* 1991;1(1):106–122.
23. Panjabi MM, Abumi K, Duranceau J, Crisco JD. Biomechanical evaluation of spinal fixation devices: stability provided by eight internal fixation devices. *Spine* 1988;13:1135–1140.
24. Hanley EN, Starr JK. Junctional burst fractures. *Spine* 1991;15.
25. Edwards CC. The Edwards modular system for three-dimensional control of the lumbar spine. In: Hanley X, Belfus Y (eds). *Spine: State of the Art Review.* Philadelphia: WB Saunders, 1992:235.
26. Levine AM, Edwards CC. Low lumbar burst fractures: reduction and stabilization using the modular spine fixation system. Orthopaedics 1988;11:1427–1432.
27. Edwards CC, Rhyne A. Late treatment of posttraumatic kyphosis. *Semin Spine Surg* 1990;2:63–69.
28. Edwards CC, Levine AM. Fractures of the lumbar spine. In: Evarts CM (ed). *Surgery of the Musculoskeletal System,* 2nd ed. New York: Churchill Livingstone, 1990;2237.
29. Edwards CC. Spinal screw fixation of the lumbar spine: early results treating the first 50 cases. *Orthop Trans* 1987;180:179–181.
30. Nicoll EA. Fractures of the dorsolumbar spine. *J Bone Joint Surg* 1949;31B:376–394.
31. Shirado O, Kaneda K. Lumbosacral fracture-subluxation associated with bilateral fractures of the first sacral pedicles: a case report and review of the literature. *J Orthop Trauma* 1995;9(4):354–358.

Surgery of Spinal Trauma,
edited by J.M. Cotler, J.M. Simpson, H.S. An, and C.P. Silveri.
Lippincott Williams & Wilkins, Philadelphia © 2000.

CHAPTER 13

Surgical Considerations of Posttraumatic Spinal Deformity

Raymond S. Kirchmier, Jr. and Francis Denis

The surgical management of posttraumatic spinal deformity is complex and offers significant challenges to even the most experienced of spine surgeons. Treatment goals for spine trauma in the acute setting include preservation and improvement of neurologic function and the achievement of spinal stability. A "stable" spine should be able to resist resulting compressive, tensile, and rotational forces, prevent progressive deformity from occurring, and protect the neural structures. Posttraumatic spine deformity arises when there has been a failure in the primary treatment of the initial injury. Causes include an underestimation of the severity of acute injury, a lack of sound understanding of biomechanics of the spine, inadequate primary treatment of the injury, and poor surgical technique or judgment. Occasionally, a seemingly stable injury may become problematic with time.

The treatment of posttraumatic spine deformities depends on its clinical manifestations. Potential sequelae include pain, progression of deformity, development of a new neurologic deficit, progression of a preexisting deficit, and poor cosmesis.

POSTTRAUMATIC CERVICAL SPINE DEFORMITY

The normal resting posture of the cervical spine is a smooth, slightly lordotic curvature. Inherent stability depends on the

R. S. Kirchmier Jr: Medical College of Virginia, Virginia Commonwealth University; Tuckahoe Orthopaedic Associates, Richmond, Virginia 23226.
F. Denis: Minnesota Spine Center, Minneapolis, Minnesota 55454.

competent interaction between the bone and soft tissues—the vertebral bodies, neural arches, intervertebral discs, the interfacet joints, the facet capsules, and the multiple ligaments. Traumatic instability with the development of deformity can arise by disruption of any of these structures and usually is due to a combination of injuries. The most common inevitable deformity that occurs is cervical kyphosis, the usual mechanism of injury being hyperflexion and axial loading. Kyphosis occurs when there is disruption of the anterior structures under compression and/or the posterior elements under tension (1). Heightened clinical awareness and a better understanding of the biomechanical principles of spinal trauma have improved our ability to treat these injuries appropriately. Unfortunately, however, the spine surgeon is still faced with the challenges of posttraumatic deformity.

Posttraumatic cervical kyphosis can present with pain, neural compression, progressive neural deficit, or progressive deformity. As cervical kyphosis progresses, the biomechanics of the region are altered. Without osteoligamentous stability, the posterior cervical paraspinous muscles are placed at a poor mechanical advantage. Etiology of pain is probably multifactorial. Pain can develop from muscular fatigue while trying to hold the head in an erect and functional position (2). With any kyphotic deformity the tendency is for kyphosis to progress with time, given an alteration in weight-bearing axis and potentials for degeneration (3,4). Pain can also be caused by the development of posttraumatic degenerative changes to the disc or joints, subtle instability (especially in cases of previous laminectomy), or occult neural compression. Zdeblick and Bohlman (5) have shown how the cervical spinal cord becomes draped over the posterior aspect of the vertebral bodies in kyphosis, increasing tension within the spinal cord itself. This tensioning can produce neural dysfunction and potentially pain by direct neural damage or by causing ischemia from vasoconstriction of the anterior spinal vessels (6). Etiology of pain in many of these situations frequently cannot be isolated by the clinician.

Subaxial cervical posttraumatic cervical deformity is much more common than atlantoaxial deformities. This discussion focuses predominantly on the occurrence of cervical kyphosis as the result of trauma. The multiple causes of posttraumatic kyphosis include progressive anterior collapse of vertebral body burst fractures, unrecognized facet joint capsular or posterior ligamentous injuries, and iatrogenic postlaminectomy cases (7–10). The indications for cervical laminectomy for treatment of acute surgical trauma are extremely rare, limited mostly to lamina or facet fractures with isolated posterior compression. If laminectomy is carried out, as many as 68% of patients will need a later fusion procedure for instability (9).

Failure to recognize posterior ligamentous disruption is the most common cause of posttraumatic cervical kyphosis (Fig. 1). The ligament complex frequently does not heal adequately to resist the usual posterior tensile stresses. Bohlman (11) has shown that progressive kyphosis can develop despite treatment of these injuries with rigid external immobilization. Stauffer and Kelly (10) have also docu-

mented progressive kyphosis in 16 patients who underwent anterior stabilization for cervical trauma, and on review of the preoperative radiographs were found to have evidence of posterior ligamentous disruption. Injuries that include a vertebral body burst fracture and associated posterior ligamentous instability are markedly unstable and have a high propensity to develop kyphotic deformity without surgical treatment. McAfee and Bohlman (12) have described excellent results in ten patients treated with simultaneous anterior decompression/stabilization and posterior stabilization for this particular injury associated with incomplete neurologic deficit. Other less common deformities that can develop subsequent to cervical spine trauma include a rotatory deformity from a unilateral facet injury (13), torticollis from traumatic C1-2 rotatory subluxation, and upper cervical kyphosis from malunited odontoid fractures or type III hangman's fracture with posterior ligamentous disruption (14,15).

Neural compression is frequently associated with posttraumatic cervical kyphosis. Clinical manifestations include pain, the development of a new neurologic deficit, worsening of a preexisting neurologic deficit, and persistence of a potentially reversible incomplete neurologic deficit. Detailed neurologic examinations on a consistent time basis should be carried out to detect what can sometimes be subtle changes. Most neurologic deficits will be caused by anterior compression of the spinal cord. Retropulsed bone fragments,

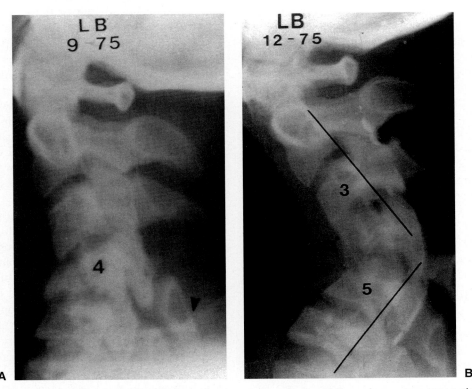

FIG. 1. A: This patient sustained a C4 burst fracture with splaying of the spinous processes signifying posterior instability at the C3-4 level. **B:** Unfortunately, severe kyphosis developed as the fracture was left to heal, now requiring anterior and posterior reconstruction. (From ref. 5, with permission.)

disc material, posterior osteophytes, and calcified ligamentous tissue can all lead to anterior cord impingement (5). Altered neural function has been shown to probably occur from a mechanical neuropraxic standpoint with disruption of normal axoplasmic flow, and from impaired blood flow to the anterior cord circulation (6,16). As many clinicians have noted, anterior decompression is the recommended treatment for anterior cervical spine compression (5,11,12,17–19). In cases of fixed kyphotic deformity, anterior decompression in addition to correction of the underlying kyphosis is necessary for optimal results. Varying degrees of neurologic recovery can be expected to occur in anterior decompressions for incomplete spinal cord or nerve root injuries, and nerve root "escape" can occur with decompression in the patient with complete quadriplegia, greatly enhancing overall function (17).

Evaluation/Surgical Indications

Evaluation begins with the history, concentrating on the mechanism of injury, previous treatment, and current symptoms. Physical examination focuses on the location of the deformity and the detailed neurologic examination. Comparisons made with previous neurologic examination should aid in detecting changes or progression of neurologic dysfunction.

Cervical imaging begins with plain radiographs to identify the injury pattern and to localize and quantify the deformity. Old radiographs are used for comparison to document progression of deformity. Swimmer's view may be necessary for viewing the cervicothoracic junction. Flexion/extension lateral radiographs should be taken to assess whether the deformity is fixed and if mechanical instability is present. Greater than 3.5 mm of vertebral body translation or greater than 11 degrees of adjacent intervertebral rotation denotes instability according to White et al. (1). The open mouth odontoid view assesses the occipitocervical and atlantoaxial articulations. Plain computed tomography (CT) with sagittal reconstruction images especially helps in evaluating upper cervical deformities and trauma.

Intraspinal assessment of the neural elements is essential in planning the appropriate treatment for traumatic cervical deformity. This is accomplished either with magnetic resonance imaging (MRI) or myelography supplemented with CT. CT usually allows better resolution of bony structures, while MRI has the advantage of being noninvasive, and direct sagittal imaging is possible. Dynamic imaging can be accomplished with both MRI and CT myelograms. The severity and localization of spinal cord and nerve root compression is identified. Frequently, compression may span multiple intervertebral segments. In the spinal cord injured patient with progressive neurologic deterioration and pain, MRI is superior to myelography for diagnosing posttraumatic syringomyelia and other intrinsic cord abnormalities (20,21).

The surgical indications for posttraumatic cervical spine deformity include the following:

1. Documented progressive cervical deformity
2. Evidence of mechanical instability
3. Pain that cannot be controlled with the usual nonoperative modalities
4. Evidence of neural compression with the presence of either an incomplete traumatic cord lesion, plateau of recovery from initial neural function, or progressive neural deficit.

Surgical Treatment

Two key factors determining the optimal surgical treatment of posttraumatic cervical kyphosis are the rigidity of the deformity and the degree of neurologic involvement. In the few cases without neural compression, treatment can be limited to correction of the deformity with stabilization. Flexible deformities may be reduced with traction maneuvers and stabilized with a posterior arthrodesis. A fixed kyphosis will have to be addressed with an anterior release/arthrodesis and probable posterior stabilization procedure depending on the integrity of the posterior structures. More commonly, neural dysfunction (myelopathy or radiculopathy) will be present with posttraumatic kyphosis requiring anterior cord decompression in addition to the reduction of the deformity (Fig. 2). Anterior approaches have been recommended by multiple authors as the treatment of choice for cervical kyphosis (5,12,17,22–25). In general, multiple anterior corpectomies are performed followed by anterior strut grafting, using either iliac crest or fibula. As the site of spinal cord compression is almost always anterior, preoperative imaging studies determine which vertebral bodies need to be removed. Careful planning is important to ensure that all of the offending vertebral bodies, osteophytes, and discs are addressed in the decompression. One- and two-level corpectomies are usually spanned with autologous iliac crest. Longer decompressions are spanned using fibula graft, either autograft or allograft. Intraoperative evoked potential neurologic monitoring should be used to help prevent iatrogenic neural injury.

Fielding and Tolli (23) reported successful results in treating postlaminectomy kyphosis first with preoperative traction, followed by multilevel corpectomies and strut grafting with postoperative halo immobilization. Recently developed anterior cervical plating systems can offer enough immediate stability to avoid the use of halo immobilization (26–28). These implants can be difficult to insert correctly and to avoid neurovascular complications. Whitecloud and La Rocca (29) showed satisfactory results in 23 of 26 patients undergoing fibular strut grafting for reconstructive cervical kyphosis cases. There were, however, three postoperative graft dislodgments.

The authors' procedure of choice for posttraumatic cervical kyphosis with myelopathy is combined anterior cord decompression/arthrodesis with posterior stabilization/arth-

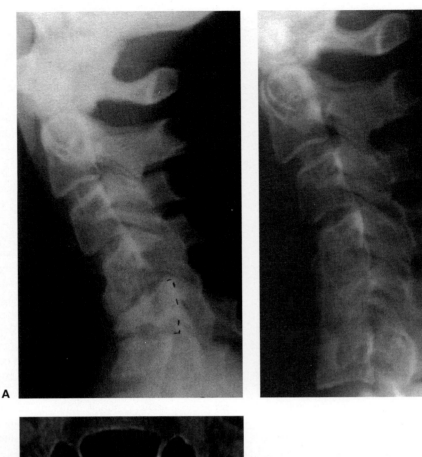

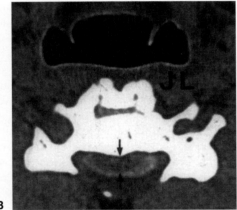

FIG. 2. A: This 3-month postinjury radiograph demonstrates an unstable C5 burst fracture with posterior instability and progressive kyphosis and neurologic deterioration. **B:** A myelogram computed tomography (CT) shows significant distortion of the spinal cord at the C5 body level secondary to bone retropulsion and kyphosis. **C:** Treatment included C5 corpectomy, cord decompression, anterior strut fusion, and posterior stabilization with appropriate correction of the kyphosis. (From ref. 24, with permission.)

rodesis. The cause of kyphotic deformity is usually deficiency of the posterior ligamentous structures, and these injuries require posterior stabilization to prevent late kyphotic collapse, which can also offer increased stability to prevent extrusion of anterior strut grafts (5,22). Late collapse and kyphosis has been reported in patients undergoing anterior interbody fusions for traumatic lesions and unidentified posterior ligamentous disruption (10). McAfee and Bohlman (12) reported on ten patients with a fixed kyphosis and an incomplete neurologic deficit secondary to burst fracture and posterior ligamentous disruptions treated with circumferential stabilization. The average kyphosis correction was 54 degrees to 13 degrees. There were no nonunions, and substantial neurologic recovery was documented in eight of the ten patients. Zdeblick and Bohlman (5) showed good results in 14 patients with cervical kyphosis and myelopathy treated with anterior corpectomy and strut grafting. Five of these patients had posttraumatic kyphosis, and four of these five were treated with posterior fusion in addition to the index procedure. Kyphosis correction averaged approximately 70%. There was 100% union rate and 13 of the 14 patients experienced significant neurologic improvement.

The technique for anterior multilevel corpectomy and strut graft fusion is shown in Figs. 3 and 4. After induction of general anesthesia, leads for electrophysiologic monitoring are placed and 10 to 15 lb of traction is applied. A Smith and Robinson (30) anterior cervical exposure is performed at the appropriate level. Discectomies are completed rostral and

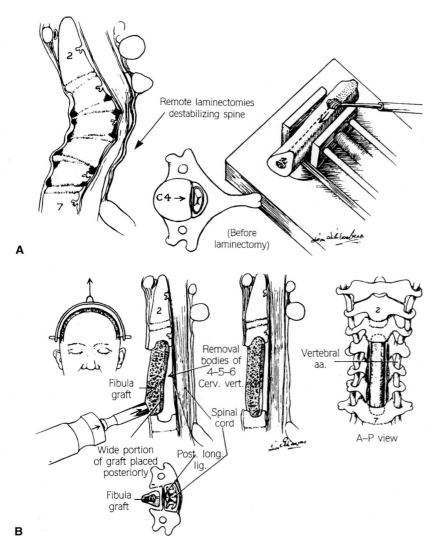

A

B

FIG. 3. A: Drawing of multilevel spinal cord compression due to kyphosis and posterior osteophytes with a previous laminectomy. The fibula strut graft is contoured and sized. **B:** After corpectomies of C4, C5, and C6, increased traction helps to reduce the kyphosis, and seating holes are created into the superior and inferior endplates. The graft is tamped into place, and when fraction is released, soft tissue tension should lock the graft into place. (From ref. 5, with permission.)

caudal to each vertebral body to be resected. It is important to identify the uncovertebral joints bilaterally to ensure complete decompression and to avoid injury to the vertebral arteries. The posterior longitudinal ligament is identified at each disc space. The central portion of each vertebral body is removed with rongeurs, and a trough is created with a burr in the central portion of the body preserving the lateral cortex and protecting the vertebral arteries. A diamond tip burr may be used as the posterior body cortex is approached. When adequately thinned, the remaining bone fragments and osteophytes are swept anteriorly with small-angle curettes away from the posterior longitudinal ligament and decompressing the spinal canal. Concave seating holes are then made with the burr in the central portion of the bony endplates at the rostral and caudal ends of the decompression. Traction is gradually increased to 40 lb and a lateral radiograph is taken to check the reduction. In cases involving compression isolated to the disc space(s), anterior release and decompression is performed only at the appropriate disc spaces. The use of a Cobb elevator as a wedging device or an intervertebral dis-

tractor between the vertebral bodies at the apex of the kyphosis may aid in obtaining correction (Fig. 5).

Strut graft reconstruction is achieved with iliac crest or fibula. Traditionally iliac crest grafts span one- and two-level corpectomies; fibula struts are used for longer decompressions. The appropriate graft length is determined and the ends of the grafts are rounded with the burr. The graft is then tamped into the concave seating holes under direct vision and then traction is returned to 5 to 10 lb. Soft tissue tensioning should lock the graft into place. A Kocher clamp can be used to check graft stability. Radiographs are repeated to check graft position and kyphosis reduction. More recently, many authors have described stabilizing anterior strut fusions with anterior cervical plating systems. This is not discussed in detail in this chapter.

With evidence of posterior ligamentous insufficiency, posterior stabilization and arthrodesis should follow the anterior procedure, typically under the same anesthetic. Turning frames greatly ease the transition to a prone position and lessen the chance of anterior graft displacement. Standard

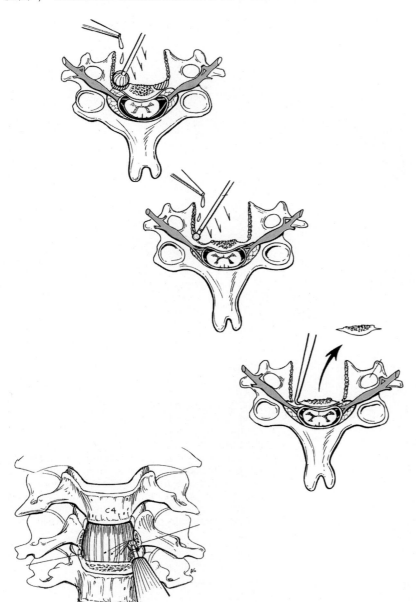

FIG. 4. Technique of anterior corpectomy with decompression. After a ronguer is used to remove the anterior half the vertebral body, burrs and curettes are used to remove the remaining bone, osteophytes, and disc tissue away from the canal. The lateral extent of decompression is the uncinate process; further lateral undermining can jeopardize the vertebral artery. (From ref. 54, with permission.)

posterior cervical arthrodesis is performed *in situ.* Stabilization is usually obtained via the Bohlman triple-wire technique (Fig. 6). Recently developed posterior plating systems are another good option, especially for treating postlaminectomy cases and cases involving multiple levels over a long fusion span (31). Advantages of the lateral mass plate fixation include improved immediate stability and more secure fixation and less reliance on rigid postoperative immobilization. Surgeon familiarity with this technique and attention to anatomic details are required to prevent neurovascular injuries during screw insertion. Flexible postlaminectomy deformities that reduce well with preoperative traction are best treated with passive correction and *in situ* posterior plating and arthrodesis. An alternate treatment for postlaminectomy kyphosis is facet wiring and arthrodesis, as described by

Callahan et al. (32). For this procedure to be effective, the kyphosis needs to be flexible, and there should be no evidence of anterior (spinal) cord impingement. A potential disadvantage of this procedure is the reliance on an autogenous rib for strut graft stability.

The postoperative management includes the use of a cervical orthosis, which is typically worn for 8 to 12 weeks or until clinical and radiographic union is complete.

POSTTRAUMATIC THORACOLUMBAR SPINE DEFORMITY

The acute treatment of thoracolumbar spine trauma, particularly unstable injuries, continues to evolve and remains controversial. The end result should be a stable spine to maxi-

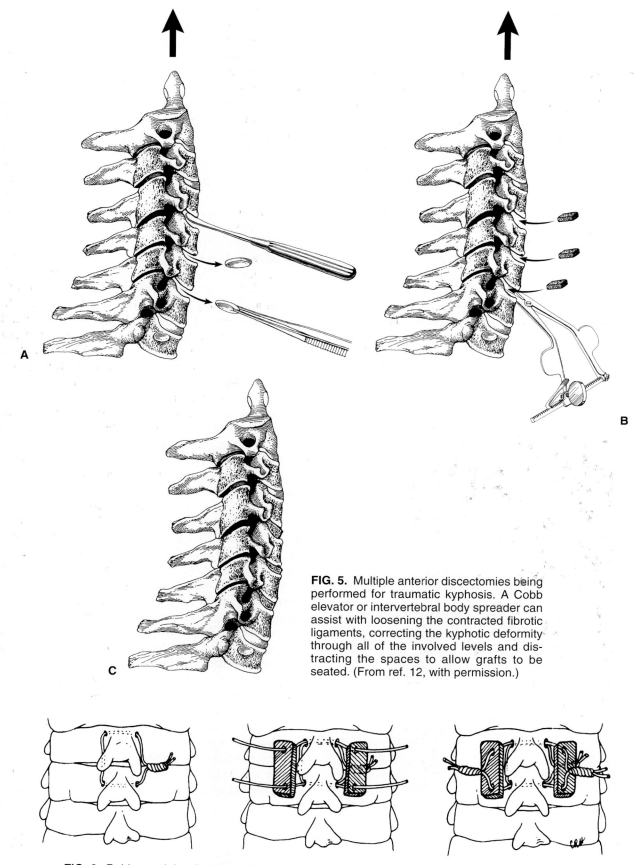

FIG. 5. Multiple anterior discectomies being performed for traumatic kyphosis. A Cobb elevator or intervertebral body spreader can assist with loosening the contracted fibrotic ligaments, correcting the kyphotic deformity through all of the involved levels and distracting the spaces to allow grafts to be seated. (From ref. 12, with permission.)

FIG. 6. Bohlman triple-wire interspinous process wiring technique. (From ref. 54, with permission.)

mize neurologic function and to prevent late deformity and pain. Failures of treatment occur, and symptomatic posttraumatic deformity can develop (Fig. 7). This section focuses mainly on posttraumatic kyphotic deformities, given their higher prevalence and the potential for neurologic sequelae.

The sagittal alignment of the thoracolumbar spine changes as it proceeds from the upper thoracic to the lower lumbar regions. The normal kyphosis of the thoracic spine is 15 to 40 degrees; the thoracolumbar junction approximates a neutral alignment, and the lumbar spine shifts to lordosis. Balance between the anterior and posterior elements and osseous and ligamentous structures maintains this resting posture. Abnormal traumatic kyphosis occurs when there is disruption either of the elements under tension (posterior), or compression (anterior), or both. In the thoracic spine, the laminae and ligamentum flavum are the main structures resisting tension. In the lumbar spine, the interfacet joint capsules and interspinous ligaments are the primary resistive structures to tension. As kyphosis progresses, the moment arm from the center line of gravity to the spine increases, deforming forces leading to worsening angulation. With more angulation, and a given load over time, the stress increases the deformity, causing greater bending (1). According to Kostuik (33) lumbar kyphosis greater than 30 degrees is usually symptomatic and leads to "flat back" syndrome. Progressive posttraumatic

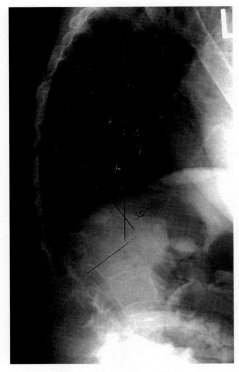

FIG. 7. This lateral radiograph demonstrates a 4-month postinjury film of an L1 burst fracture in a 55-year-old woman. This patient was initially treated elsewhere by her primary physician with observation and now presents with chronic, incapacitating pain with a normal neurologic exam. She refused surgical treatment.

kyphosis is usually a consequence of the following injuries: unstable burst fractures, flexion-rotation fracture-dislocations, flexion-distraction ligamentous injuries, or multiple contiguous compression fractures. Fractures at the thoracolumbar junction have the highest propensity to develop late deformity (8).

Many contributing factors have been associated with the development of posttraumatic kyphosis. Nonoperative treatment of unstable acute injuries frequently leads to persistent kyphosis (34,35). Several series have shown the incidence of localized pain in these cases to vary between 40% and 90% (35–38). Postmenopausal women are at increased risk for progressive kyphosis given underlying metabolic bone changes. As in the cervical spine, previous laminectomy is a significant risk factor for the formation of progressive angulation. Multiple authors have documented the inability of this procedure to improve neurologic function in acute spinal injuries, coupled with its destabilizing effect on the posterior elements (9,35,39,40). Underestimation of the severity of an unstable acute injury with inadequate follow-up can frequently lead to late deformity. Lastly, errors in surgical technique in fracture management are another source of posttraumatic morbidity. Fusions that are performed but do not address all kyphotic segments can "add on," leading to an increased kyphosis. Causes of instrumentation-related failures include poor insertional technique, the wrong levels being stabilized, and the incorrect use of distraction, compression, and bending forces (Fig. 8). Increase in angulation in the face of previous fusion always suggests underlying pseudoarthrosis.

The clinical manifestations of posttraumatic kyphosis are usually classified as mechanical or neurologic. Mechanical sequelae include pain, fatigue, progression of deformity, instability, and sitting/standing balance difficulties in neurologically impaired patients. Neurologic sequelae include occurrence of a new or progressive deficit in the presence of a persistent, potentially reversible, incomplete deficit coupled with anterior neurologic compression. Back pain is the most common symptom and is usually the main indication for reconstructive surgery in posttraumatic deformity. As in cervical deformities, it frequently is difficult to identify the exact cause of pain. Pain usually localizes to the apex of the deformity and is mechanical in nature. Bending, lifting, twisting, and prolonged erect posture are aggravating factors; the recumbent position lessens symptoms usually. Malcolm et al. (36) found pain radiating into the buttocks to be common in patients with thoracolumbar posttraumatic deformities. Potential sources of pain include segmental instability, abnormal stresses placed through the soft tissues, particularly the posterior tensile structures, muscle fatigue of the spinal extensor mechanism, and posttraumatic degenerative changes of the joints and disc. Compensatory lumbar hyperlordosis caudal to a kyphotic deformity can also elicit pain, usually caudal to the deformity apex. On occasion, neural compression presents only with localized pain, and without obvious neurologic signs.

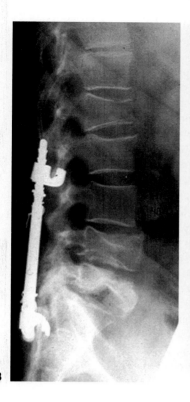 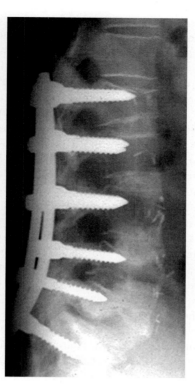

A,B

FIG. 8. A: This 40-year-old man fell off a house roof and sustained burst fractures of L4 and L5 and a compression fracture of L1. He was referred from another institution after undergoing posterior spine fusion L2-S1 with distraction instrumentation. He presented with lumbar flat-back syndrome and chronic lumbar pain. **B:** Surgical treatment required multilevel anterior fusions, posterior osteotomies, restoration of lumbar lordosis, and posterior reconstruction with instrumentation.

The development of a new kyphosis-induced neurologic deficit or progression of a preexisting deficit is an absolute indication for surgical decompression, realignment, and stabilization (8,33,41). Causes of neurologic deterioration include progression of kyphotic deformity (42), cord ischemia secondary to anterior compression, and peridural fibrosis from local instability (36). Traumatic neurologic deficits of the thoracolumbar and lumbar region are usually incomplete, frequently a mixed cord/nerve root lesion, especially for injuries at the level of the conus medullaris. The neuropraxic effect on the nerve rootlets allows for varying degrees of recovery following decompression. Treatment must be instituted to relieve ongoing compression and to lessen the "stretch" effect inherent as the cord/roots are draped over the kyphotic segment. Burst fractures can lead to late development of central or lateral recess canal stenosis with symptoms of neurogenic claudication or isolated nerve root dysfunction. Posttraumatic syringomyelia needs to be excluded as cause of a new neurologic deficit or pain in any patient with previous spinal cord injury. MRI assists in this diagnosis.

Evaluation/Surgical Indications

The preoperative evaluation again begins with a history and physical examination. Assessment for spinal deformity, tenderness, gait disturbances, and soft tissue spasms are included. Detailed neurologic exam must include testing for rectal tone and sensory deficits. Plain radiographs identify the level of injury and resulting deformities; comparison should be made with previous films to assess for progression. Bending films are a clue to the rigidity of the deformity and the presence of segmental instability.

Spinal canal imaging is performed by MRI or contrast-enhanced CT scan. MRI is the procedure of choice because of its ability to characterize spinal cord tissue. Previous spinal instrumentation presents artifacts that could complicate interpretation. Both MRI and myelogram CT should delineate whether decompression is necessary and exactly which levels need to be addressed.

Surgical indications for posttraumatic thoracolumbar kyphosis include the following:

1. Neurologic deficit
2. Progressive neurologic deficit
3. Pain not controlled with the usual conservative nonoperative modalities
4. Documented progression of kyphosis
5. Poor cosmesis (relative indication)

Surgical Treatment

In general the surgical treatment of posttraumatic thoracolumbar spine deformity entails combined anterior/posterior stabilization and arthrodesis. The four goals of surgery are to decrease pain, to improve or prevent neurologic dysfunction, to safely correct deformity, and to stabilize the spine. The presence of neurologic compression on preoperative imaging studies associated with neurologic signs and/or pain requires complete decompression of the neural elements. In the overwhelming majority of these cases compression occurs from anterior structures. The surgeon has to be familiar with anterior decompression techniques, and several series have shown better results with these procedures than with posterior approaches (36,41,43–45). In the absence of neurologic embarrassment, efforts are concentrated on obtaining spinal stability with deformity correction, instrumentation, and fusion.

Dynamic bending radiographs help assess the flexibility of the kyphotic deformity. Generally thoracic curves less than 60 degrees that are flexible and without neurologic compression can be addressed solely by posterior instrumentation and fusion. A good example of this scenario is kyphosis developing from multiple thoracic compression fractures. A correction of the deformity is afforded by using the principles of posterior tension band (46). The entire length of the kyphotic curve is included in the fusion to prevent the "adding on" phenomenon. Any of the many available segmental instrumentation systems can be used. Multiple claw constructs above and below the apex of the curve should be employed, applied in compression mode, and combined with three-point bending principles (Fig. 9).

More commonly posttraumatic kyphoses are fixed deformities and require anterior release and fusion combined with posterior fusion. Isolated posterior fusions for severe kyphosis lead to high pseudoarthrosis and failure rates (1,47,48). Reasons for failure include large bending moments and high tensile forces being placed on the posterior graft, which leads to a thin posterior fusion mass, slow incorporation, and a propensity for the fusion mass to bend as it matures. Anterior fusions are under compression and of-

fer improved biomechanical advantages for severe kyphosis. For rigid curves greater than 60 degrees, it is best to proceed with anterior release and fusion, followed by posterior instrumentation and fusion. Curve correction is not as important in offering pain relief as is the achievement of solid fusion with spinal stability (46). If anterior decompression is not required, multiple discectomies are carried out, and the choices of anterior fusion are interbody, inlay, or structural strut grafts. The contracted and fibrotic anterior longitudinal ligament have to be sectioned before correction is possible. When used, anterior strut grafts should be placed as far anterior as possible to decrease the moment arm to the neutral axis (1). Kostuik (33) has shown success in 37 patients with posttraumatic thoracolumbar kyphosis treated with isolated anterior deformity correction and instrumentation and fusion. He obtained a union rate of 97%, with mild loss of correction and good pain relief and neurologic recovery. Kaneda et al. (49) have shown good results with anterior decompression, realignment, and stabilization with instrumentation without the need for posterior stabilization in 27 patients with thoracolumbar burst fractures with neurologic deficit. Eight of these cases entailed late deformity, and better outcomes were observed with Kaneda instrumentation than Zielke instrumentation. Because most posttraumatic deformities have inherent posterior column instability, however, most authors recommend a combined anterior/posterior approach.

Malcolm et al. (36) reviewed 48 patients treated surgically for posttraumatic thoracolumbar kyphosis. Fusion was successful in all posterior and circumferential procedures, but

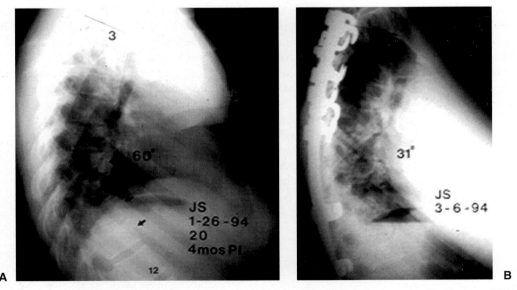

FIG. 9. A: This 20-year-old woman sustained multiple compression fractures at T8, T9, T10, and T11 in an automobile accident. She developed progressive kyphosis to 60 degrees and chronic pain over the ensuing 4 months, refractory to conservative treatment. **B:** Relative flexibility of her kyphosis allowed her surgical treatment to be limited to posterior fusion and stabilization from T3-T12. Instrumentation included multiple claws above and below the kyphotic apex, and the principles of compression and three-point bending were employed to correct the kyphosis to an acceptable 31 degrees.

there was a 50% failure rate in isolated anterior fusions. The deformity correction averaged only 25%, but complete pain relief was noted in 67% and was significantly lower in another 31%. The indications for anterior fusion included kyphosis greater than 50 degrees, previous laminectomy, anterior column insufficiency, and the need for anterior decompression. Bradford and Moe (50) reported results of anterior strut grafting for structural kyphosis in 48 patients, six of them posttraumatic. Curve correction averaged 32%, and considerations were made to include posterior stabilization and possible vascularized rib graft to decrease the pseudoarthrosis rate and to prevent anterior graft fracture or dislodgment. Roberson and Whitesides (41) have also shown good results in 32 patients with traumatic kyphosis treated with combined anterior and posterior fusion or anterior fusion alone. The isolated anterior fusions were efficacious as long as no posterior instability was present. Harms and Stoltze (45) recommended a combined approach for three reasons:

1. to immobilize and release fibrotic anterior and posterior elements for correction;
2. structurally to restore the anterior column and the posterior column tension band;
3. to shorten the length of constructs and preserve motion segments, especially important in the lumbar spine.

With proven neural compression, anterior decompression of the spinal cord/cauda equina is usually the first step in the surgical management. Occasionally for lower lumbar fractures and deformities (L4 and L5), decompression may be plausible with standard laminectomy, nerve root retraction, and bone resection. Certainly this is the case from old burst fractures that present predominantly with foraminal stenosis. Larson et al. (51) described a posterolateral decompression and fusion, but this approach has its limitations in severe deformities in placing the structural graft, and can potentially destabilize the posterior elements and lead to worsening neurologic function.

The author's technique of anterior decompression/fusion is as follows. The spine can be exposed from either the left or right side, depending on the surgeon's experience and personal preference. In general, the left exposure is not compromised by the liver, and it is easier to control the aorta and its segmental branches than those of the vena cava and azygous systems. The surgical approach depends on the spinal level involved. Transthoracic and thoracolumbar approaches may require take-down of the diaphragm for exposure of the thoracic spine and thoracolumbar spine. A retroperitoneal approach is useful for middle and lower lumbar exposures. The same principles apply to all three regions. Removing the rib one level above the level of maximal compression, usually at the apex of the kyphosis, allows the most direct approach for the decompression in thoracic cases. The segmental vessels throughout the entire length of the kyphosis are ligated near the midline to avoid disrupting the collateral circulation of the cord near the neuroforamina. The spine is then exposed by subperiosteal dissection, as described by Bradford and Moe (50). A periosteal flap is created beginning at the rib heads posteriorly and then reflecting this anteriorly after making transverse incisions at the root and caudal limits of the planned fusion. The dissection proceeds to the far side of the kyphosis. The anterior longitudinal ligament usually has to be sectioned to obtain correction after the decompression. The rib heads at the apex are removed and then all the discs within the deformity are excised back to the posterior longitudinal ligament.

At each level requiring decompression, the pedicle is identified and removed with a burr or Kerrison rongeur. A burr or larger rongeur is used to remove bone from the midportion of vertebral bodies to create a large cavity, extending to the opposite cortex, but preserving the posterior cortices. Bone wax helps control cancellous bone bleeding. The posterior cortex is then thinned with a burr until the spinal canal can be identified and entered with a small curette. The dural sac is then decompressed by pulling the remaining bone and disc material away from the neural structures into the cavity created in the vertebral body. Decompression needs to span from the near to the far pedicle. It is best to remove the bone from the far side first so the cord does not sag into the viewing area, making it very difficult then to safely place instruments back to the far side. If the decompression encompasses several levels, the apical region should be the last section addressed.

Anterior fusion is then accomplished, usually with strut grafts. In those deformities of moderate severity, which are reasonably flexible and not requiring decompression, anterior interbody fusion is performed with cancellous chips from rib, iliac crest, or allograft, and correction of the deformity obtained from posterior instrumentation. Tricortical structural iliac crest allograft bone can also be used to help create a lordosing effect. In the majority of cases where decompression has been carried out, a 1- to 2-cm hole is burred into the anterior aspect of the uppermost and lowermost vertebral bodies in the deformity in preparation for receiving the strut graft. The appropriate strut graft (rib, fibula, or iliac crest) is selected and cut to length. The deformity is gradually corrected by manual pressure over the apex and if possible by one of the commercially available anterior distractors. Spinal cord monitoring is essential during the correction phase. The graft is then tamped into the upper and lowermost vertebral bodies. Multiple strut grafts may be required in very severe rigid curves (Fig. 10). Cancellous bone chips are then packed into the space between the strut grafts and the vertebral bodies. More recently, developed anterior spinal plates and cages have become available and may aid in anterior stabilization, but long-term data are not available on their use for posttraumatic spine deformities. Anterior spinal cages packed with cancellous bone can potentially offer more immediate anterior

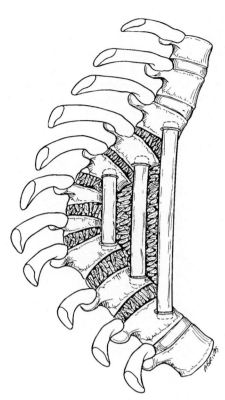

FIG. 10. A drawing of multiple anterior strut grafts being placed for severe rigid kyphosis. After discectomy and/or corpectomy is completed, an anterior distractor is placed, seating holes are developed in the superior and inferior endplates, and the most posterior strut graft is placed first into the respective vertebrae. Larger strut grafts are then sequentially inserted moving more anterior. (From ref. 54, with permission.)

column stability and lessen the time for graft incorporation (Fig. 11). After anterior stabilization, the chest/retroperitoneum is then closed in routine fashion.

Posterior arthrodesis and stabilization increase the rate of obtaining solid fusion and decrease the risk for anterior strut graft dislodgment. The posterior tension band is usually restored by placing segmental instrumentation in compression along with three-point bending. All the levels involved in the deformity need to be included in the fusion from neutral disc to neutral disc. Any of the many available spine systems can be used depending on the surgeon's experience. Multiple claw constructs above and below the deformity should be used, as the posterior column is in effect shortened as compression is applied (Fig. 12). No hook should be placed at the apex of the deformity. For deformities of the thoracolumbar junction and lumbar spine, pedicle screw systems can shorten the length of fusion and construct, and help preserve the important lumbar motion segments. In all cases of previous laminectomy, posterior spinal fusion should be performed in addition to the anterior stabilization. Postoperative

immobilization consists of either a body cast or molded thoracolumbar spinal orthosis (TLSO) until radiographic and clinical union is complete. With rigid fixation, early mobilization in the patient is possible, avoiding recumbency-related complications.

A rare phenomenon that is occasionally seen in the patient with complete traumatic paralysis is a neurotrophic spine. The radiographic appearance is typically that of bone destruction and fragmentation associated with hypertrophic bone formation, eventually leading to a massive pseudoarthrosis. Sobel et al. (52) described the clinical sequelae of five patients with Charcot spine. The presentation is usually pain with progressive kyphosis in the thoracolumbar spine, audible crepitus due to instability, and the loss of normal sitting balance. Treatment is surgical and requires sagittal plane realignment and rigid, long construct, spinal fixation and fusion. Devin et al. (53) reported satisfactory results in ten patients treated with combined anterior fusion and posterior fusion with instrumentation. Isolated posterior fusion was found to be effective in cases of single-level involvement only. Vascularized bone grafts may also help augment the fusion in these difficult cases (Fig. 13).

COMPLICATIONS

Cervical Spine

Surgical reconstruction for posttraumatic cervical kyphosis has a high relative complication rate, but this rate can be minimized with careful preoperative planning and attention to surgical detail. Complications can be classified into approach-related problems, vascular injuries, neurologic deterioration, and bone graft and instrumentation failures.

The anterior cervical approach has potential for multiple complications given the proximity of the carotid and vertebral arteries, internal jugular vein, trachea, esophagus, laryngeal nerves, and the thoracic duct. Knowledge of appropriate tissue planes is vital to prevent injury to these structures. The use of blunt retractors and the avoidance of overzealous retraction should prevent neurovascular and esophageal injuries. Hoarseness can develop postoperatively from edema or injury to the superior or recurrent laryngeal nerves. The vertebral artery can be traumatized if bony decompression is extended lateral to the uncinate processes; therefore, bony anatomic landmarks are important during the passage of instruments.

Despite several series' absent neurologic complication rates (5,12), the spinal cord is at significant risk during decompression and fusion for cervical kyphosis. Potential causes of neurologic deterioration included extreme patient positioning, the surgical approach, inadvertent passage of instruments into the spinal canal, neural compression secondary to graft placement or displacement, and vascular injury to the anterior spinal artery. Emergent reexploration is warranted in cases of hematoma or bone graft extrusion into

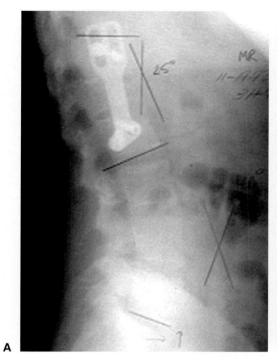

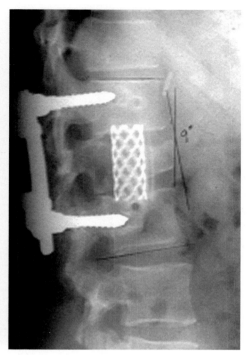

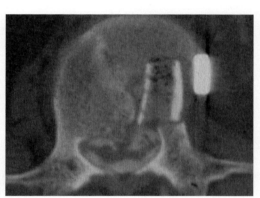

FIG. 11. A: This 31-year-old man sustained an L1 burst fracture in a motor vehicle accident and elsewhere underwent acute L1 anterior corpectomy and stabilization with plate fixation. On presentation 6 months postinjury, he complained of chronic back pain and lower extremity dysesthesias and deformity and had evidence of mixed lumbar root bilateral radiculopathies. Lateral radiograph reveals 25-degree kyphosis. **B:** Lumbar myelogram CT shows incomplete anterior L1 vertebral body decompression, significant spinal cord and cauda equina compression and apparent pseudoarthrosis. **C:** Surgical treatment included repeat complete L1 corpectomy, cord decompression, anterior reconstruction with Harms cage and nonstructural bone graft, and posterior limited fusion with pedicle screw instrumentation. His kyphosis improved to 9 degrees and he became pain-free and returned to employment.

the canal. Spinal cord monitoring can potentially detect cord dysfunction earlier and allow appropriate measures to be taken.

Anterior graft–associated complications include extrusion, collapse, fracture, and nonunions. Most extrusions are anterior and from the caudal insertion point of the graft. Graft extrusion may cause dysphagia or airway obstruction, increased kyphosis and potentially worsen neurologic status. Zdeblick and Bohlman (5) described a 21% dislodgment rate overall and experienced an increased incidence in patients with previous laminectomy. They recommended burring the inferior seating hole at least 5 mm deep in the central aspect of the bony endplate. Posterior stabilization and fusion is also recommended in any case of coexisting posterior instability. Posterior graft extrusions can be prevented by leaving a posterior lip in the bony endplate when preparing for the graft. An intraoperative lateral radiograph and exploration

with a blunt nerve hook should always be performed after graft placement to ensure proper graft positioning. Instrumentation-related complications usually occur as a result of insertion malposition or failure of fusion. Foraminal narrowing can occur from overzealous compression of lateral mass plates or overtightening of interspinous wiring. Familiarity with vertebral anatomy is critical in placing lateral mass plates to avoid injury to the spinal cord, nerve roots or the vertebral artery. Plate/screw breakage or loosening may occur in instances of pseudoarthrosis or graft collapse and may require revision surgery.

Thoracolumbar Spine

Complications of surgical treatment for posttraumatic thoracolumbar kyphosis are similar to those of the cervical spine and are similarly classified. There are some differ-

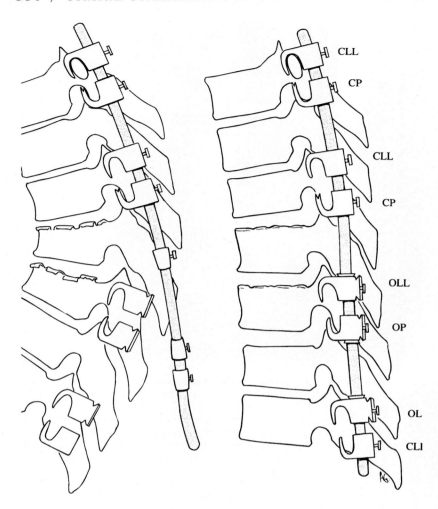

FIG. 12. The principle of multiple claws being placed above and below the kyphotic apex. The rod should be undercontoured to allow correction as it is placed into the lower hooks using three-point bending. Posterior column shortening is created by the sequential compression between hooks. (From ref. 54, with permission.)

ences, however, due to anatomic differences. The incidence of wound infection is higher in thoracolumbar procedures, especially in posterior procedures associated with instrumentation. Malcolm et al. (36) reported an overall 40% complication rate related directly to the treatment of these deformities. Due to the violation of the pleural cavity, with many anterior approaches, there is a higher incidence of respiratory insufficiency, pneumonia, pneumothorax, and recurrent pleural effusion, particularly if the diaphragm is detached. Thromboembolic phenomenon can occur as a result of prolonged recumbency; therefore, all efforts should be made to mobilize the patient as soon as possible. Postthoracotomy incisional pain along the intercostal nerve innervation can be quite limiting and may respond to intercostal nerve blocks. Arterial and venous injuries are rare and can usually be avoided by maintaining subperiosteal dissection.

Neurologic deterioration following corrective surgery for thoracolumbar kyphosis has been reported to be as high as 8%. Malcolm et al. (36) identified the thoracic spinal cord from T5 to T9 to be especially vulnerable to injuries during anterior decompression. They concluded that intraoperative hypotension and the ligation of segmental vessels too close to the neuroforamina were the most likely etiologies of postoperative spinal cord dysfunction. Inadvertent instrument passage into the spinal canal and strut graft malposition again may also lead to worsening neurologic function.

Anterior strut graft complications include fracture, collapse, extrusion, loss of correction, and delayed union. Bradford (50) and Moe found a higher incidence of graft fracture when the distance between the graft and the front of the apical vertebra was greater than 4 cm. This can be prevented by using multiple strut grafts and/or rigid posterior fixation. Multiple authors have shown that with the addition of posterior arthrodesis, the incidence of pseudarthrosis, graft dislodgment, and graft collapse with loss of correction can be significantly decreased. Posterior instrumentation complications include screw, rod, or plate breakage or loosening in conjunction with failed fusions and neurovascular injuries secondary to malposition. Posterior hooks should never be placed at the apex of a posttraumatic kyphosis.

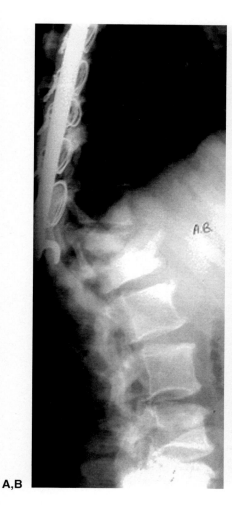
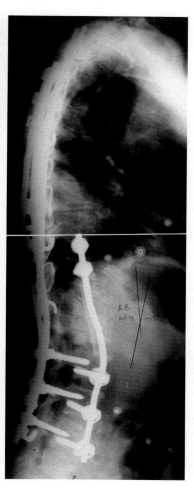

A,B

FIG. 13. A: Supine lateral radiograph of a 45-year-old woman midthoracic level paraplegic following a motor vehicle accident who was treated 10 years prior with Harrington rod sublaminar wiring stabilization. The chief complaint was lack of sitting balance in her wheelchair due to spinal instability at the thoracolumbar junction. Her kyphosis increased from 15 to 52 degrees with sitting posture and audible crepitus was detected with spinal mobility. **B:** Surgical treatment entailed anterior debridement of the pseudoarthrosis, fibular strut graft, and long construct anterior instrumentation; the second stage entailed extension of posterior instrumentation and fusion into the lower lumbar spine.

REFERENCES

1. White A, Panjabi M, Thomas C. The clinical biomechanics of kyphotic deformities. *Clin Orthop Rel Res* 1977;128:8–17.
2. Levine A, Edwards C. Complications in the treatment of acute spinal injury. *Orthop Clin North Am* 1986;17:183–203.
3. Saito T, Yamamuro T, Shikata J, Tsutsumi S. Analysis and prevention of spinal column deformity following cervical laminectomy. *Spine* 1991;16:494–502.
4. Sim F, Svier H, Janes J. Swan-neck deformity following extensive cervical laminectomy. *J Bone Joint Surg* 1974;56A:564–580.
5. Zdeblick T, Bohlman H. Cervical kyphosis and myelopathy: treatment by anterior corpectomy and strut-grafting. *J Bone Joint Surg* 1989;71A:170–182.
6. Breig A. Adverse mechanical tension in the central nervous system: an analysis of cause and effect. In: *Relief by Functional Neurosurgery.* New York: Wiley, 1978.
7. Bohlman H. Complications of treatment of fractures and dislocations of the cervical spine. In: Epps C (ed). *Complications in Orthopaedic Surgery,* 2nd ed. Philadelphia: JB Lippincott, 1986.
8. Bohlman H. Treatment of fractures and dislocations of the thoracic and lumbar spine. *J Bone Joint Surg* 1985;67A:165–169.
9. Morgan T, Wharton G, Austin G. The results of laminectomy in patients with incomplete spinal cord injuries. *J Bone Joint Surg* 1970;52:822.
10. Stauffer E, Kelly E. Fracture dislocations of the cervical spine: instability and recurrent deformity treatment by interbody fusion. *J Bone Joint Surg* 1977;59A:45–48.
11. Bohlman H. Acute fractures and dislocations of the cervical spine. *J Bone Joint Surg* 1979;61A:1119–1142.
12. McAfee P, Bohlman H. One-stage anterior cervical decompression and posterior stabilization with circumferential arthrodesis. *J Bone Joint Surg* 1989;71A:78–88.
13. Whitehill R, Richman J, Glaser J. Failure of immobilization of the cervical spine by the halo vest: a report of 5 cases. *J Bone Joint Surg* 1986;68A:326–332.
14. Ersmark H, Kalen R. Injuries of the atlas and axis: a follow-up study of 85 axis and 10 atlas fractures. *Clin Ortho Rel Res* 1987;217:257–260.
15. Levine A, Edwards C. The management of traumatic spondylolisthesis of the axis. *J Bone Joint Surg* 1985;67A:217–226.
16. Brain W, Northfield D, Wilkinson M. The neurologic manifestations of cervical spondylosis. *Brain* 1952;75:187–225.
17. Bohlman H, Anderson P. Anterior decompression and arthrodesis of the cervical spine: long-term motor improvement, part I. *J Bone Joint Surg* 1992;74A:671–682.
18. Bohlman H, et al. Mechanical factors affecting recovery from incomplete cervical spinal cord injury. *Johns Hopkins Med J* 1979;145:115–125.
19. Maiman D, Barolat G, Larson S. Management of bilateral locked facets of the cervical spine. *Neurosurgery* 1986;18:542–547.
20. Bosley T, Sergott R, et al. Comparison of metrizamide computed tomography and MRI in evaluation of lesions at the cervicomedullary junction. *Neurology* 1985;35:485–492.
21. Gabriel K, Crawford A. Identification of acute post traumatic spinal cord cysts by MRI. *J Pediatr Orthop* 1988;8:710–714.

22. Bohlman H. Surgical management of cervical spine fracture and dislocations. *Instr Course Lect* 1985;34:163–187.
23. Fielding J, Tolli T. Surgical management of post laminectomy kyphosis. *Semin Spine Surg* 1989;1:271–275.
24. McAfee P. Cervical spine trauma. In: Frymoyer J (ed). *The Adult Spine: Principles and Practice.* New York: Raven Press, 1991.
25. Zdeblick T. Cervical kyphosis. In: An H, Simpson J (eds). *Surgery of the Cervical Spine.* London: Martin Dunitz, 1994.
26. Bremer A, Nyugen T. Internal metal plate fixation combined with anterior fusion in cases of cervical spine injury. *Neurosurgery* 1983;12:649–653.
27. Capen D, Garland D, Waters R. Surgical stabilization of the cervical spine: a comparative analysis of anterior and posterior spine fusions. *Clin Ortho Rel Res* 1985;196:229–237.
28. Caspar W. Anterior stabilization with trapezoidal osteosynthetic plate technique in cervical spine injuries. In: Kehr, Weidner (eds). *Cervical Spine,* vol 1. New York: Springer-Verlag, 1987:198–204.
29. Whitecloud T, LaRocca J. Fibular strut graft in reconstructive surgery of the cervical spine. *Spine* 1976;1:33–43.
30. Smith G, Robinson R. Treatment of certain cervical spine disorders by anterior removal of the intervertebral interbody fusion. *J Bone Joint Surg* 1958;40A:607–623.
31. An H, Gordin R, Renner K. Anatomic considerations for plate-screw fixation of the cervical spine. *Spine* 1991;16(10 suppl):S548–S551.
32. Callahan R, Southwick W, et al. Cervical facet fusion for control of instability following laminectomy. *J Bone Joint Surg* 1977;59A:991–1002.
33. Kostuik J. Adult kyphosis. In: Frymoyer J (ed). *The Adult Spine: Principles and Practice.* New York: Raven Press, 1991.
34. Jodoin A, Dupuis P, Fraser M, Beumont P. Unstable fractures of the thoracolumbar spine. *J Trauma* 1985;25:197–202.
35. Roberts J, Curtiss P. Stability of the thoracic and lumbar spine in traumatic paraplegia following fracture or fracture-dislocation. *J Bone Joint Surg* 197;52A:1115–1130.
36. Malcolm B, Bradford D, Winter R, Cou S. Post-traumatic kyphosis. *J Bone Joint Surg* 1981;63A:891–899.
37. Nicoll E. Fractures of the dorsal—lumbar spine. *J Bone Joint Surg* 1949;31B:376–394.
38. Weinstein J, Collalto P, Lehmann T. Long-term follow-up of non-operatively treated thoracolumbar spine fractures. *J Orthop Trauma* 1987;1:152–159.
39. Bradford D, Alcbarnia B, Winter R, Seljescog E. Surgical stabilization of fracture and fracture-dislocation of the thoracic spine. *Spine* 1977;2:185–196.
40. Malcolm B. Spinal deformity secondary to spinal injury. *Orthop Clin North Am* 1979;10:943–952.
41. Roberson J, Whitesides T. Surgical reconstruction of late post-traumatic thoracolumbar kyphosis. *Spine* 1985;10:307–312.
42. Lonstein J. Neurologic deficits secondary to spinal deformity. *Spine* 1980;5:331–338.
43. Anderson P, Bohlman H. Late anterior decompression of thoracolumbar fractures. *Semin Spine Surg* 1990;2:54–62.
44. Bradford D, Winter R, Lonstein J, Moe J. Techniques of anterior spine surgery for management of kyphosis. *Clin Orthop Rel Res* 1977;128:129–139.
45. Harms J, Stoltze D. The indications and principles of correction of posttraumatic deformities. *Eur Spine J* 1992;1:142–152.
46. Denis F. Thoracolumbar spine trauma. In: Lonstein, Bradford, Winter, Ogilvie (eds). *Moe's Textbook of Scoliosis and Other Spinal Deformities,* 3rd ed. Philadelphia: WB Saunders, 1995.
47. Bradford D, Moe J, Montalvo F, Winter R. Scheurmann's kyphosis, results of surgical treatment by posterior spine arthrodesis in 22 patients. *J Bone Joint Surg* 1975;57A:439–447.
48. Hall J. The anterior approach to spinal deformities. *Orthop Clin North Am* 1972;3:1–15.
49. Kaneda K, Abumi K, Fujiya M. Burst fractures with neurologic deficits of the thoracolumbar-lumbar spine: results of anterior decompression and stabilization with anterior instrumentation. *Spine* 1984;9:788–795.
50. Bradford D, Moe J. Anterior strut grafting for the treatment of kyphosis. *J Bone Joint Surg* 1982;64A:680–690.
51. Larson Holst R, Hemmy D, Sauces A. Lateral extra-cavitory approach to traumatic lesions of the thoracic and lumbar spine. *J Neurosurg* 1976;45:628–637.
52. Sobel J, Bohlman H, Freehafer A. Charcot's arthropathy of the spine following spinal cord injury. *J Bone Joint Surg* 1985;67A:771–776.
53. Devin V, Ogilvie J, Transfeldt E, Bradford D. Surgical treatment of neuropathic spinal arthropathy. *J Spinal Disord* 1991;4:319–327.
54. Winter R, Lonstein J, Denis F, Smith M. *Atlas of Spine Surgery.* Philadelphia: WB Saunders, 1995.
55. An H, Simpson J (eds). *Surgery of the Cervical Spine.* London: Martin-Dunitz, 1994.
56. Anderson P, Henley B, Grady S, Winn R. Posterior cervical arthrodesis with AO reconstruction plates and bone graft. *Spine* 1991;16(3 suppl):572–579.
57. Benzel E, Larson S. Functional recovery after decompressive spine operation for cervical spine fractures. *Neurosurgery* 1987;20:742–746.
58. Bohlman H. Late progressive paralysis and pain following fractures of the thoracolumbar spine. *J Bone Joint Surg* 1976;58A:728–736.
59. Bolesta M, Bohlman H. Late sequelae of thoracolumbar fractures and fracture dislocations: surgical treatment. In: Frymoyer J (ed). *The Adult Spine.* New York: Raven Press, New York, 1991.
60. Denis F. Spinal instability as defined by the three-column spine concept in acute spinal trauma. *Clin Ortho Rel Res* 1984;189:65–76.
61. Gill K, Paseehal S, Conin J, Ashman R, Bucholz R. Posterior plating of the cervical spine: a biomechanical comparison of different posterior fusion techniques. *Spine* 1988;13:813–816.
62. Guttman L. Spinal deformities in traumatic paraplegics and tetraplegics following surgical procedures. *Paraplegia* 1969;7:38–58.
63. Kostuik J. Anterior Kostuik-Harrington distraction systems for the treatment of kyphotic deformities. *Iowa Orthop J* 1988;69:77.
64. Kostuik J. Combined single stage anterior and posterior osteotomy for correction of iatrogenic lumbar kyphosis. *Spine* 1988;13:257–266.
65. Lagrone M, Bradford D, Ogilvie J, et al. Treatment of symptomatic flat back after spinal fusion. *J Bone Joint Surg* 1988;70A:569–580.
66. Roy-Camille R, Saillant G, Mazel C. Internal fixation of the unstable cervical spine by posterior osteosynthesis with plates and screws. In: Sherk H (ed). *The Cervical Spine.* Philadelphia: JB Lippincott, 1989.
67. Sutterlin C, McAfee P, Warden K, Rey R, Farey I. A biomechanical evaluation of cervical spinal stabilization methods in a bovine model. *Spine* 1988;13:795–802.
68. Whitesides T. Traumatic kyphosis of the thoracolumbar spine. *Clin Orthop Rel Res* 1977;128:78–92.
69. Winter R. The treatment of spinal kyphosis—current concepts. *Int Orthop* 1991;15:265–271.

Surgery of Spinal Trauma,
edited by J.M. Cotler, J.M. Simpson, H.S. An, and C.P. Silveri.
Lippincott Williams & Wilkins, Philadelphia © 2000.

CHAPTER 14

Injuries of the Pediatric Cervical Spine

Peter D. Pizzutillo and Martin J. Herman

Anatomy of the Immature Cervical Spine
Clinical Presentation
Radiologic Evaluation
Spinal Cord Injury without Radiographic Abnormality
Atlantooccipital Dislocations
    Atlantooccipital Arthrodesis without Internal Fixation
    Atlantooccipital Arthrodesis with Internal Fixation
    Atlantooccipital Arthrodesis Using Wires and a
        Contoured Graft
    Atlantooccipital Fusion by Luque Loop Rod
        Instrumentation
Fracture of the Atlas (C1)

Atlantoaxial Injuries
    Traumatic Ligamentous Disruption
    Atlantoaxial Rotatory Subluxation and Dislocation
    Odontoid Separation (Synchondrosis Fracture)
    Os Odontoideum
    Atlantoaxial Posterior Cervical Arthrodesis
C2 Spondylolisthesis (Hangman's Fracture)
Subaxial Cervical Injuries (C3 to C7)
    Physeal Injuries
    Wedge-Compression Fractures
    Facet Dislocation
    Posterior Ligamentous Injuries

The care of traumatic cervical spine injuries in the child and adolescent is different from that in adults. The immature, growing cervical spine of the child presents a challenge to the treating physician. Emergency management, radiologic assessment, types of injuries sustained, and definitive treatment of these acute injuries reflect the fundamental anatomic and biologic differences in the child compared to the adult. The surgeon caring for these patients must appreciate these differences in order to provide safe, effective care of cervical spine injuries in this age group.

Cervical spine injuries in the child and adolescent are relatively rare, accounting for 2% to 3% of all traumatic injuries of the spine (1–5). The age- and sex-adjusted incidence of these injuries is estimated to be 7.41/100,00 per year (4). The majority of these injuries occur in motor vehicle accidents, in falls, and in sports activities (6). Associated neurologic injuries occur in 43% to 50% of patients (1,4,7).

The site of cervical spine injuries in children and adolescents is age-dependent. Children younger that 11 years of age generally sustain injuries to the upper cervical spine, while older children and adolescents sustain injuries to the subaxial cervical spine (1,3,4,8,9). In this younger subgroup,

a disproportionately large head, underdeveloped neck musculature, relative horizontal orientation of the upper cervical facets, and intrinsic hypermobility of the developing spine contribute to an increased incidence of upper cervical injuries (2,10). After age 8, the child's cervical spine begins to take on an adult-like configuration, with completion of this maturation by early adolescence (10,11). The cervical facets are more vertical. The ossification centers, with few exceptions, have appeared and fused, and the elasticity of the spinal column is reduced. The increased incidence of adult-type lower cervical spine injuries in the older child and adolescent reflects the changing spinal biomechanics and anatomy, as well as behavioral aspects, of the maturing child.

Arthrodesis for acute cervical spine injuries in the child and adolescent is indicated in 7% to 43% of patients in several series (1,7,12–16). The difficulties in achieving fusion seen in the adult are not seen in the child. Extension of the fusion mass beyond grafted levels and graft donor site pain and dysethesias are the most commonly reported complications; nonunion of grafted levels, neurologic complications related to surgery, late deformity, and late osteoarthrosis have also been reported (3,7,14–16).

The necessity of internal fixation in children and adolescents has not been reviewed in great detail in the literature. Success of fusion has not been correlated with use of internal fixation. Furthermore, internal fixation has been associ-

---

P. D. Pizzutillo and M. J. Herman: Orthopaedic Center for Children, St. Christopher's Hospital for Children, Philadelphia, Pennsylvania 19134.

ated with neurologic injuries, particularly in patients with ongoing spinal cord compression, fixed dislocations, and chronic instability (14,16,17).

ANATOMY OF THE IMMATURE CERVICAL SPINE

The atlas (C1) is composed of three ossification centers at birth: one for the body, and one for each of the two neural arches (lateral masses) (18). The anterior ring of C1 is unossified in children younger than 1 year of age, but ossifies and enlarges thereafter through age 6 to 9 years (10,19). The atlantal body fuses with the neural arches through the neurocentral synchondroses by age 7 years (10,19). The posterior arch usually closes by age 3 years (10) (Fig. 1).

The developing axis (C2) has four ossification centers: one for each neural arch, one for the body (occasionally two), and one for the dens (10,19). The basilar synchondrosis, between the dens and the body, fuses at age 3 to 6 years; the remnant of this fusion can persist as the subdental syn-

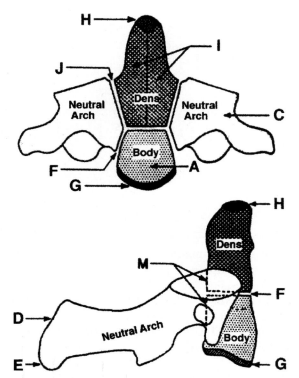

FIG. 2. Diagram of C2 (atlas). The body *(A)* in which one center (occasionally two) appears by the fifth fetal month. Neural arches *(C)* appear bilaterally by the seventh fetal month. Neural arches fuse *(D)* posteriorly by the second or third year. Bifid tip *(E)* of spinous process (occasionally a secondary center is present in each tip). Neurocentral and basinar synchondroses *(F)* fuse at 3 to 6 years. The inferior epiphyseal ring *(G)* appears at puberty and fuses at about 25 years. The summit ossification center *(H)* for the odontoid appears at 3 to 6 years and fuses with the odontoid by 12 years. Odontoid (dens) *(I)*. Two separate centers appear by the fifth fetal month and fuse with each other by the seventh fetal month. Neurocentral and basinar synchondroses (F) fuse at 3 to 6 years. Posterior surface of the body and odontoid *(M)*. (From ref. 10, with permission.)

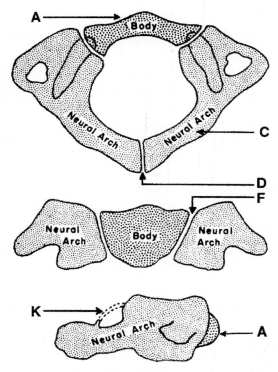

FIG. 1. Diagram of C1 (atlas). The body *(A)* is not ossified at birth, and its ossification center appears during the first year of life. The body may fail to develop, and forward extension of neural arches *(C)* may take its place. Neural arches appear bilaterally about the seventh week *(D)*, and the most anterior portion of the superior articulating surface is usually formed by the body. Synchondrosis of spinous processes unite by the third year. Union may rarely be preceded by the appearance of the secondary center within the synchondrosis. Neurocentral synchondrosis *(F)* fuses about the seventh year. The ligament surrounding the superior vertebral notch (K) may ossify, especially in later life. (From ref. 10, with permission.)

chondrosis scar (19). A summit ossification center seen at the cephalad tip of the odontoid appears at age 3 to 6 years, fusing with the main portion of the odontoid at approximately age 12 years (10,19). Persistence of this ossification center (ossiculum terminale) can be a normal anatomic variant (20) (Fig. 2).

The subaxial vertebrae, C3 to C7, ossify from three centers: a body and two neural arches (10,19). The posterior ring formed by the two neural arches fuses by 2 to 3 years of age. The neurocentral synchondroses, between the body and the neural arches anterolaterally, fuse between ages of 3 and 6 years. The ossified portion of the body, as seen from the lateral view, appears wedge-shaped because of asymmetric cephalad-caudad and anterior-posterior progression of ossification. The body appears square by age 7 years upon completion of this primary ossification. The superior and inferior epiphyseal rings (ring apophyses) appear at puberty. These

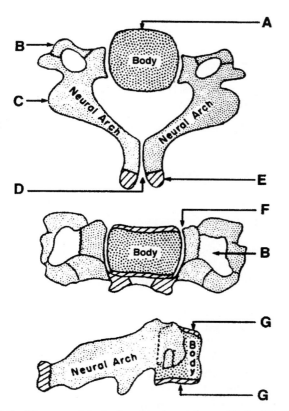

FIG. 3. Diagram of typical cervical vertebrae, C3 to C7. The body *(A)* appears by the fifth fetal month. The anterior (costal) portion of the transverse process *(B)* may develop from a separate center that appears by the sixth fetal month and joins the arch by the sixth year. Neural arches *(C)* appear by the seventh to ninth fetal week. Synchondrosis between spinous processes *(D)* usually unites by the second or third year. Secondary centers for bifid spine *(E)* appear at puberty and unite with spinous process at 25 years. Neurocentral synchondrosis *(F)* fuses at 3 to 6 years. Superior and inferior epiphyseal rings *(G)* appear at puberty and unite with the body at about 25 years. The seventh cervical vertebra differs slightly because of a long, powerful nonbifid spinous process. (From ref. 10, with permission.)

structures represent secondary ossification centers and fuse with the vertebral body by age 25 years (Fig. 3).

CLINICAL PRESENTATION

Injury to the cervical spine must be considered in the child or adolescent after trauma who is unconscious, has head or facial lacerations, or respiratory difficulties. In the conscious patient, complaints of occipital or neck pain, numbness or weakness in the extremities, and changes in bowel and bladder sensation and function indicate spinal injury until proven otherwise. In the outpatient setting, neck or occipital pain, changes in exercise tolerance or gait pattern, and transient neurologic symptoms are suggestive of progressive subacute cervical spine instability.

Emergency management of the young patient with a suspected cervical spine injury should focus initially on the ABCs, i.e., airway, breathing, and circulation. With primary assessment and resuscitation, effective immobilization of the potentially unstable spine must be carried out. Placement of an appropriately sized hard cervical collar limits effectively the motion of the cervical spine. However, if such a device is unavailable, rolled towels or sandbags, and tape, have been shown to be effective in immobilizing the cervical spine in an emergency situation (21).

Positioning of the child with a potential cervical spine injury on a backboard warrants special attention. A backboard with an occipital recess or elevated thoracic pad is required in a child younger than 8 years of age. This design prevents flexion of the cervical spine as the disproportionately large head of the child is allowed to rest with the spine in slight extension (22). Even with appropriate equipment, achieving neutral spinal alignment can often be difficult in children (23). In the patient with suspected progressive subacute instability, placement of a hard cervical collar at initial presentation provides sufficient protection while further evaluation is done.

Physical examination, especially in the young child, requires careful observation and patience. Inspection and palpation of the spine and paraspinal muscles, noting deformity, tenderness, and spasm, are done initially. Active range of motion is assessed. Assessment of passive range of motion in the acute setting, or in the unconscious patient, is contraindicated and potentially dangerous. A thorough neurologic evaluation, including testing for strength, sensation, proprioception, and reflexes, must be documented.

RADIOLOGIC EVALUATION

In the acute setting, the cross-table lateral cervical spine film is indicated until a complete cervical spine evaluation can be safely performed. Standard radiologic evaluation of the child's cervical spine should include anteroposterior, lateral, and open-mouth (odontoid) views. If no obvious patterns of instability are seen on these initial films, supervised lateral cervical spine flexion-extension views are indicated in the alert, cooperative patient with complaints of pain or neurologic findings. For the unconscious patient, other imaging modalities, such as computed tomography (CT) or magnetic resonance imaging (MRI), may be necessary to rule out acute ligamentous or bony cervical spine injuries. Passive flexion-extension views in the unconscious child are not indicated because of the risk of possible iatrogenic spinal cord injury. Additionally, an unconscious patient, or any child with a documented cervical spine injury, should have a complete radiologic evaluation of the entire spine. Approximately 25% of children with a cervical spine injury have additional, noncontiguous spinal injuries (4,24). Effective immobilization with a collar, and spinal precautions, such as log-rolling with transfers, should be maintained throughout the evaluation in all patients with suspected spinal injury.

Interpretation of the cervical spine radiograph in the growing child can be confusing. Common misinterpretations of normal radiographic findings include (10,19,25):

1. Summit ossification center of the odontoid, and tips of the transverse and spinous processes, appearing as avulsion fractures.
2. Persistent basilar (subdental) synchondrosis interpreted as an acute fracture of the odontoid.
3. Anterior wedging of the vertebral bodies simulating compression fractures.
4. Pseudosubluxation of C2 on C3, and less commonly C3 on C4, appearing as anterior instability on lateral flexion radiographs.
5. Atlantodens interval of 4.5 mm on lateral flexion cervical spine view interpreted as C1-2 instability. Up to 4.5 mm of translation can be normal in young children (6,26).
6. Physiologic variations in the width of the prevertebral soft tissues due to crying misinterpreted as soft tissue edema (27).
7. Absence of ossification of the anterior arch of C1 in the first year of life interpreted as posterior instability of C1 on C2.
8. Reversal of lordosis of the cervical spine interpreted as cervical paraspinal spasm.
9. Congenital anomalies, such as fusions and spina bifida, interpreted as acute abnormalities.

Because of the difficulties in interpreting plain radiographs of the pediatric cervical spine, special imaging studies are needed for complete, definitive evaluation in 50% of patients (28). Tomography is effective, particularly in the atlantoaxial region, to further evaluate the odontoid and lateral masses. Thin section axial CT scanning, with three-dimensional (3D) reconstruction when necessary, provides excellent images of the bony anatomy. Positioning the child's neck in flexion and extension or with right and left rotation adds a dynamic or stress component to the study and may be helpful in evaluating subtle instability or fixed rotation. CT scanning requires sedation or general anesthesia in the very young child.

Magnetic resonance imaging is helpful in evaluating both bony and soft tissue injury. The greatest value of MRI imaging is in evaluating the neural elements, particularly the spinal cord. Prevertebral soft tissue edema and signal changes within the spinal cord may be the only evidence of acute vertebral injury, particularly in the unconscious patient. Images done with the child's cervical spine positioned in flexion and extension can help elucidate the effect of subtle instability on the spinal cord, and thus may aid in treatment decision making (29). Like CT scanning, MRI requires sedation or general anesthesia in younger children.

Cineradiographic evaluation of the cervical spine is another useful modality for demonstrating subtle patterns of instability in the cervical spine. The examination, which can be recorded on video tape for later analysis, allows for evaluation in flexion and extension as well as rotation and tilt. The procedure is done under physician supervision in the awake patient using real-time imaging. Because of relatively high-dose radiation exposure, the child should be shielded during the examination.

SPINAL CORD INJURY WITHOUT RADIOGRAPHIC ABNORMALITY

Spinal cord injury without radiographic abnormality (SCIWORA) is unique to children. Incidence of this type of injury varies from 4% to 66% of all children with spinal cord injuries (30–32). Children younger than 8 years of age more commonly have severe, complete neurologic injury in the upper cervical spine; older children generally have incomplete subaxial injuries (1,33,34). Theories on etiology include traction injury to the spinal cord due to hyperelasticity of the spinal column, transient disc herniation, vertebral endplate separation, and immature cord vascularity (1,5,32,35). Delayed onset of paraplegia has been reported up to 4 days postinjury (5,34).

In the child with abnormalities on the neurologic examination but normal screening radiographs, SCIWORA must be suspected. In the awake, cooperative patient, lateral flexion-extension spine radiographs may be helpful in detecting evidence of vertebral column instability. In the unconscious patient, or the child with no obvious abnormalities on flexion-extension views, CT or MRI is indicated to define the potential spinal column injury pattern. Epidural hematoma, soft tissue swelling, and spinal cord compression or disruption may be the only signs of the acute spinal injury. Appropriate immobilization is required for presumed spinal instability in any child with SCIWORA. Surgical decompression is indicated for known compressive lesions, but otherwise is routinely not required (32). Stabilization and arthrodesis are indicated in the acute, unstable injury, for posttraumatic subacute instability, or for progressive deformity (32).

ATLANTOOCCIPITAL DISLOCATIONS

Traumatic atlantooccipital dislocation is commonly a fatal injury. Bucholz and Burkhead (36,37) reported an incidence of 8% in fatal motor vehicle accidents, with children sustaining the injury more than twice as frequently as adults. Sudden deceleration of the head likely causes acute cranialvertebral dislocation, often with spontaneous reduction (38). Lethal injury to the cervicomedullary junction of the spinal cord and vertebral arteries are the immediate causes of death (36,39).

Cases of survival after atlantooccipital dislocation are being reported with increasing frequency (40–44). Emergency care, particularly cardiopulmonary resuscitation at the scene of injury, as well as heightened awareness of potential spinal injuries, are possible explanations for the increased reporting. The degree of neurologic injury varies. Two patients with minimal weakness and hyperreflexia and one patient with unilateral extremity weakness only have been reported (43). Other neurologic abnormalities reported include respiratory distress, cranial nerve dysfunction, and varying degrees of paralysis (40–42,44).

The radiographic diagnosis of atlantooccipital dislocation is not always readily apparent because of spontaneous reduction likely occurring at the time injury, or with realignment of the head for transportation or resuscitation. The basion-dens distance should not exceed 10 mm in children, as seen on the lateral cervical spine film (45). Overdistraction after gentle traction may be the only sign of this injury. The dimension-less Powers ratio is quite sensitive to anterior atlantooccipital dislocations (46). This ratio is not valid if the atlas is fractured or if a congenital anomaly of foramen mag-

num exists (38,47), and is insensitive to posterior dislocation (48). Translation of the basion relative to the dens in flexion-extension should not exceed 1 mm in adults (49). However, this number has not been validated in children (Fig. 4).

Initial management of the acute injury includes anatomic realignment of the dislocation with gentle positioning of the head. This is followed immediately by application of a halo vest, Minerva cast, or other form of immobilization at the time of diagnosis. Cervical traction should be used with caution. Overdistraction, even with low weight, can occur. Definitive treatment after initial realignment and immobilization is posterior occipital-cervical fusion. Many surgical

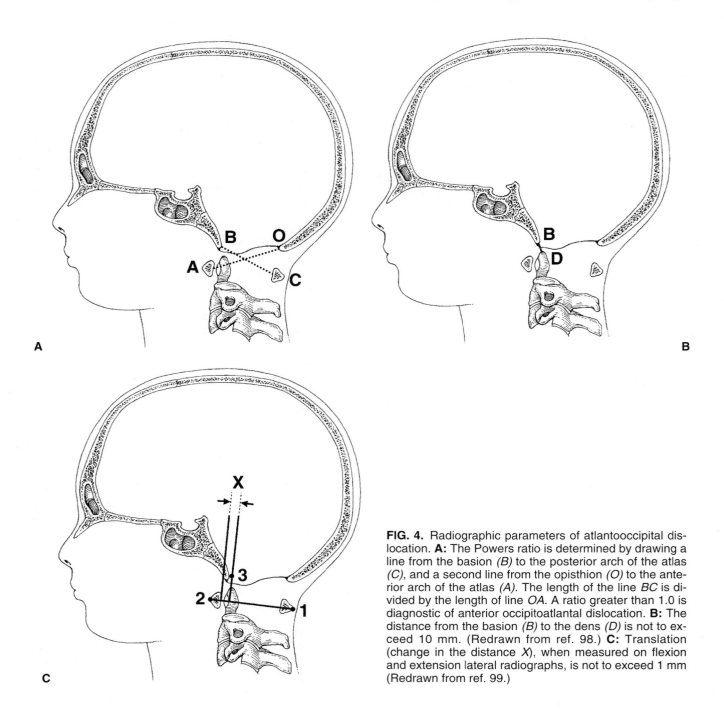

FIG. 4. Radiographic parameters of atlantooccipital dislocation. **A:** The Powers ratio is determined by drawing a line from the basion (B) to the posterior arch of the atlas (C), and a second line from the opisthion (O) to the anterior arch of the atlas (A). The length of the line BC is divided by the length of line OA. A ratio greater than 1.0 is diagnostic of anterior occipitoatlantal dislocation. **B:** The distance from the basion (B) to the dens (D) is not to exceed 10 mm. (Redrawn from ref. 98.) **C:** Translation (change in the distance X), when measured on flexion and extension lateral radiographs, is not to exceed 1 mm (Redrawn from ref. 99.)

techniques has been described (14,17,42,50–52). While the majority of the cases in these series underwent arthrodesis for atlantooccipital instability from nontraumatic etiologies, the operative principles are applicable to the unstable, traumatic atlantooccipital dislocation.

Atlantooccipital Arthrodesis without Internal Fixation

A halo is applied after induction of general anesthesia. The patient is then placed prone on a frame or modified operating table. Alternatively, a Mayfield head rest may be used to position the head and align the occiput and cervical spine. A lateral cervical spine radiograph is taken to confirm adequate cervical alignment.

A straight posterior midline incision is made from the occiput to the spinous process of C2. Infiltration of the midline dermis and subcutaneous tissue with epinephrine solution enhances hemostasis. Deep exposure is achieved by splitting the avascular midline ligamentum nuchae. The occipital protuberance (inion) as well as the spinous processes of C1 and C2 are identified. Careful subperiosteal dissection of C1 is carried out laterally. The extent of the dissection should be no greater than 1 cm from the midline to minimize the risk of injury to the vertebral arteries at this distance. The posterior occiput is subperiosteally dissected 1.5 to 2 cm laterally from the midline. The surface of the occiput is then decorticated with a curette or high-speed burr. Strips of corticocancellous iliac crest bone graft are placed across the exposed area, spanning only the levels of fusion desired. Care should be taken not to expose the laminae of more caudad vertebrae as this will increase the chances of extension of the fusion (Fig. 5). The wound is then carefully closed in layers.

Postoperatively, a halo jacket or Minerva cast is applied. Immobilization is maintained until adequate fusion is seen radiographically, usually after 8 to 12 weeks of immobilization. Lateral flexion-extension cervical spine views are required postoperatively to document stability of the fusion.

Koop et al. (14) and MacEwen (personal communication, 1997) describe a modification of this technique for use in patients with a defect in the posterior arch of C1. Exposure is achieved as above, but is extended distally to C2 or C3 beyond the defect. After extraperiosteal exposure of the occiput, a periosteal flap is turned down, covering the defect. This flap provides a bed for bone graft while protecting the dura exposed beneath the defect of C1 (Figs. 6 and 7).

Atlantooccipital Arthrodesis with Internal Fixation

Triple-Wire Technique

Positioning is done as described above. A midline subperiosteal dissection is made from the occipital protuberance, approximately 2 cm above the rim of the foramen magnum, to the level of C2. A trough is then created on either side of the protuberance using a high-speed burr. A towel clip is used to make a hole through the outer table of the skull at the protuberance. An 18- or 20-gauge wire is looped through this hole. A second wire is placed beneath the arch of C1 and looped on itself. Next, a hole is made at the base of the spinous process of C2 using a drill and a towel clip. A third wire is looped on itself through this hole. A premeasured corticocancellous graft is harvested from the iliac crest and divided in two halves. Three drill holes are placed in line through each half of the graft. After decortication of the occiput, the graphs are secured by passing the wires through the drill holes in the graft. The wires are twisted on themselves and tightened down over the grafts. Additional bone is added around and between the two corticocancellous grafts (Fig. 8). The wound is closed in layers.

Postoperative immobilization and aftercare are as described above.

This particular procedure technique is recommended in the older child and adolescent with a well-developed occipital protuberance (52). A modification of this technique, for younger children with a less developed occipital protuberance, eliminates the occipital wire (53).

Atlantooccipital Arthrodesis Using Wires and a Contoured Graft

Positioning and exposure are as described above. Two pairs of holes, aligned transversely 1.5 cm from the midline, are created in the outer table of the skull just below the transverse sinuses; a 1-cm bridge is maintained between the holes of each pair. A trough is created in the base of the occiput. A premeasured, rectangular corticocancellous graft is harvested. A caudad midline notch is fashioned in the graft to fit around the spinous process of the most caudad spinous process to be fused. An 18- to 20-gauge wire is then looped through the burr holes in the occiput. Wisconsin button wires are passed through the bases of the spinous processes of C2 and C3. The graft is locked in place by precise contouring. The wires are then passed through caudad arms of the graft, crossed over the graft, and tightened down (Fig. 9). The wound is closed in layers.

Postoperative immobilization and aftercare are as described above.

Dormans et al. (17) reported successful atlantooccipital arthrodesis in 15 of 16 cases using this technique. The authors concluded that this technique was safe, effective, and potentially a more stable construct than other previously described atlantooccipital arthrodesis techniques.

Atlantooccipital Fusion by Luque Loop Rod Instrumentation

Positioning and exposure are as described as above. Two burr holes are created and wires are passed on each side of the midline below the transverse sinuses in a fashion similar to that described above. Sublaminar wires are then passed

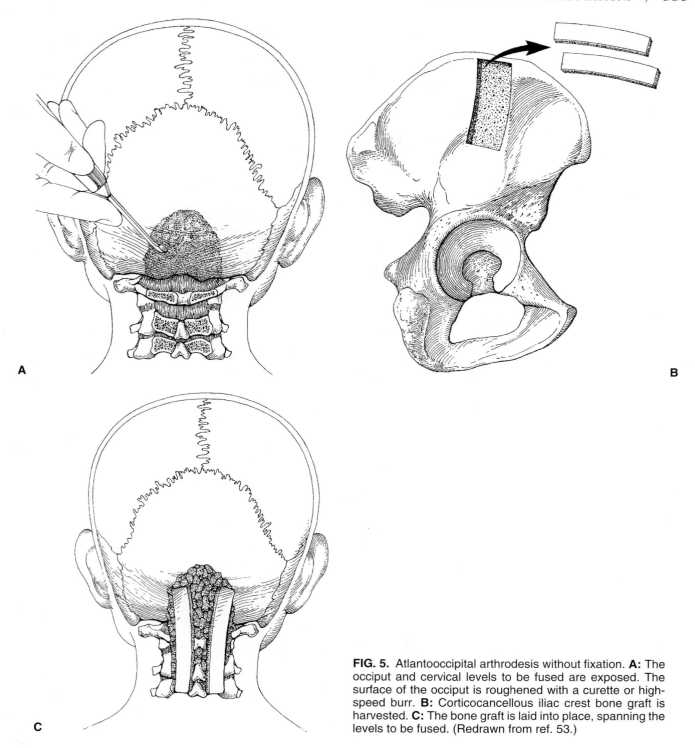

FIG. 5. Atlantooccipital arthrodesis without fixation. **A:** The occiput and cervical levels to be fused are exposed. The surface of the occiput is roughened with a curette or high-speed burr. **B:** Corticocancellous iliac crest bone graft is harvested. **C:** The bone graft is laid into place, spanning the levels to be fused. (Redrawn from ref. 53.)

under the arch of C1 and the laminae of all levels to be included in the fusion; at least two cervical levels are required to achieve stable fixation. A ³/₁₆-inch stainless steel or titanium rod, in a hairpin configuration, is contoured precisely in the sagittal plane and cut to the length of the fusion levels. The rod is laid in place and the wires are tensioned and crimped, or twisted, over the rod. Corticocancellous bone

graft is placed around the instrumentation, spanning the desired fusion levels.

Postoperative immobilization and aftercare are as described above. Alternatively, a hard cervical collar can be used if fixation is adequate.

This technique has been used successfully in adults (54–56). Advantages include the ability to achieve fixation

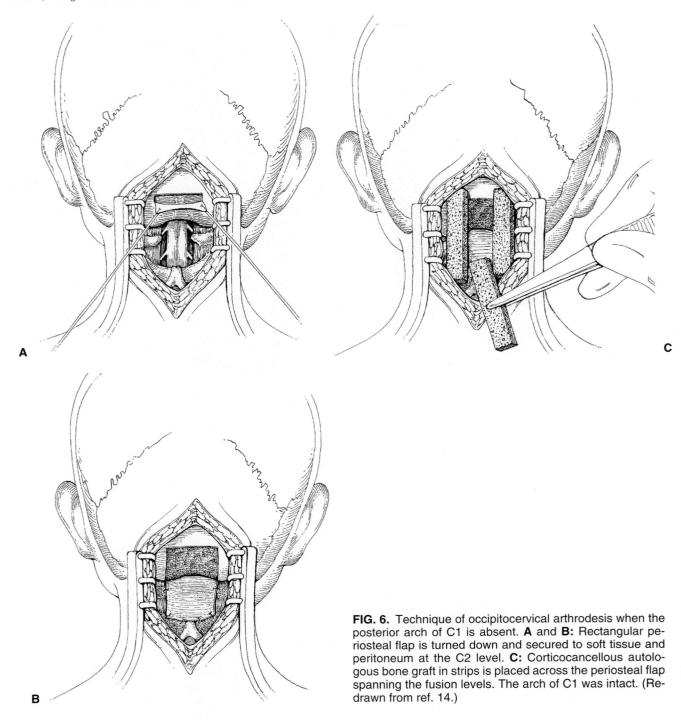

FIG. 6. Technique of occipitocervical arthrodesis when the posterior arch of C1 is absent. **A** and **B:** Rectangular periosteal flap is turned down and secured to soft tissue and peritoneum at the C2 level. **C:** Corticocancellous autologous bone graft in strips is placed across the periosteal flap spanning the fusion levels. The arch of C1 was intact. (Redrawn from ref. 14.)

around large defects, as may be created after tumor excision or decompression, and the ability to span multiple levels. Higo et al. (57) reported four successful occipitocervical fusions in children with Down syndrome; all children were immobilized postoperatively in a hard collar only. The authors site the rigidity of the construct, and thus the lack of need for a halo or other types of postoperative immobilization, as another major advantage of this technique.

FRACTURE OF THE ATLAS (C1)

Fracture of C1 is a relatively rare injury in children (4,58–60). The mechanism of injury is likely an axial load applied to the head, with forces transmitted to the lateral masses of C1 through the occipital condyles (61). The bony ring of C1 is often fractured in several places. However, in children, single fractures have been reported; the ring

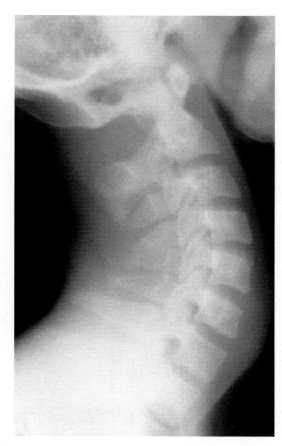

FIG. 7. Occipitocervical fusion using onlay bone graft and a Minerva cast at 4 years follow-up.

may hinge or plastically deform through the synchondroses (59). Rupture or avulsion of the transverse atlantal ligament, with separation of the lateral masses, can result in C1-C2 instability.

Plain radiographs, particularly the odontoid open-mouth view, are helpful in establishing the diagnosis. Overhang of the lateral masses of greater than 7 mm total is indicative of transverse ligament disruption, and potential atlantoaxial instability, in the adult (62). While the equivalent value indicative of instability in children has not been established in the literature, transverse ligament rupture can occur with atlas fractures in children (59). Thin-section axial CT imaging provides useful information regarding fracture displacement and fracture pattern acutely. CT imaging is also helpful for following progression of fracture healing with treatment.

Treatment of fracture of C1 generally consists of Minerva cast or halo immobilization for 8 to 12 weeks. Allen and Ferguson (63) recommended skull traction for 4 to 6 weeks followed by halo immobilization, if initial displacement of the lateral masses as seen on the odontoid radiograph exceeded a value of 4 mm. Upon removal of immobilization, flexion-extension lateral cervical spine views are performed to assess stability of the C1-C2 articulation. Posterior C1-C2 arthrodesis is indicated for persistent instability. Surgery is rarely indicated at the time of acute injury.

ATLANTOAXIAL INJURIES

Acute injuries to the C1-C2 articulation in children are generally one of three types:

1. traumatic ligamentous disruptions

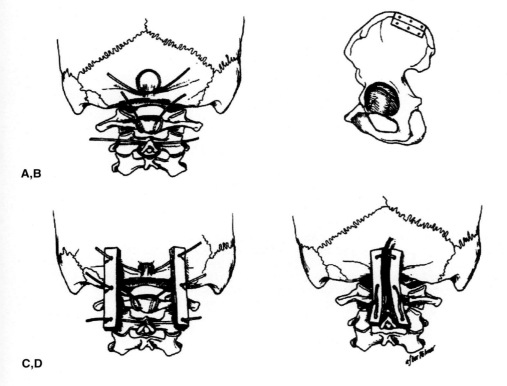

A,B

C,D

FIG. 8. Technique of atlantooccipital arthrodesis with internal fixation. **A:** A wire is looped around the external occipital protuberance at a level 2 cm above the foramen magnum. A towel clip is then used to create a hold in the ridge, and an 18-gauge wire is passed through the hole and twisted over the ridge. A second wire loop is passed around the arch of C1 and a third is passed through and around the base of the spinous process of C2. **B:** The outer table of the iliac crest is used for bone graft. **C:** Drill holes are made in the corticocancellous grafts, and wires are passed through the holes. **D:** The wires are tightened. (From ref. 100, with permission.)

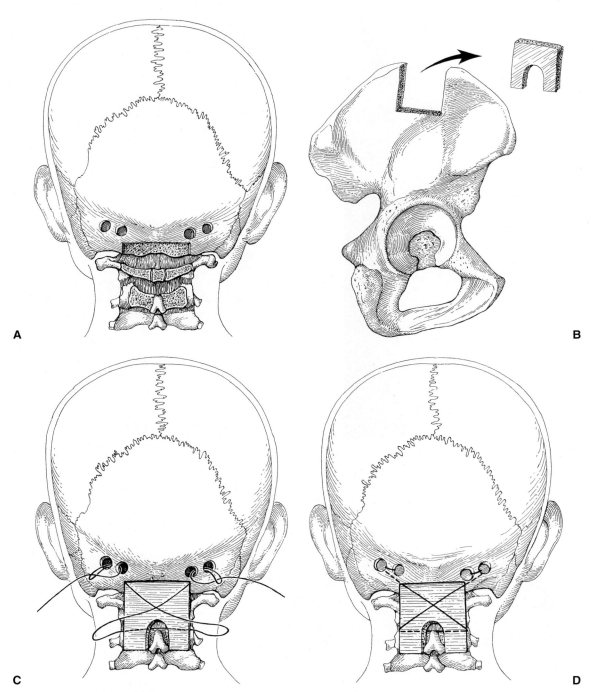

FIG. 9. Atlantooccipital arthrodesis using wires and a contoured graft. **A:** Four burr holes are placed into the occiput in transverse alignment, with two on each side of the midline, leaving a 1-cm osseous bridge between the two holes of each pair. A trough is fashioned into the base of the occiput. **B:** A corticocancellous graft is harvested from the iliac crest and shaped into a rectangle, with a notch created in the base to fit around the spinous process of the second or third cervical vertebra. **C:** Looped 16- or 18-gauge Luque wires are passed through the burr holes and looped on themselves. Wisconsin button wires are passed through the base of the spinous process of either the second or the third cervical vertebra. The graft is positioned into the occipital through and around the spinous process of the cervical vertebra at the caudad extent of the arthrodesis. The graft is locked into place by precise contouring of the bone. **D:** The wires are subsequently crossed, twisted, and cut. (Redrawn from ref. 17.)

2. rotatory atlantoaxial subluxation and dislocation
3. odontoid synchondrosis separations

Cervical flexion and extension, lateral bending, and half of all cervical rotation occur through the atlantoaxial articulation. Stability of this joint is dependent almost entirely on ligaments (64). The spinal canal is large enough at C1 to accommodate this extreme mobility without cord compromise. Steel's (65) rule of thirds states that the canal is occupied equally by the odontoid, the spinal cord, and free space. Encroachment upon this free space by displacement of the atlas a distance equal to the width of the odontoid potentially jeopardizes the spinal cord. The atlas-dens interval is commonly used to quantify the mobility of the atlantoaxial articulation, with 4.5 mm or less considered the normal range in children (6). Mobility of this articulation is also quantified by measuring the space available for the spinal cord (SAC) with flexion and extension of the cervical spine, a value more reflective of the potential for neurologic compromise (66) (Fig. 10). In addition to direct encroachment on the spinal cord, C1-C2 instability can compromise flow in the vertebral arteries, which are fixed in the transverse foramina of C1 and C2; an ischemic injury to the upper cervical cord and cerebellum may result (67,68).

Traumatic Ligamentous Disruption

Isolated transverse atlantal ligament disruption with acute C1-C2 instability is rare (6). CT scanning may be helpful in identifying transverse ligament bony avulsion as well as associated fractures. Initial treatment is reduction in extension followed by immobilization in a Minerva cast or halo vest. Immobilization is continued for 8 to 12 weeks. Upon removal of immobilization, flexion-extension radiographs are performed to document stability. If instability persists, posterior atlantoaxial fusion is indicated.

Atlantoaxial Rotatory Subluxation and Dislocation

Rotational subluxation and dislocation of the C1-2 articulation generally do not occur with significant, acute injury. Instead, this process is more commonly seen after minor trauma associated with upper respiratory or pharyngeal in-

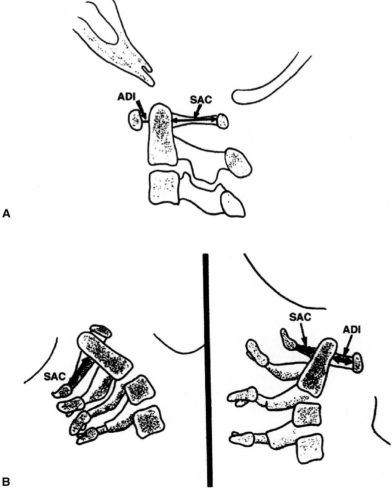

A

B

FIG. 10. Atlantoaxial articulation. **A:** Atlantodens interval (ADI) and the space available for the spinal cord (SAC). **B:** Flexion-extension lateral views of the cervical spine when atlantoaxial instability is present. Note increase in ADI and decrease in SAC with flexion.

fections. Pharyngovertebral veins drain the nasopharynx directly into an epidural and periodontoidal venous plexus. Inflammatory exudate from nasopharyngeal infections creates a hyperemic state about the supporting ligaments and capsule of the atlantoaxial complex. A secondary inflammatory process results. This inflammation may cause capsular and ligamentous laxity, as well as weakening of the fibroosseous attachment of the stabilizing ligaments (69–71). A rotatory subluxation can then easily occur with minor trauma. While most resolve with treatment and resolution of the inciting inflammatory process, some of these subluxations become fixed; entrapment of meniscus-like synovial folds (72) or fixed contracture about this articulation secondary to sustained muscle spasm (73) are possible etiologies of fixed atlantoaxial subluxation. Concomitant atlantoaxial instability may result from progressive laxity and weakening of the transverse atlantal ligament insertion (71).

The typical child with rotatory subluxation presents acutely with painful torticollis. The head is held in the cock-robin position, with the head tilted to one side and rotated to the opposite side. Muscle spasm is noted in the long sternocleidomastoid muscle, i.e., on the side to which the chin is rotated. The child resists attempts to move the head actively or passively. Neurologic findings are rare, unless significant instability is seen. If the subluxation becomes fixed, the deformity and decreased range of motion persist with subsidence of pain. Long-term rotatory fixation can lead to skull and facial asymmetry.

Plain radiographs are often difficult to interpret in patients with atlantoaxial rotatory subluxation because of difficulty in positioning of the head and neck. On the odontoid view, the lateral mass of C1 that is rotated forward appears wider and closer to the midline, while the contralateral lateral mass appears more narrow and laterally offset. Thin-section axial CT scan, done with the child's head maximally rotated to the right and left, is helpful in confirming the diagnosis by documenting loss of rotation between C1 and C2 (74,75). Three-dimensional reconstruction of axial CT images demonstrates the locking of the inferior facet of C1 anteriorly on one side and posteriorly on the opposite side (76). Flexion-extension lateral cervical spine radiographs are necessary to rule out atlantoaxial instability in the sagittal plane.

Fielding and Hawkins (73) classified atlantoaxial rotatory subluxation (Fig. 11). This classification is based on the

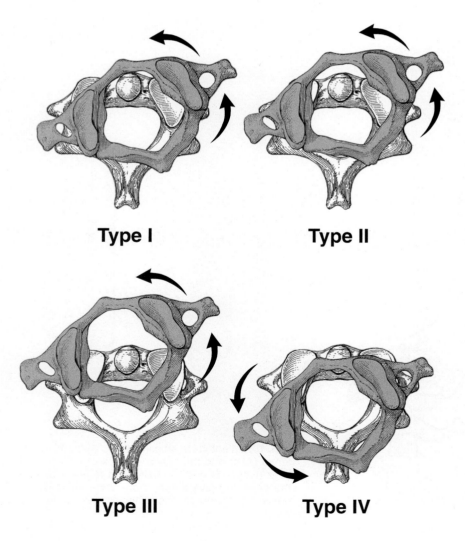

Type I

Type II

Type III

Type IV

FIG. 11. The four types of atlantoaxial rotatory displacement. (Redrawn from ref. 73.)

amount and direction of displacement of the atlas on the axis in the face of rotatory subluxation of C1 on C2. Type I, the most common type, rarely has neurologic complications and responds well to conservative means. Types II, III, and IV are less common. However, the associated atlantoaxial sagittal plane instability increases the potential for neurologic injury.

In children diagnosed with atlantoaxial rotary subluxation within a week of onset of symptoms, treatment with a soft collar and bed rest is sufficient to resolve spasm and deformity. If symptoms persist up to 4 weeks, head halter or tong cervical traction is indicated to effect reduction. The period of traction is followed by a stiff cervical collar for 4 to 6 weeks. If atlantoaxial instability is present, a Minerva cast or halo is recommended for a 6 to 8 weeks to prevent recurrence of deformity and stabilize the C1-C2 articulation (75). Flexion-extension cervical spine views are required posttreatment to document stability of the atlantoaxial complex.

Posterior C1-C2 arthrodesis is indicated for atlantoaxial rotatory subluxation or dislocation (73,75,77) for the following:

1. Persistent instability in the sagittal plane after traction and immobilization.
2. Recurrent rotational deformity after sufficient immobilization.
3. Fixed deformity present longer than 3 months.
4. Progressive neurologic findings.

Odontoid Separation (Synchondrosis Fracture)

Fracture through the odontoid synchondrosis is one of the most common injuries of the cervical spine in children, oc-curring at an average age of 4 years (78). This injury is uncommonly seen after age 7 years, i.e., the approximate age of synchondrosis closure. The mechanism of injury is most commonly a fall from a height or motor vehicle accident (79), but may occur with minor cervical spine trauma. The child often presents complaining of occipital or neck pain, and resists active and passive range of motion of the cervical spine. Neurologic injury is rare, except when a concomitant head injury is present (79,80).

Lateral cervical spine radiograph demonstrates anterior displacement and apex posterior angulation of the odontoid fragment (81). Tomography, sagittal MRI images or thin-section axial CT scan with lateral reconstruction can often detect subtle findings indicative of fracture with minimal displacement. Flexion-extension views of the cervical spine, or flexion-extension MRI evaluation, may be helpful in demonstrating fracture displacement when static images appear normal (82,83).

Treatment of acute odontoid synchondrosis separations is reduction by positioning in extension, followed by immobilization. A Minerva jacket or halo vest is then applied for 6 to 8 weeks (80,84). After removal of immobilization, flexion-extension cervical spine lateral radiographs are performed to document healing and stability of the odontoid separation. Nonunion of the separation and growth disturbance about the basilar synchondrosis are rare complications; the majority of these injuries heal without long-term sequelae (80) (Fig. 12).

Os Odontoideum

Untreated fracture of the odontoid in a child is the likely etiology of the os odontoideum. While not definitively proven,

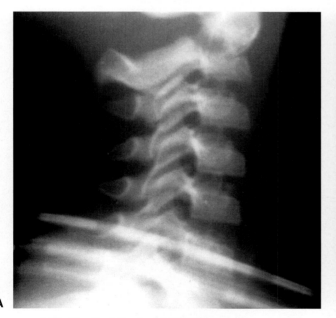
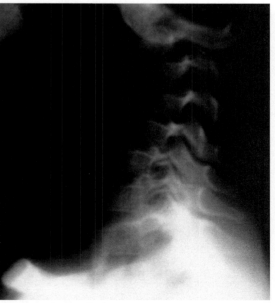

A   **B**

FIG. 12. A: A 7-year-old boy involved in a vehicle accident. Lateral cervical spine view shows C2 synchondrosis fracture. A halo was applied. **B:** At 10 weeks postinjury flexion cervical spine view shows healed synchondrosis fracture. Subaxial instability (C3–C4) is now evident. Posterior subaxial cervical fusion was performed.

it is believed that his lesion represents nonunion of an odontoid fracture, and not a congenital anomaly or failure of fusion of the odontoid summit ossification center (20,85,86) (Fig. 13).

The presence of an os odontoideum may lead to progressive C1-C2 instability. This instability may become symptomatic, manifesting as neck or occipital pain, decreased exercise tolerance, and myelopathy. Posterior C1 and C2 fusion is indicated in the symptomatic patient with instability. In the asymptotic patient with documented radiographic instability greater than 4.5 mm, treatment recommendations are unclear. Flexion-extension MRI (29), or neurophysio-

logic studies done with the child's cervical spine in flexion and extension, may be helpful in documenting subclinical, but potentially dangerous, cord impingement. Posterior cervical fusion is recommended if subclinical cord compression is noted in the face of a normal examination. Careful discussion with the family of the risks and benefits of observation versus immediate fusion is necessary.

Atlantoaxial Posterior Cervical Arthrodesis

The most commonly used techniques for atlantoaxial posterior fusion are the Gallie technique (87), with modifications,

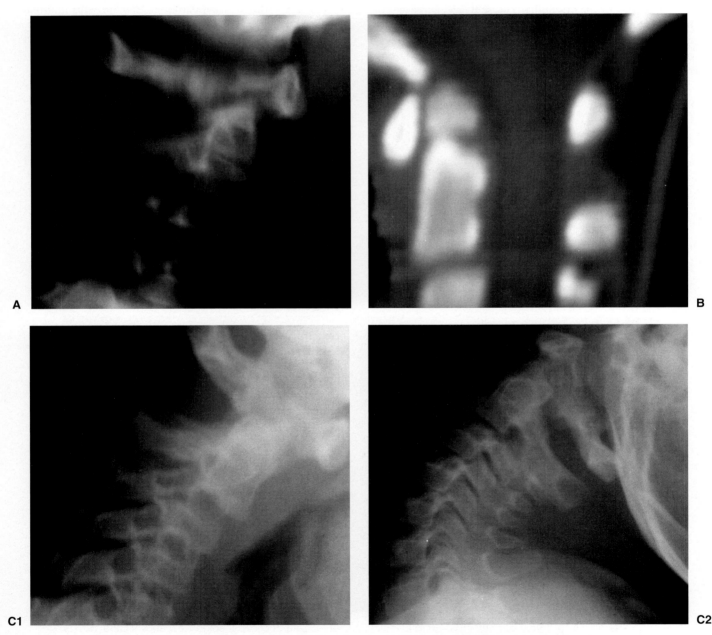

FIG. 13. A: An 11-year-old boy with 8 months of neck pain. Lateral view of the cervical spine shows os odontoideum. **B:** Lateral reconstruction of axial computed tomography (CT) scan image of same patient. **C:** Flexion *(1)* and extension *(2)* lateral cervical spine views show instability at C1–C2.

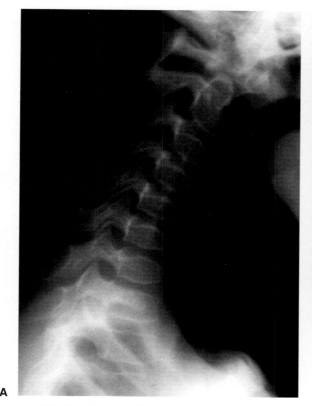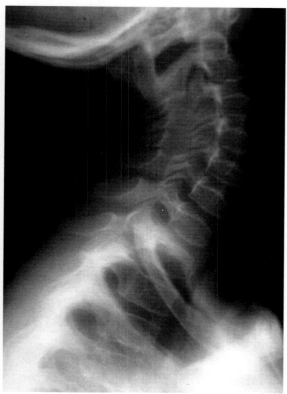

FIG. 14. Flexion **(A)** and extension **(B)** lateral cervical spine views 1 year after C1–C2 posterior spinal fusion using onlay bone graft and halo fixation.

and the Brooks-Jenkins technique (88). The Gallie technique may present less risk to the neural elements because the C2 spinous process is used for fixation instead of sublaminar wiring. The Brooks technique requires passage of sublaminar wires at C1 and C2, but theoretically provides better rotational stability (89). In younger children, i.e., less than 4 to 6 years of age, passage of sublaminar wires may be difficult because of limited space available. Overly aggressive wire tightening must be avoided to prevent cut-out of the wires through small laminae. In this younger age group, onlay bone graft followed by immobilization may be all that is required to achieve fusion (Fig. 14).

Gallie Technique

A halo is applied after induction of general anesthesia. The patient is then placed prone on a frame or modified operating table. Alternatively, a Mayfield headrest may be used to position the head and align the cervical spine. A lateral cervical spine radiograph is taken to confirm adequate cervical alignment.

Through a midline posterior incision, the lower occiput to C2 are identified; only those levels to be included in the fusion are exposed. Infiltration of the midline dermis and subcutaneous tissue with epinephrine solution enhances homeostasis. Deep exposure is achieved by splitting the avascular midline ligamentum nuchae. The posterior arch of C1 and the lamina of C2 are exposed subperiosteally; the dissection is extended no more than approximately 1 cm laterally from the midline. An 18- to 20-gauge wire loop is placed under the arch of C1 from caudad to cephalad. A corticocancellous graft is harvested and placed on the arch of C1 and the lamina of C2, beneath the wire. The wire is then looped around the C2 spinous process and the ends are tightened down over the bone graft (Fig. 15). The wound is closed in layers.

A Minerva cast or halo jacket is applied for 8 to 12 weeks postoperatively. After removal of the immobilization, lateral cervical spine flexion-extension views are recommended to document atlantoaxial stability and solid fusion.

Brooks-Jenkins Technique

Positioning and exposure are as above. Two 18- to 20-gauge sublaminar wires are passed cephalad to caudad under the laminae of C1 and C2 sequentially. Two premeasured, rectangular-shaped iliac crest full-thickness grafts are then harvested. The grafts are shaped to fit between the laminae of C1 and C2, so as to prevent hyperextension of the ring of C1 on C2. The wires on each side of the midline are twisted over the grafts and tightened (Fig. 16).

Immobilization and aftercare are as described above.

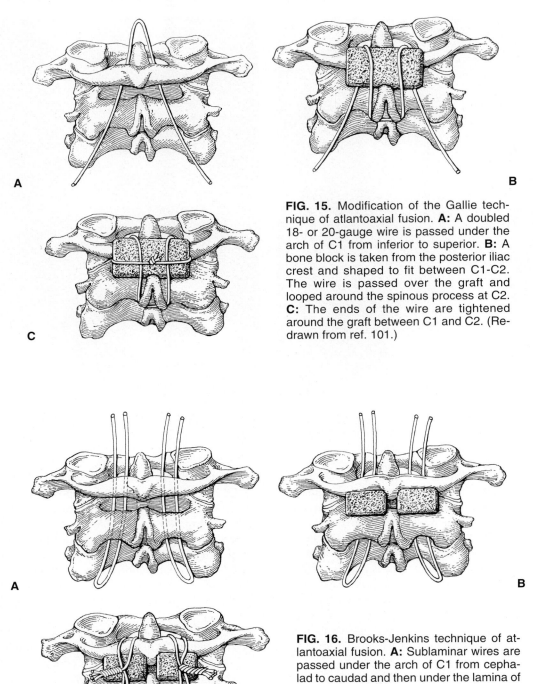

FIG. 15. Modification of the Gallie technique of atlantoaxial fusion. **A:** A doubled 18- or 20-gauge wire is passed under the arch of C1 from inferior to superior. **B:** A bone block is taken from the posterior iliac crest and shaped to fit between C1-C2. The wire is passed over the graft and looped around the spinous process at C2. **C:** The ends of the wire are tightened around the graft between C1 and C2. (Redrawn from ref. 101.)

FIG. 16. Brooks-Jenkins technique of atlantoaxial fusion. **A:** Sublaminar wires are passed under the arch of C1 from cephalad to caudad and then under the lamina of C2. **B:** Rectangular-shaped iliac crest bone grafts are harvested and contoured to fit between the arch of C1 and the lamina of C2. **C:** The wires are tightened over the grafts (Redrawn from ref. 101.)

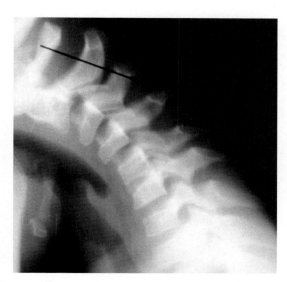

FIG. 17. Normal lateral flexion view of the cervical spine in a 7-year-old. Swischuk's line is drawn. Note pseudosubluxation at C2-C3, and incomplete ossification of vertebral bodies.

C2 SPONDYLOLISTHESIS (HANGMAN'S FRACTURE)

Spondylolisthesis of C2 has been reported uncommonly in young children (29,90). In the largest series, five bilateral C2 pedicle fractures in children 6 to 18 months of age were reported with no neurologic injuries seen (90). The mechanism of injury is likely similar to that in the adult, i.e., hyperextension.

Radiographic evaluation of a suspected C2 pedicle fracture may be difficult in the immature spine. The neurocentral synchondroses of C2 persist through approximately age 7 years. This structure, when viewed obliquely, can mimic an acute pedicle fracture (91).

Differentiation of physiologic hypermobility, i.e., pseudosubluxation, from true subluxation accompanying C2 pedicle fractures can be challenging. Swischuk's posterior laminar line, drawn from C1 to C3, is a helpful guide (Fig. 17). With cervical flexion, the body of C2 moves anteriorly on C3. In the normal child with physiologic hypermobility, Swischuk's line passes within 1 mm of the C2 lamina, despite the anterior displacement of C1 on C2. If this line passes greater than 2 mm anterior to the C2 lamina, pathologic subluxation secondary to a C2 pedicle fracture must be considered (25) (Fig. 18).

Treatment of the Hangman's fracture in the child and adolescent is similar to that in the adult. Gentle reduction, followed by immobilization in a Minerva cast, halo jacket, or custom orthosis for a 6- to 8-week period, is recommended. Fracture healing and stability of the C1-C2 articulation is documented by flexion-extension lateral cervical radiographs. In the rare case of acute instability, progressive neurologic deterioration, or chronic instability following appropriate immobilization, posterior cervical C1-C2 fusion is indicated.

SUBAXIAL CERVICAL INJURIES (C3 TO C7)

Injuries below C3 in young children are much less common than in adults (2,4,7). The cervical spine achieves an adult anatomic configuration at approximately age 8 years. Adult-like injuries to the subaxial spine occur in children older than 8 years of age, as behavioral patterns, spinal anatomy, and biomechanical properties approach those of the adult (4). With the exception of physeal injuries of the vertebral bodies, traumatic subaxial cervical spine injuries in older children and adolescents are approached in a fashion similar to those seen in adults.

Physeal Injuries

Physeal injuries through the cervical vertebral endplates are unique to the skeletally immature cervical spine. Salter-Harris I fractures of the inferior cervical endplate occur in infants and young children, associated with high-energy trauma or abuse; Salter-Harris III fractures of the vertebral endplates occur most commonly in adolescents (92). The incidence of these type of injuries is unknown, as spontaneous reduction of these physeal fractures likely occurs. Aufdermaur (33) demonstrated this injury in 12% of juvenile autopsy specimens by applying distraction to the cadaver spine. Aside from subtle widening of the vertebral interspace, plain radiographs appear normal.

Treatment of physeal vertebral injuries, if stable, is immobilization in a Minerva cast or halo jacket. The more stable type III injuries heal after 4 to 6 weeks of immobilization. Type I injuries are generally unstable. In the child who survives this injury, operative stabilization has been advocated (61).

Wedge-Compression Fractures

Wedge-compression fractures are the most common fractures of the subaxial pediatric spine (4,6). Cervical flexion, combined with axial loading, results in compression of the vertebral body anteriorly, sparing injury to the more resilient vertebral disc. Radiographic findings include loss of vertebral body height and cervical kyphosis. This injury is often not diagnosed because the wedge-compression fracture is interpreted as a normal finding in the younger child with incompletely ossified, wedge-shaped vertebral bodies. Associated injuries, including anterior teardrop fracture, lamina fracture, and spinous process fracture with widening, are suggestive of posterior ligamentous injury and potential instability.

Treatment of simple wedge-compression fractures is immobilization in a rigid collar for a 4- to 6-week period. Upon removal of immobilization, flexion-extension lateral cervical radiographs are recommended to confirm stability. If associated injuries are seen and potential instability is suspected at the time of acute injury, a halo jacket or Minerva cast is recommended. Posterior spinal fusion is indicated only for significant acute instability or residual instability postimmobilization.

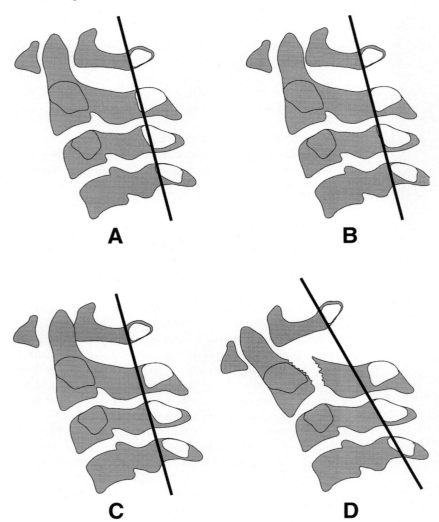

FIG. 18. Posterior laminar line of Swischuk. The normal posterior laminar line on flexion radiograph can **(A)** pass through or just behind the anterior cortex at the arch of C2, **(B)** touch the anterior aspect of the cortex at the arch of C2, **(C)** come within 1 mm of the anterior aspect of the cortex at the arch of C2. **D:** Displacement of this line greater than 2 mm anterior to the anterior aspect of the cortex at the arch of C2 is indicative of instability associated with fracture of the C2 pedicle. (Redrawn from ref. 25.)

Facet Dislocation

Unilateral and bilateral facet dislocations are the second most common significant injuries seen in the subaxial spine after compression fractures (4,6). Most of these injuries occur in the adolescent. The mechanism and injury patterns are similar to those seen in adults. Most unilateral facet dislocations, with or without fracture, can be reduced manually, or with traction. Bilateral facet dislocations represent a more severe structural injury and are frequently associated with neurologic complications. Closed reduction by traction is indicated initially. Postreduction immobilization with a halo jacket or Minerva cast is recommended. Irreducible unilateral and bilateral facet dislocations, and those injuries with significant instability or progressive neurologic findings postreduction, require open reduction and posterior cervical fusion.

Posterior Ligamentous Injuries

Flexion injuries to the subaxial spine rarely result in isolated posterior ligamentous disruption in the immature cervical spine (4). The child or adolescent with lower cervical tenderness and normal initial radiographs of the cervical spine should be immobilized in a hard collar. Repeat physical examination with flexion-extension lateral cervical spine views, after the initial cervical paraspinal spasm has subsided, is indicated to rule out instability secondary to ligamentous disruption. Documented instability requires posterior cervical fusion, as the healing potential of the posterior ligaments is limited.

Subaxial Cervical Fusion

Posterior subaxial cervical fusion is indicated for instability in the lower cervical spine. Modifications of wire fixation techniques are used commonly in the child and adolescent (93–95). Anterior decompression prior to posterior fusion is indicated only in patients with associated vertebral disc herniation or severe anterior instability, such as that seen after tumor resection or severe compression fractures. Anterior decompression with anterior fusion is a consideration in rare cases (96).

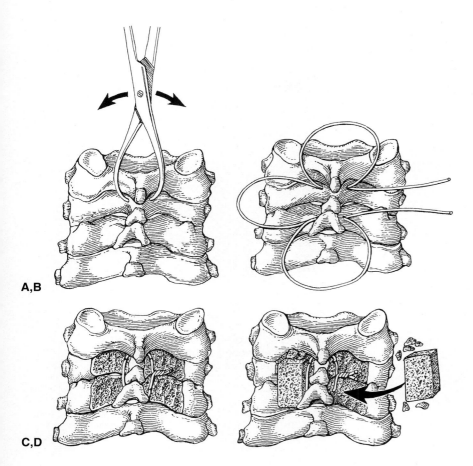

FIG. 19. Technique of subaxial cervical fusion. **A:** Holes are made in the base of the spinous processes to be fused. **B:** Wires are passed through the holes and around each spinous process. **C:** The wires are twisted together. **D:** Corticocancellous graft is placed, spanning the levels to be fused. (Redrawn from ref. 95.)

Subaxial Posterior Fusion with Wire Fixation

A halo is applied after induction of general anesthesia. The patient is then placed prone on a frame or modified operating table. Alternatively, a Mayfield head rest may be used to position the head and align the cervical spine. A lateral cervical spine radiograph is taken to confirm adequate cervical alignment.

Through a midline incision, the spinous processes and laminae are exposed subperiosteally to the facet joints laterally. Care is taken to expose only those levels to be included in the fusion. A towel clip is used to make a hole in the base of the cephalad spinous process. An 18- to 20-gauge wire is passed through this hole, looped around the spinous process,

and then back through the hole. A similar hole is created in the base of the adjacent spinous process to be fused. The end of the wire is passed through this second hole, looped around the spinous process at this level, and then passed back through this second hole. The wire ends are then twisted together and tightened. Corticocancellous iliac crest bone graft is placed on the exposed laminae and spinous processes (Fig. 19). Alternatively, a second and third wire are passed through the holes in the base of the spinous processes and through drill holes in the corticocancellous graft to secure the graft in place (Fig. 20).

A rigid cervical collar, halo vest, or Minerva cast is applied postoperatively for a 6- to 8-week period. Flexion-extension lateral radiographs are recommended upon removal

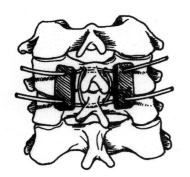
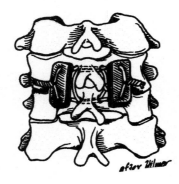

FIG. 20. Modification of subaxial fusion technique using three wires. The levels are wired together as described (see Fig. 19). A second and third wire are passed through the holes in the base of the spinous processes. The wires are then passed through drill holes in the corticocancellous graft and twisted together to secure the grafts in place. (From ref. 101.)

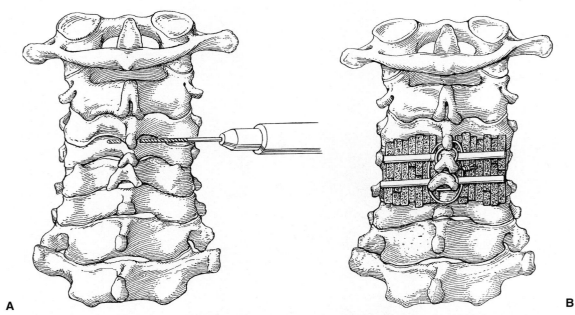

FIG. 21. Subaxial cervical fusion using supplemental fixation. **A:** Drill holes are placed through the base of the spinous processes. Kirschner wires are then placed. **B:** Wires are then looped around the spinous processes, using the Kirschner wires for additional stability. A corticocancellous graft is then placed around the construct, spanning the fusion levels. (Redrawn from ref. 94.)

of immobilization to document the stability of the levels fused.

As an alternative method, a Kirschner wire is placed through the base of the spinous processes to be fused. A 16- to 18-gauge wire is looped around the Kirschner wires in a figure-eight configuration (94,97) (Fig. 21). For younger children with small spinous processes, *in situ* fusion can be done using onlay bone graft without internal fixation. Fusion is readily achieved; care must be taken to place bone graft only over the desired fusion levels to prevent extension of the fusion.

REFERENCES

1. Hadley MN, Zabramski JM, Browner CM, Rekate H, Sonntag VKH. Pediatric spinal trauma: review of 122 cases of spinal cord vertebral column injuries. *J Neurosurg* 1988;68:18–24.
2. Henrys P, Lyne ED, Lifton C, Salciccioli G. Clinical review of cervical spine injuries in children. *Clin Orthop* 1977;129:172–176.
3. Kewalramani LS, Kraus JF, Sterling HM. Acute spinal-cord lesions in a pediatric population: epidemiological and clinical features. *Paraplegia* 1980;18:206–219.
4. McGrory BJ, Klassen RA, Chao EY, et al. Acute fracture and dislocations of the cervical spine in children and adolescents. *J Bone Joint Surg* 1993;75A:988–995.
5. Pang D, Wilberger JE. Spinal cord injury without radiologic abnormalities in children. *J Neurosurg* 1982;57:114–129.
6. Jones ET, Hensinger RN. *Injuries of the Cervical Spine in Fractures in Children*. Philadelphia: Lippincott-Raven, 1996.
7. Birney TJ, Hanley EN. Traumatic cervical spine injuries in childhood and adolescence. *Spine* 1989;14:1277–1282.
8. Apple JS, Kirks DR, Merten DF, Martinez S. Cervical spine fractures and dislocations in children. *Pediatr Radiol* 1987;17:45–49.
9. McPhee IB. Spinal fractures and dislocations in children and adolescents. *Spine* 1981;6:533–537.
10. Bailey DK. The normal cervical spine in infants and children. *Radiology* 1952;59:712–719.
11. Sherk HH, Schut L, Lane JM. Fractures and dislocations of the cervical spine in children. *Orthop Clin North Am* 1976;7:593–604.
12. Evans DL, Bethem D. Cervical spine injuries in children. *J Pediatr Orthop* 1989;9:563–568.
13. Hubbard DD. Injuries of the spine in children and adolescents. *Clin Orthop* 1974;100:56–65.
14. Koop SE, Winter RB, Lonstein JE. The surgical treatment of instability of the upper part of the cervical spine in children and adolescents. *J Bone Joint Surg* 1984;66A:403–411.
15. McGrory BJ, Klassen RA. Arthrodesis of the cervical spine for fractures and dislocations in children and adolescents. *J Bone Joint Surg* 1994;76A:1606–1616.
16. Smith MD, Phillips PA, Hensinger RA. Fusion of the upper cervical spine in children and adolescents: an analysis of 17 patients. *Spine* 1991;16:695–701.
17. Dormans JD, Drummond DS, Sutton LN, et al. Occipitocervical arthrodesis in children. *J Bone Joint Surg* 1995;77A:1234–1240.
18. Ogden JA. Radiology of postnatal skeletal development: XII. The first cervical vertebra. *Skeletal Radiol* 1984;12:12–20.
19. Cattell HS, Filtzer DL. Pseudosubluxation and other normal variations in the cervical spine in children. *J Bone Joint Surg* 1965;47A:1295–1309.
20. Fielding JW, Hensinger RN, Hawkins RJ. Os odontoideum. *J Bone Joint Surg* 1980;62A:376–383.
21. Huerta C, Griffith R, Joyce SM. Cervical spine stabilization in pediatric patients: evaluation of current techniques. *Ann Emerg Med* 1987;16:1121–1126.
22. Herzenberg JE, Hensinger RN, Dedrick DK, Phillips WA. Emergency transport and positioning of young children who have an injury of the cervical spine: the standard backboard may be hazardous. *J Bone Joint Surg* 1989;71A: 15–22.
23. Curran C, Dietrich AM, Bowman MJ, et al. Pediatric cervical spine immobilization: achieving neutral position. *J Trauma* 1995;39(4):729–732.
24. Hadden WA, Gillespie WJ. Multiple level injuries of the cervical spine. *Injury* 1985;16:628–633.
25. Swischuk LE. Anterior displacement of C2 in children: physiologic or pathologic? *Radiology* 1977;122(suppl 2):759–763.

26. Locke GR, Gardner JI, Van Epps EF. Atlas-dens interval (ADI) in children: a survey based on 200 normal cervical spines. *AJR Radium Ther Nucl Med* 1966;97:135–140.

27. Ardan GM, Kemp FH. The mechanisms of changes in form of the cervical airway in infancy. *Med Radiogr Photogr* 1968;44:26–38.

28. Anderson LD, Smith BL, DeTorre J, et al. The role of polytomography in the diagnosis and treatment of cervical spine injuries. *Clin Orthop Rel Res* 1982;165:64–68.

29. Weng MS, Haynes RJ. Flexion and extension cervical MRI in a pediatric population, *J Pediatr Orthop* 1996;16:359–363.

30. Dickman CA, Zambranski JM, Hadley M, et al. Pediatric spinal cord injury without radiographic abnormalities: report of 26 cases and review of the literature. *J Spinal Disord* 1991;4:296–305.

31. Osenbach RK, Menezes AH. Spinal cord injury without radiographic abnormality in children. *Pediatr Neurosci* 1989;15:168–175.

32. Yngve DA, Harris WP, Herndon WA, Sullivan JA, Gross RH. Spinal cord injury without osseous spine fracture. *J Pediatr Orthop* 1988;8:153–159.

33. Aufdermaur M. Spinal injuries in juveniles: necropsy findings in twelve cases. *J Bone Joint Surg* 1974;56B:513–519.

34. Ruge JR, Sinson GP, McLone DG, Cerullo LJ. Pediatric spinal injury: the very young. *J Neurosurg* 1988;68:25–30.

35. Walsh JW, Stevens DB, Young AB. Traumatic paraplegia in children without contiguous spinal fracture or dislocation. *Neurosurgery* 1983;12:439–445.

36. Bucholz RW, Burkhead WZ. Pathological anatomy of fatal atlanto-occipital dislocations. *J Bone Joint Surg* 1979;61A:248–250.

37. Bucholz RW, Burkhead WZ, Graham W, Petty C. Occult cervical spine injuries in fatal traffic accidents. *J Trauma* 1979;19:768–771.

38. Collalto PM, DeMuth WW, Schwentker EP, Boal DK. Traumatic atlanto-occipital dislocation. *J Bone Joint Surg* 1986;68A:1106–1109.

39. Davis D, Bohlman H, Walker AE, Fisher R, Robinson R. The pathological findings in fatal cranio-spinal injuries. *J Neurosurg* 1971;34:603–613.

40. Donahue DJ, Muhlbauer MS, Kaufman RA, et al. Childhood survival of atlanto-occipital dislocation: underdiagnosis, recognition, treatment and review of the literature. *Pediatr Neurosurg* 1994;21:105–111.

41. Evarts CM. Traumatic occipito-atlantal dislocation: report of a case with survival. *J Bone Joint Surg* 1970;52A:1653–1660.

42. Georgopoulos G, Pizzutillo PD, Lee MS. Occipito-atlantal instability in children. *J Bone Joint Surg* 1987;69A:429–436.

43. Montane I, Eismont FJ, Green BA. Traumatic occipito-atlantal dislocation. *Spine* 1991;16:112–116.

44. Zigler JE, Waters RL, Nelson RW, et al. Occipito-cervico-thoracic spine fusion in a patient with occipito-cervical dislocation with survival. *Spine* 1986;11:645–646.

45. Wholey MH, Bruwer AJ, Baker HL Jr. The lateral roentgenogram of the neck, with comments on the atlanto-odontoid-basion relationship. *Radiology* 1958;71:350–356.

46. Powers B, Miller MD, Kramer RS, Martinez S, Gehweiler JA Jr. Traumatic anterior atlanto-occipital dislocation. *Neurosurgery* 1979;4:12–17.

47. Price AE. *Unique Aspects of Pediatric Spine Injuries in Spinal Trauma*. Philadelphia: JB Lippincott, 1991.

48. Eismont FJ, Bohlman HH. Posterior atlanto-occipital dislocation with fractures of the atlas and odontoid process. *J Bone Joint Surg* 1978;60A:397–399.

49. Weisel SW, Rothman RH. Occipito-atlantal hypermobility. *Spine* 1979;4:187–191.

50. Grantham SA, Dick HM, Thompson RC Jr, Stinchfield FE. Occipito-cervical arthrodesis: indications, technique and results. *Clin Orthop* 1969;65:118–129.

51. Hamblem DL. Occipito-cervical fusion. Indications, technique and results. *J Bone Joint Surg* 1967;49B:33–45.

52. Wertheim SB, Bohlman HH. Occipitocervical fusion. Indications, technique, and long-term results in thirteen patients. *J Bone Joint Surg* 1987;69A:833–836.

53. Letts M, Slutsky O. Occipito-cervical arthrodesis in children. *J Bone Joint Surg* 1990;72A:1166–1170.

54. Ito T, Tsuji H, Katoh Y, et al. Occipito-cervical fusion reinforced by Luque's segmental spinal instrumentation for rheumatoid diseases. *Spine* 1988;13:1234–1238.

55. Malcolm GF, Ransford AO, Crockard HA. Treatment of non-rheumatoid occipitocervical instability: internal fixation with the Hartshill-Ransford loop. *J Bone Joint Surg* 1994;76B:357–366.

56. Ransford AO, Crokard HA, Pozo JL, Thomas NP, Nelson IW. Craniocervical instability treated by contoured loop fixation. *J Bone Joint Surg* 1986;68B:173–178.

57. Higo M, Sakov J, Taketoni E, Kojyo T. Occipitocervical fusion by Luque loop rod instrumentation in Down syndrome. *J Pediatr Orthop* 1995;15:539–542.

58. Marlin AE, Gayle RW, Lee JF. Jefferson fractures in children. *J Neurosurg* 1983;58:277–279.

59. Mikawa Y, Watanabe R, Yamano Y, Ishii K. Fractures through a synchondrosis of the anterior arch of the atlas. *J Bone Joint Surg* 1987;69B:483.

60. Tolo VT, Weiland AJ. Unsuspected atlas fractures and instability associated with oropharyngeal injury: case report. *J Trauma* 1979;19:278–280.

61. Ogden JA. *Skeletal Injury in the Child*. Philadelphia: WB Saunders, 1990.

62. Spence KF, Decker S, Sell KW. Bursting atlantal fracture associated with rupture of the transverse ligament. *J Bone Joint Surg* 1970;52A:543–549.

63. Allen BL, Ferguson RL. Cervical spine trauma in children. In: Bradford DS, Hensinger RN, eds. *The Pediatric Spine*. New York: Thieme, 1985:89–104.

64. Fielding JW, Cochran GVB, Lawsing JF III, Hohl M. Tears of the transverse ligament of the atlas: a clinical and biomechanical study. *J Bone Joint Surg* 1974;56A:1683–1691.

65. Steel HH. Anatomical and mechanical consideration of the atlanto-axial articulation. In: Proceedings of the American Orthopaedic Association. *J Bone Joint Surg* 1968;50A:1481–1482.

66. Hensinger RN. Osseous anomalies of the craniovertebral junction. *Spine* 1986;11:323.

67. Dommisse GF. *The Arteries and Veins of the Human Spinal Cord from Birth*. New York: Churchill-Livingstone, 1975.

68. Gabrielsen TO, Maxwell JA. Traumatic atlanto-occipital dislocation, with case report of a patient who survived. *AJR* 1966;97:624–629.

69. Lippmann RK. Arthropathy due to adjacent inflammation. *J Bone Joint Surg* 1953;35A:967–979.

70. Parke WW, Rothman RH, Brown MD. The pharyngovertebral veins: an anatomical rationale for Grisel's syndrome. *J Bone Joint Surg* 1984;66A:568–574.

71. Watson-Jones R. Spontaneous hyperemic dislocation of atlas. *Proc R Soc Med* 1932;25:586–590.

72. Kawabe N, Hirotani MH, Tanaka O. Pathomechanism of atlantoaxial rotatory fixation in children. *J Pediatr Orthop* 1989;9:569–574.

73. Fielding JW, Hawkins RJ. Atlanto-axial rotatory fixation. *J Bone Joint Surg* 1977;59A:37–44.

74. Fielding JW, Stillwell WT, Chynn KY, Spyropoulos EC. Use of computed tomography for the diagnosis of atlanto-axial rotatory fixation. *J Bone Joint Surg* 1978;60A:1102–1104.

75. Phillips WA, Hensinger RN. The management of rotatory atlanto-axial subluxation in children. *J Bone Joint Surg* 1989;71A:664–668.

76. Scapinelli R. Three-dimensional computed tomography in infantile atlantoaxial rotatory fixation. *J Bone Joint Surg* 1994;76B:367–370.

77. Nerubay J, Lin E, Weiss J, Level A, Katznelson A, Tadmor R. Post-traumatic atlantoaxial rotatory fixation. *J Pediatr Orthop* 1985;5:734–736.

78. Seimon LP. Fracture of the odontoid process in young children. *J Bone Joint Surg* 1977;59A:943–948.

79. Dunn ME, Seljeskog EL. Experience in the management of odontoid process injuries: an analysis of 128 cases. *Neurosurgery* 1986;18:306–310.

80. Sherk HH, Nicholson JT, Chung SMK. Fractures of the odontoid process in young children. *J Bone Joint Surg* 1978;60A:921–924.

81. Bhattacharya SK. Fracture and displacement of the odontoid process in a child. *J Bone Joint Surg* 1974;56A:1071–1072.

82. McAfee PC, Bohlman HH, Han JS, Salvagno RT. Comparison of nuclear magnetic resonance imaging and computed tomography in the diagnosis of upper cervical spinal cord compression. *Spine* 1986;11:295–304.

83. Roach JW, Duncan D, Wenger DR, Maravilla A. Atlanto-axial instability and spinal cord compression in children: diagnosis by computed tomography. *J Bone Joint Surg* 1984;66A:708–714.

84. Grogono BJS. Injuries of the atlas and axis. *J Bone Joint Surg* 1954;36B:397–410.

85. Fielding JW, Griffin PP. Os odontoideum: an acquired lesion. *J Bone Joint Surg* 1974;56A:187–190.

86. Hawkins RJ, Fielding JW, Thompson WJ. Os odontoideum: congenital or acquired? *J Bone Joint Surg* 1976;58A:413–414.

87. Gallie WE. Fractures and dislocations of the cervical spine. *Am J Surg* 1939;46:495–499.

88. Brooks AL, Jenkins EB. Atlantoaxial arthrodesis by wedge compression method. *J Bone Joint Surg* 1978;60A:279–284.

89. Montesano P, Juach E. Anderson P, et al. Biomechanics of cervical spine fixation. *Spine* 1991;16(suppl 3):510–516.

90. Pizzutillo PD, Rocha EF, D'Astous J, Kling TF, McCarthy RE. Bilateral fractures of the pedicle of the second cervical vertebra in the young child. *J Bone Joint Surg* 1986;68A:892–896.

91. Swischuk LE, Hayden CK Jr, Sarwar M. The dens-arch synchondrosis versus the hangman's fracture. *Pediatr Radiol* 1979;8: 100–102.

92. Lawson JP, Ogden JA, Bucholz RW, Hughes SA. Physeal injuries of the cervical spine. *J Pediatr Orthop* 1987;7:428–435.

93. Bohlman HH. Acute fractures and dislocations of the cervical spine. *J Bone Joint Surg* 1979;61A:1119–1142.

94. Hall JE, Simmons ED, Danylchuk K, et al. Instability of the cervical spine and neurological involvement in Klippel-Feil syndrome: a case report. *J Bone Joint Surg* 1990;72A:460–462.

95. Weiss JC, McAfee PC. Lower cervical spine arthrodesis: Wiring technique. In: *The Cervical Spine*, the Cervical Spine Research Society. Philadelphia: Lippincott-Raven, 1998:487–498.

96. Shacked I, Ram Z, Haddon M. The anterior cervical approach for traumatic injuries to the cervical spine in children. *Clin Orthop Rel Res* 1993;292:144–150.

97. Davey JR, Rorabeck CH, Bailey SI, et al. A technique of posterior cervical fusion for instability of the cervical spine. *Spine* 1985;10:722–728.

98. Bulas DI, Fitz H, Roberts JM, et al. Chronic atlantoaxial instability in Down's syndrome. *J Bone Joint Surg* 1985;67A:1356.

99. Gabriel K, Mason D, Carang P. Occipito-atlantal translation in Down's Syndrome. *Spine* 1990;15:997–1002.

100. An H. Internal fixation of the cervical spine: current indications and techniques. *J Am Acad Orthop Surg* 1995;3:194–206.

Surgery of Spinal Trauma,
edited by J.M. Cotler, J.M. Simpson, H.S. An, and C.P. Silveri.
Lippincott Williams & Wilkins, Philadelphia © 2000.

CHAPTER 15

Injuries of the Pediatric Thoracolumbar Spine

Randall T. Loder

Injuries of the thoracic and lumbar spine in children are rare compared to adults, and pediatric spine fractures account for 2% to 5% of all spinal injuries (1–5). The actual incidence of pediatric thoracolumbar spine injuries may be greater than reported since the statistics are skewed toward the more severe injuries; many children with mild injuries are never admitted to the hospital (6,7). The mechanism of injury often varies with the age of the child. Thoracolumbar spine fractures in infancy are frequently due to abuse. In the first decade of life they are typically from motor vehicle accidents or falls from heights (8–12). In the second decade of life they typically occur from sports or recreational activities (e.g., bicycles, motorcycles, and motor vehicle accidents (13–18). Injuries due to gunshot wounds are also increasing (19).

Anatomic and biomechanical differences in the pediatric spine influence both the radiographic appearance of the spine as well as the type of fractures that occur. The anatomic differences are an increased cartilage-bone ratio and the presence of secondary ossification centers; the biomechanical differences are soft tissue hyperelasticity and more mineralized bone in the vertebral bodies of children compared to older adults.

In the infant horizontal conical shadows of lessened density extend inward from both the anterior and posterior walls of the vertebral bodies. These shadows represent vascular spaces and can be confused with a fracture (Fig. 1) (20). The posterior indentation represents the foramen for the posterior arteries and veins in the vertebral wall; it is present in all vertebrae and at all ages. The more noticeable anterior conical shadow represents a large sinusoidal space within the vertebra. This anterior notch usually disappears by age 1 year with ossification of the anterior and lateral walls of the vertebral bodies. In infancy and early childhood, the vertebral bodies are largely cartilaginous and the intervertebral disc spaces radiographically appear larger than they are (Fig. 1). With maturation the ossification center of the centrum enlarges and the cartilage-vertebral body ratio reverses.

The vertebral apophyses are secondary centers of ossification that develop in the cartilaginous endplates at the superior and inferior surfaces of the vertebral bodies. They radiographically appear between 8 and 12 years of age, and normally fuse with the vertebral bodies by age 21. They are thicker at the periphery than at the center, and thus appear as a ring with early ossification; hence they are called "ring" apophyses. These apophyses are equivalent to the epiphyses of a long bone, separated from the vertebral body by a narrow cartilaginous physis; vertical growth of the vertebral body occurs at these physes. They can be radiographically confused with an avulsion fracture.

In children the elasticity of the discs and vertebral bodies far exceeds that of the neural elements. This elasticity partially accounts for the occurrence of the SCIWORA syndrome (spinal cord injury without objective radiographic abnormality) in younger children (2,7,9,12,13,21–23). By age

R. T. Loder: Section of Orthopaedic Surgery, University of Michigan School of Medicine, Ann Arbor, Michigan 48109-0328.

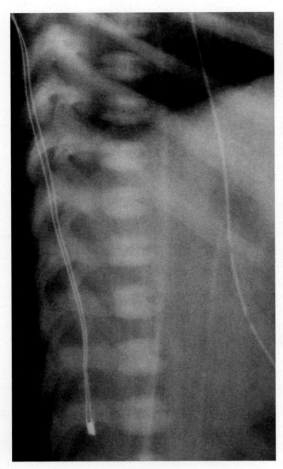

FIG. 1. The lateral radiograph of a normal spine of an infant born prematurely at 36 weeks of gestation. Since the superior and inferior vertebral endplates and vertebral apophyses are cartilaginous, there is an apparent widening of the intervertebral spaces relative to the ossific portion of the vertebrae. The anterior and posterior notching of the walls of the vertebral body are due to normal vascular channels and may be confused with fracture.

10 years, the mechanical and anatomic characteristics of the bony thoracolumbar spine approach that of the adult, and the fracture patterns become the same.

CLASSIFICATION OF INJURIES TO THE PEDIATRIC THORACOLUMBAR SPINE

Fractures and Dislocations

Injury Mechanism

The three main mechanisms are flexion with or without compression, distraction, and shear. Compression injuries due to hyperflexion are more common than distraction, shear, or subluxation/dislocation injuries (11,24). In the immature spine, the intact disc is more resistant to vertical compression than the vertebral body. During compression of the immature spine, the vertebral body always breaks before the normal discs fail. This is supported clinically by the fact that

there are few children with posteriorly herniated discs, and only after significant loading injuries (25,26).

With slow vertebral loading, the major distortion is a bulge in the endplate, with only a slight change in the annulus and no change in the shape of the nucleus pulposus (27). This endplate bulging squeezes blood out of the cancellous bone, acting as a shock-absorbing mechanism. With continuing compression of the endplate fractures, nuclear material ruptures into the vertebral body, and the two vertebrae come closer.

In older children, the nucleus polposus is no longer fluid, and compression forces are transmitted through the annulus. This results in either tearing of the annulus with collapse of the vertebral body, or a marginal plateau fracture (27). When larger forces are applied more rapidly, a bursting type injury may occur, similar to that in adults (Fig. 2). The vertebral disc of a child is more elastic and transmits the force through multiple levels (7,18,24,27). This is reflected by the clinical fact that multiple compression fractures are more common in children (Fig. 3) than adults (4,10,24,28). These usually occur in the midthoracic to midlumbar areas (10,11,29). In children who have suffered violent accidents, such as being hit by a car, thoracolumbar spine injuries are primarily of the shear type (1) (Fig. 4). The vertebrae typically fracture through the endplate apophysis. These injuries may also be associated with flexion and rotation, which leads to shearing and often traumatic spondylolisthesis.

A specific injury is the Chance fracture, named after its description by Chance (30) in 1948. Smith and Kaufer (31) clarified it as an injury to the lumbar spine associated with seat belts; forward flexion over the belt distracts the posterior vertebral elements, leading to a ligamentous disruption of the interspinous ligaments, ligamentum flavum, and facet capsules. The middle and anterior columns may fail through either soft tissues (posterior longitudinal ligament and disc) or bone (vertebral body or endplate). If the fulcrum of rotation is slightly posterior to the anterior margin of the vertebral body, there may be a slight component of anterior vertebral body compression. This injury, previously uncommon in children (32), is increasing with the more frequent use of lap belts in children due to seat-belt restraint laws (33,34). A reverse Chance fracture, i.e., a hyperextension injury, has also been described in children (35–37), often infants. A fracture through the posterior elements alone without lumbar body fracture has also been reported in children and adults (38).

Physical Examination

In the alert and cooperative child, complaints of pain suggest a spinal injury. In older children, pain and tenderness of the spine is usually present. Inability to walk and muscle spasms are often present with unstable injuries of the spine. In the multiply injured child a significant vertebral fracture can be easily overlooked, and a high index of suspicion must be maintained at all times for the possibility of vertebral injury

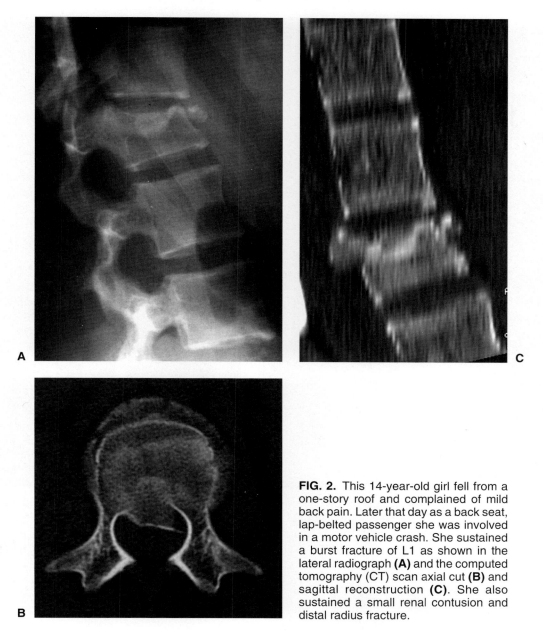

FIG. 2. This 14-year-old girl fell from a one-story roof and complained of mild back pain. Later that day as a back seat, lap-belted passenger she was involved in a motor vehicle crash. She sustained a burst fracture of L1 as shown in the lateral radiograph **(A)** and the computed tomography (CT) scan axial cut **(B)** and sagittal reconstruction **(C)**. She also sustained a small renal contusion and distal radius fracture.

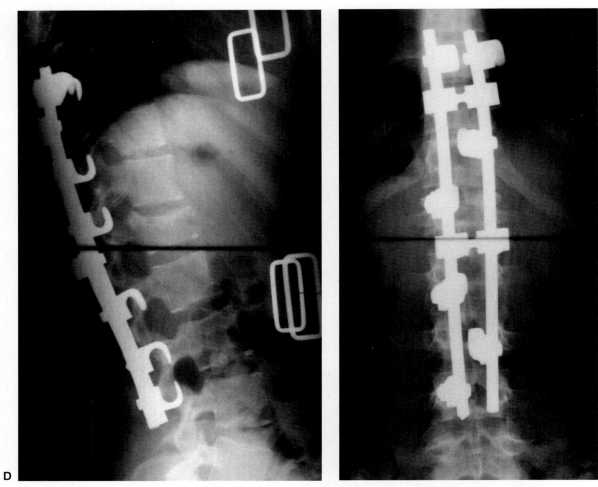

FIG. 2. *Continued.* Three days later she underwent posterior spinal fusion and instrumentation: lateral radiograph **(D)** and posteroanterior radiograph **(E)**. Note the correction of the traumatic kyphosis and partial restoration of vertebral body height.

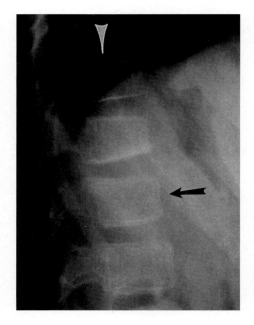

FIG. 3. This 7-year, 4-month-old girl fell 8 feet from a jungle gym, landing on her back. She complained of significant back pain but initial radiographs were normal. Three weeks after her fall she was entirely asymptomatic; a repeat lateral radiograph demonstrates minimal compression fractures at T12 *(white arrowhead)* and L1. Also note the flattening of the vertebral endplates at L2 *(arrow)* and L3, with slight irregularity of the cortical margins, which also represents minimal compression deformities.

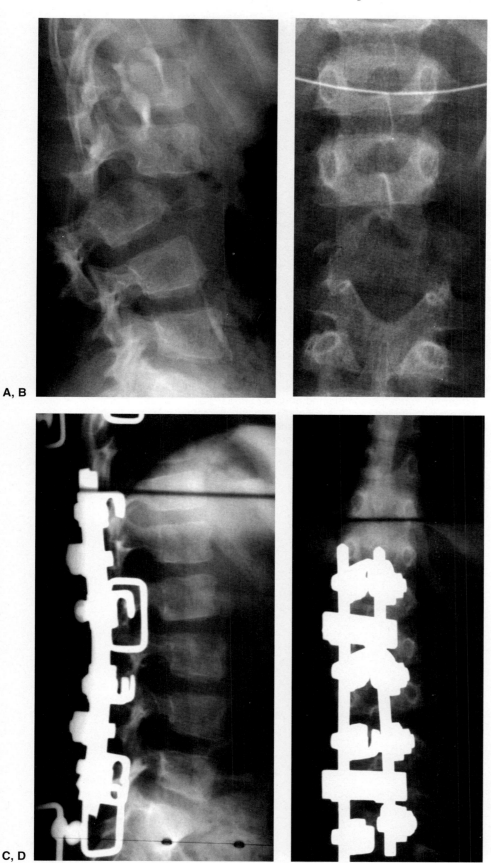

FIG. 4. This 6-year, 8-month-old girl was a seat belt–restrained passenger involved in a head-on motor vehicle crash. She sustained a fracture-dislocation at the L2-3 level [lateral radiograph **(A)** and anteroposterior radiograph **(B)**] with complete and permanent paraplegia. She also sustained facial injuries and a mesenteric hematoma. Three days after injury an open reduction, posterior instrumentation, and spinal fusion was performed: lateral radiograph **(C)** and posteroanterior radiograph **(D)**. By 1 year after injury she had 3+ power in her right quadriceps and 4+ power in her left quadriceps muscles and was developing paresthesias in the feet.

A, B

C, D

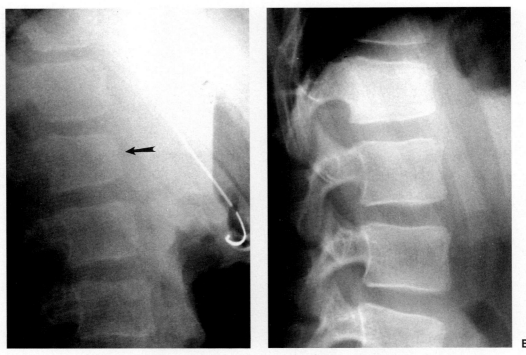

FIG. 5. This 13-year-old boy fell 12 feet from a tree, landing on a sidewalk. He sustained a left parietal skull fracture and subdural hematoma and a contusion of the left frontal region. His initial Glasgow Coma Score was 7. Upon awakening from the coma, he complained of upper lumbar pain. The lateral radiograph demonstrates subtle compression anteriorly at L2 *(arrow)* **(A)**. He was immobilized with a thoracolumbar spinal orthosis (TLSO). The lateral radiograph 8 weeks after injury **(B)** demonstrates the same vertebral body compression; also, healing callus with its increased radiodensity is now seen. This increased sclerosis is frequently the only sign of a subtle pediatric compression fracture involving the thoracolumbar spine.

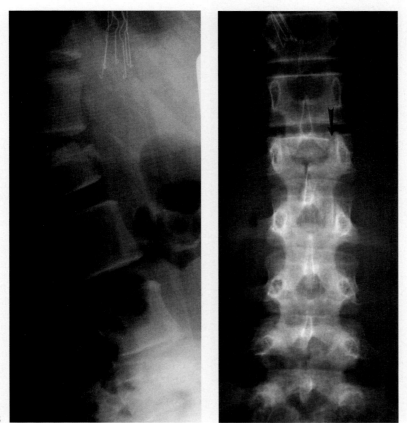

FIG. 6. This 16-year-old girl was an unrestrained passenger involved in a motor vehicle crash and ejected from the car. She sustained bilateral femur fractures, compression fractures at L1 and L5, and a burst fracture at L2: lateral radiograph **(A)** and posteroanterior radiograph **(B)**. Note the widening of the interpedicular distance **(B)**; the fracture and compression of the superior vertebral endplate can also be seen *(arrow)*.

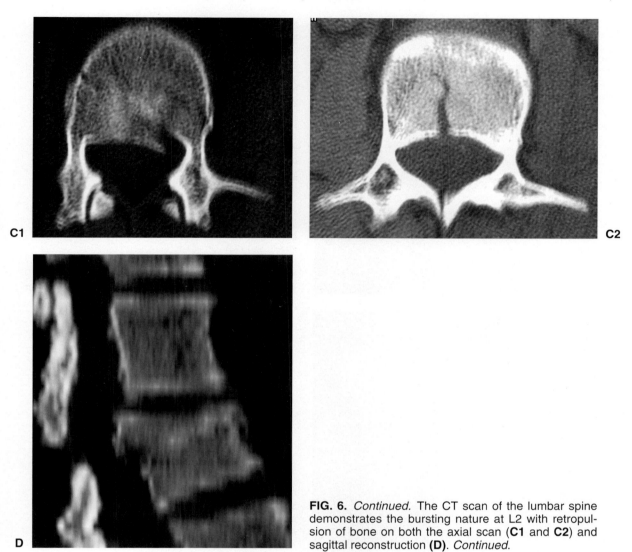

FIG. 6. *Continued.* The CT scan of the lumbar spine demonstrates the bursting nature at L2 with retropulsion of bone on both the axial scan (**C1** and **C2**) and sagittal reconstruction (**D**). *Continued.*

when dealing with seriously injured children (39,40) (Figs. 5 and 6). The possibility of multiple, noncontiguous, vertebral fractures must also be remembered in the severely injured patient (41–44) (Fig. 6). Fractures of the lumbar or thoracic transverse processes, although innocuous appearing, are often associated with serious abdominal injury (20%), particularly to the spleen and liver, pelvis, urinary tract, or chest (39,45–51). In children with lap-belt injuries, 50% to 90% have intraabdominal pathology (33,52,53), especially small bowel ruptures and traumatic pancreatitis (Fig. 7). Ecchymosis in a lap-belt distribution should always alert the clinician to search for a Chance fracture (54). In some series (53,55), the abdominal injuries are so severe that they dominate the early clinical picture with late detection of the spinal injury. These children often have marked soft tissue swelling, bruising, and tenderness along the posterior spinal area.

Neurologic Injury

From 9% to 15% of all spinal cord injuries occur in children, with males predominating (2:1) (7,11,56). In the young child

the lesion is more often at the cervicothoracic junction (23) and the neurologic injury is more likely permanent. The teenager is more likely to have a transient or an incomplete neurologic deficit that resolves or improves (4). Delayed onset of paraplegia (2 hours to 4 days) may represent a vascular insult to the spinal cord (57). Vascular insults are typically at the midportion of the thoracic spine (watershed area), and usually associated with a blow to the chest or abdomen, resulting in shock or profound hypotension from internal injuries. Complete and permanent paraplegia is the typical outcome. In the older child a vertebral fracture is the most common cause of neurologic injury (83%) (7). Fracture-dislocations are most common, usually at the thoracolumbar junction (36%), with the remainder between T4 and L2 (4,7,10,11,24,58). The risk of neurologic injury increases with canal narrowing: spinal canal stenosis of 35% at T11-12, 45% at L1, and 55% at L2 and below are significant factors for neurologic impairment (59). In Chance fractures, neurologic injuries are typically uncommon, although in one series 3 of 10 children had a paraplegia (53). This may be re-

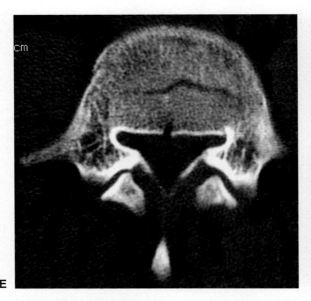

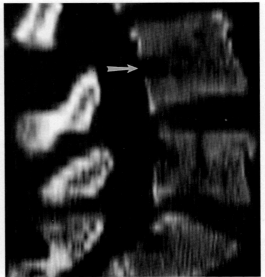

E   F

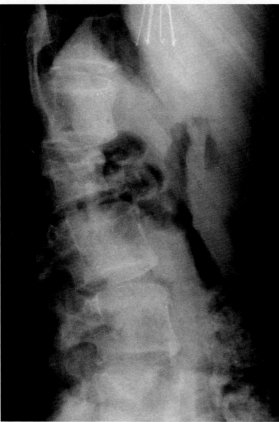

G

FIG. 6. *Continued.* Similarly, the compression fracture of L5 without bony retropulsion is also demonstrated on both the axial scan **(E)** and sagittal reconstruction **(F)**. On the sagittal reconstruction **(F)** also note the comminuted, nondisplaced fracture of the L4 vertebral body *(white arrow)*, which was not appreciated on the plain radiographs. She was neurologically intact. Within the first 24 hours of injury severe adult respiratory distress syndrome (ARDS) developed and subsequently pulmonary emboli occurred, which resulted in a prolonged course of ventilatory support with placement of an inferior venal caval filter. By the time her respiratory status had stabilized, significant healing of the spine fractures had occurred. Thus only orthotic management was prescribed for mobilization. At age 18 follow-up radiographs demonstrate healed fractures with no change in the lumbar kyphosis **(G)**. She was asymptomatic regarding her back and had no neurologic symptoms.

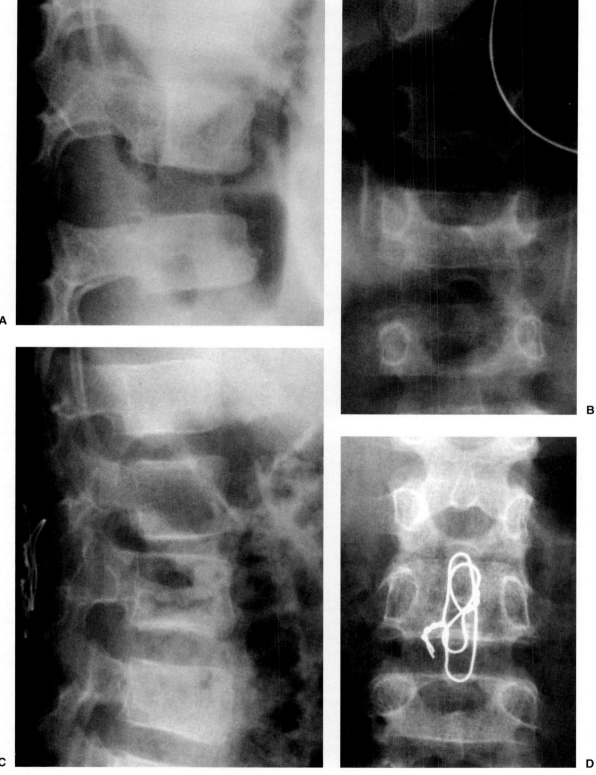

FIG. 7. This 5-year, 3-month-old boy was on the passenger side of a pick-up truck, sitting on his mother's lap. The lap belt was across his abdomen. The truck was involved in a motor vehicle crash. He complained of back pain; the radiographs demonstrate a ligamentous Chance injury: lateral radiograph **(A)** and anteroposterior radiograph **(B)**. A posterior spinal fusion with interspinous process wiring was performed with supplementary pantaloon spica cast immobilization. Radiographs 4 years later demonstrate solid fusion: lateral **(C)** and posteroanterior **(D)**.

lated to the higher center of gravity in children (34), resulting in an increased moment arm and greater distraction, contributing to the development of paraplegia.

Several problems peculiar to children may result in diagnostic errors unless careful clinical and radiographic examinations are performed. The most serious is failure to recognize paralysis, either complete or partial. This may prove difficult in a frightened, hurt, uncooperative child. Gross flexion or reflex withdrawal of the limbs may mislead the clinician into thinking that voluntary movement is present. Serial observations over time may be necessary to determine the true neurologic status of the patient. Somatosensory evoked potentials may be helpful in the difficult case (60).

Many children have been reported (particularly those under age 10) with SCIWORA (2–4,7,9,12,13,21–23,58,61–65). SCIWORA occurs in 5% to 55% of all pediatric spinal cord injuries (64,22). The immature and elastic pediatric spine is much more deformable than that of an adult. Momentary displacement from external forces may endanger the spinal cord without disrupting bone or ligaments. The injury is a combination of hyperextension, flexion, distraction, and spinal cord ischemia. Ischemia may arise from direct cord contusion or vascular insufficiency (66). The neurologic deficit may range from complete cord transection to partial cord deficits; the cervical and thoracic spine are nearly equal in incidence (64). Neurologic loss is more often complete in younger children (0–8 years). Thoracic lesions tend to be neurologically complete in younger children (92%) compared to adolescents (50%). Lumbar lesions are quite rare and tend to be incomplete in all age groups (27). By definition no disruption, malalignment, or other abnormalities are seen on plain radiographs. Physiologic disruption of the spinal cord is not necessarily associated with anatomic disruption. The exact pathoanatomy is unknown; magnetic resonance imaging (MRI) does not always show cord transection, and myelography often shows only cord edema.

Imaging Studies

Compression is the most common finding, ranging from slight flattening of the normally convex endplates (Fig. 3) to frank wedging of the vertebra (Figs. 5 and 6). Compression fractures in children are classified by their appearance as wedge-shaped or beak-shaped, with upper or lower prominent anterior contours (10). Both types may be asymmetric on the sagittal view as well as the frontal view. There may be a zone of increased density in the vertebral body due to compression and overlapping of the trabecular bone (10,11). Multiply damaged vertebrae are common (Fig. 3), but clinically observable kyphosis is uncommon without a fracture-dislocation (Fig. 4) (10). True fracture lines are seldom seen in the prepubertal child. Avulsed vertebral corners, commonly seen in the adult, are rarely seen in children (62). If the amount of force is significant, the endplate ruptures and the disc is extruded into the vertebral body, forming a Schmorl's node, typically in the lower thoracic and upper lumbar vertebrae (67).

Adult fracture patterns, such as subluxation or fracture-dislocation, are less common in children, and more common in adolescents. As in the adult, computed tomography (CT) scans and sagittal reconstructions are more accurate in detecting posterior arch fractures and retropulsed bone with spinal canal narrowing (68,69) (Figs. 2 and 6). The CT cuts must be at right angles to the vertebral bodies, or the lesion will be confused with a pseudofracture (68).

Pediatric Chance fractures are more frequent in the midlumbar spine (L1–L3) compared to the thoracolumbar junction in adults. This may be related to the higher center of gravity in children (34). Routine lateral radiographs are the best way of making the diagnosis (Fig. 7). All children thought to have an abdominal injury in association with a seat belt should have lateral spine radiographs (70). There are four types of pediatric Chance fractures (Fig. 8) (53). Avulsion of spinous processes often extends over several vertebral levels, often with anterior compression fractures. Posteriorly, facet dislocations are more common than laminar fracture. CT scans do not usually demonstrate the presence of this injury, since the cuts are in the same plane as the hori-

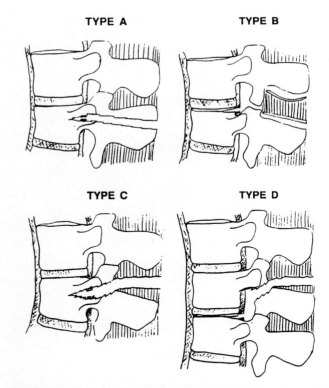

FIG. 8. Seat-belt fracture patterns in skeletally immature children. Type A is a bony disruption of the posterior column extending just into the middle column. Type B is an avulsion of the posterior elements with facet joint disruption or fracture and extension into the apophysis of the vertebral body. Type C is a posterior ligamentous disruption with a fracture line entering the vertebra close to the pars interarticularis and extending into the middle column. Type D is a posterior ligamentous disruption with a fracture line traversing the lamina and extending into the apophysis of the adjacent vertebral body. (From ref. 53, with permission.)

zontal fracture and dislocations, and should only be used when further information is needed regarding bony fragments within the canal or injury to the osseous posterior arch. If there is concern for the gastrointestinal tract, appropriate imaging is advised.

Magnetic resonance imaging is the study of choice in imaging the cord or cauda equina for injury (23,34,57,71–76). The presence of internal fixation is not a contraindication to the MRI scan. However, false-negative and false-positive MRI scans may occur. There are three types of MRI patterns on the T2-weighted images seen in acute spinal cord injuries. Type I is a decreased signal consistent with acute intraspinal hemorrhage; type II is a bright signal consistent with acute cord edema, and type III is a mixed signal of central hypointensity and peripheral hyperintensity, consistent with contusion. Type I patients show no improvement in Frankel class, whereas types II and III frequently improve at least one Frankel grade (72).

Spondylolysis

Spondylolysis at L5-S1 has an anatomic incidence of 5% in the general population. There are supporting data to favor both a developmental and congenital origin for its etiology. Congenital deficiency of the sacrum and lack of integrity of the posterior structures, on a genetic basis, may predispose to spondylolysis. Developmental factors such as trauma, posture, or certain repetitive activities may lead to a stress fracture of the pars interarticularis.

Only one infant has been discovered to have a pars interarticularis defect (77). However, there are other factors that support a congenital origin (78–80). An increase among family members and certain ethnic groups has been reported by numerous authors, with an incidence of 27% to 69% in near relatives, versus an expected frequency of 4% to 8% in the general population (81,82). There is a racial and gender difference, with the lowest incidence in black females, and the highest (6.4%) in white males. People with spondylolysis have an increased incidence of sacral spina bifida (28% to 42%) and congenital lack of development of the proximal sacrum and superior sacral facets (81–83).

Since spondylolysis usually occurs in children after walking age (most typically at 7 or 8 years), trauma is a likely etiologic factor (78,84–86). In the laboratory spondylolysis can be produced only by a high degree of forced hyperflexion (87). The pars interarticularis lesion is not produced in infant cadavers despite vigorous flexion and extension (78). Although minor trauma is common (50% of males and 25% of females) and often initiates the onset of symptoms, seldom is the injury severe (83,88–90). Rather, the onset of symptoms coincides closely with the adolescent growth spurt (83,90,91).

Spondylolysis likely represents a "stress" or fatigue fracture of the pars interarticularis (86,92). A fatigue fracture can occur at physiologic loads during cyclic flexion-extension motion of the lumbar spine (92). Lumbar lordosis, accentu-ated by the normal hip flexion contractures of childhood (93), focuses the force of weight bearing on the pars interarticularis, leading to gradual disruption (94). Anatomic studies suggest that shear stresses are greater on the pars interarticularis when the spine is extended (92,94). In young people, the pars interarticularis is thin, the neural arch has not reached its maximum strength, and the intervertebral disc is less resistant to shear (95). These stresses may be further accentuated by lateral flexion movements on the extended spine, as in gymnastics (92,94). Spondylolysis is four times more frequent (11%) in female gymnasts than in nongymnasts (5); many initially have normal x-rays and later develop spondylolysis. The connection of spondylolisthesis with human activities that increase physiologic lumbar lordosis, such as gymnastics and football, is supported by the unusual finding and prevalence of spondylolisthesis seen in children with myelomeningocele. The prevalence increased from 1.5% for children at the L1-2 level to 15.6% for children at the L5-S1 level (96). This increasing prevalence with increasing neurologic function reflects the higher functional demands at the lumbosacral articulation as the child's ambulatory capability increases. It also reflects the increasing lordotic posture seen in these lower level myelomeningocele children.

Acute spondylolysis may also occur with sudden and uncustomarily heavy loads (86,93). The defect may either heal or develop into a pseudarthrosis with persistent symptoms and the radiographic appearance of spondylolysis. An increased incidence has been noted in teenagers with thoracolumbar Scheuermann's disease, a condition believed to be caused by excessive and repetitive mechanical loading on the immature spine (97). Similarly, thoracolumbar kyphosis is often associated with a compensatory increase in lumbar lordosis. An increased incidence has been noted in those performing heavy physical work, such as weight lifters, lumbermen, and football linemen (98,99).

Spondylolysis commonly occurs in late childhood or early adolescence, yet symptoms are relatively uncommon in children or teenagers (88,100). Only 13% of children known to have spondylolysis develop symptoms before 18 years of age (100). For the occasional child who may develop symptoms, the onset usually coincides with the adolescent growth spurt (88,90).

Although pain is the major complaint in adults, a significant number of children do not have pain and seek medical attention only because of a postural deformity or gait abnormality due to hamstring tightness. When present, pain is generally localized to the low back and, to a lesser, extent, the posterior buttocks and thighs (88,90). Symptoms are usually initiated or aggravated by strenuous activity of the spine common to many different sporting activities. They can also be aggravated by incorrect sporting technique or too rapid an advancement in the sport. Symptoms are usually decreased by rest and activity limitation (5,88,92,101).

Physical examination may demonstrate some tenderness to palpation in the region of the low back. There may be

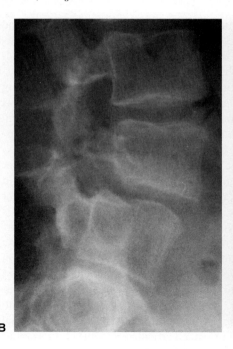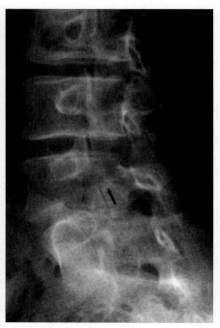

A, B

FIG. 9. This 12-year, 7-month-old boy had a progressive history of low back pain and intermittent leg pain. The lateral radiograph **(A)** demonstrates a grade I spondylolisthesis at the L5-S1 level. The oblique radiograph **(B)** profiles the lytic isthmic defect *(arrow),* or break in the neck of the "Scotty dog."

some splinting, guarding, and restriction of side-to-side motion in the low back, particularly if the condition is of acute onset. Children, unlike adults, seldom have objective signs of nerve root compression such as motor weakness, reflex changes, or sensory deficits (91), although a careful search for sacral anesthesia and bladder dysfunction should be performed. Children with spondylolysis rarely have myelographic evidence of disc protrusion; in those children explored for herniation, none was found (88,91,102). Hamstring tightness (so-called spasm) is commonly found in the symptomatic patient (80%) with diminished forward flexion of the hips, and may be found in patients with spondylolysis or with all grades of spondylolisthesis. It is thought by some to be a sign of nerve root irritation. However, there is no evidence to support this contention (84,91, 103). Hamstring tightness is seldom accompanied by neurologic signs (84,88,90).

Spondylolysis, the radiolucent defect in the pars interarticularis, can be seen on nearly all x-rays of the lumbar spine when large. If unilateral, as it occurs in 20% of patients, or not accompanied by spondylolisthesis, it can be a very subtle finding (85,104), and oblique views of the lumbar spine are often necessary. If oblique views are not obtained in young symptomatic patients, the diagnosis will be missed 20% of the time (104). The "Scotty dog" of Lachapele with the defect appearing at the terrier's neck is a helpful visual aid to those inexperienced with oblique x-rays (Fig. 9). In an acute injury, the gap is narrow with irregular edges, whereas in the long-standing lesion the edges are smooth and rounded, suggesting a pseudarthrosis. The width of the gap depends on the amount of bone resorption following the fracture and the degree of spondylolisthesis.

Less commonly, children may have poorly developed pos-

terior structures, or the dysplastic type of spondylolysis [type I of Wiltse et al. (80)]. This is a common type in symptomatic children (26% to 35%) (105). Because of anomalous development, the posterior facets appear to subluxate on the sacral facets. In children with the dysplastic type, the pars interarticularis becomes attenuated like pulled taffy rather than as a gap or defect in the pars interarticularis. This type has been termed the "greyhound" of Hensinger et al. (88); a defect may later appear in the center. Both the dysplastic and spondylolytic types likely represent the same disease process, as both lesions are present in members of the same family (85,82). The spondylolytic type is likely an acute stress fracture of the par interarticularis, and the dysplastic or elongated type a chronic stress reaction with gradual attenuation of the pars.

Deficiency of the posterior elements is common in spondylolysis. Dysraphic or malformed laminae have been found in 32% to 94% of these patients, and if discovered on routine lumbosacral views, should prompt a more detailed radiographic investigation (82). CT scanning is rarely indicated in an acute fracture of the pars interarticularis, as a combination of bone scan and oblique films will more reliably detect the lesion (106). Similarly, spondylolysis at L4 or L3 is more difficult to diagnose with CT scans because the plane of scanning is parallel to the fracture (107). An MRI should be considered if the patient's symptoms or neurologic signs do not resolve with bed rest. Bladder or bowel dysfunction or perineal hypesthesia also warrants an MRI scan.

Sherman et al. (108) described the unusual appearance of reactive sclerosis and hypertrophy of the pedicle and lamina and contralateral spondylolysis in the same vertebral segment. They appearance suggest that this condition represents a physiologic response to stress, the result of repeated trauma in the presence of an unstable neural arch. This condition responds to conservative measures and symptomatic treatment. Radiologically, this condition may be confused with the reactive sclerosis of an osteoid osteoma, which is important because excision of a sclerotic pedicle that is associated with a contralateral spondylolysis may increase instability. The presence of a nidus on the CT scan should confirm the diagnosis of an osteoid osteoma. A bone scan is not helpful in differentiating between the two, as both exhibit increased uptake due to the presence of increased bone activity.

When the diagnosis is suspected clinically, but cannot be confirmed radiographically (particularly those in the stress reaction stage before fracture), a bone scan is helpful, especially the single photon emission computed tomography (SPECT) scan (29,109). Bone scans always demonstrate an area of increased bone turnover due to the healing fracture. Positive bone scans are found to be associated with the short clinical history and may demonstrate increased uptake in those patients whose symptoms are of only 5 to 7 days' duration (106,110). The bone scan is also helpful in distinguishing between those with an established nonunion and those in whom healing is still progressing and who may benefit from immobilization (92,110). The bone scan is not recommended in those whose symptoms are of more than 1 year's duration or for those who do not have symptoms (110). The bone scan is particularly helpful to those caring for the young athlete whose activities are highly associated with spondylolysis, such as gymnastics (5). Early detection of the stress reaction may lead to appropriate treatment measures, and, as a consequence, shorten the recovery period. Similarly, the bone scan can be used to assess recovery and can be performed before the athlete returns to competition (5).

Lumbar Apophyseal Injury

The slipped vertebral apophysis, unique only to adolescents, probably represents a pure compression injury. These patients are usually adolescent boys with traumatic displacement of a lumbar vertebral ring apophysis into the spinal canal and associated disc protrusion (111–115). The displacement typically arises from the posterior inferior rim of L4, and less commonly the inferior rim of L3 or L5. The age and circumstances under which this injury occurs are analogous to the slipped capital femoral epiphysis (116), suggesting that the vertebral endplate is more susceptible during the phases of rapid growth. Both chronic and acute forms have been described, and the problem is often erroneously diagnosed as a herniated disc due to the similarity of symptoms (117,118). There is a high association (38%) with lumbar Scheuermann's disease (117); the preexisting marginal Schmorl's node may weaken the edge and lead to a slip of the apophysis (118).

Slipped vertebral apophysis typically follows a traumatic incident such as weight lifting, gymnastics, or shoveling (116). Acutely these children have signs and symptoms of a central herniated nucleus pulposus, including neurologic findings such as muscle weakness, absent reflexes, and positive straight leg raising (118). Late findings are similar to that of spinal stenosis.

In children with slipped vertebral apophysis, a small bony fragment (the edge of the vertebral endplate) is seen within the spinal canal. CT has proven to be an excellent technique to confirm the diagnosis (117–119). The fracture can be classified into three types (Fig. 10) (120). Type I is a separation of the posterior rim of the involved vertebra and a calcified arc on CT scan with no evidence of associated large bony fracture. Type II is an avulsion fracture of part of the vertebral body, annular rim, and cartilage. Type

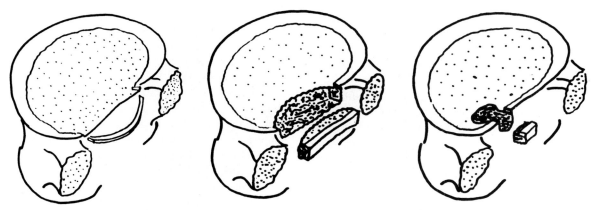

FIG. 10. Schematic representation of the three types of avulsion fractures. In type I *(left)*, an arcuate fragment is found, but no osseous defect is seen at the posterior rim of the vertebral body. Type II *(middle)* is an avulsion fracture of the posterior rim of the vertebral body that includes a rim of bone. The fragment is not arcuate, and it is thicker than in type I. The sharply avulsed osseous edge is recognized on CT. Type III *(right)* is a localized fracture posterior to an irregularity of the cartilage endplate. The osseous defect anterior to the fragment, as depicted on CT, is larger than the fragment. (From ref. 120, with permission.)

III is more localized and includes smaller posterior irregularities of the cartilaginous endplate. These patients are typically 11 to 13 years of age for type I, 13 to 18 for type II, and older than 18 for type III. MRI shows a large anterior extradural impression (or rarely even a complete block) from the slipped apophysis and protruded disc (116,121). Recently, a type IV has been described, which spans the entire length and breadth of the posterior vertebral margin between the endplates (122,123).

Herniated Nucleus Pulposus

Herniated lumbar nucleus pulposus in children and adolescents is quite rare. The first series was described in 1950 (124), and since then there have been several more reports (26,116,125–132). The quoted incidence of surgically proven lumbar disc prolapse in non-Asian children and adolescents ranges from 0.5% (26) to 3.2% (20) of all patients; in a very large series of 9,991 discectomies, 50 (0.5%) occurred in those ≤16 years of age. The incidence is higher in Japanese children (6.7%); in one series, 31 of 456 patients involved children <16 years of age (129).

In the series of children and adolescents (26,126,129.133) with herniated nucleus polposus, excluding slipped vertebral apophysis, the average age was approximately 16 years; the youngest child was 8 years of age. There is a male predominance, ranging from 1.5:1 (126) to 3.6:1 (129). The patients are often taller and heavier for their age (25). The vast majority of patients complain of sciatica (70% to 100%) and low back pain (60% to 100%), with an average symptom duration of 6 to 12 months. Approximately one-third to one-half have a history of trauma; sports are involved in up to 64% [45 of 70 patients in one series (129)].

Although the symptoms are extremely similar in children and adolescents compared to adults, physical findings may be different. A positive straight leg raising test is quite common (85% to 98%); decreased deep tendon reflexes are not as frequent as in adults (45% to 64%). Likewise, muscle motor weakness is less common [~30% in three series (26,126,133)]. Sensory loss is also less frequent compared to the adult population, ranging from 10% to 25% (26,126, 133).

Radiographic findings are usually not present, although minor structural abnormalities were present in 30% of patients in one series (26). A loss of disc space height has been seen as frequently as 33% (129); mild scoliosis due to muscle spasm can be occasionally seen. Most authors have noted an equal distribution of herniation between the L4-5 and L5-S1 disc spaces. However, one series noted a much higher prevalence of the L4-5 level (87%) (129).

TREATMENT OPTIONS AND SURGICAL TECHNIQUES

Permanent disc space narrowing and spontaneous interbody fusion following injury is uncommon in children, as the healthy intervertebral discs typically transmit the force to the vertebral bodies (28). This finding, along with the presence of the rib cage in the thoracic spine, makes a stronger case for nonoperative treatment in the management of pediatric spine injuries when compared to adults. Approximately two-thirds of children have stable injuries.

Flexion

Simple compression fractures heal quickly with little tendency for further progression. Symptomatic treatment is usually sufficient for the mild injury, with a short period of bed rest or immobilization with a cast or corset/orthosis (Figs. 3 and 5). Many can be treated at home with minimal hospitalization. In those reports comparing casts with bed rest, the specific type of treatment did not affect the outcome, and the children were generally asymptomatic in 1 to 2 weeks (11,24,28) (Fig. 3). Posterior tenderness in the area of the fracture occasionally persists, but usually does not pose any serious problem (11). Symptoms may persist for some time with endplate fracture and disc herniation into the vertebral body, but usually resolve with symptomatic treatment.

Distraction and Shear

Unstable injuries such as vertebral subluxation or fracture-dislocation should be reduced (24,28,134–136) (Fig. 4). The child should be kept on a turning frame or at complete bed rest with log rolling until the acute symptoms subside, and then proceed to operative reduction and fixation. In children with neurologic injury, the fracture should be reduced promptly, especially if the neurologic injury involves the conus medullaris and nerve roots. Children with burst fractures that result in spinal canal narrowing (>25%) and kyphosis are at increased risk of further canal compromise and should be considered for early correction and decompression (134) (Fig. 2).

As a rule these are adult fracture patterns occurring in adolescents. Spontaneous interbody fusion seldom occurs, and should not be depended on to provide long-term stability (24,28). The spinal canal and vertebral elements are the same size as in adults, and adult instrumentation for reduction and stabilization is used (130,137–139). All instrumentations must be at least one level above and below the level(s) of injury and accompanied by a posterior spinal fusion. In older children with severe neurologic deficits, extending the fusion to the sacrum as a guard against the late onset of paralytic scoliosis (139) has been rarely advocated.

Certain stable injuries in the adult may progress in children. Severe crushing of the vertebral body and endplate (burst fractures) is analogous to a Salter IV injury of the vertebral epiphysis. Growth arrest leads to progressive kyphosis (28). Early recognition, reduction, stabilization, and fusion prevent late deformity and neurologic injury.

The indications for immediate surgical decompression (2,6) are the same as in the adult: progressive neurologic deficit or the extremely rare open fracture. Reduction of an unstable fracture-dislocation is a relative indication. Laminectomy is seldom helpful, particularly in the child without bony injury (4,58,135,140,141). It accentuates an already unstable condition that may lead to progressive deformity (142) such as kyphosis, which is difficult to manage (58,139,140,142,143). If laminectomy is deemed necessary, it should be accompanied by a short segment fusion.

The outcome of SCIWORA is determined mostly by the initial neurologic status. Approximately one-fourth of the children may have a late deterioration in neurologic function. Treatment is controversial. Brace immobilization for 3 months has been recommended by Pang and Pollack (64), with complete avoidance of all sports. However, in their series no instability was noted in any of the children at initial evaluation, and only one child later developed instability on flexion/extension radiographs. Without documented radiographic instability, I believe the biomechanical usefulness of brace immobilization is questionable. Pang and Pollack, however, denote this as treating "incipient instability." Regardless of whether or not the child is braced, close follow-up is needed regarding neurologic function. Flexion/extension radiographs after 3 months of bracing should be taken; any late development of instability requires surgical stabilization.

Chance Fractures

If the injury is completely osseous in all columns, then closed reduction with reconstitution of lordosis and cast immobilization is recommended. In older, heavier adolescents the cast can be problematic, in which case posterior spinal fusion and instrumentation can be considered (Fig. 11). If the injury is ligamentous, operative reduction with fusion is indicated, since ligamentous disruptions do not usually heal without instability. [In one series, only those with an initial kyphosis of > 20 degrees failed brace treatment, and those authors advocate immobilization for all injuries if the kyphosis is < 20 degrees (52). All successfully brace-treated children had a decrease in kyphosis over time, as the potential for anterior growth remained in these young children]. The type of fixation depends on the child's age. In small children simple interspinous wiring supplemented by postoperative cast immobilization is used (Fig. 7); in the adolescent standard compression types of instrumentation can be used.

Spondylolysis and Spondylolisthesis

Some children and young adults may heal the spondylolytic defect with a cast or brace [thoracolumbar spinal orthosis (TLSO)] if there is an acute, clearly documented onset with injury (86,91,93,101,110,144,145). Healing is more likely with unilateral defects (144) than bilateral defects. Unfortunately, not all heal with immobilization (86), but immobilization should be considered if the injury can be documented

to be of recent origin. The bone scan may be helpful to indicate a continuing process versus one of a long duration (92).

In children with long-standing spondylolysis, healing is unlikely, but the symptoms usually respond to conservative measures (88). Restriction of vigorous activities and back and abdominal strengthening exercises are usually successful in controlling those patients with mild backache and hamstring tightness (105). Patients with more severe or persistent complaints may require bed rest, cast or brace immobilization, and nonnarcotic analgesics (146). Hamstring tightness is an excellent clinical guide to the success or failure of the treatment. The majority of affected children have excellent relief of symptoms or only minimal discomfort on long-term follow-up (85,91).

Any child or adolescent with symptoms due to spondylolysis, especially if under 10 years of age, should be closely followed for progression to spondylolisthesis (85,86). Those with asymptomatic spondylolysis or those with minimal symptoms do not need to restrict their activities since 7.2% of asymptomatic young men aged 18 to 30 years have the pars defect with relatively few having persistent symptoms (147). Thus, limitation of activity in a growing child does not seem justified (101,105). It must be emphasized that it is quite uncommon for spondylolysis to be symptomatic in adolescence, and one should be particularly cautious with the child whose symptoms do not respond to bed rest or who has objective neurologic findings. In this situation, other studies (e.g., MRI, electromyography) should be considered.

A small percentage of young people with spondylolysis who do not respond to conservative measures or who are unwilling to curtail their activities may require surgical stabilization. A posterolateral fusion from L5-S1 with autogenous bone graft is usually sufficient. In those who have a spondylolisthesis of grade III or greater, the fusion is usually extended to L4 (88). Nachemson (148) reported solid healing of the defect using a bone graft coupled with an intertransverse process fusion. The role of instrumentation as a means of reduction is controversial.

In those patients in whom the defect is small (6 to 7 mm) and the degree of spondylolisthesis is slight, a variety of techniques have been described to directly reduce the defect. These include wiring of the transverse process or screw placement across the pars, coupled with a bone graft (e.g., a pseudarthrosis repair) (149–153). These procedures are usually recommended for the older teenager and young adult <30 years of age with a minimal degree of displacement and degenerative change (148,152). The best candidates for this method of treatment are those with defects between L1 and L4 or in situations with multiple defects (149,152); it is an attractive alternative to the traditional transverse process fusion because it repairs the defect at one vertebral level rather than involving a second unaffected vertebrae (149,153). In properly selected patients, 80% to 90% obtain a solid fusion, with 80% good to excellent results. In children the Gill procedure or laminectomy is never indicated without an associated fusion (88). Removal of the posterior elements may in

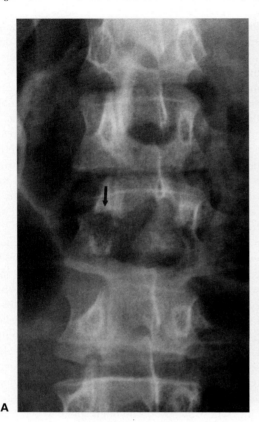

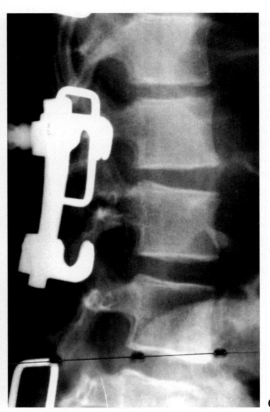

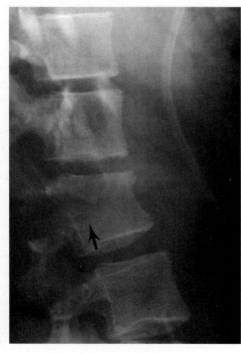

FIG. 11. This 15-year-old girl was a passenger in the back seat (right side) of a car involved in a motor vehicle crash, being hit by the other vehicle from the left side at a high rate of speed. She was restrained by the lap belt. She sustained a contusion of the cervical spine at C1 resulting in a C2-level Brown-Séquard syndrome. Radiographs of the cervical spine were normal; however, radiographs of the lumbar spine demonstrated a bony Chance fracture at L2: anteroposterior (A) and lateral (B). Note the distraction of the posterior bony elements *(arrow)*. Due to her associated injuries (traumatic pancreatitis), age, neurologic deficit (Brown-Séquard syndrome), and body size (63 kg), it was felt that closed reduction and pantaloon spica cast immobilization would be problematic if elected as the method of treatment for the L2 Chance fracture. It was therefore elected to proceed with posterior spinal fusion and compression instrumentation. The postoperative lateral radiograph (C) demonstrates closure of the distracted posterior elements and reconstitution of the anterior vertebral body compression.

fact be harmful, leading to increased instability and spondylolisthesis in the postoperative period.

A rare type of spondylolisthesis, the acute spondylolytic spondylolisthesis, has been recently described (154). It is the result of high-energy trauma and is an unstable spine injury, similar to a fracture/dislocation. The pars interarticularis of L5 is typically involved; thus it is not the so-called traumatic spondylolisthesis (type IV) caused by a fracture in areas of the bony hook other than the pars interarticularis, differentiating these two acute types of spondylolistheses. The deformity typically progresses, with some developing neurologic compromise. Due to its unstable nature, high risk of progression, and possibility of developing neurologic compromise, it should be treated operatively. Grade I deformities may be adequately treated with a posterior arthrodesis; more severe deformities may need both anterior and posterior arthrodesis, due to the greater disruption of secondary ligamentous restraints.

Slipped Vertebral Apophysis

There is no role for nonoperative treatment. Laminectomy and decompression with removal of the bony ridge gives excellent results (116,118). Disc removal alone is not sufficient to relieve the nerve root impingement (118).

Herniated Nucleus Pulposus

Treatment should initially consist of a brief trial of rest, antiinflammatory agents, and physiotherapy. Appropriate discal imaging (e.g., MRI or myelogram) should be performed if there is a persistent neurologic deficit or positive nerve tension signs remain after 2 to 4 weeks of conservative treatment (126,127,129,133,155). Once the diagnosis is confirmed and the anatomic level localized, surgical treatment should be considered. Most authors advocate simple discectomy without fusion (125,129,133,156).

Although all patients should be initially treated conservatively (except for the extremely rare cauda equina syndrome), the success rate and results of conservative treatment are believed by many authors to be less satisfactory than surgical treatment (126,129,133). Zamani and MacEwen (132) found that in the absence of neurologic deficits, conservative treatment is quite adequate. However, the overall results of conservative treatment were 25% to 30% good or excellent in two series (126,133). Surgical treatment typically demonstrates good or excellent results in 75% to 90% of children and adolescents (20,133,155). In some series the best surgical results were in those patients offered surgery early (125,126). Prolonged conservative therapy in a child or adolescent with a herniated nucleus pulposus and having a scoliosis secondary to spasm may result in the scoliosis becoming fixed, or even worse in magnitude (133).

COMPLICATIONS

The Fracture Itself

Progression of the deformity is uncommon in children (157), unless the injury is unstable, such as with a fracture-dislocation, or if there is a neurologic deficit. There is a great propensity for the vertebral body to restructure related to stimulation of vertebral growth and overgrowth (10,11,24, 158) (Fig. 12). In the child under age 10 years the vertebral body tends to return to its normal shape, even with multiple compression fractures, and kyphosis is uncommon (11,24, 40,159). However, complete reconstitution is possible only if there is no protrusion of the nucleus pulposus into the vertebra (11,157,159). The vertebral endplate is the area of active growth, and if damaged, there will be little subsequent correction of the deformity. Asymmetric growth of a damaged vertebra, particularly in the thoracolumbar area, is usually compensated by the undamaged adjacent vertebra and seldom results in a significant scoliosis (11,157). Spontaneous interbody fusion is rare in children and is believed to be blocked by the interposed, undamaged, intervertebral disc (7,18,24,27).

Neurologic Injury

The most devastating problem for a child with a thoracolumbar spine injury is paraplegia. The spinal cord–injured child can be expected to have all the problems found in the adult: increased susceptibility to long-bone fractures, hip dislocation, pressure sores, joint contractures, and genitourinary complications (8,13,160). In addition, the child will likely develop progressive spinal deformity (scoliosis, kyphosis, and lordosis) (Fig. 13). In immature children (girls <12, boys <14 years of age) the incidence of progressive spinal deformity following traumatic paraplegia is 86% to 100% (13,21,39,141,160). The onset of curvature has been reported as early as 3 years of age (13). Scoliosis erodes the child's ability to sit easily, and in the young child pelvic obliquity may lead to subluxation of the hip and ischial pressure sores (143,161).

Progression of the spinal curvature is directly related to the age of the child, spasticity, and the level of the lesion (139,141). Children with more proximal injuries are more likely to have a progressive deformity than those injured at or below the level of the conus medullaris (8,13,162). The fracture seldom determines the direction of spinal curvature; rather, the majority develop a long paralytic thoracolumbar curve due to the influence of gravity and asymmetric spasticity (139,143). Lumbar lordosis is reversed with the development of a long thoracolumbar kyphosis (139,143). Increased lumbar lordosis is less common (18%) and usually associated with hip flexion contractures in the ambulatory patient (141,143,162).

In adolescents near skeletal maturity at the time of injury, spinal deformity is more often due to the fracture-dislocation itself (141). Progressive kyphosis and pain at the fracture site

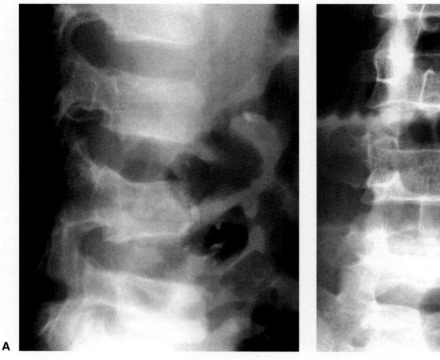

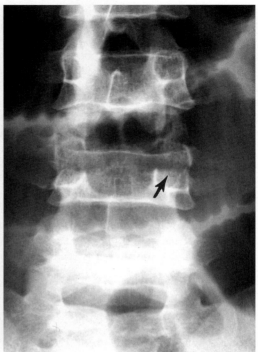

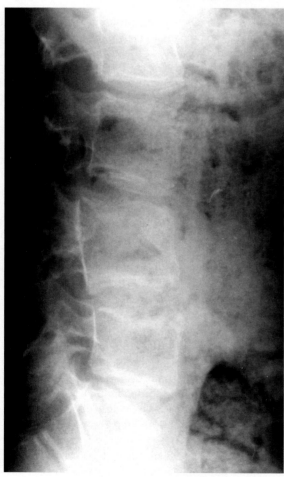

FIG. 12. This 10-year-old boy was involved in a motor vehicle crash (near head on collision). He was a passenger in the back seat of a vehicle and restrained by a lap belt. He sustained a bony Chance fracture at L4 [lateral radiograph **(A)** and posteroanterior radiograph **(B)**] with complete paraplegia; he also sustained a jejunal perforation with intestinal necrosis that required laparotomy and resection shortly after injury. Note that the fracture line is easily seen on the anteroposterior radiograph with fracture and separation of the lumbar pedicle *(arrow)*. This is often the only hint of an osseous Chance fracture on the posteroanterior radiograph. Due to prolonged bed rest and hyperalimentation needed for the abdominal injuries, and after discussion with the parents regarding both cast immobilization and surgical stabilization as treatment methods, it was elected to treat this fracture nonoperatively with cast immobilization. At age 13 years, 6 months, the fracture is solidly healed **(C)**. Note the increased vertebral height of L4 due to overgrowth and healing in a slightly distracted position.

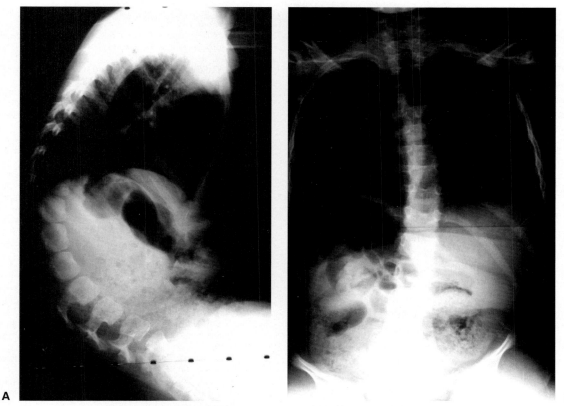

FIG. 13. This girl sustained a SCIWORA (spinal cord injury without objective radiographic abnormality) at the T4 level at 8 months of age. By age 9 years, 6 months, a paralytic thoracolumbar kyphosis of 91 degrees from T8 to L5 had developed **(A)**; a mild paralytic scoliosis of 18 degrees from T4 to T12 had also developed **(B)**.

is common (42%), particularly in those with a laminectomy (58,141,143,161). If the kyphosis is progressive, long-term neurologic sequelae may develop with further loss of function from tenting of the neural structures over the kyphus. This is another reason for early surgical stabilization of these fractures in adolescents (141).

Scoliosis treatment should be initiated soon after the injury, prior to developing a severe curve. Total-contact underarm plastic orthoses have been helpful in controlling the collapsing paralytic curve, at least for some period of time (8). Treatment recommendations are similar to those for idiopathic scoliosis. Curves less than 40 to 45 degrees may be controlled by bracing, or at least surgery can be delayed until further spinal growth has occurred and the child is of optimal age (139,161,163). For curves greater than 45 to 50 degrees, surgical stabilization should be undertaken. In one series (141), 68% required surgical correction. Children with severe or rigid curves may also need an anterior release. Segmental instrumentation, such as Harrington/Luque rods with sublaminar wiring or the newer rotational systems (e.g., Cotrel-Dubousset) are used, along with spinal arthrodesis. The child should be quickly mobilized after surgery to avoid the problems associated with long periods of bed rest (e.g., pneumonia, decubiti in insensate areas).

With the advent of MRI, the "rare" posttraumatic syringomyelia is being discovered with increasing frequency (76). Symptoms can develop many years after injury (4.5 years average), even more than 15 years later (21,164). Pain is the initial symptom in over half of the children, followed by progressive neurologic loss as demonstrated by sweating below the level of the original lesion, loss of motor function, and changes in the deep tendon reflexes (164). The best method to detect the lesion is MRI. An initial baseline MRI has been advocated in these children to later facilitate detection (76,165).

SPECIAL PEDIATRIC FRACTURES IN THE THORACOLUMBAR SPINE

Repetitive Stress Fractures

A fatigue fracture is due to abnormal or repetitive loading of normal bone. It typically occurs in young, active individuals, usually in the metatarsals and tibia in children (166). Fatigue stress fractures of the sacrum in children have been described (167). These children present with pelvic pain and positive FABER (flexion-abduction-external rotation) tests. The diagnosis is confirmed on CT scan. Treatment is conservative.

Abuse and Violence

Vertebral injuries due to child abuse are less common than those of the extremities (168,169). The injuries are usually due to hyperflexion, and may be simple compression of the vertebral bodies, avulsion of the secondary centers of ossification of the spinous processes, and less frequently herniation of the nucleus polposus into the vertebral body. Fracture-dislocations or kyphosis secondary to severe disruptions are quite rare (168–173), although there are striking examples of T12-L1 subluxation/dislocation with complete paraplegia from spanking (170,171); these represent a circumferential growth plate fracture of the thoracolumbar spine (174). There are no radiographic vertebral changes specific for the battered child syndrome. Kleinman and Marks (175) found three main patterns: (a) compression, usually no more than 25% of the anterior half of the vertebral body; (b) fracture of the anterosuperior aspect of the vertebral body with extension into the anterior aspect of the endplate; and (c) combined lesions. Similarly, the classic corner fractures of the long bones are present in only 15% of abused children (176). A high index of suspicion is more helpful than a specific radiographic finding. The children may exhibit other signs of neglect, such as poor nutrition and poor hygiene.

Spinal injuries from gunshot wounds are increasing. At the Rancho Los Amigos Medical Center, gunshot wounds in children accounted for an equal number of spinal injuries as motor vehicle accidents during the period 1985 to 1989 (38%), compared to 6% prior to 1970 (19). Laminectomy is rarely needed (177–179), has no influence on the outcome of complete lesions, and is detrimental to those with incomplete lesions (180), resulting in cerebrospinal fluid fistulas, infection, and late instability. The only indication for surgery is a progressive neurologic deficit (181). One exception may be a motor lesion between T12-L4, where one series showed a significantly better motor recovery with bullet removal (182).

REFERENCES

1. Aufdermaur M. Spinal injuries in juveniles. Necropsy findings in twelve cases. *J Bone Joint Surg* 1974;56B:513–519.
2. Babcock JL. Spinal injuries in children. *Pediatr Clin North Am* 1975; 22:487–500.
3. Hachen HJ. Spinal cord injury in children and adolescents: diagnostic pitfalls and therapeutic considerations in the acute stage. *Paraplegia* 1977–78;15:55–64.
4. Hadley MN, Zabramski JM, Browner CM, Rekate H, Sonntag VH. Pediatric spinal trauma: review of 122 cases of spinal cord and vertebral column injuries. *J Neurosurg* 1988;68:18–24.
5. Jackson DW, Wiltse LL, Cirincione RJ. Spondylolysis in the female gymnasts. *Clin Orthop* 1976;117:68–73.
6. Anderson M, Schutt AH. Spinal injury in children. A review of 156 cases seen from 1950 through 1978. *Mayo Clin Proc* 1980;55:499–504.
7. Kewalramani LS, Tori JA. Spinal cord trauma in children: neurologic patterns, radiologic features, and pathomechanics of injury. *Spine* 1980;5:11–18.
8. Campbell J, Bonnett C. Spinal cord injury in children. *Clin Orthop* 1975;112:114–123.
9. Glasauer FE, Cares HL. Traumatic paraplegia in infancy. *JAMA* 1972;219:38–41.
10. Hegenbarth R, Ebel KD. Roentgen findings in fractures of the vertebral column in childhood. Examination of 35 patients and its results. *Pediatr Radiol* 1976;5:34–39.
11. Horal J, Nachemson A, Scheller S. Clinical and radiological long term follow-up of vertebral fractures in children. *Acta Orthop Scand* 1972; 43:491–503.
12. Scher AT. Trauma of the spinal cord in children. *S Afr Med J* 1976; 50:2023–2025.
13. Banniza Von Vazan UK, Paeslack V. Scoliotic growth in children with acquired paraplegia. *Paraplegia* 1977–78;15:65–73.
14. Herkowitz HN, Samberg C. Vertebral column injuries associated with tobogganing. *J Trauma* 1978;18:806–810.
15. Kewalramani LS, Kraus JF, Sterling HM. Acute spinal-cord lesions in a pediatric population: epidemiological and clinical features. *Paraplegia* 1980;18:206–219.
16. Odom JA, Brown CW, Messner DG. Tubing injuries. *J Bone Joint Surg* 1976;58A:733.
17. Paulson JA. The epidemiology of injuries in adolescents. *Pediatr Ann* 1988;17:84–96.
18. Shrosbree RD. Spinal cord injuries as a result of motorcycle accidents. *Paraplegia* 1978;16:102–112.
19. Haffner DL, Hoffer MM, Wiedbusch R. Etiology of children's spinal injuries at Rancho Los Amigos. *Spine* 1993;18:679–684.
20. O'Connell JEA. Intervertebral disc lesions in childhood and adolescence. *Br J Surg* 1960;47:611–616.
21. Melzak J. Paraplegia among children. *Lancet* 1969;2:45–48.
22. Pang D, Wilberger Jr JE. Spinal cord injury without radiographic abnormalities in children. *J Neurosurg* 1982;57:114–129.
23. Yngve DA, Harris WP, Herndon WA, Sullivan JA, Gross RH. Spinal cord injury without osseous spine fracture. *J Pediatr Orthop* 1988;8: 153–159.
24. Hubbard DD. Injuries of the spine in children and adolescents. *Clin Orthop* 1974;100:56–65.
25. Bulos S. Herniated intervertebral lumbar disc in the teenager. *J Bone Joint Surg* 1973;55B:273–278.
26. DeOrio JK, Bianco AJ Jr. Lumbar disc excision in children and adolescents. *J Bone Joint Surg* 1982;64A:991–996.
27. Roaf R. A study of the mechanics of spinal injuries. *J Bone Joint Surg* 1960;42B:810–823.
28. McPhee IB. Spinal fractures and dislocations in children and adolescents. *Spine* 1981;6:533–537.
29. Mandell GA, Harcke HT. Scintigraphy of spinal disorders in adolescents. *Skeletal Radiol* 1993;22:393–401.
30. Chance GQ. Note on a type of flexion fracture of the spine. *Br J Radiol* 1948;21:432–433.
31. Smith WS, Kaufer H. Patterns and mechanisms of lumbar injuries associated with lap seat belts. *J Bone Joint Surg* 1969;51A:239–254.
32. Blasier RD, LaMont RL. Chance fracture in a child: a case report with nonoperative treatment. *J Pediatr Orthop* 1985;5:92–93.
33. Anderson A, Henley MB, Rivara FP, Maier RV. Flexion distraction and Chance injuries to the thoracolumbar spine. *J Orthop Trauma* 1991;5:153–160.
34. Kerslake RW, Jaspan T, Worthington BS. Magnetic resonance imaging of spinal trauma. *Br J Radiol* 1991;64:386–402.
35. Ferrandez L, Usabiaga J, Curto JM, Alonso A, Martin F. Atypical multivertebral fracture due to hyperextension in an adolescent girl. *Spine* 1989;14:645–646.
36. Miller JA, Smith TH. Seatbelt induced chance fracture in an infant. *Pediatr Radiol* 1991;21:575–577.
37. Rodger RM, Missiuna P, Ein S. Entrapment of bowel within a spine fracture. *J Pediatr Orthop* 1991;11:783–785.
38. Abel MS. Transverse posterior element fractures associated with torsion. *Skeletal Radiol* 1989;17:556–560.
39. LeGay DA, Petrie DP, Alexander DI. Flexion-distraction injuries of the lumbar spine and associated abdominal trauma. *J Trauma* 1990; 30:436–444.
40. Lim LH, Lam LK, Moore MH, Trott JA, David DJ. Associated injuries in facial fractures: review of 839 patients. *Br J Plast Surg* 1993;46:635–638.
41. Henderson RL, Reid DC, Saboe LA. Multiple noncontiguous spine fractures. *Spine* 1991;16:128–131.
42. Korres DS, Katsaros A, Pantazopoulos T, Hartofilakidis-Garofalidis G. Double or multiple level fractures of the spine. *Injury* 1981;13: 147–152.
43. Pal JM, Mulder DS, Brown RA, Fleiszer DM. Assessing multiple trauma: is the cervical spine enough? *J Trauma* 1988;28:1282–1284.

44. Powell JN, Waddell JP, Tucker WS, Transfeldt EE. Multiple-level noncontiguous spinal fractures. *J Trauma* 1989;29:1146–1150.
45. Agran PF, Dunkle DE, Winn DG. Injuries to a sample of seatbelted children evaluated and treated in a hospital emergency room. *J Trauma* 1987;27:58–64.
46. Hoffman MA, Spence LJ, Wesson DE, Armstrong PF, Williams JI, Filler RM. The pediatric passenger: trends in seatbelt use and injury patterns. *J Trauma* 1987;27:974–976.
47. Reid AB, Letts RM, Black GB. Pediatric Chance fractures: association with intra-abdominal injuries and seatbelt use. *J Trauma* 1990;30:384–391.
48. Sclafani SJA, Florence LO, Phillips TF, et al. Lumbar arterial injury: radiologic diagnosis and management. *Radiology* 1987;165:709–714.
49. Sturm JT, Hines JT, Perry JF Jr. Thoracic spinal fractures and aortic rupture: a significant and fatal association. *Ann Thorac Surg* 1990;50:931–933.
50. Sturm JT, Perry JF Jr. Injuries associated with fractures of the transverse processes of the thoracic and lumbar vertebrae. *J Trauma* 1984;24:597–599.
51. Woelfel GF, Moore EE, Cogbill TH, VanWay CW III. Severe thoracic and abdominal injuries associated with lap-harness seatbelts. *J Trauma* 1984;24:166–167.
52. Glassman SD, Johnson JR, Holt RT. Seatbelt injuries in children. *J Trauma* 1992;33:882–886.
53. Rumball K, Jarvis J. Seat-belt injuries of the spine in young children. *J Bone Joint Surg* 1992;74B:571–574.
54. Sivit CJ, Taylor CA, Newman KD, et al. Safety-belt injuries in children with lap-belt ecchymosis: CT findings in 61 patients. *AJR* 1991;157:111–114.
55. Gumley G, Taylor TKF, Ryan MD. Distraction fractures of the lumbar spine. *J Bone Joint Surg* 1982;64B:520–525.
56. Dickman CA, Rekate HL, Sonntag VKH, Zabramski JM. Pediatric spinal trauma: vertebral column and spinal cord injuries in children. *Pediatr Neurosci* 1989;15:237–256.
57. Choi JU, Hoffman HJ, Hendrick EB, Humphreys RP, Keith WS. Traumatic infarction of the spinal cord in children. *J Neurosurg* 1986;65:608–610.
58. Burke DC. Traumatic spinal paralysis in children. *Paraplegia* 1974;11:268–276.
59. Hashimoto T, Kaneda K, Abumi K. Relationship between traumatic spinal canal stenosis and neurologic deficits in thoracolumbar burst fractures. *Spine* 1988;13:1268–1272.
60. Bell HJ, Dykstra DD. Somatosensory evoked potentials as an adjunct to diagnosis of neonatal spinal cord injury. *J Pediatr* 1985;106:298–301.
61. Burke DC. Spinal cord trauma in children. *Paraplegia* 1971;9:1–14.
62. Glasauer FE, Cares HL. Biomechanical fractures of traumatic paraplegia in infancy. *J Trauma* 1973;13:166–170.
63. LeBlanc HJ, Nadell J. Spinal cord injuries in children. *Surg Neurol* 1974;2:411–414.
64. Pang D, Pollack IF. Spinal cord injury without radiographic abnormality in children—the SCIWORA syndrome. *J Trauma* 1989;29:654–664.
65. Ruge JR, Sinson GP, McClone DG, Cerullo LJ. Pediatric spinal injury: the very young. *J Neurosurg* 1988;68:25–30.
66. Linssen WHJ, Praamstra P, Gabreëls FJM, Rotteveel JJ. Vascular insufficiency of the cervical cord due to hyperextension of the spine. *Pediatr Neurol* 1990;6:123–125.
67. Begg AC. Nuclear herniations of the intervertebral disc. *J Bone Joint Surg* 1954;36B:180–193.
68. Boechat MI. Spinal deformities and pseudofractures. *AJR* 1987;148:97–98.
69. Gellad FE, Levine AM, Joslyn JN, Edwards CC, Bosse M. Pure thoracolumbar facet dislocation: clinical features and CT appearance. *Radiology* 1986;161:505–508.
70. Taylor GA, Eggli KD. Lap-belt injuries of the lumbar spine in children. A pitfall in CT diagnosis. *AJR* 1988;150:1355–1358.
71. Betz RR, Gelman AJ, DeFilipp GJ, Mesgarzadeh M, Clancy M, Steel HH. Magnetic resonance imaging (MRI) in the evaluation of spinal cord injured children and adolescents. *Paraplegia* 1987;25:92–99.
72. Bondurant FJ, Cotler HB, Kulkarni MV, McArdle CB, Harris Jr JH. Acute spinal cord injury. A study using physical examination and magnetic resonance imaging. *Spine* 1990;15:161–168.
73. Brightman RP, Miller GA, Rea GL, Chkeres DW, Hunt WE. Magnetic resonance imaging of trauma to the thoracic and lumbar spine. The im-

portance of the posterior longitudinal ligament. *Spine* 1992;17:541–550.
74. McArdle CB, Crofford MJ, Mirfakhraee M, Amparo EG, Calhoun JS. Surface coil MR of spinal trauma: preliminary experience. *AJNR* 1986;7:885–893.
75. Prenger EC. Magnetic resonance imaging of the pediatric spine. *Semin Ultrasound CT MRI* 1991;12:410–428.
76. Tarr RW, Drolshagen LF, Kerner TC, Allen JH, Partain CL, James AE. MR imaging of recent spinal trauma. *J Comput Assist Tomogr* 1987;11:412–417.
77. Borkow SE, Kleiger B. Spondylolisthesis in the newborn. *Clin Orthop* 1971;81:73–76.
78. Rowe GG, Roche MB. The etiology of separate neural arch. *J Bone Joint Surg* 1953;35A:102–110.
79. Wertzberger KL, Peterson HA. Acquired spondylolysis and spondylolisthesis in the young child. *Spine* 1980;5:422–437.
80. Wiltse LL, Newman PH, MacNab I. Classification of spondylolysis and spondylolisthesis. *Clin Orthop* 1976;117:23–29.
81. Kettelkamp DB, Wright DG. Spondylolysis in the Alaskan eskimo. *J Bone Joint Surg* 1971;53A:563–566.
82. Wynne-Davies R, Scott JHS. Inheritance and spondylolisthesis. A radiographic family survey. *J Bone Joint Surg* 1979;61B:301–305.
83. Dandy DJ, Shannon MJ. Lumbosacral subluxation (group I spondylolisthesis). *J Bone Joint Surg* 1971;53B:578–595.
84. Baker DR, McHollick W. Spondyloschisis and spondylolisthesis in children. *J Bone Joint Surg* 1956;38A:933–934.
85. Wiltse LL. Spondylolisthesis in children. *Clin Orthop* 1961;21:156–163.
86. Wiltse LL, Widell EH, Jackson DW. Fatigue fracture: the basic lesion in isthmic spondylolisthesis. *J Bone Joint Surg* 1975;57A:17–22.
87. Hitchcock HH. Spondylolisthesis. Observations on its development, progression, and genesis. *J Bone Joint Surg* 1940;22:1–16.
88. Hensinger RN, Lang JR, MacEwen GD. Surgical management of spondylolisthesis in children and adolescents. *Spine* 1976;1:207–216.
89. McKee BW, Alexander WJ, Dunbar JS. Spondylolysis and spondylolisthesis in children: a review. *J Can Assoc Radiol* 1971;22:100–109.
90. Sherman FC, Rosenthal RK, Hall JC. Spine fusion for spondylolysis and spondylolisthesis in children. *Spine* 1979;4:59–67.
91. Turner RH, Bianco AJ Jr. Spondylolysis and spondylolisthesis in children and teen-agers. *J Bone Joint Surg* 1971;53A:1298–1306.
92. Letts M, Smallman T, Afanasiev R, Gouw G. Fracture of the pars interarticularis in adolescent athletes: a clinical-biomechanical analysis. *J Pediatr Orthop* 1986;6:40–46.
93. Newman PH. The etiology of spondylolisthesis. *J Bone Joint Surg* 1963;45B:39–59.
94. Krenz J, Troup JDG. The structure of the pars interarticularis of the lower lumbar vertebrae and its relation to the etiology of spondylolysis. *J Bone Joint Surg* 1973;55B:735–741.
95. Cyron BM, Hutton WC. Variations in the amount and distribution of cortical bone across the pars interarticulars of L5. *Spine* 1979;4:163–167.
96. Stanitski CL, Stanitski DF, LaMont RL. Spondylolisthesis in myelomeningocele. *J Pediatr Orthop* 1994;14:568–591.
97. Ogilvie JW, Sherman J. Spondylolysis in Scheuermann's disease. *Spine* 1987;12:251–253.
98. Ferguson RJ. Low-back pain in college football linemen. *J Bone Joint Surg* 1974;56A:1300.
99. Libson E, Bloom RA, Shapiro Y. Scoliosis in young men with spondylolysis or spondylolisthesis. *Spine* 1984;9:445–447.
100. Fredrickson BE, Baker D, McHolick WJ, Yuan HA, Lubicky JP. The natural history of spondylolysis and spondylolisthesis. *J Bone Joint Surg* 1984;66A:699–707.
101. Micheli LJ. Low back pain in the adolescent: differential diagnosis. *Am J Sports Med* 1979;7:362–364.
102. Stauffer RN, Coventry MB. Posterolateral lumbar-spine fusion. *J Bone Joint Surg* 1972;54A:1195–1204.
103. Phalen GS, Dickson JA. Spondylolisthesis and tight hamstrings. *J Bone Joint Surg* 1961;43A:505–512.
104. Libson E, Bloom RA, Dinari G, Robin GC. Oblique lumbar spine radiographs: importance in young patients. *Radiology* 1984;151:89–90.
105. Hensinger RN. Spondylolysis and spondylolisthesis in children. *Instr Course Lect* 1983;32:132–150.
106. Papanicolaou N, Wilkinson RH, Emans JB, Treves S, Mitchell LJ. Bone scintigraphy and radiography in young athletes with low back pain. *AJR* 1985;145:1039–1044.

107. Rothman SLG. Computed tomography of the spine in older children and teenagers. *Clin Sports Med* 1986;2:247–270.

108. Sherman FC, Wilkinson RH, Hall JE. Reactive sclerosis of a pedicle and spondylolysis in the lumbar spine. *J Bone Joint Surg* 1977;59A: 49–54.

109. Bellah RD, Summerville DA, Treves ST, Micheli LJ. Low-back pain in adolescent athletes: detection of stress injury to the pars interarticularis. *Radiology* 1991;180:509–512.

110. Van Den Oever M, Merrick MV, Scott JHS. Bone scintigraphy in symptomatic spondylolysis. *J Bone Joint Surg* 1987;69B:453–456.

111. Handel SF, Twiford FW, Reigel DHL, Kaufman HH. Posterior lumbar apophyseal fractures. *Radiology* 1979;130:629–633.

112. Keller RH. Traumatic displacement of the cartilaginous vertebral rim: a sign of intervertebral disc prolapse. *Radiology* 1974;110:21–24.

113. Lippitt AB. Fracture of a vertebral body endplate and disk protrusion causing subarachnoid block in an adolescent. *Clin Orthop* 1976;116: 112–115.

114. Lowrey JJ. Dislocated lumbar vertebral epiphysis in adolescent children. Report of three cases. *J Neurosurg* 1973;38:232–234.

115. Techakapuch S. Rupture of the lumbar cartilage plate into the spinal canal in an adolescent. A case report. *J Bone Joint Surg* 1981;63A: 481–482.

116. Callahan DJ, Pack LL, Bream RC, Hensinger RN. Intervertebral disc impingement syndrome in a child, report of a case and suggested pathology. *Spine* 1986;11:402–404.

117. Dietemann JL, Runge M, Badoz A, et al. Radiology of posterior lumbar apophyseal ring fractures: report of 13 cases. *Neuroradiology* 1988;30:337–344.

118. Sovio OM, Bell HM, Beauchamp RD, Tredwell SJ. Fracture of the lumbar vertebral apophysis. *J Pediatr Orthop* 1985;5:550–552.

119. Wagner A, Albeck MJ, Madsen FF. Diagnostic imaging in fracture of the lumbar vertebral ring apophyses. *Acta Radiol* 1992;33:72–75.

120. Takata K, Inoue S, Takahashi K, Ohtsuka Y. Fracture of the posterior margin of a lumbar vertebral body. *J Bone Joint Surg* 1988;70A:589–594.

121. Rothfus WE, Goldberg AL, Deeb ZL, Daffner RH. MR recognition of posterior lumbar vertebral ring fracture. *J Comput Assist Tomogr* 1990;14:790–794.

122. Epstein NE, Epstein JA. Limbus lumbar vertebral fractures in 27 adolescents and adults. *Spine* 1991;16:962–966.

123. Epstein NE, Epstein JA, Mauri T. Treatment of fractures of the vertebral limbus and spinal stenosis in five adolescents and five adults. *Neurosurgery* 1989;24:595–604.

124. Key JA. Intervertebral-disc lesions in children and adolescents. *J Bone Joint Surg* 1950;32A:97–102.

125. Beks JWF, terWeeme CA. Herniated lumbar discs in teenagers. *Acta Neurochir* 1975;31:195–199.

126. Clarke NMP, Cleak DK. Intervertebral lumbar disc prolapse in children and adolescents. *J Pediatr Orthop* 1983;3:202–206.

127. Epstein JA, Lavine LS. Herniated lumbar intervertebral discs in teenage children. *J Neurosurg* 1964;21:1070–1075.

128. Hashimoto K, Fujita K, Kojimoto H, Shimomura Y. Lumbar disc herniation in children. *J Pediatr Orthop* 1990;10:394–396.

129. Kurihara A, Kataoka O. Lumbar disc herniation in children and adolescents. *Spine* 1980;5:443–451.

130. Rugtveit A. Juvenile lumbar disc herniations. *Acta Orthop Scand* 1966;37:348–356.

131. Taylor TKF. Intervertebral disc prolapse in children and adolescents. *J Bone Joint Surg* 1971;53B:357.

132. Zamani MH, MacEwen GD. Herniation of the lumbar disc in children and adolescents. *J Pediatr Orthop* 1982;2:528–533.

133. DeLuca PF, Mason DE, Weiand R, Howard R, Bassett GS. Excision of herniated nucleus pulposus in children and adolescents. *J Pediatr Orthop* 1994;14:318–322.

134. Bradford DS, McBride GG. Surgical management of thoracolumbar spine fractures with incomplete neurologic deficits. *Clin Orthop* 1987;218:201–216.

135. Jackson RW. Surgical stabilization of the spine. *Paraplegia* 1975;13: 71–74.

136. Westerborn A, Olsson O. Mechanics, treatment and prognosis of fractures of the dorso-lumbar spine. *Acta Chir Scand* 1953;102:59–83.

137. Bryant CE, Sullivan JA. Management of thoracic and lumbar spine fractures with Harrington distraction rods supplemented with segmental wiring. *Spine* 1983;8:532–537.

138. Crawford AH. Operative treatment of spine fractures in children. *Orthop Clin North Am* 1990;21:325–339.

139. Lancourt JE., Dickson JH, Carter RE. Paralytic spinal deformity following traumatic spinal-cord injury in children and adolescents. *J Bone Joint Surg* 1981;63A:47–53.

140. Flesch JR, Leider LL, Erickson DL, Chou SN, Bradford DS. Harrington instrumentation and spine fusion for unstable fractures and fracture-dislocations of the thoracic and lumbar spine. *J Bone Joint Surg* 1977;59A:143–153.

141. Mayfield JK, Erkkila JC, Winter RB. Spine deformity subsequent to acquired childhood spinal cord injury. *J Bone Joint Surg* 1981;63A: 1401–1411.

142. Yasuoka S, Peterson HA, MacCarty CS. Incidence of spinal column deformity after multilevel laminectomy in children and adults. *J Neurosurg* 1982;57:441–445.

143. Kilfoyle RM, Foley JJ, Norton PL. Spine and pelvic deformity in childhood and adolescent paraplegia. A study of 104 cases. *J Bone Joint Surg* 1965;47A:659–682.

144. Lafond G. Surgical treatment of spondylolisthesis. *Clin Orthop* 1962;22:175–179.

145. Rabushka SE, Apfelback H, Love L. Spontaneous healing of spondylolysis of the fifth lumbar vertebra: case report. *Clin Orthop* 1973;93: 256–259.

146. Steiner ME, Micheli LJ. Treatment of symptomatic spondylolysis and spondylolisthesis with the modified Boston brace. *Spine* 1985;10: 937–943.

147. Moreton RD. So-called normal backs. *Ind Med Surg* 1969;38:216–219.

148. Nachemson A. Repair of the spondylolisthesis defect and intertransverse fusion for young patients. *Clin Orthop* 1976;117:101–105.

149. Bradford DS, Iza J. Repair of the defect in spondylolysis or minimal degrees of spondylolisthesis by segmental wire fixation and bone grafting. *Spine* 1985;10:673–679.

150. Buck JE. Direct repair of the defect in spondylolisthesis. *J Bone Joint Surg* 1970;52B:432–437.

151. Eingorn D, Pizzutillo PD. Pars interarticularis fusion of multiple levels of lumbar spondylolysis. *Spine* 1985;10:250–252.

152. Nicol RO, Scott JHS. Lytic spondylolysis: repair by wiring. *Spine* 1986;11:1027–1030.

153. Pedersen AK, Hagen R. Spondylolysis and spondylolisthesis. Treatment by internal fixation and bone grafting the defect. *J Bone Joint Surg* 1988;70A:15–24.

154. Hilibrand AS, Urquhart AG, Graziano GP, Hensinger RN. Acute spondylolytic spondylolisthesis. Risk for progression and neurlogic complications. *J Bone Joint Surg* 1995;77A:190–196.

155. Børgesen SE, Vang PS. Herniation of the lumbar intervertebral disk in children and adolescents. *Acta Orthop Scand* 1974;45:500–549.

156. Bradford DS, Garcia A. Herniations of the lumbar intervertebral disk in children and adolescents. *JAMA* 1969;210:2045–2051.

157. Ruckstuhl J, Morscher E, Jani L. Behandlung und prognose von wirbelfrakturen im kindes-und jugendlichen. *Chirurg* 1976;47:458–467.

158. Hubbard DD. Fractures of the dorsal and lumbar spine. *Orthop Clin North Am* 1976;7:605–614.

159. Povaz F. Behandlungsergebnisse und prognose von wirbelbruchen bei kindern. *Chirurg* 1969;40:30–33.

160. Audic B, Maury M. Secondary vertebral deformities in childhood and adolescence. *Paraplegia* 1969;7:11–16.

161. Bedbrook GM. Correction of scoliosis due to paraplegia sustained in paediatric age-group. *Paraplegia* 1977–78;15:90–96.

162. McSweeney T. Spinal deformity after spinal cord injury. *Paraplegia* 1969;6:212–221.

163. Koch BM, Eng GM. Neonatal spinal cord injury. *Arch Phys Med Rehabil* 1979;60:378–381.

164. Williams B, Terry AF, Jones HWF, McSweeney T. Syringomyelia as a sequel to traumatic paraplegia. *Paraplegia* 1981;19:67–80.

165. Lyons BM, Brown DJ, Calvert JM, Woodward JM, Wriedt CHR. The diagnosis and management of post traumatic syringomyelia. *Paraplegia* 1987;25:340–350.

166. Devas MB. Stress fractures in children. *J Bone Joint Surg* 1963;45B: 528–541.

167. Grier D, Wardell S, Sarwark J, Poznaski AK. Fatigue fractures of the sacrum in children: two case reports and a review of the literature. *Skeletal Radiol* 1993;22:515–518.

168. Cullen JC. Spinal lesions in battered babies. *J Bone Joint Surg* 1975;57B:364–366.

169. Swischuk LE. Spine and spinal cord trauma in the battered child syndrome. *Radiology* 1969;92:733–738.
170. Diamond P, Hansen CM, Christofersen MR. Child abuse presenting as a thoracolumbar spinal fracture dislocation: a case report. *Pediatr Emerg Care* 1994;10:83–86.
171. Dickson RA, Leatherman KD. Spinal injuries in child abuse: case report. *J Trauma* 1978;18:811–812.
172. Kleinman PK, Zito JL. Avulsion of the spinous processes caused by infant abuse. *Radiology* 1984;151:389–391.
173. Renard M, Tridon P, Kuhnast M, Renauld JM, Dollfus P. Three unusual cases of spinal cord injury in childhood. *Paraplegia* 1978–79; 16:130–134.
174. Carrion WV, Dormans JP, Drummond DS, Christofersen MR. Circumferential growth plate fracture of the thoracolumbar spine from child abuse. *J Pediatr Orthop* 1996;16:210–214.
175. Kleinman PK, Marks SC. Vertebral body fractures in child abuse: radiologic-histopathologic correlates. *Invest Radiol* 1992;27:715–722.
176. Kogutt MS, Swischuk LE, Fagan GJ. Patterns of injury and significance of uncommon fractures in the battered child syndrome. *AJR Radium Ther Nucl Med* 1974;121:143–149.
177. Cybulski GR, Stone JL, Kant R. Outcome of laminectomy for civilian gunshot injuries of the terminal spinal cord and cauda equina: review of 88 cases. *Neurosurgery* 1989;24:392–397.
178. Six E, Alexander Jr E, Kelly DL, Davis Jr CH, McWhorter JM. Gunshot wounds to the spinal cord. *South Med J* 1979;72:699–702.
179. Yashon D, Jane JA, White RJ. Prognosis and management of spinal cord and cauda equina bullet injuries in sixty-five civilians. *J Neurosurg* 1970;31:163–170.
180. Stauffer ES, Wood RW, Kelly EG. Gunshot wounds of the spine: the effects of laminectomy. *J Bone Joint Surg* 1979;61A:389–392.
181. Heiden JS, Weiss MH, Rosenberg AW, Kurze T, Apuzzo MLJ. Penetrating gunshot wounds of the cervical spine in civilians. *J Neurosurg* 1975;42:575–579.
182. Waters RL, Adkins RH. The effects of removal of bullet fragments retained in the spinal canal: a collaborative study by the National Spinal Cord Injury model systems. *Spine* 1991;16:934–939.

Subject Index

Note: Page numbers followed by f indicate figures; those followed by t indicate tables.

function of components of, 75–77, 77f, 78f
innervation of, 5, 5f, 6f, 8
instability of, 119, 119t, 223, 223t
ligamentous injuries of, radiographic
   evaluation of, 131–132, 133f
load tolerance of, 77–80, 79f–81f
muscle groups of, 76, 77f
normal motion of, 75–77, 77f, 78f
osseous structures and articulations of, 10–12,
   10f, 12f–13f
posttraumatic kyphosis of, 317–322
   clinical manifestations of, 317–318
   etiology of, 317–319, 318f
   evaluation of, 318
   surgical treatment of, 318–322, 320f–323f
      complications of, 328–329
      indications for, 319
progressive posttraumatic myelopathy of,
   radiographic evaluation of, 142–145,
   144f, 145f
radiographic evaluation of, 117–118, 117f,
   131–145, 159, 161t, 220–223, 222f, 223f
reduction and immobilization of, 119–124,
   120f–123f, 224
residual stability of, 80–81, 82f, 119, 119t
torticollis of
   radiographic evaluation of, 134–137
   treatment of, 191–192
vertical compression injuries of, 228–229,
   229f
   radiographic evaluation of, 137–138, 137f
Cervical spine injuries
   in children, 333–352
      clinical presentation of, 335
      epidemiology of, 333
      without radiographic abnormality, 336
      radiologic evaluation of, 335–336
      site of, 333
   classification of, 226–232, 226t
   corticosteroids for, 225
   early management of, 118–119, 223–225,
      223t
   goals with, 163t
   initial assessment of, 219–220, 221f, 222t
   mechanism of, 77–80, 79f–81f
   missed, 114, 220
   prevention of complications of, 224–225
   spinal cord damage due to, radiographic
      evaluation of, 142, 143f
   subaxial, in children, 349–352, 351f, 352f
   surgical treatment of, 21–25, 225–243
      anesthesia for, 232–233
      anterior approach in, 23–25, 25f, 26f
      by anterior cervical plate fixation, 241–243
      by anterior decompression and fusion,
         237–241, 240f–241f
      by cervical spine locking plate, 242f, 243
      by foraminectomy, 234–235, 234f
      general principles of, 225
      by interspinous wire technique, 235–236,
         235f–237f
      by laminectomy, 233–234, 233f, 234f
      lateral approach in, 25, 27f
      by lateral mass plate fixation, 236–237,
         238f, 239f
      posterior approach in, 21–22, 22f, 24f
      by posterior cervical fusion, 235

by posterior decompression, 233
timing of, 225
Cervical spine locking plate, 242f, 243
Cervical spondylosis, 116
Cervical traction, 52, 119
Cervical vertebrae, 10–12, 10f, 12f–13f
   dimensions of, 63, 66f
Cervicothoracic injuries, 247–255
   assessment of, 247–250, 248f–250f, 248t
   challenges in treating, 247, 248t
   closed reduction of, 251
   definitive treatment of, 251
   early treatment of, 251
   radiographic evaluation of, 247–250,
      248f–250f, 248t
   surgical treatment of, 251–255
      approaches to, 27–30, 28f, 29f, 251–253
      methods for, 253–254, 254f
      results of, 255
Cervicothoracic junction
   anatomy of, 12–13
      surgical, 252–253
   lymphatic structures of, 252
   neurologic structures of, 252
   vascular structures of, 252
Cervicothoracic plate, 254, 254f
Chance fractures, 149f
   biomechanics of, 88, 90f, 148–149, 311
   in children
      diagnosis of, 361, 363f, 364–365, 364f
      mechanism of, 356
      treatment of, 369, 370f, 372f
   classification of, 272
   reverse, 356
   treatment of, 290–291, 290f–291f
Charcot spine, 328, 331f
Children
   atlantoaxial injuries in, 341–347, 343f–348f
   atlantooccipital dislocations in, 336–340,
      337f, 339f, 342f
   atlas fractures in, 340–341
   C2 spondylolisthesis in, 349, 349f, 350f
   cervical spine in, anatomy of, 334–335, 334f,
      335f
   cervical spine injuries in, 333–352
      atlantoaxial posterior cervical arthrodesis
         for, 346–347, 347f, 348f
      atlantooccipital arthrodesis for, 338–340,
         339f–342f
      clinical presentation of, 335
      epidemiology of, 333
      without radiographic abnormality, 336
      radiologic evaluation of, 335–336
      site of, 333
      subaxial, 349–352, 351f, 352f
      subaxial cervical fusion for, 350
      subaxial posterior fusion with wire fixation
         for, 351–352, 351f, 352f
   facet dislocation in, 350
   hangman's fracture in, 349, 349f, 350f
   herniated nucleus pulposus in, 368, 371
   lumbar apophyseal injury in, 367–368, 367f,
      371
   odontoid fractures in, 197
   odontoid separation in, 345, 345f
   os odontoideum in, 345–346, 346f
   physeal injuries in, 349

posterior ligamentous injuries in, 350
spine board for, 114
synchondrosis fracture in, 345, 345f
thoracolumbar spine in, anatomy of, 355–356,
   356f
thoracolumbar spine injuries in, 355–374
   due to abuse and violence, 374
   classification of, 356–368
   complications of, 371–373, 372f, 373f
   fractures and dislocations, 356–365
      Chance (seat belt), 356, 361, 363f,
         364–365, 364f, 369, 370f, 372f
      complications of, 371, 372f
      imaging studies of, 364–365
      mechanism of, 356, 357f–359f
      neurologic injury due to, 361–364,
         371–373, 373f
      physical examination of, 356–361,
         360f–363f
      repetitive stress, 373
      treatment options for, 368–369, 370f
   spondylolysis and spondylolisthesis,
      365–367, 366f, 369–371
      treatment options for, 368–371, 370f
   wedge-compression fractures in, 349
Circulatory status, assessment of, 115
Clay shoveler's fracture, 132
Clivus baseline, 183, 184f
Clonazepam (Klonopin), for pain, 173t
Clonidine, for spasticity, 170
Closed reduction, 119–120, 120f–122f
   of cervical spine, 224
   of cervicothoracic spine, 251
Coccyx
   osseous structures of, 15
   posterior surgical approaches to, 33
Cock robin position, 188
Cold rolled rod, for anterior middle posterior
   column injuries, 107f
Columns, of spine, 89, 91f, 148, 271, 272f
Comminution, amount of, 286, 286f
Community reintegration outings, 176
Complete injury, 59, 116, 158
Compression flexion injuries, 229–231, 230f
   in children, 368
Compression fractures
   simple, 132
   of thoracic spine, 258–259, 259t, 265, 265f
   of thoracolumbar junction, 271–272,
      272f–275f, 273
   of thoracolumbar spine, in children, 356,
      358f, 360f–362f, 364, 368
   vertical, 137–138, 137f
Compressive forces, 61
Computed tomography (CT)
   of cervical spine, 222
   in initial evaluation, 118
   quantitative, 63, 67f
   of thoracolumbar junction, 269–270, 270f,
      271f
Concussion, of spinal cord, 116
Connectors, in Edwards modular system, 302,
   303f
Consciousness, level of, 115
Contractures, 174
Contusion, cord, 141f
Conus medullaris, 1